Pediatric Cardiology for Practitioners

Fifth Edition

Pediatric Cardiology for Practitioners

Myung K. Park, MD, FAAP, FACC

Professor Emeritus (Pediatrics)
University of Texas Health Science Center
San Antonio, Texas

Clinical Professor of Pediatrics
College of Medicine, Texas A&M University System
Health Science Center
College Station, Texas

Attending Cardiologist
Driscoll Children's Hospital
Corpus Christi, Texas

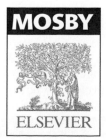

MOSBY

ELSEVIER

MOSBY
ELSEVIER

1600 John F. Kennedy Blvd.
Ste 1800
Philadelphia, PA 19103-2899

PEDIATRIC CARDIOLOGY FOR PRACTITIONERS   ISBN: 978-0-323-04636-7

Notice

Knowledge and best practice in this field are constantly changing. As new research and experience broaden our knowledge, changes in practice, treatment, and drug therapy may become necessary or appropriate. Readers are advised to check the most current information provided (i) on procedures featured or (ii) by the manufacturer of each product to be administered, to verify the recommended dose or formula, the method and duration of administration, and contraindications. It is the responsibility of the practitioner, relying on their own experience and knowledge of the patient, to make diagnoses, to determine dosages and the best treatment for each individual patient, and to take all appropriate safety precautions. To the fullest extent of the law, neither the Publisher nor the Author assumes any liability for any injury and/or damage to persons or property arising out or related to any use of the material contained in this book.

The Publisher

Library of Congress Cataloging-in-Publication Data
Park, Myung K. (Myung Kun), 1934–
  Pediatric cardiology for practitioners / Myung K. Park.—5th ed.
      p. ; cm.
  Includes bibliographical references and index.
  ISBN 978-0-323-04636-7
  1. Pediatric cardiology. I. Title.
  [DNLM: 1. Heart Diseases. 2. Child. 3. Heart Defects, Congenital. 4. Infant.
WS 290 P235p 2008]
  RJ421.P37 2008
  618.92'12—dc22

                                                                            2007002639

Acquisitions Editor: Judith Fletcher
Developmental Editor: Colleen McGonigal
Publishing Services Manager: Frank Polizzano
Project Manager: Rachel Miller
Book Designer: Ellen Zanolle

Printed in the United States of America

Last digit is the print number: 9 8 7 6 5 4 3 2 1

This book is affectionately dedicated to my wife, Issun,
our sons (Douglas, Christopher, and Warren),
our grandchildren (Natalie and Audrey),
and their mother (Jin-Hee).

FOREWORD
TO FIRST EDITION

I was very honored by Dr. Park's request that I review his manuscript and write a foreword. Having carefully read it, I am even more pleased to be able to write a foreword with unqualified praise and to recommend this book to my colleagues in pediatrics and family medicine. I think that it is so well organized and logical that serious students and even pediatric cardiologists in training will find it useful.

One of the more obvious difficulties encountered by a busy house officer or a practitioner is that most textbooks are organized to be useful to the individual who already knows the diagnosis. This "Catch-22" is resolved by Dr. Park's presentation, which permits scanning and rapid identification of the problem area, and then progresses stepwise to the clinical diagnosis, the medical management of the problem, and the general potential of surgical assistance.

This book is both concise and thorough, a relatively rare combination in the medical literature. It spares the practitioner the great detail usually found in a cardiology textbook on esoteric details of the echocardiogram, catheterization, angiocardiogram, and surgical procedures. The presentations are practical, giving drug dosages, intervals, and precautions. Although he presents alternative views where appropriate, Dr. Park is courageous in presenting his own recommendations, which are well thought out and, above all, logical.

It is easy for me to see the impact of Dr. Park's career in this excellent book.

He had a thorough general pediatric training, followed by several years in pediatric cardiology and cardiovascular physiology in this country. After some years in academic pediatric cardiology in Canada, he returned to this country and served as a family practitioner in a small community in the state of Washington. He learned well the problems of practicing in an area where consultants were not convenient for the practitioner, nor was it easy to transport a patient quickly to a major center. He returned to a research fellowship in pharmacology, and consequently knows more about the dynamics of cardiovascular drugs than anyone I can think of in the field of pediatric cardiology. For the past several years he has actively taught and practiced pediatric cardiology in a university setting and has learned the process of transmitting the information and the skills that he has acquired in his career. This book reflects all of these experiences, and the balance between science and practical considerations is reflected in every page, with the particular clarity of a natural teacher.

I am proud of my earlier association with Dr. Park, and particularly proud of his present contribution to pediatric cardiology.

Warren G. Guntheroth, MD
Professor of Pediatrics
Head, Division of Pediatric Cardiology
University of Washington School of Medicine
Seattle, Washington

PREFACE
TO FIRST EDITION

Since teaching pediatric cardiology, I have felt that there was a need for a book that was written primarily for noncardiologists, such as medical students, house staff, and practitioners. Although many excellent pediatric cardiology textbooks are available, they are not very helpful to the noncardiologist, because they are filled with many details that are beyond the need or comprehension of practitioners. In addition, these books are not very effective in teaching practitioners how to approach children with potential cardiac problems; they are usually helpful only when the diagnosis is known. This book is intended to meet the needs of noncardiologist practitioners for improving their skills in arriving at clinical diagnoses of cardiac problems, using basic tools available in their offices and community hospitals. This book will also serve as a quick reference in the area of pediatric cardiology. Although echocardiograms, cardiac catheterization, and angiocardiograms provide more definite information about the problem, these tools are not discussed at length in this book because they are not routinely available to practitioners, and their use requires special skills.

In writing a small yet comprehensive book, occasional oversimplification was unavoidable. Major emphasis was placed on the effective utilization of basic tools: history taking, physical examination, ECGs, and chest roentgenograms. Significance of abnormal findings in each of these areas is discussed, with differential diagnoses whenever applicable. A section is provided for pathophysiology, for in-depth understanding of clinical manifestations of cardiac problems. Accurate but succinct discussion of congenital and acquired cardiac conditions is presented for quick reference. Indications, timing, procedures, risks, and complications for surgical treatment of

cardiac conditions are also briefly discussed for each condition. Common cardiac arrhythmias are presented, with brief discussions of descriptions, causes, significance, and management of each arrhythmia. A special section addresses cardiac problems of the neonate; another is devoted to special problems, such as congestive heart failure, systemic hypertension, pulmonary hypertension, chest pain, and syncope.

I would like to thank my teachers and my colleagues, past and present, who directly and indirectly influenced me and taught me how to teach pediatric cardiology, and those students and house staff who gave me valuable suggestions during the early stages of this book. My special thanks are due Dr. Warren G. Guntheroth, who encouraged me to write this book, read the entire manuscript, and gave me many helpful suggestions. I gratefully acknowledge Mrs. Linda Barragan for her expert secretarial assistance, Mr. Ronald Reif for careful proofreading, and the Department of Educational Resources, University of Texas Health Science Center at San Antonio, for their superb art and photographic works, and especially Mrs. Deborah Felan for her excellent art work.

Finally, it is impossible to express adequately my debt to my brother, Young Kun, and my sister, Po Kun, who provided me with powerful stimulus, encouragement, and hearty support throughout my schooling and who maintained confidence in me. Most of all, I am deeply indebted to my lovely wife and our wonderful boys, who accepted with understanding the inconvenience associated with my long preoccupation with this book.

Myung K. Park, MD

PREFACE
TO FIFTH EDITION

Since the publication of the fourth edition of *Pediatric Cardiology for Practitioners* in 2002, important advances have been made not only in the diagnosis but also in the medical and surgical management of children with congenital and acquired heart diseases. These advances make it necessary to update this book. Extensive updating and revisions have been made throughout the book at the level that is appropriate for cardiology fellows, primary care physicians, residents, and medical students. Despite extensive revision, the book maintains its original goal of providing practitioners with fundamental and practical information for the management of children with cardiac problems. Thus, the general layout of the book has been preserved to serve as a small reference book, avoiding excessive theoretical discussions or detailed surgical descriptions commonly found in subspecialty textbooks.

Although revisions have been made throughout the book, special emphasis was placed in the area of cardiac surgery, where not only have new procedures been introduced but also the timing of old procedures has changed to earlier ages, making some earlier descriptions of surgical management no longer appropriate or somewhat incorrect for certain conditions. The revision includes illustrations of several new surgical procedures and diagrams of surgical options for most cyanotic heart defects. No major attempts were made to summarize surgical mortality rates, complications, or the results of long-term follow-up, because such data are institution dependent, continually changing, and easily accessible through electronic media.

For the chapter on electrocardiography, new normative data are presented based on the recently revised edition of *How to Read Pediatric ECGs,* 4th edition (which I coauthored with Dr. Warren G. Guntheroth). The number of two-dimensional echocardiographic diagrams has been greatly increased, and more detailed normative values of both M-mode and two-dimensional echocardiography have been included in the appendices.

Sections dealing with blood pressure and systemic hypertension have been extensively rewritten because of the controversies that exist with regard to children's blood pressure standards. To be specific, the age- and height-percentile–based standards published by the National High Blood Pressure Education Program are scientifically and logically unsound and impractical for busy practitioners to use. This is an important issue, because blood pressure standards will clearly influence the diagnosis and management of hypertension. As such, this important topic is discussed and normative blood pressure data obtained from the San Antonio Children's Blood Pressure Study are presented: The data by the High Blood Pressure Education Program are presented in the appendices for completeness.

Although every topic and chapter has been updated, certain topics were given more extensive revision, including cyanotic heart defects, infective endocarditis, cardiomyopathies, Kawasaki disease, long QT syndrome, supraventricular tachycardia, ventricular arrhythmias, implantable cardioverter-defibrillators, syncope, and pulmonary hypertension. Two new chapters, Palpitation and Athletes with Cardiac Problems, have been added. A major expansion has been made in the chapter Dyslipidemia and Other Cardiovascular Risk Factors in order to emphasize the need for practitioners' attention to preventive cardiology. In this chapter, the diagnosis and management of dyslipidemia, obesity, physical inactivity, and smoking are discussed.

I wish to acknowledge contributions of the following individuals to the revision. My colleagues at the Driscoll Children's Hospital provided constructive suggestions. In particular, I am much indebted to Mehrdad Salamat, MD, attending cardiologist at the Driscoll Children's Hospital and Clinical Assistant Professor at the Texas A&M University Health Science Center, for his enthusiastic support for the revision; he read through the old edition and provided me with many helpful and constructive suggestions. Becky Melton, MLS, and Paula Scott, PhD, MLS, librarians at the Driscoll Children's Hospital, helped me with literature searches throughout the project. Linda Lopez, a cardiac sonographer (and the manager of Driscoll's McAllen Cardiology Clinic) has provided me with helpful suggestions on the echocardiographic illustrations. Marnie Palacios, microcomputer application specialist at Multimedia and Web Services, the University of Texas Health Science Center, has been instrumental in producing superb graphics for this edition. Most of all, I thank my wife for her understanding during my long period of preoccupation with this project.

Myung K. Park, MD

FREQUENTLY USED ABBREVIATIONS

AR	aortic regurgitation	MVP	mitral valve prolapse
AS	aortic stenosis	PA	pulmonary artery or arterial
ASA	atrial septal aneurysm	PAPVR	partial anomalous pulmonary
ASD	atrial septal defect		venous return
AV	atrioventricular	PBF	pulmonary blood flow
BDG	bidirectional Glenn operation	PDA	patent ductus arteriosus
BP	blood pressure	PFO	patent foramen ovale
BVH	biventricular hypertrophy	PPHN	persistent pulmonary
CAD	coronary artery disease		hypertension of newborn
CHD	congenital heart disease	PR	pulmonary regurgitation
	(or defect)	PS	pulmonary stenosis
CHF	congestive heart failure	PVC	premature ventricular
COA	coarctation of the aorta		contraction
DORV	double outlet right ventricle	PVOD	pulmonary vascular
ECD	endocardial cushion defect		obstructive disease
ECG	electrocardiograph or	PVR	pulmonary vascular resistance
	electrocardiographic	RA	right atrium or atrial
echo	echocardiography or	RAD	right axis deviation
	echocardiographic	RAH	right atrial hypertrophy
EF	ejection fraction	RBBB	right bundle branch block
HCM	hypertrophic cardiomyopathy	RPA	right pulmonary artery
HOCM	hypertrophic obstructive	RV	right ventricle or ventricular
	cardiomyopathy	RVH	right ventricular hypertrophy
HLHS	hypoplastic left heart	RVOT	right ventricular outflow tract
	syndrome	S1	first heart sound
ICD	implantable cardioverter-	S2	second heart sound
	defibrillator	S3	third heart sound
IVC	inferior vena cava	S4	fourth heart sound
LA	left atrium or left atrial	SBE	subacute bacterial endocarditis
LAD	left axis deviation	SEM	systolic ejection murmur
LAH	left atrial hypertrophy	SVC	superior vena cava
LBBB	left bundle branch block	SVT	supraventricular tachycardia
LPA	left pulmonary artery	TAPVR	total anomalous pulmonary
LV	left ventricle or ventricular		venous return
LVH	left ventricular hypertrophy	TGA	transposition of the great
LVOT	left ventricular outflow tract		arteries
MAPCAs	multiple aortopulmonary	TOF	tetralogy of Fallot
	collateral arteries	TR	tricuspid regurgitation
MPA	main pulmonary artery	VSD	ventricular septal defect
MR	mitral regurgitation	WPW	Wolff-Parkinson-White
MS	mitral stenosis		

CONTENTS

Part I

BASIC TOOLS IN ROUTINE EVALUATION OF CARDIAC PATIENTS

Initial office evaluation of a child with possible cardiac abnormalities is usually accomplished by history taking; physical examination that includes inspection, palpation, and auscultation; electrocardiogram (ECG); and chest roentgenogram.

The weight of the information gained from these different techniques varies with the type and severity of the disease. For example, if a mother had diabetes during her pregnancy, a macrosomic infant has an increased chance of having cardiac problems. The prevalence of congenital heart defects in infants of diabetic mothers is three to four times that found in the general population. Ventricular septal defect, transposition of the great arteries, and coarctation of the aorta are more common defects. Congenital malformations of all types are increased in these infants. Hypertrophic cardiomyopathy with or without obstruction occurs in 10% to 20% of these infants, and they also have an increased risk of persistent pulmonary hypertension of the newborn. The physician should look for these defects when examining the child. Auscultation may be the most important source of information in the diagnosis of acyanotic heart disease such as ventricular septal defect or patent ductus arteriosus. However, auscultation is rarely diagnostic in cyanotic congenital heart disease such as transposition of the great arteries, in which heart murmur is often absent. Careful palpation of the peripheral pulses is more important than auscultation in the detection of coarctation of the aorta. Measurement of blood pressure is the most important diagnostic tool in the detection of hypertension. The ECG and chest x-ray films have strengths and weaknesses in their utility for assessing the severity of heart disease. The ECG detects hypertrophy well and therefore detects conditions of pressure overload, but it is less reliable at detecting dilatation from volume overload. Chest x-ray films are most reliable in establishing volume overload, but they demonstrate hypertrophy without dilatation poorly.

The next five chapters discuss these basic tools (history, physical examination, ECG, chest roentgenogram) in depth and provide flow diagrams to help correctly diagnose pediatric cardiac problems.

Chapter 1

History Taking

As in the evaluation of any other system, history taking is a basic step in cardiac evaluation. Maternal history during pregnancy is often helpful in the diagnosis of congenital heart disease (CHD) because certain prenatal events are known to be teratogenic. Past history, including the immediate postnatal period, provides more direct information relevant to the cardiac evaluation. Family history also helps link a cardiac problem to other medical problems that may be prevalent in the family. Box 1–1 lists important aspects of history taking for children with potential cardiac problems.

Gestational and Natal History

Infections, medications, and excessive alcohol intake may cause CHD, especially if they occur early in pregnancy.

INFECTIONS

1. Maternal rubella infection during the first trimester of pregnancy commonly results in multiple anomalies, including cardiac defects.
2. Infections by cytomegalovirus, herpesvirus, and coxsackievirus B are suspected to be teratogenic if they occur in early pregnancy. Infections by these viruses later in pregnancy may cause myocarditis.
3. Human immunodeficiency virus infection (in illicit drug users) has been associated with infantile cardiomyopathy.

MEDICATIONS, ALCOHOL, AND SMOKING

1. Several medications are suspected teratogens.
   a. Amphetamines have been associated with ventricular septal defect (VSD), patent ductus arteriosus (PDA), atrial septal defect (ASD), and transposition of the great arteries (TGA).
   b. Anticonvulsants are suspected of causing CHD. Phenytoin (Dilantin) has been associated with pulmonary stenosis (PS), aortic stenosis (AS), coarctation of the aorta (COA), and PDA. Trimethadione (Tridione) has been associated with TGA, tetralogy of Fallot (TOF), and hypoplastic left heart syndrome.
   c. Lithium has been associated with Ebstein's anomaly.
   d. Retinoic acid may cause conotruncal anomalies.
   e. Valproic acid may be associated with various heart defects such as ASD, VSD, AS, pulmonary atresia with intact ventricular septum, and COA.
   f. Other medications suspected of causing CHD include progesterone and estrogen (VSD, TOF, TGA).

BOX 1–1	SELECTED ASPECTS OF HISTORY TAKING

GESTATIONAL AND NATAL HISTORY
Infections, medications, excessive smoking or alcohol intake during pregnancy
Birth weight

POSTNATAL, PAST AND PRESENT HISTORY
Weight gain, development, and feeding pattern
Cyanosis, "cyanotic spells," and squatting
Tachypnea, dyspnea, puffy eyelids
Frequency of respiratory infection
Exercise intolerance
Heart murmur
Chest pain
Syncope
Palpitations
Joint symptoms
Neurologic symptoms
Medications

FAMILY HISTORY
Hereditary disease
Congenital heart defect
Rheumatic fever
Sudden unexpected death
Diabetes mellitus, arteriosclerotic heart disease, hypertension, and so on

2. Excessive alcohol intake during pregnancy has been associated with VSD, PDA, ASD, and TOF (fetal alcohol syndrome).

3. Although cigarette smoking has not been proved to be teratogenic, it does cause intrauterine growth retardation.

MATERNAL CONDITIONS

1. There is a high incidence of cardiomyopathy in infants born to diabetic mothers. In addition, these babies have a higher incidence of structural heart defects (e.g., TGA, VSD, PDA).

2. Maternal lupus erythematosus and mixed connective tissue disease have been associated with a high incidence of congenital heart block in offspring.

3. The incidence of CHD increases from about 1% in the general population to as much as 15% if the mother has CHD, even if it is postoperative (see Table A–2 in Appendix A).

BIRTH WEIGHT

Birth weight provides important information about the nature of the cardiac problem.

1. If an infant is small for gestational age, this may indicate intrauterine infections or use of chemicals or drugs. Rubella syndrome and fetal alcohol syndrome are typical examples.

2. Infants with high birth weight, often seen in offspring of diabetic mothers, show a higher incidence of cardiac anomalies. Infants with TGA often have a birth weight higher than average; these infants arc cyanotic.

Postnatal History

WEIGHT GAIN, DEVELOPMENT, AND FEEDING PATTERN

Weight gain and general development may be delayed in infants and children with congestive heart failure (CHF) or severe cyanosis. Weight is affected more significantly than height. If weight is severely affected, physicians should suspect a more general dysmorphic condition. Poor feeding of recent onset may be an early sign of CHF in infants, especially if the poor feeding is the result of fatigue and dyspnea.

CYANOSIS, "CYANOTIC SPELLS," AND SQUATTING

The presence of cyanosis should be assessed. If the parents think that their child is cyanotic, the physician should ask them about the onset (at birth, several days after birth?), severity of cyanosis, permanent or paroxysmal nature, parts of the body that were cyanotic (e.g., fingers, toes, lips), and whether the cyanosis becomes worse after feeding. Evanescent acrocyanosis is normal in the neonate.

A "cyanotic spell" is seen most frequently in infants with TOF and requires immediate attention. Physicians should ask about the time of its appearance (e.g., in the morning on awakening, after feeding), duration of the spell, and frequency of the spells. Most important is whether infants were breathing *fast* and *deep* during the spell or were holding their breath. This helps differentiate between a true cyanotic spell and a breath-holding spell.

The physician should ask whether the child squats when tired or has a favorite body position (such as knee-chest position) when tired. A history of squatting or assuming a knee-chest position strongly suggests cyanotic heart disease, particularly TOF.

TACHYPNEA, DYSPNEA, AND PUFFY EYELIDS

Tachypnea, dyspnea, and puffy eyelids are signs of CHF. Left-sided heart failure produces tachypnea with or without dyspnea. Tachypnea becomes worse with feeding and eventually results in poor feeding and poor weight gain. A sleeping respiratory rate of more than 40 breaths/minute is noteworthy. A rate of more than 60 breaths/minute is abnormal, even in a newborn.

Wheezing or persistent cough at night may be an early sign of CHF. Puffy eyelids and sacral edema are signs of systemic venous congestion. Ankle edema, which is commonly seen in adults, is not found in infants.

FREQUENCY OF RESPIRATORY INFECTIONS

CHDs with a large left-to-right shunt and increased pulmonary blood flow predispose to lower respiratory tract infections. Frequent upper respiratory tract infections are not related to CHD, although children with vascular rings may sound as if they have a chronic upper respiratory tract infection.

EXERCISE INTOLERANCE

Decreased exercise tolerance may result from any significant heart disease, including large left-to-right shunt lesions, cyanotic defects, valvular stenosis or regurgitation, and arrhythmias. Obese children may be inactive and have decreased exercise tolerance in the absence of heart disease. A good assessment of exercise tolerance can be obtained by asking the following questions: Does the child keep up with other children? How many blocks can the child walk or run? How many flights of stairs can the child climb without fatigue? Does the weather or the time of day influence the child's exercise tolerance?

With infants who do not walk or run, an estimate of exercise tolerance can be gained from the infant's history of feeding pattern. Parents often report that the child takes naps; however, many healthy children nap regularly.

HEART MURMUR

If a heart murmur is the chief complaint, the physician should obtain information about the time of its first appearance and the circumstances of its discovery. A heart murmur heard within a few hours of birth usually indicates a stenotic lesion (AS, PS), atrioventricular (AV) valve regurgitation, or small left-to-right shunt lesions (VSD, PDA). The murmur of large left-to-right shunt lesions, such as VSD or PDA, may be delayed because of slow regression of pulmonary vascular resistance. In the case of a stenotic lesion, the onset of the murmur is not affected by the pulmonary vascular resistance, and the murmur is usually heard shortly after birth. A heart murmur that is first noticed on a routine examination of a healthy-looking child is more likely to be innocent, especially if the same physician has been following the child's progress. A febrile illness is often associated with the discovery of a heart murmur.

CHEST PAIN

Chest pain is a common reason for referral and parental anxiety. If chest pain is the primary complaint, the physician asks whether the pain is activity related (e.g., Do you have chest pain only when you are active, or does it come even when you watch television?). The physician also asks about the duration (e.g., seconds, minutes, hours) and nature of the pain (e.g., sharp, stabbing, squeezing) and radiation to other parts of the body (e.g., neck, left shoulder, left arm). Chest pain of cardiac origin is not sharp; it manifests as a deep, heavy pressure or the feeling of choking or a squeezing sensation, and it is usually triggered by exercise. The physician should ask whether deep breathing improves or worsens the pain. Pain of cardiac origin, except for pericarditis, is not affected by respiration.

Cardiac conditions that may cause chest pain include severe AS (usually associated with activity), pulmonary hypertension or pulmonary vascular obstructive disease, and mitral valve prolapse (MVP). Chest pain in MVP is not necessarily associated with activity, but there may be a history of palpitation. There is increasing doubt about the relationship between chest pain and MVP in children. Less common cardiac conditions that can cause chest pain include severe PS, pericarditis of various causes, and Kawasaki disease (in which stenosis or aneurysm of the coronary artery is common).

Most children complaining of chest pain do not have a cardiac condition (see Chapter 30); cardiac causes of chest pain are rare in children and adolescents. The three most common noncardiac causes of chest pain in children are costochondritis, trauma to the chest wall or muscle strain, and respiratory diseases with cough (e.g., bronchitis, asthma, pneumonia, pleuritis). The physician should ask whether the patient has experienced recent trauma to the chest or has engaged in activity that may have resulted in pectoralis muscle soreness.

Gastroesophageal reflux and exercise-induced asthma are other recognizable causes of noncardiac chest pain in children. Exercise-induced asthma typically occurs 5 to 10 minutes into physical activities in a child with asthma. A psychogenic cause of chest pain is also possible; parents should be asked whether there has been a recent cardiac death in the family.

SYNCOPE

Syncope is a transient loss of consciousness and muscle tone that result from inadequate cerebral perfusion. Dizziness is the most common prodromal symptom of syncope. These complaints could represent a serious cardiac condition that may result in sudden death. They may also be due to noncardiac causes (such as benign vasovagal syncope), neuropsychiatric conditions, and metabolic disorders.

A history of exertional syncope may suggest arrhythmias (particularly ventricular arrhythmias, such as seen in long QT syndrome) or severe obstructive lesions (such as severe AS or hypertrophic cardiomyopathy [HCM]). Syncope provoked by exercise, that accompanied by chest pain, or a history of unoperated or operated heart disease suggests a potential cardiac cause of syncope. Syncope while sitting down suggests arrhythmias or seizure disorders. Syncope while standing for a long time suggests vasovagal syncope without underlying cardiac disease, which is the most common syncope in children (see Chapter 31 for further discussion). Hypoglycemia is a rare cause of syncope occurring in the morning. Syncopal duration less than 1 minute suggests vasovagal syncope, hyperventilation, or syncope related to another orthostatic mechanism. A longer duration of syncope suggests convulsive disorders, migraine, or arrhythmias.

Family history should include coronary heart disease risk factors, including history of myocardial infarction in family members younger than 30 years, cardiac arrhythmia, CHD, cardiomyopathies, long QT syndrome, seizures, and metabolic and psychological disorders. A detailed discussion is presented in Chapter 31.

PALPITATION

Palpitation is a subjective feeling of rapid heartbeats. Some parents and children report sinus tachycardia as palpitation. Paroxysms of tachycardia (such as supraventricular tachycardia [SVT]) or single premature beats commonly cause palpitation (see Chapter 32). Children with hyperthyroidism or MVP may first be taken to the physician because of complaints of palpitation.

JOINT SYMPTOMS

When joint pain is the primary complaint, acute rheumatic arthritis or rheumatoid arthritis is a possibility, although the incidence of the former has dramatically decreased in this country. The number of joints involved, duration of the symptom, and migratory or stationary nature of the pain are important. Arthritis of acute rheumatic fever typically involves large joints, either simultaneously or in succession, with a characteristic migratory nature. Pain in a rheumatic joint is so severe that children refuse to walk. A history of recent sore throat (and throat culture results) or rashes suggestive of scarlet fever may be helpful. The physician should also ask whether the joint was swollen, red, hot, or tender (see Chapter 20 for further discussion).

NEUROLOGIC SYMPTOMS

A history of stroke suggests thromboembolism secondary to cyanotic CHD with polycythemia or infective endocarditis. In the absence of cyanosis, stroke can rarely be caused by paradoxical embolism of a venous thrombus through an ASD. Although rare, primary hypercoagulable states should also be considered; these include such conditions as antithrombin III deficiency, protein C deficiency, protein S deficiency, disorders of the fibrinolytic system (e.g., hypoplasminogenemia, abnormal plasminogen, plasminogen activator deficiency), dysfibrinogenemia, factor XII deficiency, and lupus anticoagulant (Schafer, 1985). There are hosts of other conditions that cause secondary hypercoagulable states. A history of headache may be a manifestation of cerebral hypoxia with cyanotic heart disease, severe polycythemia, or brain abscess in cyanotic children. Although it is claimed to occur in adults, hypertension with or without COA rarely causes headaches in children. Choreic movement strongly suggests rheumatic fever.

MEDICATIONS

Physicians should note the name, dosage, timing, and duration of cardiac and noncardiac medications. Medications may be responsible for the chief complaint of the visit or certain physical findings. Tachycardia and palpitation may be caused by cold medications or antiasthmatic drugs.

A history of tobacco and illicit drug use, which could be the cause of the chief complaints, should be asked about, preferably through a private interview with the child.

Family History

HEREDITARY DISEASE

Some hereditary diseases may be associated with certain forms of CHD. For example, Marfan's syndrome is frequently associated with aortic aneurysm or with aortic or mitral insufficiency. Holt-Oram syndrome (ASD and limb abnormalities), long QT syndrome (sudden death related to ventricular arrhythmias), and idiopathic sudden death in the family should be noted. PS secondary to a dysplastic pulmonary valve is common in Noonan's syndrome. Lentiginous skin lesion (*l*entigines, *e*lectrocardiogram abnormalities, *o*cular hypertelorism, *p*ulmonary stenosis, *a*bnormal genitalia, *r*etardation of growth, and *d*eafness [LEOPARD] syndrome) is often associated with PS and cardiomyopathy. Selected hereditary diseases in which cardiovascular disease is frequently found are listed in Table 2–1 along with other nonhereditary syndromes.

CONGENITAL HEART DISEASE

The incidence of CHD in the general population is about 1% or, more precisely, 8 to 12 of 1000 live births. This does not include PDA in premature infants. The recurrence risk of CHD associated with inherited diseases or chromosomal abnormalities is related to the recurrence risk of the syndrome.

A history of CHD in close relatives increases the chance of CHD in a child. In general, when one child is affected, the risk of recurrence in siblings is about 3%, which is a threefold increase. Having a child with hypoplastic left heart syndrome (HLHS) increases the risk of CHD in a subsequent child (to approximately 10%), and most centers perform fetal echocardiography. The risk of recurrence is related to the prevalence of particular defects. Lesions with a higher prevalence (e.g., VSD) tend to have a higher risk of recurrence, and lesions with a lower prevalence (e.g., tricuspid atresia, persistent truncus arteriosus) have a lower risk of recurrence. Table A–1 in Appendix A lists the recurrence risk figures for various CHDs, which can be used for counseling. The importance of cytoplasmic inheritance has been shown in some families, based on the observation that the recurrence risk is substantially higher if the mother is the affected parent (see Table A–2 in Appendix A)

RHEUMATIC FEVER

Rheumatic fever frequently occurs in more than one family member. There is a higher incidence of the condition among relatives of rheumatic children. Although the knowledge of genetic factors involved in rheumatic fever is incomplete, it is generally agreed that there is an inherited susceptibility to acquiring rheumatic fever.

HYPERTENSION AND ATHEROSCLEROSIS

Essential hypertension and coronary artery disease show a strong familial pattern. Therefore, when a physician suspects hypertension in a young person, it is important to obtain a family history of hypertension. Atherosclerosis results from a complex process in which hereditary and environmental factors interact. The most important risk factor for atherosclerosis is a positive family history with coronary heart disease occurring before age 55 in one's father or grandfather and before age 65 in one's mother or grandmother. Clustering of cardiovascular risk factors occurs frequently in the same individual (metabolic syndrome), which calls for investigation for other risk factors when one risk factor is found. A detailed discussion of cardiovascular risk factors is presented in Chapter 33.

Chapter 2

Physical Examination

As with the examination of any child, the order and extent of the physical examination of infants and children with potential cardiac problems should be individualized. The more innocuous procedures, such as inspection, should be done first, and the more frightening or uncomfortable parts should be delayed until later in the examination.

Supine is the preferred position for examining patients in any age group. However, if older infants and young children between 1 and 3 years of age refuse to lie down, they can be examined initially while sitting on their mothers' laps.

Growth Pattern

Growth impairment is frequently observed in infants with congenital heart diseases (CHDs). The growth chart should reflect height and weight in terms of absolute values and also in percentiles. Accurate plotting and following of the growth curve are essential parts of the initial and follow-up evaluations of a child with significant heart problems. In overweight children, acanthosis nigricans should be checked in the neck and abdomen.

Different patterns of growth impairment are seen in different types of CHD.

1. Cyanotic patients have disturbances in both height and weight.

2. Acyanotic patients, particularly those with a large left-to-right shunt, tend to have more problems with weight gain than with linear growth. The degree of growth impairment is proportional to the size of the shunt.

3. Acyanotic children with pressure overload lesions without intracardiac shunt grow normally.

Poor growth in a child with a mild cardiac anomaly or failure of catch-up weight gain after repair of the defect may indicate failure to recognize certain syndromes or may be due to the underlying genetic predisposition.

Inspection

Much information can be gained by simple inspection without disturbing a sleeping infant or frightening a child with a stethoscope. Inspection should include the following: general appearance and nutritional state; any obvious syndrome or chromosomal abnormalities; color (i.e., cyanosis, pallor, jaundice); clubbing; respiratory rate, dyspnea, and retraction; sweat on the forehead; and chest inspection.

GENERAL APPEARANCE AND NUTRITIONAL STATE

The physician should note whether the child is in distress, well nourished or undernourished, and happy or cranky. Obesity should also be noted; besides being associated with other cardiovascular risk factors such as dyslipidemia, hypertension, and hyperinsulinemia, obesity is an independent risk factor for coronary artery disease.

CHROMOSOMAL SYNDROMES

Obvious chromosomal abnormalities known to be associated with certain congenital heart defects should be noted by the physician. For example, about 40% to 50% of children with Down syndrome have a congenital heart defect; the two most common are endocardial cushion defect (ECD) and ventricular septal defect (VSD). A newborn with trisomy 18 syndrome usually has a congenital heart defect. Table 2–1 shows cardiac defects associated with selected chromosomal abnormalities, along with other hereditary and nonhereditary syndromes.

Table 2–1. **Major Syndromes Associated with Cardiovascular Abnormalities**

Disorders	CV Abnormalities: Frequency and Types	Major Features	Etiology
Alagille's syndrome (arteriohepatic dysplasia)	Frequent (85%), peripheral PA stenosis with or without complex CV abnormalities.	Peculiar facies (95%) consisting of deep-set eyes, broad forehead, long straight nose with flattened tip, prominent chin, small, low-set malformed ears. Paucity of intrahepatic interlobular bile duct with chronic cholestasis (91%), hypercholesterolemia, butterfly-like vertebral arch defects (87%), growth retardation (50%), and mild mental retardation (16%)	AD Chromosome 22q11.2
CHARGE association	Common (65%); TOF, truncus arteriosus, aortic arch anomalies (e.g., vascular ring, interrupted aortic arch)	*C*oloboma, *h*eart defects, choanal *a*tresia, growth or mental *r*etardation, *g*enitourinary anomalies, *e*ar anomalies, genital hypoplasia	Unknown
Carpenter's syndrome	Frequent (50%); PDA, VSD, PS, TGA	Brachycephaly with variable craniosynostosis, mild facial hypoplasia, polydactyly, and severe syndactyly ("mitten hands")	AR
Cockayne's syndrome	Accelerated atherosclerosis	Senile-like changes beginning in infancy, dwarfing, microcephaly, prominent nose and sunken eyes, visual loss (retinal degeneration), and hearing loss	AR
Cornelia de Lange's (de Lange's) syndrome	Occasional (30%); VSD	Synophrys and hirsutism, prenatal growth retardation, microcephaly, anteverted nares, downturned mouth, mental retardation	Unknown AD?
Cri du chat syndrome (deletion 5p syndrome)	Occasional (25%); variable CHD (VSD, PDA, ASD)	Cat-like cry in infancy, microcephaly, downward slant of palpebral fissures	Partial deletion, short arm of chromosome 5
Crouzon's disease (craniofacial dysostosis)	Occasional; PDA, COA	Ptosis with shallow orbits, premature craniosynostosis, maxillary hypoplasia	AD
DiGeorge syndrome	Frequent; interrupted aortic arch, truncus arteriosus, VSD, PDA, TOF	Hypertelorism, short philtrum, downslanting eyes, hypoplasia or absence of thymus and parathyroid, hypocalcemia, deficient cell-mediated immunity	Microdeletion of 22q11.2 (overlap with velocardiofacial syndrome)
Down syndrome (trisomy 21)	Frequent (40%–50%); ECD, VSD	Hypotonic, flat facies, slanted palpebral fissure, small eyes, mental deficiency, simian crease	Trisomy 21
Ehlers-Danlos syndrome	Frequent; ASD, aneurysm of aorta and carotids, intracranial aneurysm, MVP	Hyperextensive joints, hyperelasticity, fragility and bruisability of skin, poor wound healing with thin scar	AD
Ellis–van Creveld syndrome (chondroectodermal dysplasia)	Frequent (50%); ASD, single atrium	Short stature of prenatal onset, short distal extremities, narrow thorax with short ribs, polydactyly, nail hypoplasia, neonatal teeth	AR
Fetal alcohol syndrome	Occasional (25%–30%); VSD, PDA, ASD, TOF	Prenatal growth retardation, microcephaly, short palpebral fissure, mental deficiency, irritable infant or hyperactive child	Ethanol or its byproducts

Table 2–1. **Major Syndromes Associated with Cardiovascular Abnormalities** *(Continued)*

Disorders	CV Abnormalities: Frequency and Types	Major Features	Etiology
Fetal trimethadione syndrome	Occasional (15%–30%); TGA, VSD, TOF	Ear malformation, hypoplastic midface, unusual eyebrow configuration, mental deficiency, speech disorder	Exposure to trimethadione
Fetal warfarin syndrome	Occasional (15%–45%); TOF, VSD	Facial asymmetry and hypoplasia, hypoplasia or aplasia of the pinna with blind or absent external ear canal (microtia), ear tags, cleft lip or palate, epitubular dermoid, hypoplastic vertebrae	Exposure to warfarin
Friedreich's ataxia	Frequent; hypertrophic cardiomyopathy progressing to heart failure	Late-onset ataxia, skeletal deformities	AR
Goldenhar's syndrome (oculoauriculovertebral spectrum)	Frequent (35%);VSD, TOF	Facial asymmetry and hypoplasia, microtia, ear tag, cleft lip/palate, hypoplastic vertebra	Unknown Usually sporadic
Glycogen storage disease II (Pompe's disease)	Very common; cardiomyopathy	Large tongue and flabby muscles, cardiomegaly; LVH and short PR interval on ECG, severe ventricular hypertrophy on echocardiography; normal FBS and GTT	AR
Holt-Oram syndrome (cardiac-limb syndrome)	Frequent; ASD, VSD	Defects or absence of thumb or radius	AD
Homocystinuria	Frequent; medial degeneration of aorta and carotids, atrial or venous thrombosis	Subluxation of lens (usually by 10 yr), malar flush, osteoporosis, arachnodactyly, pectus excavatum or carinatum, mental defect	AR
Infant of diabetic mother	CHDs (3%–5%); TGA, VSD, COA; cardiomyopathy (10%–20%); PPHN	Macrosomia, hypoglycemia and hypocalcemia, polycythemia, hyperbilirubinemia, other congenital anomalies	Fetal exposure to high glucose levels
Kartagener's syndrome	Dextrocardia	Situs inversus, chronic sinusitis and otitis media, bronchiectasis, abnormal respiratory cilia, immotile sperm	AR
LEOPARD syndrome (multiple lentigenes syndrome)	Very common; PS, HOCM, long PR interval	*L*entiginous skin lesion, *E*CG abnormalities, *o*cular hypertelorism, *p*ulmonary stenosis, *a*bnormal genitalia, *r*etarded growth, *d*eafness	AD
Long QT syndrome: Jervell and Lange-Nielsen syndrome Romano-Ward syndrome	Very common; long QT interval on ECG, ventricular tachyarrhythmia	Congenital deafness (not in Romano-Ward syndrome), syncope resulting from ventricular arrhythmias, family history of sudden death (±)	AR AD
Marfan syndrome	Frequent; aortic aneurysm, aortic and/or mitral regurgitation	Arachnodactyly with hyperextensibility, subluxation of lens	AD
Mucopolysaccharidosis Hurler's syndrome (type I) Hunter's syndrome (type II) Morquio's syndrome (type IV)	Frequent; aortic and/or mitral regurgitation, coronary artery disease	Coarse features, large tongue, depressed nasal bridge, kyphosis, retarded growth, hepatomegaly, corneal opacity (not in Hunter's syndrome), mental retardation; most patients die by 10 to 20 yr of age	AR XR AR
Muscular dystrophy (Duchenne's type)	Frequent; cardiomyopathy	Waddling gait, "pseudohypertrophy" of calf muscle	XR
Neurofibromatosis (von Recklinghausen's disease)	Occasional; PS, COA, pheochromocytoma	Café-au-lait spots, multiple neurofibromas, acoustic neuroma, variety of bone lesions	AD
Noonan's syndrome (Turner-like syndrome)	Frequent; PS (dystrophic pulmonary valve), LVH (or anterior septal hypertrophy)	Similar to Turner's syndrome but may occur in phenotypic male and without chromosomal abnormality	Usually sporadic Apparent AD?

Table continued on the following page

Table 2–1. **Major Syndromes Associated with Cardiovascular Abnormalities** *(Continued)*

Disorders	CV Abnormalities: Frequency and Types	Major Features	Etiology
Pierre Robin syndrome	Occasional; VSD, PDA; less commonly ASD, COA, TOF	Micrognathia, glossoptosis, cleft soft palate	In utero mechanical constraint?
Osler-Rendu-Weber syndrome (hereditary hemorrhagic telangiectasia)	Occasional; pulmonary arteriovenous fistula	Hepatic involvement, telangiectases, hemangioma or fibrosis	AD
Osteogenesis imperfecta	Occasional; aortic dilatation, aortic regurgitation, MVP	Excessive bone fragility with deformities of skeleton, blue sclera, hyperlaxity of joints	AD/AR
Progeria (Hutchinson-Gilford syndrome)	Accelerated atherosclerosis	Alopecia, atrophy of subcutaneous fat, skeletal hypoplasia and dysplasia	Unknown Occasional AD or AR
Rubella syndrome	Frequent (>95%); PDA and PA stenosis	Triad of the syndrome: deafness, cataract, and CHDs. Others include intrauterine growth retardation, microcephaly, microphthalmia, hepatitis, neonatal thrombocytopenic purpura	Maternal rubella infection during the first trimester
Rubinstein-Taybi syndrome	Occasional (25%); PDA, VSD, ASD	Broad thumbs or toes; hypoplastic maxilla with narrow palate; beaked nose, short stature, mental retardation	Sporadic; locus at 16p13.3
Smith-Lemli-Opitz syndrome	Occasional; VSD, PDA, others	Broad nasal tip with anteverted nostrils; ptosis of eyelids; syndactyly of second and third toes; short stature, mental retardation	AR
Thrombocytopenia–absent radius (TAR) syndrome	Occasional (30%); TOF, ASD, dextrocardia	Thrombocytopenia, absent or hypoplastic radius, normal thumb; "leukemoid" granulocytosis and eosinophilia	AR
Treacher Collins syndrome	Occasional; VSD, PDA, ASD	Defects of lower lids; malar hypoplasia with downslanting palpebral fissure; malformation of auricle or ear canal defect, cleft palate	Fresh mutation AD
Trisomy 13 syndrome (Patau's syndrome)	Very common (80%); VSD, PDA, dextrocardia	Low birth weight, central facial anomalies, polydactyly, chronic hemangiomas, low-set ears, visceral and genital anomalies	Trisomy 13
Trisomy 18 syndrome (Edwards' syndrome)	Very common (90%); VSD, PDA, PS	Low birth weight, microcephaly, micrognathia, rocker-bottom feet, closed fists with overlapping fingers	Trisomy 18
Tuberous sclerosis	Frequent; rhabdomyoma	Triad of adenoma sebaceum (2–5 yr of age), seizures, and mental defect; cyst-like lesions in phalanges and elsewhere; fibrous angiomatous lesions (83%) with varying colors in nasolabial folds, cheeks, and elsewhere	AD
Turner's syndrome (XO syndrome)	Frequent (35%); COA, bicuspid aortic valve, AS, hypertension, aortic dissection later in life	Short female; broad chest with widely spaced nipples; congenital lymphedema with residual puffiness over the dorsa of fingers and toes (80%)	XO with 45 chromosomes
VATER association (VATER/VACTERL syndrome)	Common (>50%); VSD, other defects	*V*ertebral anomalies, *a*nal atresia, *c*ongenital heart defects, *t*racheoesophageal (TE) fistula, *r*enal dysplasia, *l*imb anomalies (e.g., radial dysplasia)	Sporadic
Velocardiofacial syndrome (Shprintzen's syndrome)	Very common (85%); truncus arteriosus, TOF, pulmonary atresia with VSD, interrupted aortic arch type B), VSD, and D-TGA	Structural or functional palatal abnormalities, unique facial characteristics ("elfin facies" with auricular abnormalities, prominent nose with squared nasal root and narrow alar base, vertical maxillary excess with long face), hypernasal speech, conductive hearing loss, hypotonia, developmental delay and learning disability	Unknown Chromosome 22q11 (probably the same disease as DiGeorge's syndrome)
Williams syndrome	Frequent; supravalvular AS, PA stenosis	Varying degrees of mental retardation, so-called elfin facies (consisting of some of the following: upturned nose, flat nasal bridge, long philtrum, flat malar area, wide mouth, full lips, widely spaced teeth, periorbital fullness), hypercalcemia of infancy?	Sporadic AD?

Table 2–1. **Major Syndromes Associated with Cardiovascular Abnormalities** *(Continued)*

Disorders	CV Abnormalities: Frequency and Types	Major Features	Etiology
Zellweger's syndrome (cerebrohepatorenal syndrome)	Frequent; PDA, VSD or ASD	Hypotonia, high forehead with flat facies, hepatomegaly, albuminuria	AR

AD, autosomal dominant; AR, autosomal recessive; AS, aortic stenosis; ASD, atrial septal defect; CHD, congenital heart disease; COA, coarctation of the aorta; CV, cardiovascular; ECD, endocardial cushion defect; ECG, electrocardiogram; FBS, fasting blood sugar; GTT, glucose tolerance test; HOCM, hypertrophic obstructive cardiomyopathy; LVH, left ventricular hypertrophy; MR, mitral regurgitation; MVP, mitral valve prolapse; PA, pulmonary artery; PDA, patent ductus arteriosus; PFC, persistent fetal circulation; PPHN, persistent pulmonary hypertension of newborn; PS, pulmonary stenosis; TGA, transposition of the great arteries; TOF, tetralogy of Fallot; VSD, ventricular septal defect; XR, sex-linked recessive; ±, may or may not be present.

HEREDITARY AND NONHEREDITARY SYNDROMES AND OTHER SYSTEMIC MALFORMATIONS

Congenital cardiovascular anomalies are associated with a number of hereditary or nonhereditary syndromes and malformations of other systems. For example, a child with a missing thumb or deformities of a forearm may have an atrial septal defect (ASD) or VSD (e.g., Holt-Oram syndrome [cardiac-limb syndrome]). Newborns with CHARGE association (*c*oloboma, *h*eart defects, choanal *a*tresia, growth or mental *r*etardation, *g*enitourinary anomalies, *e*ar anomalies) show a high prevalence of conotruncal abnormalities (e.g., tetralogy of Fallot, double-outlet right ventricle, persistent truncus arteriosus). A list of cardiac anomalies in selected hereditary and nonhereditary syndromes is shown in Table 2–1. Certain congenital malformations of other organ systems are associated with an increased prevalence of congenital heart defects (Table 2–2).

Table 2–2. **Prevalence of Associated Congenital Heart Defects in Patients with Other System Malformations**

Organ System and Malformation	Frequency (Range) (%)	Specific Cardiac Defects
Central Nervous System		
Hydrocephalus	6 (4.5–14.9)	VSD, ECD, TOF
Dandy-Walker syndrome	3 (2.5–4.3)	VSD
Agenesis of corpus callosum	15	No specific defects
Meckel-Gruber syndrome	14	No specific defects
Thoracic Cavity		
TE fistula and/or esophageal atresia	21 (15–39)	VSD, ASD, TOF
Diaphragmatic hernia	11 (9.6–22.9)	No specific defects
Gastrointestinal		
Duodenal atresia	17	No specific defects
Jejunal atresia	5	No specific defects
Anorectal anomalies	22	No specific defects
Imperforate anus	12	TOF, VSD
Ventral Wall		
Omphalocele	21 (19–32)	No specific defects
Gastroschisis	3 (0–7.7)	No specific defects
Genitourinary		
Renal agenesis		
Bilateral	43	No specific defects
Unilateral	17	No specific defects
Horseshoe kidney	39	No specific defects
Renal dysplasia	5	No specific defects

ASD, atrial septal defect; ECD, endocardial cushion defect; TE, tracheoesophageal; TOF, tetralogy of Fallot; VSD, ventricular septal defect.

Modified from Copel JA, Kleinman CS: Congenital heart disease and extracardiac anomalies: Association and indications for fetal echocardiography. Am J Obstet Gynecol 154:1121, 1986.

COLOR

The physician should note whether the child is cyanotic, pale, or jaundiced. In cases of cyanosis, the degree and distribution should be noted (e.g., throughout the body, only on the lower or upper half of the body). Mild cyanosis is difficult to detect. The arterial saturation is usually 85% or lower before cyanosis is detectable in patients with normal hemoglobin levels (see Chapter 11). Cyanosis is more noticeable in natural light than in artificial light. Cyanosis of the lips may be misleading, particularly in children who have deep pigmentation. The physician should also check the tongue, nail beds, and conjunctiva. When in doubt, the use of pulse oximetry is confirmatory. Children with cyanosis do not always have cyanotic congenital heart defects. Cyanosis may result from respiratory diseases or central nervous system disorders. Cyanosis that is associated with arterial desaturation is called *central cyanosis*. Cyanosis associated with normal arterial saturation is called *peripheral cyanosis*. Even mild cyanosis in a newborn requires thorough investigation (see Chapter 14).

Peripheral cyanosis may be noticeable in newborns who are exposed to cold and those with congestive heart failure (CHF) because, in both conditions, peripheral blood flow is sluggish, losing more oxygen to peripheral tissues. Cyanosis is also seen in polycythemic patients with normal O_2 saturation (see Chapter 11 for the relationship between cyanosis and hemoglobin levels). Circumoral cyanosis, cyanosis around the mouth, is found in normal children with fair skin. Isolated circumoral cyanosis is not significant. Acrocyanosis is a bluish or red discoloration of the fingers and toes of normal newborns in the presence of normal arterial oxygen saturation.

Pallor may be seen in infants with vasoconstriction from CHF or circulatory shock or in severely anemic infants. Newborns with severe CHF and those with congenital hypothyroidism may have prolonged physiologic jaundice. Patent ductus arteriosus (PDA) and pulmonary stenosis (PS) are common in newborns with congenital hypothyroidism. Hepatic disease with jaundice may cause arterial desaturation because of the development of pulmonary arteriovenous fistula (e.g., arteriohepatic dysplasia).

CLUBBING

Long-standing arterial desaturation (usually longer than 6 months in duration), even if too mild to be detected by an inexperienced person, results in clubbing of the fingernails and toenails. When fully developed, clubbing is characterized by a widening and thickening of the ends of the fingers and toes as well as by convex fingernails and loss of angle between the nail and nail bed (Fig. 2–1). Reddening and shininess of the terminal phalanges are seen in the early stages of clubbing. Clubbing appears earliest and most noticeably in the thumb. Clubbing may also be associated with lung disease (e.g., abscess), cirrhosis of the liver, and subacute bacterial endocarditis. Occasionally, clubbing occurs in healthy people, such as that seen in *familial clubbing*.

RESPIRATORY RATE, DYSPNEA, AND RETRACTION

The physician should note the respiratory rate of every infant and child. If the infant breathes irregularly, the physician should count for a whole minute. The respiratory rate

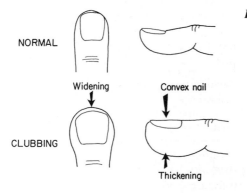

Figure 2–1. *Diagram of normal and clubbed fingers.*

is faster in children who are crying, upset, eating, or feverish. The most reliable respiratory rate is that taken during sleep. After finishing a bottle of formula, an infant may breathe faster than normal for 5 to 10 minutes. A resting respiratory rate of more than 40 breaths/minute is unusual, and more than 60 breaths/minute is abnormal at any age. Tachypnea, along with tachycardia, is the earliest sign of left-sided heart failure. If the child has dyspnea or retraction, it may be a sign of a more severe degree of left-sided heart failure or a significant lung pathology.

SWEAT ON THE FOREHEAD

Infants with CHF often have a cold sweat on the forehead. This is an expression of heightened sympathetic activity as a compensatory mechanism for decreased cardiac output.

ACANTHOSIS NIGRICANS

Acanthosis nigricans is a dark pigmentation of skin creases most commonly seen on the neck in the majority of obese children and those with type 2 diabetes. It is also found in axillae, groins, inner thighs, and on the belt line of the abdomen. Rarely, acanthosis occurs in patients with Addison's disease, Cushing's syndrome, polycystic ovary syndrome (Stein-Leventhal syndrome), hypothyroidism, and hyperthyroidism. This condition is associated with insulin resistance and a higher risk of developing type 2 diabetes. However, serum insulin levels are surprisingly low in some of these patients, suggesting a state of insulin insufficiency.

INSPECTION OF THE CHEST

Precordial bulge, with or without actively visible cardiac activity, suggests chronic cardiac enlargement. Acute dilatation of the heart does not cause precordial bulge. Pigeon chest (pectus carinatum), in which the sternum protrudes on the midline, is usually not a result of cardiomegaly.

Pectus excavatum (undue depression of the sternum) rarely, if ever, causes significant cardiac embarrassment. Rather, it may be a cause of a pulmonary systolic murmur or a large cardiac silhouette on a posteroanterior view of a chest roentgenogram, which compensates for the diminished anteroposterior diameter of the chest. As a group, children with a significant pectus excavatum have a lower endurance time than normal children.

Harrison's groove, a line of depression in the bottom of the rib cage along the attachment of the diaphragm, indicates poor lung compliance of long duration, such as that seen in large left-to-right shunt lesions.

Palpation

Palpation should include the peripheral pulses (their presence or absence, the pulse rate, the volume of the pulses) and the precordium (the presence of a thrill, the point of maximal impulse [PMI], precordial hyperactivity). Although ordinarily palpation follows inspection, auscultation may be more fruitful on a sleeping infant who might wake up and become uncooperative.

PERIPHERAL PULSES

1. The physician should count the pulse rate and note any irregularities in the rate and volume. The normal pulse rate varies with the patient's age and status. The younger the patient, the faster the pulse rate. Increased pulse rate may indicate excitement, fever, CHF, or arrhythmia. Bradycardia may mean heart block, digitalis toxicity, and so on. Irregularity of the pulse suggests arrhythmias, but sinus arrhythmia (an acceleration with inspiration) is normal.

2. The right and left arm and an arm and a leg should be compared for the volume of the pulse. Every patient should have palpable pedal pulses, either dorsalis pedis, tibialis posterior, or both. It is often easier to feel pedal pulses than femoral pulses. Attempts at palpating a femoral pulse often wake up a sleeping infant or upset a toddler. If a good pedal pulse is felt, coarctation of the aorta (COA) is effectively ruled out, especially if the blood pressure in the arm is normal.

Weak leg pulses and strong arm pulses suggest COA. If the right brachial pulse is stronger than the left brachial pulse, the cause may be COA occurring near the origin of the left subclavian artery or supravalvular aortic stenosis (AS). A weaker right brachial pulse than the left suggests an aberrant right subclavian artery arising distal to the coarctation.

3. Bounding pulses are found in aortic run-off lesions such as PDA, aortic regurgitation (AR), large systemic arteriovenous fistula, or persistent truncus arteriosus (rarely). Pulses are bounding in premature infants because of the lack of subcutaneous tissue and because many have PDA.

4. Weak, thready pulses are found in cardiac failure or circulatory shock or in the leg of a patient with COA. A systemic–to–pulmonary artery shunt (either classic Blalock-Taussig shunt or modified Gore-Tex shunt) or subclavian flap angioplasty for repair of COA may result in an absent or weak pulse in the arm affected by surgery. Arterial injuries resulting from previous cardiac catheterization may cause a weak pulse in the affected limb.

5. Pulsus paradoxus (paradoxical pulse) is suspected when there is marked variation in the volume of arterial pulses with the respiratory cycle. The term *pulsus paradoxus* does *not* indicate a phase reversal; rather, it is an exaggeration of normal reduction of systolic pressure during inspiration. When arterial blood pressure is being monitored through an indwelling arterial catheter, the presence of pulsus paradoxus is easily detected by a wide swing (>10 mm Hg) in arterial pressure. In a child without arterial pressure monitoring, accurate evaluation requires sphygmomanometry (Fig. 2–2). Pulsus paradoxus may be associated with cardiac tamponade secondary to pericardial effusion or constrictive pericarditis or to severe respiratory difficulties seen with asthma or pneumonia. It is also seen in patients who are on ventilators with high pressure settings, but in that case, the blood pressure increases with inflation.

The presence of pulsus paradoxus is confirmed by the use of a sphygmomanometer as follows.

a. The cuff pressure is raised about 20 mm Hg above the systolic pressure.
b. The pressure is lowered slowly until Korotkoff sound 1 is heard for some but not all cardiac cycles, and the reading is noted (line A on Fig. 2–2).
c. The pressure is lowered further until systolic sounds are heard for all cardiac cycles, and the reading is noted (line B on Fig. 2–2).
d. If the difference between readings A and B is greater than 10 mm Hg, pulsus paradoxus is present.

CHEST

One should palpate the following on the chest: apical impulse, PMI, hyperactivity of the precordium, and palpable thrill.

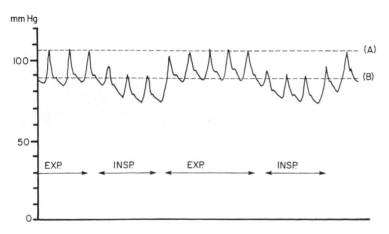

Figure 2–2. Diagram of pulsus paradoxus. Note the reduction in systolic pressure of more than 10 mm Hg during inspiration. EXP, expiration; INSP, inspiration.

Apical Impulse. Palpation of the apical impulse is usually superior to percussion in the detection of cardiomegaly. Its location and diffuseness should be noted. Percussion in infants and children is inaccurate and adds little. The apical impulse is normally at the fifth intercostal space in the midclavicular line after age 7. Before this age, the apical impulse is in the fourth intercostal space just to the left of the midclavicular line. An apical impulse displaced laterally or downward suggests cardiac enlargement.

Point of Maximal Impulse. The PMI is helpful in determining whether the right ventricle (RV) or left ventricle (LV) is dominant. With RV dominance, the impulse is maximal at the lower left sternal border or over the xiphoid process; with LV dominance, the impulse is maximal at the apex. Normal newborns and infants have RV dominance and therefore more RV impulse than older children. If the impulse is more diffuse and slow rising, it is called a *heave*. If it is well localized and sharp rising, it is called a *tap*. Heaves are often associated with volume overload. Taps are associated with pressure overload.

Hyperactive Precordium. The presence of a hyperactive precordium characterizes heart disease with volume overload, such as that seen in defects with large left-to-right shunts (e.g., PDA, VSD) or heart disease with severe valvular regurgitation (e.g., AR, mitral regurgitation [MR]).

Thrills. Thrills are vibratory sensations that represent palpable manifestations of loud, harsh murmurs. Palpation for thrills is often of diagnostic value. A thrill on the chest is felt better with the palm of the hand than with the tips of the fingers. However, the fingers are used to feel a thrill in the suprasternal notch and over the carotid arteries.

1. Thrills in the upper left sternal border originate from the pulmonary valve or pulmonary artery (PA) and therefore are present in PS, PA stenosis, or PDA (rarely).

2. Thrills in the upper right sternal border are usually of aortic origin and are seen in AS.

3. Thrills in the lower left sternal border are characteristic of a VSD.

4. Thrills in the suprasternal notch suggest AS but may be found in PS, PDA, or COA.

5. The presence of a thrill over the carotid artery or arteries accompanied by a thrill in the suprasternal notch suggests diseases of the aorta or aortic valve (e.g., COA, AS). An isolated thrill in one of the carotid arteries without a thrill in the suprasternal notch may be a carotid bruit.

6. Thrills in the intercostal spaces are found in older children with severe COA and extensive intercostal collaterals.

Blood Pressure Measurement

When possible, every child should have his or her blood pressure (BP) measured as part of the physical examination. Children's BP values are compared with an existing set of normative BP standards to determine whether the child has an abnormal level of BP. To determine whether the obtained BP level is normal or abnormal, there must be a reliable set of normative BP standards that are derived by a correct BP measuring method. Unfortunately, there have been problems and confusions regarding the proper method of measuring BP and the normative BP values for children. Scientifically unsound methods of BP measurement recommended by two National Institutes of Health (NIH) task forces (1977 and 1987) have dominated the field, and they are the sources of confusion. At this time, both the methodology and standards recommended by the NIH task forces have been abandoned. However, the most recent BP standards recommended by the Working Group of the National High Blood Pressure Education Program (NHBPEP) are still problematic. These normal standards not only are scientifically and logically unsound and not evidence based but also are impractical for use by busy practitioners (see later for further discussion).

In this subsection, the following important issues in children's BP measurement are discussed for a quick overview.

1. What is the currently recommended BP measurement method?

2. Which normal BP standards should be used and why?

   a. Why are the old NIH task forces' BP standards not acceptable?

   b. What is wrong with BP standards recommended by the Working Group of NHBPEP?

   c. Alternative BP standards derived from the San Antonio Children's Blood Pressure Study (SACBPS)

3. Are BP levels obtained by oscillometric device interchangeable with those obtained by the auscultatory method?

4. How to interpret arm and leg BP values

5. BP levels in neonates and small children

6. The important concept of peripheral amplification of systolic pressure

1. What is the currently recommended BP measuring method?

Until recently, in children, the BP cuff was chosen on the basis of the length of the arm, contrary to common practice for adult patients. Two task forces of the NIH, 1977 and 1987, have recommended this unscientific method, initially recommending that the cuff width be two thirds of the arm length and later changing it to three quarters of the length of the arm, and have provided normal BP standards based on these methods.

The BP cuff selection based on the length of the arm is scientifically unsound and violates the physical principles underlying indirect BP measurement, which were established a century ago. For adults, a Special Task Force of the American Heart Association (AHA) recommended the correct cuff selection method in 1950, and it has been in use ever since. The correct width of the BP cuff is 40% to 50% of the circumference of the limb on which the BP is being measured (Fig. 2–3). In 1988, the AHA's Special Task Force extended the same cuff selection method to children. This unified cuff selection method provides continuity from childhood to adulthood.

Differences in the methodology recommended by three national committees are summarized in Table 2–3 for quick comparison. The following summarizes current views on BP measurement techniques (of the AHA and the NHBPEP).

   a. The BP cuff width should be 40% to 50% of the circumference of the extremity with the cuff long enough to encircle the extremities completely or nearly completely (endorsed by both groups).

   b. The NHBPEP recommends Korotkoff phase 5 (K5) as the diastolic pressure, but this recommendation is debatable on the basis of a number of earlier reports. Earlier studies indicated that K4 agrees better with true diastolic pressure for children up to 12 years (endorsed by the AHA, NIH task forces, and the Bogalusa Heart Study [Hammond et al, 1995]).

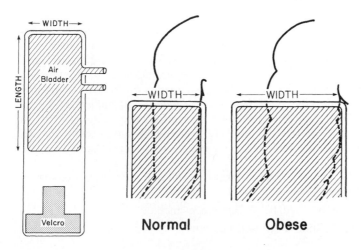

Figure 2–3. Diagram showing a method of selecting an appropriate-sized blood pressure cuff. The selection is based on the thickness rather than the length of the arm. The end of the cuff is at the top, and the cuff width is compared with the circumference or diameter of the arm. The width of the inflatable part of the cuff (bladder, crosshatched areas) should be 40% to 50% of the circumference (or 125% to 155% of the diameter) of the arm.

Table 2–3. **Comparison of Recommendations by Three National Committees**

	National Institutes of Health Task Force (1987)	American Heart Association, Special Task Force (1988)	Working Group, NHBPEP (1996, 2004)
Position	Sitting	Sitting	Sitting
Cuff width	Three quarters of arm length	40%–50% of arm circumference	Approximately 40% of arm circumference
Diastolic pressure	K4 for 3–12 yr K5 for ≥13 yr	K4 for child K5 for adult	K5 for both child and adult
Number of measurements	1	Average of 2	Average of 2 or more
Stethoscope	Bell	Bell	—
Normative standards	Yes	No	Modified from NIH (1987)

NHBPEP; National High Blood Pressure Education Program; K4; Korotkoff phase 4; K5; Korotkoff phase 5.

    c. Two or more readings should be averaged (because the averaged values are closer to the basal BP level and are more reproducible) (endorsed by both groups).

    d. The child should be in sitting position with the arm at heart level (endorsed by both groups).

2. Which normal BP standards should be used and why?

    a. Because the NIH normative data were the results of single measurements obtained by using the unscientific cuff selection method, these BP standards are no longer valid.

    b. The Working Group of the NHBPEP recommended a new set of normal BP values, which are expressed as a function of age and height percentile (NHBPEP, 2004). These BP standards are not only statistically and logically unsound but also impractical for use by busy practitioners (Park, 2005).

      1). Although the recommended methods of the NHBPEP are correct, the data presented were obtained by a methodology that is discordant with the committee's own recommendations; that is, the BP values were derived from the currently invalid methods of NIH Task Force 1987 (with BP cuff width selected by the arm length). They are single measurements, rather than the averages of multiple readings, as currently recommended.

      2). The rationale for recommending BP values according to age and height percentile is statistically and logically unsound. Partial correlation analysis in the SACBPS showed that, when auscultatory BP levels were adjusted for age and weight, the correlation coefficient of systolic BP with height was very small ($r = 0.068$ for boys; $r = 0.072$ for girls), whereas when adjusted for age and height, the correlation of systolic pressure with weight remained high ($r = 0.343$ for boys; $r = 0.294$ for girls). These findings indicate that the contribution of height to BP levels is negligible. The apparent contribution of height to BP levels may be secondary to its close correlation with weight ($r = 0.86$). A similar conclusion was reached with oscillometric BP levels in the same study. Thus, we found no rationale to use both age and height percentile to express children's normative BP standards. Although weight is a very important contributor to BP, weight cannot be used as a second variable because this would interfere with detection of high BP in obese children. Therefore, we have recommended that children's BP values be expressed as a function of age only (Park et al, 2001).

      3). A relatively complex set of BP standards requiring additional computational steps to classify the level of a child's BP, which is a highly variable measurement, is not a wise recommendation. In a busy practice, following such guidelines is impractical relative to what is to be gained by such an approach.

Although the BP standards of the NHBPEP suffer from the deficiencies previously outlined, the nationally publicized BP standards are presented in Appendix B for completeness (Tables B–1 and B–2).

c. Normative BP percentile values from the San Antonio study are recommended as alternative BP standards until nationwide data become available. These are the only available BP standards that have been obtained according to the currently recommended method. In the SACBPS, BP levels were obtained in more than 7000 schoolchildren, of three ethnic groups (African American, Mexican American, and Non-Hispanic white), enrolled in kindergarten through 12th grade. Both the auscultatory and oscillometric (Dinamap model 8100) methods were used in the study, and the data were the averages of three readings. No consistent ethnic difference was found among the three ethnic groups, but there were important gender differences. Figures 2–4 and 2–5 show normal auscultatory BP percentile curves according to age for boys and girls, respectively. Percentile BP values for these figures are presented in Appendix B (Tables B–3 and B–4).

3. Are BP levels obtained by oscillometric device interchangeable with those obtained by the auscultatory method?

The accuracy of indirect BP measurement by an oscillometric method (Dinamap model 1846) has been demonstrated. In fact, oscillometric BP levels correlated better with intra-arterial pressures than levels obtained by the auscultatory method (Park et al, 1987). The arm circumference–based cuff selection method is also appropriate for the Dinamap method. The oscillometric method also provides some advantages over auscultation: it eliminates observer-related variations and it can be used successfully in infants and small children. (see Table B–5 for normal values in

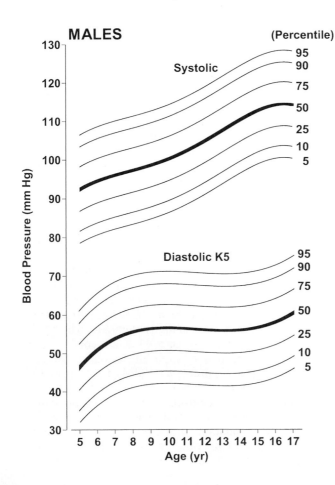

Figure 2–4. Age-specific percentile curves of auscultatory systolic and diastolic (K5) pressures in boys 5 to 17 years of age. Blood pressure values are the average of three readings. The width of the blood pressure cuff was 40% to 50% of the circumference of the arm. Percentile values for the figure are shown in Table B–3, Appendix B.

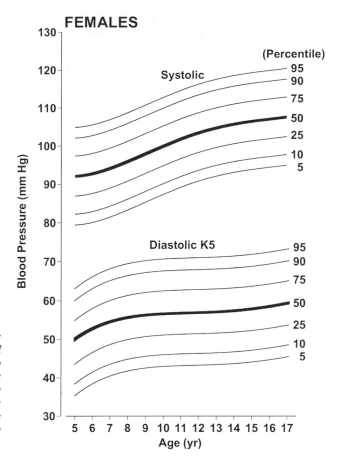

FEMALES

Figure 2–5. Age-specific percentile curves of auscultatory systolic and diastolic (K5) pressures in girls 5 to 17 years of age. Blood pressure values are the average of three readings. The width of the blood pressure cuff was 40% to 50% of the circumference of the arm. Percentile values for the figure are shown in Table B–4, Appendix B.

infants and small children.) Auscultatory BP measurements in small infants not only are difficult to obtain but also have not been shown to be accurate.

We found, however, that BP levels obtained by Dinamap (model 8100) were on average 10 mm Hg higher than levels obtained by the auscultatory method for the systolic pressure and 5 mm Hg higher for the diastolic pressure. Therefore, the auscultatory and Dinamap BPs are not interchangeable. This necessitates oscillometric specific normative BP standards so that one does not use normal auscultatory BP standards when the oscillometric method is used. Oscillometric BP percentile values (Dinamap model 8100) are presented in Appendix B (Tables B–6 and B–7).

One should not consider the auscultatory BP the gold standard; it is not. The gold standard is an intra-arterial BP. The fact that oscillometric BP readings do not agree with those obtained by the auscultatory method does not mean that they are invalid. It simply indicates that the two indirect methods give different values. Aside from the issue of accuracy, the oscillometric method is widely used in large pediatric and pediatric cardiology practices and in the setting of emergency departments. Thus, oscillometric BP values should be compared only with oscillometric specific BP standards as presented in Appendix B (see Tables B–6 and B–7).

4. How do arm BP values compare with leg BP values?

Four-extremity BP measurements are often obtained to rule out COA. The same cuff selection criterion (i.e., 40% to 50% of the circumference) applies for calf or thigh pressure determination. When using an oscillometric device, the patient should be in the supine position for BP measurements in the arm and leg. When using the auscultatory method, the thigh pressure is obtained with the stethoscope placed over the popliteal artery with the patient's legs bent and the patient in the supine or prone position.

How do BP levels in the arm and leg compare in normal children? Even when a considerably wider cuff is selected for the thigh, the Dinamap systolic pressure in the thigh or calf is about 5 to 10 mm Hg higher than that in the arm (Park et al, 1993), except in newborns, in whom the arm and calf pressures are the same (see later). This reflects in part the peripheral amplification of systolic pressure (see the later discussion of this important topic). Thus, the systolic pressure in the thigh (or calf) should be higher than or at least equal to that in the arm. If the systolic pressure is lower in the leg, COA may be present. Leg BP determinations are mandatory in a child with hypertension in the arm to rule out COA. The presence of a femoral pulse does not rule out a coarctation.

5. What are normative BP levels in neonates and small children?

Although BP is not routinely measured in healthy newborns, it must be measured when one suspects COA, hypertension, or hypotension. In contrast to the recommendations of the NHBPEP, the auscultatory method is difficult to apply in newborns and small children and obtained values are not reliable and reproducible. Therefore, the oscillometric method is frequently used instead. Abbreviated normative Dinamap BP standards for newborns and small children (younger than 5 years) are presented in Table 2–4. Full percentile values are presented in Appendix B (Table B–5). The same BP cuff selection method as used in older children applies to this age group; that is, the cuff width is approximately 50% of the circumference of the extremity. In the newborn, the systolic pressures in the arm and the calf are the same (Park et al, 1989). The absence of a higher systolic pressure in the leg in the newborn may be related to the presence of a normally narrow aortic isthmus.

6. What is peripheral amplification of systolic pressure?

Many physicians incorrectly assume that peripherally measured BP values, such as those measured in the arm, reflect central aortic pressure, which is the perfusing pressure for the brain. This assumption is incorrect in certain clinical situations. Some physicians also incorrectly think that the systolic pressure in the central aorta is higher than that in the brachial, radial, and pedal arteries. As shown schematically in Figure 2–6, systolic pressure becomes higher and higher as one moves farther peripherally, although the diastolic and mean pressures remain the same or decrease slightly (O'Rourke, 1968). If this is correct, how does blood flow distally? There is a change in the arterial pressure waveform at different levels in an arterial tree as shown in Figure 2–6, but the area under the curve decreases slightly in the peripheral sites.

It is important for physicians to understand that the peripheral systolic pressure obtained by both direct and indirect methods does not always reflect the central aortic pressure. The relationship between the peripheral and the central systolic pressures is not always predictable, and there are some clinically important situations in which the peripheral amplification becomes more prominent. The following summarizes key points of the peripheral amplification of systolic pressure.

a. The amplification is limited to systolic pressure only (not diastolic pressure).
b. The systolic amplification is greater in children (with more reactive arteries) than in older adults, who may have degenerative arterial disease.

Table 2–4. Normative Blood Pressure Levels by Dinamap Monitor in Children

Age	Mean BP Levels (mm Hg)	90th Percentile	95th Percentile
1–3 days	64/41 (50)	75/49 (50)	78/52 (62)
1 mo–2 yr	95/58 (72)	106/68 (83)	110/71 (86)
2–5 yr	101/57 (74)	112/66 (82)	115/68 (85)

Dinamap model 1846SX was used.
Blood pressure (BP) levels are systolic/diastolic, with the mean in parentheses.
Modified from Park MK, Menard SM: Normative oscillometric blood pressure values in the first 5 years in an office setting. Am J Dis Child 143:860, 1989.

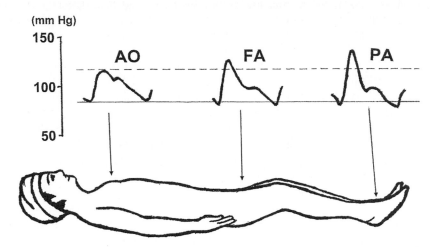

Figure 2–6. *Schematic diagram of pulse wave changes at different levels of the systemic arteries. AO, aorta; FA, femoral artery; PA, pedal artery. (Modified from Geddes LA: Handbook of Blood Pressure Measurement. Clifton, NJ, Humana Press, 1991.)*

    c. Pedal artery systolic pressures are higher than the radial artery pressures, which is a reflection of this phenomenon.

    d. The amplification is more marked in vasoconstricted states, many of them clinically important.

        1). Impending circulatory shock in which a high level of circulating catecholamines exists. Early diagnosis of an impending circulatory shock can be missed if one pays attention only to systolic pressure; the mean arterial and diastolic pressures should be low in this situation.

        2). A child in CHF (in which peripheral vasoconstriction exists) may exhibit an exaggerated systolic amplification.

        3). Arm systolic pressure in subjects running on a treadmill can be markedly higher than the central aortic pressure. A dramatic illustration of this phenomenon is shown in Figure 6–13 (section of exercise stress test) in a young adult running on treadmill with catheters in the ascending aorta and the radial artery.

        4). Subjects receiving catecholamine infusion or other vasoconstrictors in the setting of critical care units

    e. Less amplification of systolic pressure is noted in vasodilated states.

        1). Subjects receiving vasodilators

        2). Subjects who have received a contrast dye injection (which has vasodilating effects) during cardiac catheterization

Auscultation

Although auscultation of the heart requires more skill, it also provides more valuable information than other methods of heart examination. The bell-type chest piece is better suited for detecting low-frequency events, whereas the diaphragm selectively picks up high-frequency events. When the bell is firmly pressed against the chest wall, it acts like the diaphragm by filtering out low-frequency sounds or murmurs and picking up high-frequency events. Physicians should ordinarily use both the bell and the diaphragm, although using the bell both lightly and firmly pressed against the chest may be equally effective, especially in sleeping infants. Using only the diaphragm may result in missing some important low-frequency murmurs or sounds, such as mid-diastolic rumble, pulmonary regurgitation (PR) murmur, and faint Still's innocent heart murmurs. One should not limit examination to the four traditional auscultatory areas. The entire precordium, as well as the sides and back of the chest, should be explored with the stethoscope. Systematic attention should be given to the following aspects:

1. Heart rate and regularity: Heart rate and regularity should be noted in every child. Extremely fast or slow heart rates or irregularity in the rhythm should be evaluated by an ECG and a long rhythm strip (see Chapters 24 and 25).

2. Heart sounds: Intensity and quality of the heart sounds, especially the second heart sound (S2), should be evaluated. Abnormalities of the first heart sound (S1) and the third heart sound (S3) and the presence of a gallop rhythm or the fourth sound (S4) should be noted. Muffled heart sounds should also be noted.

3. Systolic and diastolic sounds: An ejection click in early systole provides a clue to aortic or pulmonary valve stenosis. A midsystolic click provides important clues to the diagnosis of mitral valve prolapse. An opening snap in diastole (present in mitral stenosis) should be noted, but it is extremely rare in pediatrics.

4. Heart murmurs: Heart murmurs should be evaluated in terms of intensity, timing (systolic or diastolic), location, transmission, and quality.

HEART SOUNDS

The heart sound should be identified and analyzed before the analysis of heart murmurs (Fig. 2–7). Muffled and distant heart sounds are present in pericardial effusion and heart failure.

First Heart Sound. The S1 is associated with closure of the mitral and tricuspid valves. It is best heard at the apex or lower left sternal border. Splitting of the S1 may be found in normal children, but it is infrequent. Abnormally wide splitting of S1 may be found in right bundle branch block (RBBB) or Ebstein's anomaly. Splitting of S1 should be differentiated from ejection click or S4.

1. Ejection click is more easily audible at the upper left sternal border in PS. In a bicuspid aortic valve, the click may be louder at the lower left sternal border or apex than at the upper right sternal border.

2. S4 is rare in children.

Second Heart Sound. The S2 in the upper left sternal border (i.e., pulmonary valve area) is of critical importance in pediatric cardiology. The S2 must be evaluated in terms of the degree of splitting and the intensity of the pulmonary closure component of the second heart sound (P2) in relation to the intensity of the aortic closure component of the second heart sound (A2). Although best heard with the diaphragm of a stethoscope, both components are readily audible with the bell. Abnormalities of splitting of the S2 and the intensity of the P2 are summarized in Box 2–1.

Splitting of the S2. In every normal child, with the exception of occasional newborns, two components of the S2 should be audible in the upper left sternal border. The first is the A2; the second is the P2.

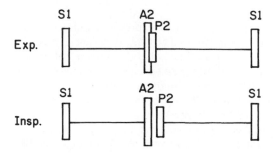

Figure 2–7. Diagram showing the relative intensity of A2 and P2 and the respiratory variation in the degree of splitting of the S2 at the upper left sternal border (pulmonary area). Exp., expiration; Insp., inspiration.

BOX 2–1	SUMMARY OF ABNORMAL S2

ABNORMAL SPLITTING

Widely Split and Fixed S2

Volume overload (e.g., ASD, PAPVR)
Pressure overload (e.g., PS)
Electrical delay (e.g., RBBB)
Early aortic closure (e.g., MR)
Occasional normal child

Narrowly Split S2

Pulmonary hypertension
AS
Occasional normal child

Single S2

Pulmonary hypertension
One semilunar valve (e.g., pulmonary atresia, aortic atresia, persistent truncus arteriosus)
P2 not audible (e.g., TGA, TOF, severe PS)
Severe AS
Occasional normal child

Paradoxically Split S2

Severe AS
LBBB, WPW syndrome (type B)

ABNORMAL INTENSITY OF P2

Increased P2 (e.g., pulmonary hypertension)
Decreased P2 (e.g., severe PS, TOF, TS)

AS, aortic stenosis; ASD, atrial septal defect; LBBB, left bundle branch block; MR, mitral regurgitation; PAPVR, partial anomalous pulmonary venous return; PS, pulmonary stenosis; RBBB, right bundle branch block; TGA, transposition of the great arteries; TOF, tetralogy of Fallot; TS, tricuspid stenosis; WPW, Wolff-Parkinson-White.

Normal Splitting of the S2. The degree of splitting of the S2 varies with respiration, increasing with inspiration and decreasing or becoming single with expiration (see Fig. 2–7). Although a new theory regarding the cause of normal respiratory variation in the splitting of the S2 is based on the vascular impedance of systemic and pulmonary circuits, the traditional explanation relates these events to the closure of the aortic and pulmonary valves. During inspiration, because of a greater negative pressure in the thoracic cavity, there is an increase in systemic venous return to the right side of the heart. This increased volume of blood in the RV prolongs the duration of RV ejection time, which delays the closure of the pulmonary valve, resulting in a wide splitting of the S2. The absence of splitting (i.e., single S2) or a widely split S2 usually indicates an abnormality.

Abnormal Splitting of the S2. Abnormal splitting may be in the form of wide splitting, narrow splitting, a single S2, or paradoxical splitting of the S2 (rarely).

1. A widely split and fixed S2 is found in conditions that prolong the RV ejection time or that shorten the LV ejection. Therefore, it is found in:

   a. ASD or partial anomalous pulmonary venous return (PAPVR) (conditions in which the amount of blood ejected by the RV is increased; *volume overload*).

   b. PS (the valve stenosis prolongs the RV ejection time; *pressure overload*).

   c. RBBB (a delay in *electrical* activation of the RV) delays the completion of the RV ejection.

   d. MR (a decreased forward output seen in this condition shortens the LV ejection time, making aortic closure occur earlier than normal).

   e. An occasional normal child, including "prolonged hangout time" seen in children with dilated PA (a condition called *idiopathic dilatation of the PA*). In dilated PA, the increased capacity of the artery produces less recoil to close the pulmonary valve, which delays closure.

2. A narrowly split S2 is found in conditions in which the pulmonary valve closes early (e.g., pulmonary hypertension) or the aortic valve closure is delayed (e.g., AS). This is occasionally found in a normal child.

3. A single S2 is found in the following situations.
   a. When only one semilunar valve is present (e.g., aortic or pulmonary atresia, persistent truncus arteriosus)
   b. When the P2 is not audible (e.g., transposition of the great arteries [TGA], tetralogy of Fallot [TOF], severe PS)
   c. When aortic closure is delayed (e.g., severe AS)
   d. When the P2 occurs early (e.g., severe pulmonary hypertension)
   e. In an occasional normal child

4. A *paradoxically split S2* is found when the aortic closure (A2) follows the pulmonary closure (P2) and therefore is seen when the LV ejection is greatly delayed (e.g., severe AS, left bundle branch block [LBBB], sometimes Wolff-Parkinson-White [WPW] preexcitation).

Intensity of the P2. The *relative* intensity of the P2 compared with the A2 must be assessed in every child. In the pulmonary area, the A2 is usually louder than the P2 (see Fig. 2–7). The A2 is *not* the second heart sound at the aortic area; rather, it is the first (or aortic closure) component of the second heart sound at the pulmonary area (i.e., upper left sternal border). Judgment as to normal intensity of the P2 is based on experience. There is no substitute for listening to the hearts of many normal children. Abnormal intensity of the P2 may suggest a pathologic condition. Increased intensity of the P2, compared with that of the A2, is found in pulmonary hypertension. Decreased intensity of the P2 is found in conditions with decreased diastolic pressure of the PA (e.g., severe PS, TOF, tricuspid atresia).

Third Heart Sound. The S3 is a somewhat low-frequency sound in early diastole and is related to rapid filling of the ventricle (Fig. 2–8). It is best heard at the apex or lower left sternal border. It is commonly heard in normal children and young adults. A loud S3 is abnormal and is audible in conditions with dilated ventricles and decreased ventricular compliance (e.g., large-shunt VSD or CHF). When tachycardia is present, it forms a "Kentucky" gallop.

Fourth Heart Sound or Atrial Sound. The S4 is a relatively low-frequency sound of late diastole (i.e., presystole) and is rare in infants and children (see Fig. 2–8). When present, it is always pathologic and is seen in conditions with decreased ventricular compliance or CHF. With tachycardia, it forms a "Tennessee" gallop.

Gallop Rhythm. A gallop rhythm is a rapid triple rhythm resulting from the combination of a loud S3, with or without an S4, and tachycardia. It generally implies a pathologic condition and is commonly present in CHF. A summation gallop represents tachycardia and a superimposed S3 and S4.

SYSTOLIC AND DIASTOLIC SOUNDS

1. An ejection click (or ejection sound) follows the S1 very closely and occurs at the time of the ventricular ejection's onset. Therefore, it sounds like a splitting of the S1. However, it is usually audible at the base (either side of the upper sternal border), whereas the split S1 is usually audible at the lower left sternal border (exception with

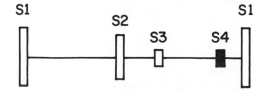

Figure 2–8. Diagram showing the relative relationship of the heart sounds. Filled bar shows an abnormal sound.

an aortic click, discussed in a later section). If the physician hears what sounds like a split S1 at the upper sternal border, it may be an ejection click (Fig. 2–9).

The pulmonary click is heard at the second and third left intercostal spaces and changes in intensity with respiration, being louder on expiration. The aortic click is best heard at the second right intercostal space but may be louder at the apex or mid-left sternal border. It usually does not change its intensity with respiration.

The ejection click is most often associated with:

a. Stenosis of semilunar valves (e.g., PS or AS).
b. Dilated great arteries, which are seen in systemic or pulmonary hypertension, idiopathic dilatation of the PA, TOF (in which the aorta is dilated), and persistent truncus arteriosus.

2. Midsystolic click with or without a late systolic murmur is heard at the apex in mitral valve prolapse (MVP) (see Fig. 2–9 and Chapter 21).

3. Diastolic opening snap is rare in children and is audible at the apex or lower left sternal border. It occurs somewhat earlier than the S3 during diastole and originates from a stenosis of the atrioventricular (AV) valve, such as mitral stenosis (MS) (see Fig. 2–9).

EXTRACARDIAC SOUNDS

1. A pericardial friction rub is a grating, to-and-fro sound produced by friction of the heart against the pericardium. The sound is similar to that of sandpaper rubbed on wood. Such a sound usually indicates pericarditis. The intensity of the rub varies with the phase of the cardiac cycle rather than the respiratory cycle. It may become louder when the patient leans forward. Large accumulation of fluid (pericardial effusion) may result in disappearance of the rub.

2. A pericardial knock is an adventitious sound associated with chronic (i.e., constrictive) pericarditis. It rarely occurs in children.

HEART MURMURS

Each heart murmur must be analyzed in terms of intensity (grade 1 to 6), timing (systolic or diastolic), location, transmission, and quality (musical, vibratory, blowing, and so on).

Intensity

Intensity of the murmur is customarily graded from 1 to 6.

Grade 1	Barely audible
Grade 2	Soft, but easily audible
Grade 3	Moderately loud, but not accompanied by a thrill
Grade 4	Louder and associated with a thrill
Grade 5	Audible with the stethoscope barely on the chest
Grade 6	Audible with the stethoscope off the chest

Figure 2–9. Diagram showing the relative position of ejection click (EC), midsystolic click (MC), and diastolic opening snap (OS). Filled bars show abnormal sounds.

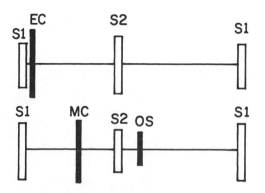

The difference between grades 2 and 3 or grades 5 and 6 may be somewhat subjective. The intensity of the murmur may be influenced by the status of cardiac output. Thus, any factor that increases the cardiac output (e.g., fever, anemia, anxiety, exercise) intensifies any existing murmur or may even produce a murmur that is not audible at basal conditions.

Classification of Heart Murmurs

Based on the timing of the heart murmur in relation to the S1 and S2, the heart murmur is classified as a systolic, diastolic, or continuous murmur.

Systolic Murmurs. Most heart murmurs are systolic in timing in that they occur between the S1 and S2. Systolic murmurs were classified by Aubrey Leatham in 1958 into two subtypes according to the time of onset: (1) ejection type and (2) regurgitant type (Fig. 2–10). Joseph Perloff classified systolic murmurs according to their time of onset and termination into four subtypes: (1) midsystolic (or ejection), (2) holosystolic, (3) early systolic, or (4) late systolic (Fig. 2–11). The holosystolic murmur and early systolic murmur of Perloff are the same as the regurgitant murmur of Leatham. The types of murmurs (as described previously) and the location of the maximum intensity of the murmur are important in the assessment of a systolic murmur. Transmission of the murmur to a particular direction and the quality of the murmur also help in deciding the cause of the murmur. These aspects are discussed in detail in the following.

Types of Systolic Murmurs.

Midsystolic (or Ejection Systolic) Murmurs. A midsystolic murmur (or ejection-type murmur) begins after S1 and ends before S2. Midsystolic murmurs coincide with turbulent flow through the semilunar valves and occur in the following settings: (1) flow of blood through stenotic or deformed semilunar valves (such as AS or PS); (2) accelerated systolic flow through normal semilunar valves, such as seen during pregnancy, fever,

Types of Systolic Murmurs (Leatham)

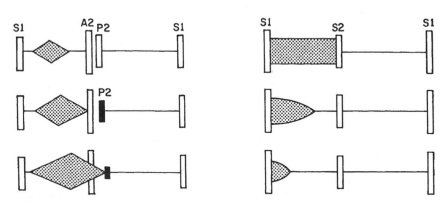

Ejection Systolic Murmurs   **Regurgitant Systolic Murmurs**

Figure 2–10. *Diagram of Leatham's classification of systolic murmurs. This classification is based primarily on the relationship of the S1 to the onset of the murmur. Short ejection-type murmur with the apex of the diamond in the early part of systole is found with mild stenosis of semilunar valves (top, left). With increasing severity of stenosis, the murmur becomes longer and the apex moves toward the S2 (middle, left). In severe pulmonary stenosis, the murmur may go beyond the A2 (bottom, left). A regurgitant systolic murmur is most often due to ventricular septal defect (VSD) and is usually holosystolic, extending all the way to the S2 (top, right). The regurgitant murmur may end in middle or early systole (not holosystolic) in some children, especially in those with small-shunt VSD and in some neonates with VSD (middle and bottom, right). Regardless of the length or intensity of the murmur, all regurgitant systolic murmurs are pathologic.*

Types of Systolic Murmurs (Perloff)

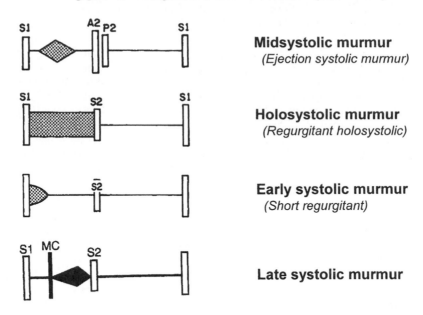

Figure 2–11. *Diagram of Perloff's classification of systolic murmurs. Midsystolic murmur is the same as ejection systolic murmur of Leatham. Holosystolic and early systolic murmurs are both regurgitant murmurs of Leatham. Late systolic murmur is typically audible with mitral valve prolapse.*

anemia, or thyrotoxicosis; and (3) innocent (normal) midsystolic murmurs (see Innocent Heart Murmurs later in this section). There is an interval between the S1 and the onset of the murmur, which coincides with the isovolumic contraction period. The intensity of the murmur increases toward the middle and then decreases during systole (crescendo-decrescendo or diamond shaped in contour). The murmur usually ends before the S2 (see Fig. 2–10, left). The murmur may be short or long and is audible at the second left or second right intercostal space.

Holosystolic Murmurs. Holosystolic murmurs begin with S1 and occupy all of systole up to the S2. No gap exists between the S1 and the onset of the murmur. Analysis of the presence or absence of a gap between the S1 and the onset of the systolic murmur is of utmost importance in distinguishing between midsystolic murmurs and holosystolic or early systolic murmurs. Holosystolic and early systolic murmurs of Perloff are included in regurgitant systolic murmurs of Leatham. The intensity of holosystolic murmurs usually levels off all the way to the S2. Holosystolic murmurs are caused by the flow of blood from a chamber that is at a higher pressure throughout systole than the receiving chamber, and they usually occur while the semilunar valves are still closed. These murmurs are associated with *only* the following three conditions: VSD, MR, and tricuspid regurgitation (TR). None of these ordinarily occurs at the base (i.e., second left or right intercostal space).

Early Systolic Murmurs. Early systolic murmurs (or short regurgitant murmurs) begin with the S1, diminish in decrescendo, and end well before the S2, generally at or before midsystole (see Fig. 2–11). Only the three conditions that cause holosystolic murmurs (VSD, MR, and TR) are the causes of an early systolic murmur. An early systolic murmur is a feature of TR with normal RV systolic pressure. When the RV systolic pressure is elevated, a holosystolic murmur results. Early systolic murmurs may occur in a neonate with a large VSD and in children or adults with a very small VSD or with a large VSD and pulmonary hypertension.

Late Systolic Murmurs. The term "late systolic" applies when a murmur begins in middle to late systole and proceeds up to the S2 (see Fig. 2–11). The late systolic murmur of mitral valve prolapse is prototypical (see Chapter 21).

Location of Systolic Murmurs. In addition to the type of systolic murmurs, the location of maximal intensity of the murmur is important when diagnosing the heart murmur's origin. The following four locations are important: (1) upper left sternal border (pulmonary valve area), (2) upper right sternal border (aortic valve area), (3) lower left sternal border, and (4) the apex. For example, a holosystolic murmur heard maximally at the lower left sternal border is characteristic of a VSD. A midsystolic murmur maximally audible at the second left intercostal space is usually pulmonary in origin. The location of the heart murmur often helps differentiate between a midsystolic murmur and a holosystolic murmur. For example, a long PS murmur may sound like the holosystolic murmur of a VSD; however, because the maximal intensity is at the upper left sternal border, it is unlikely that a VSD caused the murmur. Although rare, a subarterial infundibular VSD murmur may be maximally heard at the upper left sternal border. Differential diagnosis of systolic murmurs according to the location is discussed in detail in this section (see Tables 2–5 to 2–8; Fig. 2–12).

Transmission of Systolic Murmurs. The transmission of systolic murmurs from the site of maximal intensity may help determine the murmur's origin. For example, an apical systolic murmur that transmits well to the left axilla and lower back is characteristic of MR, whereas one that radiates to the upper right sternal border and the neck is more likely to originate in the aortic valve. A systolic ejection murmur at the base that transmits well to the neck is more likely to be aortic in origin; one that transmits well to the back is more likely to be of pulmonary valve or PA origin.

Quality of Systolic Murmurs. The quality of a murmur may help diagnose heart disease. Systolic murmurs of MR or of a VSD have a uniform, high-pitched quality, often described as blowing. Midsystolic murmurs of AS or PS have a rough, grating quality. A common innocent murmur in children, which is best audible between the lower left sternal border and apex, has a characteristic "vibratory" or humming quality.

Differential Diagnosis of Systolic Murmurs at Various Locations. Systolic murmurs that are audible at the four locations are presented in Figure 2–12. More common conditions

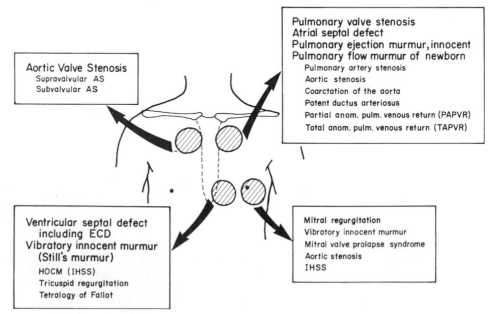

Figure 2–12. *Diagram showing systolic murmurs audible at various locations. Less common conditions are shown in smaller type (see Tables 2–5 to 2–8). AS, aortic stenosis; ECD, endocardial cushion defect; HOCM, hypertrophic obstructive cardiomyopathy; IHSS, idiopathic hypertrophic subaortic stenosis.*

Table 2–5. **Differential Diagnosis of Systolic Murmurs at the Upper Left Sternal Border (Pulmonary Area)**

Condition	Important Physical Findings	Chest X-ray Films	ECG Findings
Pulmonary valve stenosis	SEM, grade 2 to 5/6 *Thrill (±) S2 may be split widely when mild *Ejection click (±) at 2LICS Transmit to the back	*Prominent MPA (poststenotic dilatation) Normal PVM	Normal if mild RAD *RVH RAH if severe
ASD	SEM, grade 2 to 3/6 *Widely split and fixed S2	*Increased PVM *RAE, RVE	RAD RVH *RBBB (rsR′)
Pulmonary flow murmur of newborn	SEM, grade 1 to 2/6 No thrill *Good transmission to the back and axilla Newborns	Normal	Normal
Pulmonary flow murmur of older children	SEM, grade 2 to 3/6 No thrill Poor transmission	Normal Occasional pectus excavatum or straight back	Normal
PA stenosis	SEM, grade 2 to 3/6 Occasional continuous murmur P2 may be loud *Transmits well to the back and both lung fields	Prominent hilar vessels (±)	RVH or normal
AS	SEM, grade 2 to 5/6 *Also audible in 2RICS *Thrill (±) at 2RICS and SSN *Ejection click at apex, 3LICS, or 2RICS (±) Paradoxically split S2 if severe	Absence of prominent MPA Dilated aorta	Normal or LVH
TOF	*Long SEM, grade 2 to 4/6, louder at MLSB Thrill (±) Loud, single S2 (= A2) Cyanosis, clubbing	*Decreased PVM *Normal heart size Boot-shaped heart Right aortic arch (25%)	RAD *RVH or BVH RAH (±)

COA	SEM, grade 1 to 3/6
	*Loudest at left interscapular area (back)
	*Weak or absent femorals
	Hypertension in arms
	Frequent associated AS, bicuspid aortic
	  valve, or MR
		*Classic "3" sign on plain
		  film or "E" sign on
		  barium esophagogram
		Rib notching (±)
			LVH in children
			RBBB (or RVH)
			  in infants

PDA	*Continuous murmur at left
	  infraclavicular area
	Occasional crescendic systolic only
	Grade 2 to 4/6
	Thrill (±)
	Bounding pulses
		*Increased PVM
		*LAE, LVE
			Normal,
			  LVH, or BVH

TAPVR	SEM, grade 2 to 3/6 Widely split and fixed S2 (±) *Quadruple or quintuple rhythm *Diastolic rumble at LLSB *Mild cyanosis (↓PO₂) and clubbing (±)	*Increased PVM RAE and RVE Prominent MPA "Snowman" sign	RAD RAH *RVH
PAPVR	Physical findings similar to those of ASD *S2 may not be fixed unless associated with ASD	*Increased PVM *RAE and RVE "Scimitar" sign (±)	Same as in ASD

*Findings that are characteristic of the condition.

AS, aortic stenosis; ASD, atrial septal defect; BVH, biventricular hypertrophy; COA, coarctation of the aorta; ECG, electrocardiogram; LAE, left atrial enlargement; 2LICS, second left intercostal space; 3LICS, third left intercostal space; LLSB, lower left sternal border; LVE, left ventricular enlargement; LVH, left ventricular hypertrophy; MLSB, mid-left sternal border; MPA, main pulmonary artery; MR, mitral regurgitation; PA, pulmonary artery; PAPVR, partial anomalous pulmonary venous return; PDA, patent ductus arteriosus; PVM, pulmonary vascular markings; RAD, right axis deviation; RAE, right atrial enlargement; RAH, right atrial hypertrophy; RBBB, right bundle branch block; 2RICS, second right intercostal space; RVE, right ventricular enlargement; RVH, right ventricular hypertrophy; SEM, systolic ejection murmur; SSN, suprasternal notch; TAPVR, total anomalous pulmonary venous return; TOF, tetralogy of Fallot; ±, may or may not be present.

*Table 2–6. **Differential Diagnosis of Systolic Murmurs at the Upper Right Sternal Border (Aortic Area)***

Condition	Important Physical Findings	Chest X-ray Films	ECG Findings
Aortic valve stenosis	SEM, grade 2 to 5/6, at 2RICS, may be loudest at 3LICS *Thrill (±), URSB, SSN, and carotid arteries *Ejection click *Transmits well to neck S2 may be single	Mild LVE (±) Prominent ascending aorta or aortic knob	Normal or LVH with or without "strain"
Subaortic stenosis	SEM, grade 2 to 4/6 *AR murmur almost always present in discrete stenosis No ejection click	Usually normal	Normal or LVH
Supravalvular aortic stenosis	SEM, grade 2 to 3/6 Thrill (±) No ejection click *Pulse and BP may be greater in right than left arm *Peculiar facies and mental retardation (±) Murmur may transmit well to the back (PA stenosis)	Unremarkable	Normal, LVH or BVH

*Findings that are characteristic of the condition.
AR, aortic regurgitation; BP, blood pressure; BVH, biventricular hypertrophy; ECG, electrocardiogram; 3LICS, third left intercostal space; LVE, left ventricular enlargement; LVH, left ventricular hypertrophy; PA, pulmonary artery; 2RICS, second right intercostal space; SEM, systolic ejection murmur; SSN, suprasternal notch; URSB, upper right sternal border; ±, may or may not be present.

*Table 2–7. **Differential Diagnosis of Systolic Murmurs at the Lower Left Sternal Border***

Condition	Important Physical Findings	Chest X-ray Films	ECG Findings
VSD	*Regurgitant systolic, grade 2 to 5/6 May not be holosystolic Well localized at LLSB *Thrill often present P2 may be loud	*Increased PVM *LAE and LVE (cardiomegaly)	Normal LVH or BVH
ECD, complete	Similar to findings of VSD *Diastolic rumble at LLSB *Gallop rhythm common in infants	Similar to large VSD	*Superior QRS axis, LVH or BVH
Vibratory innocent murmur (Still's)	SEM, grade 2 to 3/6 *Musical or vibratory with midsystolic accentuation *Maximum between LLSB and apex	Normal	Normal
HOCM or IHSS	SEM, grade 2 to 4/6 Medium pitched Maximum at LLSB or apex Thrill (±) *Sharp upstroke of brachial pulses May have MR murmur	Normal or globular LVE	LVH Abnormally deep Q waves in leads V5 and V6
TR	*Regurgitant systolic, grade 2 to 3/6 *Triple or quadruple rhythm (in Ebstein's) Mild cyanosis (±) Hepatomegaly with pulsatile liver and neck vein distention when severe	Normal PVM RAE if severe	RBBB, RAH, and first-degree AV block in Ebstein's
TOF	Murmurs can be louder at ULSB	(see Table 2–5)	(see Table 2–5)

*Findings that are characteristic of the condition.
AV, atrioventricular; BVH, biventricular hypertrophy; ECD, endocardial cushion defect; ECG, electrocardiogram; HOCM, hypertrophic obstructive cardiomyopathy; IHSS, idiopathic hypertrophic subaortic stenosis; LAE, left atrial enlargement; LLSB, lower left sternal border; LVE, left ventricular enlargement; LVH, left ventricular hypertrophy; MR, mitral regurgitation; PVM, pulmonary vascular markings; RAE, right atrial enlargement; RAH, right atrial hypertrophy; RBBB, right bundle branch block; SEM, systolic ejection murmur; TR, tricuspid regurgitation; TOF, tetralogy of Fallot; ULSB, upper left sternal border; VSD, ventricular septal defect; ±, may or may not be present.

Table 2–8. **Differential Diagnosis of Systolic Murmurs at the Apex**

Condition	Important Physical Findings	Chest X-ray Films	ECG Findings
MR	*Regurgitant systolic, may not be holosystolic, grade 2 to 3/6 Transmits to left axilla (less obvious in children) May be loudest in the mid-precordium	LAE and LVE	LAH and LVH
MVP	*Midsystolic click with/without late systolic murmur *High frequency of thoracic skeletal anomalies (pectus excavatum, straight back) (85%)	Normal	Inverted T wave in lead aVF
Aortic valve stenosis	The murmur and ejection click may be best heard at the apex rather than at 2RICS	Mild LVE (±) Prominent ascending aorta or aortic knob	Normal or LVH with or without "strain"
HOCM or IHSS	The murmur of IHSS may be maximal at the apex (may represent MR)	Normal or globular LVE	LVH Abnormally deep Q waves in leads V5 and V6
Vibratory innocent murmur	This innocent murmur may be loudest at the apex	Normal	Normal

*Findings that are characteristic of the condition.
ECG, electrocardiogram; HOCM, hypertrophic obstructive cardiomyopathy; IHSS, idiopathic hypertrophic subaortic stenosis; LAE, left atrial enlargement; LAH, left atrial hypertrophy; LVE, left ventricular enlargement; LVH, left ventricular hypertrophy; MR, mitral regurgitation; MVP, mitral valve prolapse; 2RICS, second right intercostal space.

are listed in larger type and less common conditions in smaller type. For quick reference, characteristic physical, ECG, and x-ray findings that are helpful in differential diagnoses are listed in Tables 2–5 through 2–8.

1. Upper left sternal border (or pulmonary area): In many conditions both pathologic and physiologic (i.e., innocent murmur), a systolic murmur is most audible at the upper left sternal border. Audible systolic murmurs at this location are usually midsystolic murmurs and may be the result of one of the following:

   a. PS
   b. ASD
   c. Innocent (normal) pulmonary flow murmur of newborns
   d. Innocent pulmonary flow murmur of older children
   e. PA stenosis
   f. AS
   g. TOF
   h. COA
   i. PDA with pulmonary hypertension (a continuous murmur of a PDA is usually loudest in the left infraclavicular area)
   j. Total anomalous pulmonary venous return (TAPVR)
   k. PAPVR

   Conditions a through d are more common than the other listed conditions. Table 2–5 summarizes other clinical findings that are useful in the differential diagnosis of systolic murmurs audible at the upper left sternal border.

2. Upper right sternal border or aortic area: Systolic murmurs at the upper right sternal border are also midsystolic type. They are caused by narrowing of the aortic valve or its neighboring structures. The murmur transmits well to the neck. Often it transmits with a thrill over the carotid arteries. The midsystolic murmur of AS may be heard with equal clarity at the upper left sternal border (i.e., "pulmonary area") as well as at the apex. However, the PS murmur does not transmit well to the upper right sternal border and the neck; rather, it transmits well to the back and the sides of the chest. Systolic murmurs in the upper right sternal border are caused by the following:

   a. AS
   b. Subvalvular AS (subaortic stenosis)
   c. Supravalvular AS

Characteristic physical, ECG, and x-ray findings that help in the differential diagnosis of these conditions are presented in Table 2–6.

3. Lower left sternal border: Systolic murmurs that are maximally audible at this location may be either holosystolic, early systolic, or midsystolic type and may result from one of the following conditions:

   a. VSD murmur is either a holosystolic or early systolic murmur (a small muscular VSD murmur may be heard best between the lower left sternal border and the apex).

   b. Vibratory or musical innocent murmur (e.g., Still's murmur); this murmur may be equally loud or even louder toward the apex, and the maximal intensity may be in the mid-precordium.

   c. Hypertrophic obstructive cardiomyopathy (HOCM) (formerly known as idiopathic hypertrophic subaortic stenosis)

   d. TR

   e. TOF

Characteristic physical, ECG, and x-ray findings that help in the differential diagnosis of these conditions are presented in Table 2–7.

4. Apical area: Systolic murmurs that are maximally audible at the apex may be holosystolic, midsystolic, or late systolic murmurs and result from one of the following conditions:

   a. MR (holosystolic)

   b. MVP (late systolic murmur, usually preceded by a midsystolic click)

   c. AS (midsystolic)

   d. HOCM (midsystolic)

   e. Vibratory innocent murmur (midsystolic)

Characteristic physical, ECG, and x-ray findings are summarized in Table 2–8.

Diastolic Murmurs. Diastolic murmurs occur between the S2 and S1. Based on timing and relation to the heart sounds, they are classified into three types: early diastolic (or protodiastolic), mid-diastolic, and late diastolic (or presystolic) (Fig. 2–13).

1. **Early diastolic decrescendo murmurs** occur early in diastole, immediately after the S2, and are caused by incompetence of the aortic or pulmonary valve (see Fig. 2–13).

Because the aorta is a high-pressure vessel, AR murmurs are high pitched and best heard with the diaphragm of a stethoscope at the third left intercostal space. The AR murmur radiates well to the apex because the regurgitation is directed toward the apex. Bounding peripheral pulses may be present if the AR is significant. AR murmurs are associated with congenital bicuspid aortic valve, subaortic stenosis, an intervention for AS (i.e., postvalvotomy or post–balloon dilatation), and rheumatic heart disease with AR. Occasionally, a subarterial infundibular VSD with prolapsing aortic cusps may cause an AR murmur.

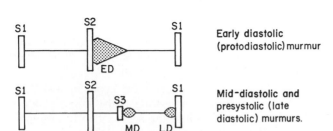

Early diastolic (protodiastolic) murmur

Mid-diastolic and presystolic (late diastolic) murmurs.

Figure 2–13. Diagram of diastolic murmurs and the continuous murmur. ED, early diastolic or protodiastolic murmur; LD, late diastolic or presystolic murmur; MD, mid-diastolic murmur.

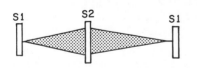

Continuous murmur

PR murmurs also occur early in diastole. They are usually medium pitched but may be high pitched if pulmonary hypertension is present. They are best heard at the third left intercostal space and radiate along the left sternal border. These murmurs are associated with postoperative TOF (because of surgically induced PR), pulmonary hypertension, postoperative pulmonary valvotomy or post–balloon valvuloplasty for PS, and mild isolated deformity of the pulmonary valve.

2. **Mid-diastolic murmurs** start with a loud S3 and are heard in early or mid-diastole but are not temporally midway through diastole (see Fig. 2–13). These murmurs are always low pitched and best heard with the bell of the stethoscope applied lightly to the chest. These murmurs are caused by turbulence in mitral or tricuspid flow secondary to anatomic stenosis or relative stenosis of these valves.

   Mitral mid-diastolic murmurs are best heard at the apex and are often referred to as an *apical rumble*, although frequently they sound more like a hum than a rumble. These murmurs are associated with MS or a large left-to-right shunt VSD or PDA, which produces relative MS secondary to a large flow across the normal-sized mitral valve.

   Tricuspid mid-diastolic murmurs are best heard along the lower left sternal border. These murmurs are associated with ASD, PAPVR, TAPVR, and ECD because they all result in relative tricuspid stenosis (TS). Anatomic stenosis of the tricuspid valve is also associated with these murmurs, but such cases are rare.

3. **Presystolic (or late diastolic) murmurs** are also caused by flow through the AV valves during ventricular diastole. They result from active atrial contraction that ejects blood into the ventricle rather than a passive pressure difference between the atrium and ventricle. These low-frequency murmurs occur late in diastole or just before the onset of systole (see Fig. 2–13) and are found with anatomic stenosis of the mitral or tricuspid valve.

Continuous Murmurs. Continuous murmurs begin in systole and continue without interruption through the S2 into all or part of diastole (see Fig. 2–13). Continuous murmurs are caused by the following:

1. Aortopulmonary or arteriovenous connection (e.g., PDA, arteriovenous fistula, after systemic-to-PA shunt surgery, persistent truncus arteriosus, rarely)
2. Disturbances of flow patterns in veins (e.g., venous hum)
3. Disturbance of flow pattern in arteries (e.g., COA, PA stenosis)

The murmur of PDA has a machinery-like quality, becoming louder during systole (crescendo), peaking at the S2, and diminishing in diastole (decrescendo). This murmur is maximally heard in the left infraclavicular area or along the upper left sternal border. With pulmonary hypertension, only the systolic portion can be heard, but it is crescendic during systole.

Venous hum is a common innocent murmur that is audible in the upright position, in the infraclavicular region, unilaterally or bilaterally. The murmur's intensity also changes with the position of the neck. When the child lies supine, the murmur usually disappears. It is usually heard better on the right side.

Less common continuous murmurs of severe COA may be heard over the intercostal collaterals. The continuous murmurs of PA stenosis may be heard over the right and left anterior chest, the sides of the chest, and in the back.

The combination of a systolic murmur (e.g., VSD, AS, or PS) and a diastolic murmur (e.g., AR or PR) is referred to as a *to-and-fro murmur* to distinguish it from a machinery-like continuous murmur.

Innocent Heart Murmurs

Innocent heart murmurs, also called *functional murmurs*, arise from cardiovascular structures in the absence of anatomic abnormalities. Innocent heart murmurs are common in children. More than 80% of children have innocent murmurs of one type or another sometime during childhood. All innocent heart murmurs (as well as pathologic murmurs) are accentuated or brought out in a high-output state, usually during a febrile illness.

Probably the only way a physician can recognize an innocent heart murmur is to become familiar with the more common forms of these murmurs by auscultating under the supervision of pediatric cardiologists. All innocent heart murmurs are associated with normal ECG and x-ray findings. When one or more of the following are present, the murmur is more likely pathologic and requires cardiac consultation:

1. Symptoms
2. Abnormal cardiac size or silhouette or abnormal pulmonary vascularity on chest roentgenograms
3. Abnormal ECG
4. Diastolic murmur
5. A systolic murmur that is loud (i.e., grade 3/6 or with a thrill), long in duration, and transmits well to other parts of the body
6. Cyanosis
7. Abnormally strong or weak pulses
8. Abnormal heart sounds

Classic Vibratory Murmur. This is the most common innocent murmur in children, first described by Still in 1909. Most vibratory murmurs are detected between 3 and 6 years of age, but the same murmur may be present in neonates and infants as well as adolescents. It is maximally audible at the mid-left sternal border or over the mid-precordium (between the lower left sternal border and the apex). It is generally of low frequency and best heard with the bell of the stethoscope with the patient in the supine position. The murmur is midsystolic (i.e., not regurgitant) in timing and of grade 2 to 3/6 in intensity. This murmur is not accompanied by a thrill or ejection click. It has a distinctive quality, described as a "twanging string," groaning, squeaking, buzzing, or vibratory sound, giving a pleasing musical character to the murmur. The murmur is generally loudest in the supine position and often changes in character, pitch, and intensity with upright positioning. The vibratory quality may disappear and the murmur may become softer when the bell is pressed harder, thereby proving its low frequency. The intensity of the murmur increases during febrile illness or excitement, after exercise, or in anemic states. The murmur may disappear briefly at a maximum Valsalva maneuver. The ECG and chest x-ray films are normal (Table 2–9; Fig. 2–14).

Table 2–9. ***Common Innocent Heart Murmurs***

Type (Timing)	Description of Murmur	Age Group
Classic vibratory murmur (Still's murmur) (systolic)	Maximal at MLSB or between LLSB and apex Grade 2 to 3/6 Low-frequency vibratory, "twanging string," groaning, squeaking, or musical	3–6 yr Occasionally in infancy
Pulmonary ejection murmur (systolic)	Maximal at ULSB Early to midsystolic Grade 1 to 3/6 in intensity Blowing in quality	8–14 yr
Pulmonary flow murmur of newborn (systolic)	Maximal at ULSB Transmits well to the left and right chest, axilla, and back Grade 1 to 2/6 in intensity	Prematures and full-term newborns Usually disappears by 3–6 mo of age
Venous hum (continuous)	Maximal at right (or left) supraclavicular and infraclavicular areas Grade 1 to 3/6 in intensity Inaudible in the supine position Intensity changes with rotation of the head and compression of the jugular vein	3–6 yr
Carotid bruit (systolic)	Right supraclavicular area and over the carotids Grade 2 to 3/6 in intensity Occasional thrill over a carotid	Any age

LLSB, lower left sternal border; MLSB, mid-left sternal border; ULSB, upper left sternal border.

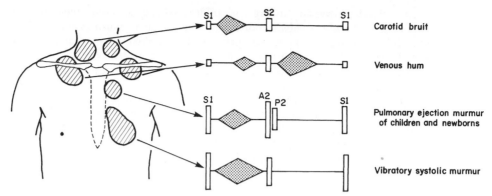

Figure 2–14. Diagram of innocent heart murmurs in children.

An inexperienced examiner may confuse this murmur with the murmur of a VSD. The murmur of a VSD is usually harsh, grade 2 to 3/6 in intensity, holosystolic starting with the S1 rather than midsystolic, and often accompanied by a palpable thrill. The ECG and x-ray films are often abnormal.

The origin of the murmur remains obscure. It is believed to be generated by low-frequency vibrations of normal pulmonary leaflets at their attachments during systole or periodic vibrations of a left ventricular false tendon.

Pulmonary Ejection Murmur (Pulmonary Flow Murmur) of Childhood. It is common in children between 8 and 14 years of age but is most frequent in adolescents. The murmur is maximally audible at the upper left sternal border. This murmur represents an exaggeration of normal ejection vibrations within the pulmonary trunk. The murmur is exaggerated by the presence of pectus excavatum, straight back, or kyphoscoliosis. The murmur is midsystolic in timing and slightly grating (rather than vibratory) in quality, with relatively little radiation. The intensity of the murmur is usually a grade 1 to 3/6. The S2 is normal, and there is no associated thrill or ejection click (see Table 2–9; Fig. 2–14). The ECG and chest x-ray films are normal.

This murmur may be confused with the murmur of pulmonary valve stenosis or an ASD. In pulmonary valve stenosis, there may be an ejection click, systolic thrill, widely split S2, right ventricular hypertrophy (RVH) on ECG, and poststenotic dilatation of the main PA segment on chest x-ray films. Important differential points of ASD include a widely split and fixed S2, a mid-diastolic murmur of relative TS audible at the lower left sternal border if the shunt is large, RBBB or mild RVH on ECG manifested by rsR' in V1, and chest x-ray films revealing increased pulmonary vascular markings and enlargement of the right atrium, RV, and main PA.

Pulmonary Flow Murmur of Newborns. This murmur is commonly present in newborns, especially those with low birth weight. The murmur usually disappears by 3 to 6 months of age. If it persists beyond this age, a structural narrowing of the pulmonary arterial tree (i.e., PA stenosis) should be suspected. It is best audible at the upper left sternal border. Although the murmur is only a grade 1 to 2/6 in intensity, it transmits impressively to the right and left chest, both axillae, and the back. There is no ejection click. The ECG and chest x-ray film are normal (see Table 2–9; Fig. 2–14).

In the fetus, the main PA trunk is large but the branches of the pulmonary artery are relatively hypoplastic because they receive a small amount of blood flow during fetal life (only 15% of combined ventricular output goes to these vessels). When the ductus closes after birth, the large dome-shaped main pulmonary artery trunk gives off two small branch pulmonary arteries. The flow through these small vessels produces turbulence with a faster flow velocity and the turbulence is transmitted along the smaller branches of the PAs. Therefore, this murmur is heard well around the chest wall. The murmur is louder in small preterm babies than the larger full-term neonates.

The murmur resembles the murmur of organic PA stenosis, which may be seen as a component of rubella syndrome, Williams' syndrome, or Alagille's syndrome.

Characteristic noncardiac findings in children with these syndromes lead physicians to suspect that the PA stenosis murmur has an organic cause. Organic PA stenosis is frequently associated with other cardiac defects (e.g., VSD and pulmonary valve stenosis), is at the site of a previous Blalock-Taussig shunt, or is seen occasionally as an isolated anomaly. The heart murmur of organic PA stenosis persists beyond infancy, and the ECG may show RVH if the stenosis is severe.

Venous Hum. This murmur is commonly audible in children between the ages of 3 and 6 years. It originates from turbulence in the jugular venous system. This is a continuous murmur in which the diastolic component is louder than the systolic component. The murmur is maximally audible at the right and/or left infraclavicular and supraclavicular areas (see Table 2–9; Fig. 2–14). The venous hum is heard only in the upright position and disappears in the supine position. It can be obliterated by rotating the head or by gently occluding the neck veins with the fingers.

It is important to differentiate a venous hum from the continuous murmur of a PDA. The murmur of a PDA is loudest at the upper left sternal border or left infraclavicular area and may be associated with bounding peripheral pulses and wide pulse pressure if the shunt is large. The systolic component is louder than the diastolic component. The x-ray films show increased pulmonary vascular markings and cardiac enlargement. The ECG may be normal (with a small shunt) or show left ventricular hypertrophy or combined ventricular hypertrophy (with a large shunt).

Carotid Bruit (or Supraclavicular Systolic Murmur). This is an early systolic ejection murmur, best heard in the supraclavicular fossa or over the carotid arteries (see Table 2–9; Fig. 2–14). It is produced by turbulence in the brachiocephalic or carotid arteries. The murmur is a grade 2 to 3/6 in intensity. Although it rarely occurs, a faint thrill is palpable over a carotid artery. This bruit may be found in children of any age.

The murmur of AS often transmits well to the carotid arteries with a palpable thrill, requiring differentiation from carotid bruits. In AS, the murmur is louder at the upper right sternal border, and a systolic thrill is often present in the upper right sternal border and suprasternal notch as well as over the carotid artery. An ejection click is often present in aortic valve stenosis. The ECG and chest x-ray film may appear abnormal.

Some Special Features of the Cardiac Examination of Neonates

The following section briefly summarizes some unique aspects of normal and abnormal physical findings in the newborn, which are different from those in older infants and children. The difference is caused by the normal RV dominance and elevated pulmonary vascular resistance seen in the early neonatal period. Premature infants in general have less RV dominance and lower pulmonary vascular resistance than full-term neonates, adding variability to this generalization.

NORMAL PHYSICAL FINDINGS OF NEONATES

The following are normal cardiovascular findings in newborn infants:

1. The heart rate generally is faster in newborns than in older children and adults (the newborn rate is usually 100 beats/minute, with a normal range of 70 to 180 beats/minute).

2. A varying degree of acrocyanosis is the rule rather than the exception.

3. Mild arterial desaturation with arterial partial pressure of oxygen (Po_2) as low as 60 mm Hg is not unusual in an otherwise normal neonate. This may be caused by an intrapulmonary shunt through an as yet unexpanded portion of the lungs or by a right atrium–to–left atrium shunt through a patent foramen ovale.

4. The RV is relatively hyperactive, with the point of maximal impulse at the lower left sternal border rather than at the apex.

5. The S2 may be single in the first days of life.

6. An ejection click (representing pulmonary hypertension) is occasionally heard in the first hours of life.

7. A newborn may have an innocent heart murmur. Four common innocent murmurs in the newborn period are pulmonary flow murmur of the newborn (see Fig. 2–14), transient systolic murmur of PDA, transient systolic murmur of TR, and vibratory innocent systolic murmur.

   a. Pulmonary flow murmur of the newborn is the most common heart murmur in newborn infants (see previous section).

   b. Transient systolic murmur of PDA is caused by a closing ductus arteriosus and is audible on the first day of life. It is a grade 1 to 2/6, only systolic, at the upper left sternal border and in the left infraclavicular area.

   c. Transient systolic murmur of TR is indistinguishable from that of VSD. It is believed that a minimal tricuspid valve abnormality produces regurgitation in the presence of high pulmonary vascular resistance (and high RV pressure), but the regurgitation disappears as the pulmonary vascular resistance falls. Therefore, this murmur is more common in infants who had fetal distress or neonatal asphyxia because they tend to maintain high pulmonary vascular resistance for a longer period.

   d. Vibratory innocent murmur is a counterpart of Still's murmur in older children (see previous section).

8. Peripheral pulses are easily palpable in all extremities, including the foot, in *every* normal infant. The peripheral pulses normally appear to be bounding in premature babies because of the lack of subcutaneous tissue.

ABNORMAL PHYSICAL FINDINGS IN NEONATES

The following abnormal physical findings suggest cardiac malformation. Repeated examination is important because physical findings change rapidly in normal infants as well as in infants with cardiac problems.

1. Cyanosis, particularly when it does not improve with the administration of oxygen, suggests a cardiac abnormality.

2. Decreased or absent peripheral pulses in the lower extremities suggest COA. Weak peripheral pulses throughout suggest hypoplastic left heart syndrome (HLHS) or circulatory shock. Bounding peripheral pulses suggest aortic runoff lesions, such as PDA or persistent truncus arteriosus.

3. Tachypnea of greater than 60 breaths/minute with or without retraction suggests a cardiac abnormality.

4. Hepatomegaly may suggest a heart defect. A midline liver suggests asplenia or polysplenia syndrome.

5. A heart murmur may be a presenting sign of a congenital heart defect, although innocent murmurs are much more frequent than pathologic murmurs. Most pathologic murmurs should be audible during the first month of life, with the exception of an ASD. However, the time of appearance of a heart murmur depends on the nature of the defect.

   a. Heart murmurs of stenotic lesions (e.g., AS, PS) and those due to AV valve regurgitation are audible immediately after birth and persist because these murmurs are not affected by the level of pulmonary vascular resistance.

   b. Heart murmurs of large VSD may not be audible until 1 to 2 weeks of age, when the pulmonary vascular resistance becomes sufficiently low to allow shunt to occur.

   c. The murmur of an ASD appears after a year or two, when the compliance of the RV improves to allow a significant atrial shunt. A newborn or a small infant with a large ASD may not have a heart murmur.

6. Even in the absence of a heart murmur, a newborn infant may have a serious heart defect that requires immediate attention (e.g., severe cyanotic heart defect such as TGA or pulmonary atresia with a closing PDA). Infants who are in severe CHF may not have a loud murmur until the myocardial function is improved through anticongestive measures.

7. Irregular cardiac rhythm and abnormal heart rate suggest a cardiac abnormality.

Chapter 3

Electrocardiography

In the clinical diagnosis of congenital or acquired heart disease, the presence of electrocardiographic (ECG) abnormalities is often helpful. Hypertrophies (of ventricles and atria) and ventricular conduction disturbances are the two most common forms of ECG abnormalities. Other ECG abnormalities such as atrioventricular (AV) conduction disturbances, arrhythmias, and ST-segment and T-wave changes are also helpful in the clinical diagnosis of cardiac problems.

Throughout this chapter, the vectorial approach is used whenever possible. The vectorial approach is preferred to "pattern reading," which has an infinite number of possibilities. The following topics are discussed in the order listed.

What is the vectorial approach?
Comparison of pediatric and adult ECGs
Basic measurements and their normal values necessary for interpretation of an ECG (which include rhythm, heat rate, QRS axis, and P and T axes)
Atrial and ventricular hypertrophy
Ventricular conduction disturbances
ST-segment and T-wave changes, including myocardial infarction

Cardiac arrhythmias and AV conduction disturbances are discussed in Chapters 24 and 25.

What Is the Vectorial Approach?

The vectorial approach views the standard scalar ECG as three-dimensional vector forces that vary with time. A vector is a quantity that possesses magnitude *and* direction; a scalar is a quantity that has magnitude only. A scalar ECG, which is routinely obtained in clinical practice, shows only the magnitude of the forces against time. However, by combining scalar leads that represent the frontal projection and the horizontal projections of the vector cardiogram, one can derive the *direction* of the force from scalar ECGs. The limb leads (leads I, II, III, aVR, aVL, and aVF) provide information about the frontal projection (reflecting superior-inferior and right-to-left forces), and the precordial leads (leads V1 through V6, V3R, and V4R) provide information about the horizontal plane that reflects forces that are right to left and anterior-posterior (Fig. 3–1). It is important for the readers to become familiar with the orientation of each scalar ECG lead. Once learned, the vectorial approach helps the readers to retain the knowledge gained and even helps them recall what has been forgotten.

HEXAXIAL REFERENCE SYSTEM

It is necessary to memorize the orientation of the hexaxial reference system (see Fig. 3–1A). The hexaxial reference system is made up by the six limb leads (leads I, II, III, aVR, aVL, and aVF) and provides information about the superoinferior

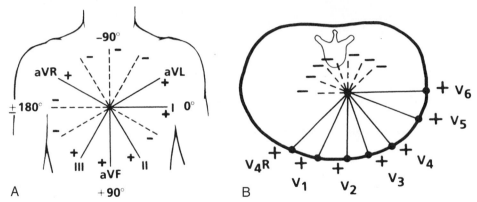

Figure 3–1. *Hexaxial reference system (**A**) shows the frontal projection of a vector loop, and horizontal reference system (**B**) shows the horizontal projection. The combination of **A** and **B** constitutes the 12-lead (or 13-lead) electrocardiogram. (From Park MK, Guntheroth WG: How to Read Pediatric ECGs, 4th ed. Philadelphia, Mosby, 2006.)*

and right-left relationships of the electromotive forces. In this system, leads I and aVF cross at a right angle at the electrical center (see Fig. 3–1A). The bipolar limb leads (I, II, and III) are clockwise with an angle between them of 60 degrees. Note that the positive poles of aVR, aVL, and aVF are directed toward the right and left shoulders and the foot, respectively. The positive limb of each lead is shown by a solid line and the negative limb by a broken line. The positive pole of each lead is indicated by the lead label. The positive pole of lead I is labeled as 0 degree and the negative pole of the same lead as ±180 degrees. The positive pole of aVF is designated as +90 degrees and the negative pole of the same lead as −90 degrees. The positive poles of leads II and III are +60 and +120 degrees, respectively, and so on. The hexaxial reference system is used in plotting the QRS axis, T axis, and P axis.

The lead I axis represents the left-right relationship with the positive pole on the left and the negative pole on the right. The aVF lead represents the superior-inferior relationship with the positive pole directed inferiorly and the negative pole directed superiorly. The R wave in each lead represents the depolarization force directed toward the positive pole; the Q and S waves are the depolarization force directed toward the negative pole. Therefore, the R wave of lead I represents the leftward force and the S wave of the same lead represents the rightward force (see Fig. 3–1A). The R wave in aVF represents the inferiorly directed force and the S wave the superiorly directed force. By the same token, the R wave in lead II represents the leftward and inferior force and the R wave in lead III represents the rightward and inferior force. The R wave in aVR represents the rightward and superior force and the R wave in aVL represents the leftward and superior force.

An easy way to memorize the hexaxial reference system is shown in Figure 3–2 by a superimposition of a body with stretched arms and legs on the X and Y axes. The hands and feet are the positive poles of electrodes. The left and right hands are the positive poles of leads aVR and aVL, respectively. The left and right feet are the positive poles of leads II and III, respectively. The bipolar limb leads I, II, and III are clockwise in sequence for the positive electrode.

HORIZONTAL REFERENCE SYSTEM

The horizontal reference system consists of precordial leads (leads V1 through V6, V3R, and V4R) (see Fig. 3–1B) and provides information about the anterior-posterior and the left-right relationship. Leads V2 and V6 cross approximately at a right angle at the electrical center of the heart. The V6 axis represents the left-right relationship and the V2 axis represents the anterior-posterior relationship. The positive limb of each lead is shown by a solid line and the negative limb by a broken line. The positive pole of each lead is indicated by the lead label (e.g., V4R, V1, V2). The precordial leads V3R

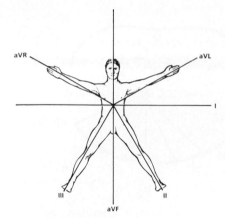

Figure 3–2. An easy way to memorize the hexaxial reference system. (From Park MK, Guntheroth WG: How to Read Pediatric ECGs, 4th ed. Philadelphia, Mosby, 2006.)

and V4R are at the mirror image points of V3 and V4, respectively, in the right chest, and these leads are quite popular in pediatric cardiology because right ventricular (RV) forces are more prominent in infants and children.

Therefore, the R wave of V6 represents the leftward force and the R wave of V2 the anterior force. Conversely, the S wave of V6 represents the rightward force and the S wave of V2 the posterior force. The R wave in V1, V3R, and V4R represents the rightward *and* anterior force and the S wave of these leads represents the leftward and posterior force (see Fig. 3–1B). The R wave of lead V5 in general represents the leftward force, and the R waves of leads V3 and V4 represent a transition between the right and left precordial leads. Ordinarily, the S wave in V2 represents the posterior and thus the left ventricular force, but in the presence of a marked right axis deviation the S wave of V2 may represent RV force that is directed rightward and posteriorly.

INFORMATION AVAILABLE ON THE 12-LEAD SCALAR ELECTROCARDIOGRAM

Three major types of information are available in the commonly available form of a 12-lead ECG tracing (Fig. 3–3).

1. The lower part of the tracing is a rhythm strip (of lead II).

2. The upper left side of the recording gives frontal plane information and the upper right side of the recording presents horizontal plane information. The frontal plane information is provided by the six limb leads (leads I, II, III, aVR, aVL, and aVF) and the horizontal plane information by the precordial leads. In Figure 3–3, the QRS vector is predominantly directed inferiorly (judged by predominant R waves in leads II, III, and aVF, so-called inferior leads) and is equally anterior and posterior, judged by the equiphasic QRS complex in V2.

3. There is also a calibration marker at the right (or left) margin, which is used to determine the magnitude of the forces. The calibration marker consists of two vertical deflections of 2.5 mm width. The initial deflection shows the calibration factor for the six limb leads, and the latter part of the deflection shows the calibration factor for the six precordial leads. With the full standardization, a 1-millivolt signal introduced into the circuit causes a deflection of 10 mm on the record. With the half standardization, the same signal produces a 5-mm deflection. The amplitude of ECG deflections is read in millimeters rather than in millivolts. When the deflections are too big to be recorded, the sensitivity may be reduced to one fourth. With half standardization, the measured height in millimeters should be multiplied by 2 to obtain the correct amplitude of the deflection. In Figure 3–3, half standardization was used for the precordial leads.

Thus, from the scalar ECG tracing, one can gain information about the frontal and horizontal orientations of the QRS (or ventricular) complexes and other electrical activities of the heart as well as the magnitude of such forces.

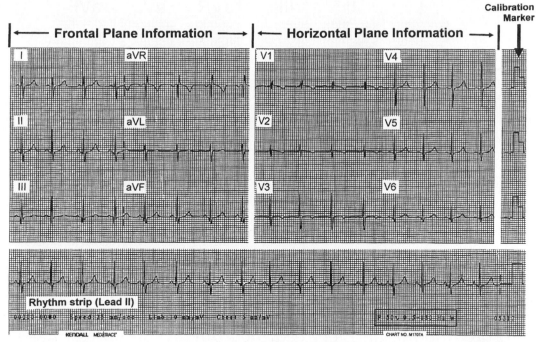

Figure 3–3. *A common form of a routine 12-lead scalar electrocardiogram. There are three types of information available on the recording. Frontal and horizontal plane information is given on the upper part of the tracing. Calibration factors are shown on the right edge of the recording. Rhythm strip (lead II) is shown at the bottom.*

Comparison of Pediatric and Adult Electrocardiograms

ECGs of normal infants and children are quite different from those of normal adults. The most remarkable difference is RV dominance in infants. RV dominance is most noticeable in newborns, and it gradually changes to left ventricular (LV) dominance of adults. By 3 years of age, the child's ECG resembles that of young adults. The age-related difference in the ECG reflects age-related anatomic differences; the right ventricle (RV) is thicker than the left ventricle (LV) in newborns and infants, and the LV is much thicker than the RV in adults.

RV dominance of infants is expressed in the ECG by right axis deviation (RAD) and large rightward and/or anterior QRS forces (i.e., tall R waves in lead aVR and the right precordial leads [V4R, V1, and V2] and deep S waves in lead I and the left precordial leads [V5 and V6]), compared with the adult ECG.

An ECG from a 1-week old neonate (Fig. 3–4) is compared with that of a young adult (Fig. 3–5). The infant's ECG demonstrates RAD (+140 degrees) and dominant R waves in the right precordial leads. The T wave in V1 is usually negative. Upright T waves in V1 in this age group suggest right ventricular hypertrophy (RVH). Adult-type R/S progression in the precordial leads (deep S waves in V1 and V2 and tall R waves in V5 and V6; as seen in Fig. 3–5) is rarely seen in the first month of life; instead, there may be *complete reversal* of the adult-type R/S progression, with tall R waves in V1 and V2 and deep S waves in V5 and V6. *Partial reversal* is usually present, with dominant R waves in V1 and V2 as well as in V5 and V6, in children between the ages of 1 month and 3 years.

The normal adult ECG shown in Figure 3–5 demonstrates the QRS axis near +60 degrees and the QRS forces directed to the left, inferiorly and posteriorly, which is manifested by dominant R waves in the left precordial leads and dominant S waves in the right precordial leads, the so-called adult R/S progression. The T waves are usually anteriorly oriented, resulting in upright T waves in V2 through V6 and sometimes in V1.

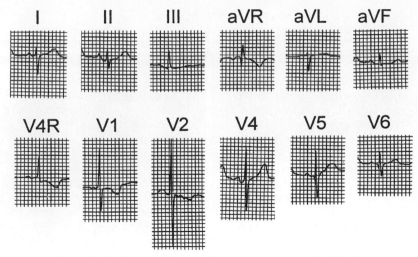

Figure 3–4. *Electrocardiogram from a normal 1-week-old infant.*

Basic Measurements and Their Normal and Abnormal Values Necessary for Routine Interpretation of an Electrocardiogram

In this section, basic measurements that are necessary for routine interpretation of an ECG are briefly discussed in the order listed. This sequence is one of many approaches that can be used in routine interpretation of an ECG. The methods of their measurements are followed by their normal and abnormal values and the significance of abnormal values.

1. Rhythm (sinus or nonsinus) by considering the P axis
2. Heart rate (atrial and ventricular rates, if different)
3. The QRS axis, the T axis, and the QRS-T angle
4. Intervals: PR, QRS, and QT

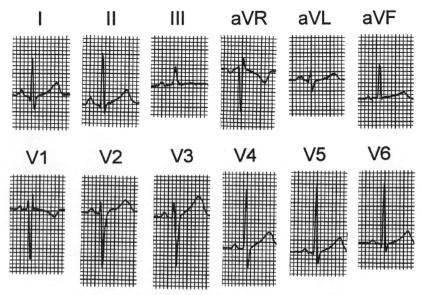

Figure 3–5. *Electrocardiogram from a normal young adult.*

5. The P-wave amplitude and duration

6. The QRS amplitude and R/S ratio; also abnormal Q waves

7. ST-segment and T-wave abnormalities

RHYTHM

Sinus rhythm is the normal rhythm at any age and is characterized by P waves preceding each QRS complex and a normal P axis (0 to +90 degrees); the latter is an often neglected criterion. The requirement of a normal P axis is important in discriminating sinus from nonsinus rhythm. In sinus rhythm, the PR interval is regular but is not necessarily normal. (The PR interval may be prolonged as seen in sinus rhythm with first-degree AV block.)

Because the sinoatrial node is located in the right upper part of the atrial mass, the direction of atrial depolarization is from the right upper part toward the left lower part, with the resulting P axis in the lower left quadrant (0 to +90 degrees) (Fig. 3–6A). Some atrial (nonsinus) rhythms may have P waves preceding each QRS complex, but they have an abnormal P axis (see Fig. 3–6B). For the P axis to be between 0 and +90 degrees, P waves must be upright in leads I and aVF or at least not inverted in these leads; simple inspection of these two leads suffices. A normal P axis also results in upright P waves in lead II and inverted P waves in aVR. A method of plotting axes is presented later for the QRS axis.

HEART RATE

There are many different ways to calculate the heart rate, but they are all based on the known time scale of ECG papers. At the usual paper speed of 25 mm/second, 1 mm = 0.04 second and 5 mm = 0.20 second (Fig. 3–7). The following methods are often used to calculate the heart rate.

1. Count the R-R cycle in six large divisions (1/50 minute) and multiply it by 50 (Fig. 3–8).

2. When the heart rate is slow, count the number of large divisions between two R waves and divide that into 300 (because 1 minute = 300 large divisions) (Fig. 3–9).

3. Measure the R-R interval (in seconds) and divide 60 by the R-R interval. The R-R interval is 0.36 second in Figure 3–8: 60 ÷ 0.36 = 166.

4. Use a convenient ECG ruler.

5. An approximate heart rate can be determined by memorizing heart rates for selected R-R intervals (Fig. 3–10). When R-R intervals are 5, 10, 15, 20, and 25 mm, the respective heart rates are 300, 150, 100, 75, and 60 beats/minute.

When the ventricular and atrial rates are different, as in complete heart block or atrial flutter, the atrial rate can be calculated using the same methods as described for the ventricular rate; for the atrial rate, the P-P interval rather than the R-R interval is used.

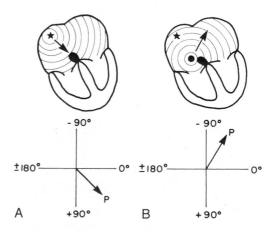

Figure 3–6. *Comparison of P axis in sinus rhythm (**A**) and low atrial rhythm (**B**). In sinus rhythm, the P waves are upright in leads I and aVF. In low atrial rhythm, the P wave is inverted in lead aVF.*

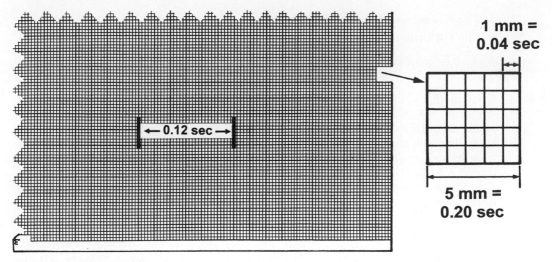

Figure 3–7. *Electrocardiogram paper. Time is measured on the horizontal axis. Each 1 mm equals 0.04 second, and each 5 mm (a large division) equals 0.20 second. Thirty millimeters (or six large divisions) equal 1.2 second or 1/50 minute. (From Park MK, Guntheroth WG: How to Read Pediatric ECGs, 4th ed. Philadelphia, Mosby, 2006.)*

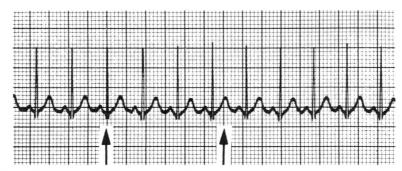

Figure 3–8. *Heart rate of 165 beats/minute. There are about 3.3 cardiac cycles (R-R intervals) in six large divisions. Therefore the heart rate is 3.3 × 50 = 165 (by method 1). By method 3, the R-R interval is 0.36 second; 60 ÷ 0.36 = 166. The rates derived by the two methods are very close.*

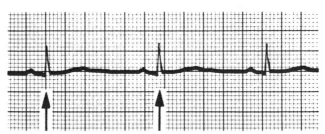

Figure 3–9. *Heart rate of 52 beats/minute. There are 5.8 large divisions between the two arrows. Therefore, the heart rate is 300 ÷ 5.8 = 52.*

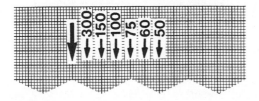

Figure 3–10. *Quick estimation of heart rate. When the R-R interval is 5 mm, the heart rate is 300 beats/minute. When the R-R interval is 10 mm, the rate is 150 beats/ minute, and so on.*

Because of age-related differences in the heart rate, the definitions of bradycardia (<60 beats/minute) and tachycardia (>100 beats/minute) used for adults do not help distinguish normal from abnormal heart rates in pediatric patients. Operationally, tachycardia is present when the heart rate is faster than the upper range of normal for that age, and bradycardia is present when the heart rate is slower than the lower range of normal. Examples of normal heart rate (and ranges) per minute recorded on the ECG for selected ages are as follows (Davignon et al, 1979/80).

Newborn	145 (90–180)
6 months	145 (105–185)
1 year	132 (105–170)
4 years	108 (72–135)
14 years	85 (60–120)

QRS AXIS, T AXIS, AND QRS-T ANGLE

QRS Axis. The most convenient way to determine the QRS axis is the successive approximation method using the hexaxial reference system (see Fig. 3–1A). The same approach is also used for the determination of the T axis (see later). For the determination of the QRS axis (as well as the T axis), one uses only the hexaxial reference system (or the six limb leads), not the horizontal reference system.

Successive Approximation Method.

Step 1. Locate a quadrant, using leads I and aVF (Fig. 3–11). In the top panel of Figure 3–11, the net QRS deflection of lead I is positive. This means that the QRS axis is in the left hemicircle (i.e., from −90 degrees through 0 to +90 degrees) from the lead I point of view. The net positive QRS deflection in aVF means that the QRS axis is in the lower hemicircle (i.e., from 0 through +90 degrees to +180 degrees) from the aVF point of view. To satisfy the polarity of both leads I and aVF, the QRS axis must be in the lower left quadrant (i.e., 0 to +90 degrees). Four quadrants can be easily identified based on the QRS complexes in leads I and aVF (see Fig. 3–11).

Step 2. Among the remaining four limb leads, find a lead with an equiphasic QRS complex (in which the height of the R wave and the depth of the S wave are equal). The QRS axis is perpendicular to the lead with an equiphasic QRS complex in the predetermined quadrant.

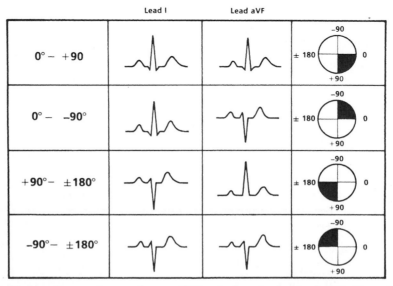

Figure 3–11. *Locating quadrants of mean QRS axis from leads I and aVF. (From Park MK, Guntheroth WG: How to Read Pediatric ECGs, 4th ed. Philadelphia, Mosby, 2006.)*

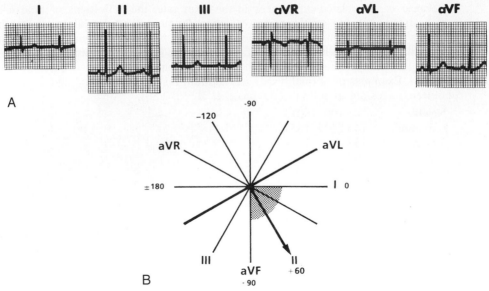

Figure 3–12. *A, Set of six limb leads.* **B,** *Plotted QRS axis is shown.*

Example. Determine the QRS axis in Figure 3–12.

Step 1. The axis is in the lower left quadrant (0 to +90 degrees) because the R waves are upright in leads I and aVF.

Step 2. The QRS complex is equiphasic in aVL. Therefore, the QRS axis is +60 degrees, which is perpendicular to aVL.

Normal QRS Axis. Normal ranges of QRS axis vary with age. Newborns normally have RAD compared with the adult standard. By 3 years of age, the QRS axis approaches the adult mean value of +50 degrees. The mean and ranges of a normal QRS axis according to age are shown in Table 3–1.

Abnormal QRS Axis. The QRS axis outside normal ranges signifies abnormalities in the ventricular depolarization process.

1. Left axis deviation (LAD) is present when the QRS axis is less than the lower limit of normal for the patient's age. LAD occurs with left ventricular hypertrophy (LVH), left bundle branch block (LBBB), and left anterior hemiblock.

2. RAD is present when the QRS axis is greater than the upper limit of normal for the patient's age. RAD occurs with RVH and right bundle branch block (RBBB).

3. "Superior" QRS axis is present when the S wave is greater than the R wave in aVF. The overlap with LAD should be noted. It may occur with left anterior hemiblock (in the range of −30 to −90 degrees, seen in endocardial cushion defect (ECD) or tricuspid atresia) or with RBBB. It is rarely seen in otherwise normal children.

T Axis. The T axis is determined by the same methods used to determine the QRS axis. In normal children, including newborns, the mean T axis is +45 degrees, with a range of 0 to +90 degrees, the same as in normal adults. This means that the T waves

Table 3–1. **Mean and Ranges of Normal QRS Axes by Age**

Age	Mean (Range)
1 wk–1 mo	+ 110° (+30 to +180)
1–3 mo	+ 70° (+10 to +125)
3 mo–3 yr	+ 60° (+10 to +110)
Older than 3 yr	+ 60° (+20 to +120)
Adult	+ 50° (−30 to +105)

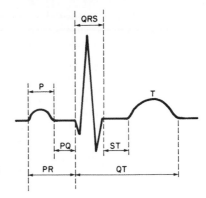

Figure 3–13. *Diagram illustrating important intervals (or durations) and segments of an electrocardiographic cycle.*

must be upright in leads I and aVF. The T waves can be flat, but must not be inverted, in these leads. The T axis outside the normal quadrant suggests conditions with myocardial dysfunction similar to those listed for abnormal QRS-T angle (see the following).

QRS-T Angle. The QRS-T angle is formed by the QRS axis and the T axis. A QRS-T angle greater than 60 degrees is unusual, and one greater than 90 degrees is certainly abnormal. An abnormally wide QRS-T angle with the T axis outside the normal quadrant (0 to +90 degrees) is seen in severe ventricular hypertrophy with "strain," ventricular conduction disturbances, and myocardial dysfunction of a metabolic or ischemic nature.

INTERVALS

Three important intervals are routinely measured in the interpretation of an ECG: PR interval, QRS duration, and QT interval. The duration of the P wave is also inspected (Fig. 3–13).

PR Interval. The normal PR interval varies with age and heart rate (Table 3–2). The older the person and the slower the heart rate, the longer is the PR interval.

Prolongation of the PR interval (i.e., first-degree AV block) is seen in myocarditis (rheumatic, viral, or diphtheric), digitalis or quinidine toxicity, certain congenital heart defects (ECD, atrial septal defect [ASD], Ebstein's anomaly), other myocardial dysfunctions, hyperkalemia, and an otherwise normal heart with vagal stimulation.

A short PR interval is present in Wolff-Parkinson-White (WPW) preexcitation, Lown-Ganong-Levine syndrome, myocardiopathies of glycogenosis, Duchenne's muscular dystrophy (or relatives of these patients), Friedreich's ataxia, pheochromocytoma, and otherwise normal children. The lower limits of normal PR interval are shown under WPW preexcitation (see later).

Variable PR intervals are seen in wandering atrial pacemaker and Wenckebach's phenomenon (Mobitz type I second-degree AV block).

QRS Duration. The QRS duration varies with age (Table 3–3). It is short in infants and increases with age.

Table 3–2. **PR Interval: Rate (and Upper Limits of Normal) for Age**

Rate	0–1 mo	1–6 mo	6 mo–1 yr	1–3 yr	3–8 yr	8–12 yr	12–16 yr	Adult
<60						0.16 (0.18)	0.16 (0.19)	0.17 (0.21)
60–80					0.15 (0.17)	0.15 (0.17)	0.15 (0.18)	0.16 (0.21)
80–100	0.10 (0.12)				0.14 (0.16)	0.15 (0.16)	0.15 (0.17)	0.15 (0.20)
100–120	0.10 (0.12)			(0.15)	0.13 (0.16)	0.14 (0.15)	0.15 (0.16)	0.15 (0.19)
120–140	0.10 (0.11)	0.11 (0.14)	0.11 (0.14)	0.12 (0.14)	0.13 (0.15)	0.14 (0.15)		0.15 (0.18)
140–160	0.09 (0.11)	0.10 (0.13)	0.11 (0.13)	0.11 (0.14)	0.12 (0.14)			(0.17)
160–180	0.10 (0.11)	0.10 (0.12)	0.10 (0.12)	0.10 (0.12)				
>180	0.09	0.09 (0.11)	0.10 (0.11)					

From Park MK, Guntheroth WG: How to Read Pediatric ECGs, 4th ed. Philadelphia, Mosby, 2006.

Table 3–3. QRS Duration According to Age: Mean (Upper Limits of Normal*)

	0–1 mo	1–6 mo	6–12 mo	1–3 yr	3–8 yr	8–12 yr	12–16 yr	Adults
Seconds	0.05 (0.07)	0.055 (0.075)	0.055 (0.075)	0.055 (0.075)	0.06 (0.075)	0.06 (0.085)	0.07 (0.085)	0.08 (0.10)

*Upper limit of normal refers to the 98th percentile.
Derived from percentile charts in Davignon A, Rautaharju P, Boisselle E, et al: Normal ECG standards for infants and
  children. Pediatr Cardiol 1:123–131, 1979/80.

The QRS duration is prolonged in conditions grouped as ventricular conduction disturbances, which include RBBB, LBBB, preexcitation (e.g., WPW preexcitation), and intraventricular block (as seen in hyperkalemia, toxicity from quinidine or procainamide, myocardial fibrosis, myocardial dysfunction of a metabolic or ischemic nature). Ventricular arrhythmias (e.g., premature ventricular contractions, ventricular tachycardia, implanted ventricular pacemaker) also produce a wide QRS duration. Because the QRS duration varies with age, the definition of bundle branch block or other ventricular conduction disturbances should vary with age (see the section on ventricular conduction disturbances).

QT Interval. The QT interval varies primarily with heart rate. The heart rate–corrected QT (QTc) interval is calculated by the use of Bazett's formula:

$$QTc = \frac{QT\,measured}{\sqrt{RR\,interval}}$$

According to Bazett's formula, the normal QTc interval (mean ± SD) is 0.40 (± 0.014) second with the upper limit of normal 0.44 second in children 6 months and older. The QTc interval is slightly longer in the newborn and small infants with the upper limit of normal QTc 0.47 second in the first week of life and 0.45 second in the first 6 months of life.

Long QT intervals may be seen in long QT syndrome (e.g., Jervell and Lange-Nielsen syndrome, Romano-Ward syndrome), hypocalcemia, myocarditis, diffuse myocardial diseases (including hypertrophic and dilated cardiomyopathies), head injury, severe malnutrition, and so on. A number of drugs are also known to prolong the QT interval. Among these are antiarrhythmic agents (especially class IA, IC, and III), antipsychotic phenothiazines (e.g., thioridazine, chlorpromazine), tricyclic antidepressants (e.g., imipramine, amitriptyline), arsenics, organophosphates, antibiotics (e.g., ampicillin, erythromycin, trimethoprim-sulfa, amantadine), and antihistamines (e.g., terfenadine).

A short QT interval is a sign of a digitalis effect or of hypercalcemia. It is also seen with hyperthermia and in short QT syndrome (a familial cause of sudden death with QTc ≤ 300 milliseconds).

The *JT interval* is measured from the J point (the junction between the S wave and the ST segment) to the end of the T wave. A prolonged JT interval has the same significance as a prolonged QT interval. The JT interval is measured only when the QT interval is prolonged or when the QRS duration is prolonged as seen with ventricular conduction disturbances. The JT interval is also expressed as a rate corrected interval (called JTc) using Bazett's formula. Normal JTc (mean ± SD) is 0.32 ± 0.02 second with the upper limit of normal 0.34 second in normal children and adolescents.

P-WAVE DURATION AND AMPLITUDE

The P-wave duration and amplitude are important in the diagnosis of atrial hypertrophy. Normally, the P amplitude is less than 3 mm. The duration of P waves is shorter than 0.09 second in children and shorter than 0.07 second in infants (see the section on criteria for atrial hypertrophy).

QRS AMPLITUDE, R/S RATIO, AND ABNORMAL Q WAVES

The QRS amplitude and R/S ratio are important in the diagnosis of ventricular hypertrophy. These values also vary with age (Tables 3–4 and 3–5). Because of the normal dominance

Table 3–4. R and S Voltages According to Lead and Age: Mean (and Upper Limit*) (in mm)

Lead	0–1 mo	1–6 mo	6–12 mo	1–3 yr	3–8 yr	8–12 yr	12–16 yr	Adults
R Voltages								
I	4 (8)	7 (13)	8 (16)	8 (16)	7 (15)	7 (15)	6 (13)	6 (13)
II	6 (14)	13 (24)	13 (27)	12 (23)	13 (22)	14 (24)	14 (24)	5 (25)
III	8 (16)	9 (20)	9 (20)	9 (20)	9 (20)	9 (24)	9 (24)	6 (22)
aVR	3 (8)	2 (6)	2 (6)	2 (5)	2 (4)	1 (4)	1 (4)	1 (4)
aVL	2 (7)	4 (8)	5 (10)	5 (10)	3 (10)	3 (10)	3 (12)	3 (9)
aVF	7 (14)	10 (20)	10 (16)	8 (20)	10 (19)	10 (20)	11 (21)	5 (23)
V3R	10 (19)	6 (13)	6 (11)	6 (11)	5 (10)	3 (9)	3 (7)	
V4R	6 (12)	5 (10)	4 (8)	4 (8)	3 (8)	3 (7)	3 (7)	
V1	13 (24)	10 (19)	10 (20)	9 (18)	8 (16)	5 (12)	4 (10)	3 (14)
V2	18 (30)	20 (31)	22 (32)	19 (28)	15 (25)	12 (20)	10 (19)	6 (21)
V5	12 (23)	20 (33)	20 (31)	20 (32)	23 (38)	26 (39)	21 (35)	12 (33)
V6	5 (15)	13 (22)	13 (23)	13 (23)	15 (26)	17 (26)	14 (23)	10 (21)
S Voltages								
I	5 (10)	4 (9)	4 (9)	3 (8)	2 (8)	2 (8)	2 (8)	1 (6)
V3R	3 (12)	3 (10)	4 (10)	5 (12)	7 (15)	8 (18)	7 (16)	
V4R	4 (9)	4 (12)	5 (12)	5 (12)	5 (14)	6 (20)	6 (20)	
V1	7 (18)	5 (15)	7 (18)	8 (21)	11 (23)	12 (25)	11 (22)	10 (23)
V2	18 (33)	15 (26)	16 (29)	18 (30)	20 (33)	21 (36)	18 (33)	14 (36)
V5	9 (17)	7 (16)	6 (15)	5 (12)	4 (10)	3 (8)	3 (8)	
V6	3 (10)	3 (9)	2 (7)	2 (7)	2 (5)	1 (4)	1 (4)	1 (13)

*Upper limit of normal refers to the 98th percentile.
Voltages measured in millimeters, when 1 mV = 10 mm paper.
Data are from three sources: (1) Percentile charts in Davignon A, Rautaharju P, Boisselle E, et al: Normal ECG standards for infants and children. Pediatr Cardiol 1:123–131, 1979/80. (2) Data for leads I, II, III, aVL, and aVF are from Guntheroth WG: Pediatric Electrocardiography. Philadelphia, WB Saunders, 1965 (used by permission). (3) Data for V4R and those for adults are from Park MK, Guntheroth WG: How to Read Pediatric ECGs, 3rd ed. St. Louis, Mosby–Year Book, 1992.

Table 3–5. R/S Ratio: Mean and Upper and Lower Limits of Normal According to Age

Lead		0–1 mo	1–6 mo	6 mo–1 yr	1–3 yr	3–8 yr	8–12 yr	12–16 yr	Adult
V1	LLN	0.5	0.3	0.3	0.5	0.1	0.15	0.1	0.0
	Mean	1.5	1.5	1.2	0.8	0.65	0.5	0.3	0.3
	ULN	19	S = 0	6	2	2	1	1	1
V2	LLN	0.3	0.3	0.3	0.3	0.05	0.1	0.1	0.1
	Mean	1	1.2	1	0.8	0.5	0.5	0.5	0.2
	ULN	3	4	4	1.5	1.5	1.2	1.2	2.5
V6	LLN	0.1	1.5	2	3	2.5	4	2.5	2.5
	Mean	2	4	6	20	20	20	10	9
	ULN	S = 0	S = 0	S = 0	S = 0	S = 0	S = 0	S = 0	S = 0

LLN, lower limits of normal; ULN, upper limits of normal.
From Guntheroth WB: Pediatric Electrocardiography. Philadelphia, WB Saunders, 1965.

Table 3–6. Q Voltages According to Lead and Age: Mean (and Upper Limit*) (in mm)

	0–1 mo	1–6 mo	6–12 mo	1–3 yr	3–8 yr	8–12 yr	12–16 yr	Adults
III	1.5 (5.5)	1.5 (6.0)	2.1 (6.0)	1.5 (5.0)	1.0 (3.5)	0.6 (3.0)	1.0 (3.0)	0.5 (4)
aVF	1.0 (3.5)	1.0 (3.5)	1.0 (3.5)	1.0 (3.0)	0.5 (3.0)	0.5 (2.5)	0.5 (2.0)	0.5 (2)
V5	0.1 (3.5)	0.1 (3.0)	0.1 (3.0)	0.5 (4.5)	1.0 (5.5)	1.0 (3.0)	0.5 (3.0)	0.5 (3.5)
V6	0.5 (3.0)	0.5 (3.0)	0.5 (3.0)	0.5 (3.0)	1.0 (3.5)	0.5 (3.0)	0.5 (3.0)	0.5 (3)

*Upper limit of normal refers to the 98th percentile.
Voltages measured in millimeters, when 1 mV = 10 mm paper.
Data are from percentile charts in Davignon A, Rautaharju P, Boisselle E, et al: Normal ECG standards for infants and
   children. Pediatr Cardiol 1:123–131, 1979/80.

of RV forces in infants and small children, R waves are taller than S waves in the right precordial leads (i.e., V4R, V1, V2) and S waves are deeper than R waves in the left precordial leads (i.e., V5, V6) in this age group. Accordingly, the R/S ratio (the ratio of the R-wave and S-wave voltages) is large in the right precordial leads and small in the left precordial leads in infants and small children.

Normal mean Q voltages and upper limits are presented in Table 3–6. The average normal Q-wave duration is 0.02 second and does not exceed 0.03 second. Abnormal Q waves may manifest themselves as deep and/or wide Q waves or as abnormal leads in which they appear. Deep Q waves may be present in ventricular hypertrophy of the "volume overload" type. Deep and wide Q waves are seen in myocardial infarction. The presence of Q waves in the right precordial leads (e.g., severe RVH or ventricular inversion) or the absence of Q waves in the left precordial leads (e.g., LBBB or ventricular inversion) is abnormal.

ST SEGMENT AND T WAVES

The normal ST segment is isoelectric. However, in the limb leads, elevation or depression of the ST segment up to 1 mm is not necessarily abnormal in infants and children. An elevation or a depression of the ST segment is judged in relation to the PR segment as the baseline. Some ST-segment changes are normal (nonpathologic) and others are abnormal (pathologic). (See a later section on nonpathologic and pathologic ST-T changes in this chapter.)

Tall peaked T waves may be seen in hyperkalemia and LVH (of the volume overload type). Flat or low T waves may occur in normal newborns or with hypothyroidism, hypokalemia, pericarditis, myocarditis, and myocardial ischemia.

Atrial Hypertrophy

RIGHT ATRIAL HYPERTROPHY

Tall P waves (>3 mm) indicate right atrial hypertrophy or "P pulmonale" (Fig. 3–14).

LEFT ATRIAL HYPERTROPHY

A widened and often notched P wave (with the P duration >0.10 second in children; >0.08 second in infants) is seen in left atrial hypertrophy or "P mitrale." In V1, the P wave is diphasic with a prolonged negative segment (see Fig. 3–14).

BIATRIAL HYPERTROPHY

In biatrial hypertrophy, a combination of increased amplitude and duration of the P wave is present (see Fig. 3–14).

Ventricular Hypertrophy

GENERAL CHANGES

Ventricular hypertrophy produces abnormalities in one or more of the following: the QRS axis, the QRS voltages, the R/S ratio, the T axis, and miscellaneous areas.

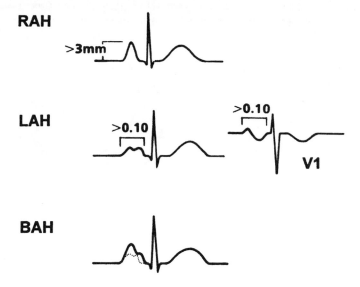

Figure 3–14. *Criteria for atrial hypertrophy. BAH, biatrial hypertrophy; LAH, left atrial hypertrophy; RAH, right atrial hypertrophy. (From Park MK, Guntheroth WG: How to Read Pediatric ECGs, 4th ed. Philadelphia, Mosby, 2006.)*

1. *Changes in the QRS axis.* The QRS axis is usually directed toward the ventricle that is hypertrophied. Although RAD is present with RVH, LAD is seen with the volume overload type, but not with the pressure overload type, of LVH. Marked LAD usually indicates ventricular conduction disturbances (e.g., left anterior hemiblock or "superior" QRS axis).

2. *Changes in QRS voltages.* Anatomically, the RV occupies the right and anterior aspect, and the LV occupies the left, inferior, and posterior aspect of the ventricular mass. With ventricular hypertrophy, the voltage of the QRS complex increases in the direction of the respective ventricle.

    In the frontal plane (Fig. 3–15A), LVH shows increased R voltages in leads I, II, aVL, aVF, and sometimes III, especially in small infants. RVH shows increased R voltages in aVR and III and increased S voltages in lead I (see Table 3–4 for normal R and S voltages).

    In the horizontal plane (see Fig. 3–15B), tall R waves in V4R, V1, and V2 or deep S waves in V5 and V6 are seen in RVH. With LVH, tall R waves in V5 and V6 and/or deep S waves in V4R, V1, and V2 are present (see Table 3–4).

3. *Changes in R/S ratio.* The R/S ratio represents the relative electromotive force of opposing ventricles in a given lead. In ventricular hypertrophy, a change may be seen only in the R/S ratio, without an increase in the absolute voltage. An increase in the R/S ratio in the right precordial leads suggests RVH; a decrease in the R/S ratio in these leads suggests LVH. Likewise, an increase in the R/S ratio in the left precordial leads suggests LVH, and a decrease in the ratio suggests RVH (see Table 3–5).

4. *Changes in the T axis.* Changes in the T axis are seen in severe ventricular hypertrophy with relative ischemia of the hypertrophied myocardium. In the presence of other criteria of ventricular hypertrophy, a wide QRS-T angle (i.e., >90 degrees) with the T axis outside the normal range indicates a strain pattern. When the T axis remains in the normal quadrant (0 to +90 degrees), a wide QRS-T angle alone indicates a *possible* strain pattern.

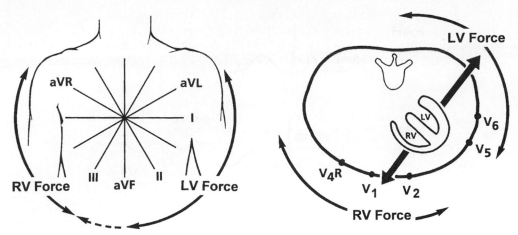

Figure 3–15. *Diagrammatic representation of left and right ventricular forces on the frontal projection or hexaxial reference system (**A**) and the horizontal plane (**B**). LV, left ventricular; RV, right ventricular. (From Park MK, Guntheroth WG: How to Read Pediatric ECGs, 4th ed. Philadelphia, Mosby, 2006.)*

5. *Miscellaneous nonspecific changes*
   a. RVH
      1). A q wave in V1 (qR or qRs pattern) suggests RVH, although it may be present in ventricular inversion.
      2). An upright T wave in V1 after 3 days of age is a sign of probable RVH.
   b. LVH

   Deep Q waves (>5 mm) and/or tall T waves in V5 and V6 are signs of LVH of volume overload type. These may be seen with a large-shunt ventricular septal defect (VSD).

CRITERIA FOR RIGHT VENTRICULAR HYPERTROPHY

In RVH, some or all of the following criteria are present.

1. RAD for the patient's age (see Table 3–1)
2. Increased rightward and anterior QRS voltages (in the absence of prolonged QRS duration) (see Table 3–4); a wide QRS complex with increased QRS voltages suggests ventricular conduction disturbances (e.g., RBBB) rather than ventricular hypertrophy.
   a. R waves in V1, V2, or aVR greater than the upper limits of normal for the patient's age
   b. S waves in I and V6 greater than the upper limits of normal for the patient's age

   In general, abnormal forces to the right *and* anteriorly are stronger criteria than abnormal forces to the right or anteriorly only.
3. Abnormal R/S ratio in favor of the RV (in the absence of bundle branch block) (see Table 3–5)
   a. R/S ratio in V1 and V2 greater than the upper limits of normal for age
   b. R/S ratio in V6 less than 1 after 1 month of age.
4. Upright T waves in V1 in patients more than 3 days of age, provided that the T is upright in the left precordial leads (V5, V6); upright T waves in V1 are not abnormal in patients older than 6 years.
5. A q wave in V1 (qR or qRs patterns) suggests RVH (the physician should ascertain that there is not a small r in an rsR' configuration).
6. In the presence of RVH, a wide QRS-T angle with T axis outside the normal range (in the 0 to −90 degree quadrant) indicates a strain pattern. A wide QRS-T angle with the T axis within the normal range suggests a *possible* strain pattern.

Figure 3–16 is an example of RVH. There is RAD for the patient's age (+150 degrees). The T axis is −10 degrees, and the QRS-T angle is abnormally wide (160 degrees) with the T axis in an abnormal quadrant. The QRS duration is normal. The R waves in leads III and aVR and the S waves in leads I and V6 are beyond the upper limits of normal, indicating an abnormal rightward force. The R/S ratios in V1 and V2 are larger than the upper limits of normal, and the ratio in V6 is smaller than the lower limits of normal, again indicating RVH. Therefore, this tracing shows RVH with strain.

The diagnosis of RVH in newborns is particularly difficult because of the normal dominance of the RV during this period of life. Helpful signs in the diagnosis of RVH in newborns are as follows.

1. S waves in lead I that are 12 mm or greater

2. Pure R waves (with no S waves) in V1 that are greater than 10 mm

3. R waves in V1 that are greater than 25 mm or R waves in aVR that are greater than 8 mm

4. A qR pattern seen in V1 (this is also seen in 10% of normal newborns)

5. Upright T waves seen in V1 after 3 days of age

6. RAD with the QRS axis greater than +180 degrees

CRITERIA FOR LEFT VENTRICULAR HYPERTROPHY

In LVH, some or all of the following abnormalities are present.

1. LAD for the patient's age (see Table 3–1)

2. QRS voltages in favor of the LV (in the absence of a prolonged QRS duration for age) (see Table 3–4)

   a. R waves in leads I, II, III, aVL, aVF, V5, or V6 greater than the upper limits of normal for age

   b. S waves in V1 or V2 greater than the upper limits of normal for age

   In general, the presence of abnormal forces to more than one direction (e.g., to the left, inferiorly, and posteriorly) is a stronger criterion than the abnormality in only one direction.

3. Abnormal R/S ratio in favor of the LV: R/S ratio in V1 and V2 less than the lower limits of normal for the patient's age (see Table 3–5)

4. Q waves in V5 and V6, greater than 5 mm, as well as tall symmetrical T waves in the same leads ("LV diastolic overload")

5. In the presence of LVH, a wide QRS-T angle with the T axis outside the normal range indicates a strain pattern; this is manifested by inverted T waves in lead I or aVF. A wide QRS-T angle with the T axis within the normal range suggests a *possible* strain pattern.

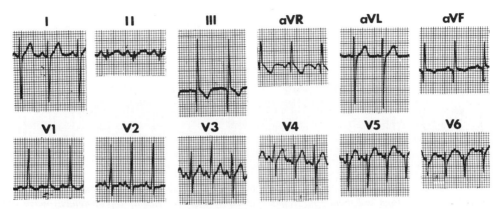

Figure 3–16. Tracing from a 10-month-old infant with severe tetralogy of Fallot.

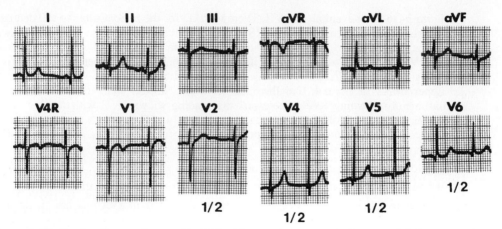

Figure 3–17. *Tracing from a 4-year-old child with a moderate ventricular septal defect. Note that some precordial leads are in half normal standardization.*

Figure 3–17 is an example of LVH. There is LAD for the patient's age (0 degrees). The R waves in leads I, aVL, V5, and V6 are beyond the upper limits of normal, indicating abnormal leftward force. The QRS duration is normal. The T axis (+55 degrees) remains in the normal quadrant. This tracing shows LVH (without strain).

CRITERIA FOR BIVENTRICULAR HYPERTROPHY

BVH may be manifested in one of the following ways.

1. Positive voltage criteria for RVH and LVH in the absence of bundle branch block or preexcitation (i.e., with normal QRS duration)

2. Positive voltage criteria for RVH or LVH and relatively large voltages for the other ventricle

3. Large equiphasic QRS complexes in two or more of the limb leads and in the mid-precordial leads (i.e., V2 through V5), called the Katz-Wachtel phenomenon (with normal QRS duration)

Figure 3–18 is an example of BVH. It is difficult to plot the QRS axis because of large diphasic QRS complexes in limb leads. The R and S voltages are large in some limb leads and in the mid-precordial leads (Katz-Wachtel phenomenon). The S waves in leads I and V6 are abnormally deep (i.e., abnormal rightward force), and the R wave in V1 (i.e., rightward and anterior force) is also abnormally large, suggesting RVH.

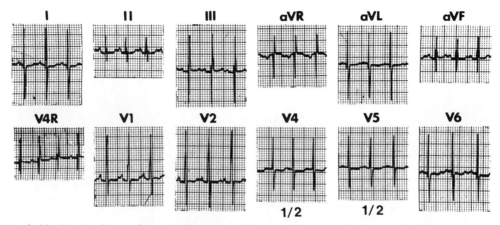

Figure 3–18. *Tracing from a 2-month-old infant with large-shunt ventricular septal defect, patent ductus arteriosus, and severe pulmonary hypertension.*

The R waves in leads I and aVL (i.e., leftward force) are also abnormally large. Therefore, this tracing shows BVH.

Ventricular Conduction Disturbances

Conditions that are grouped together as ventricular conduction disturbances have abnormal prolongation of the QRS duration in common. Ventricular conduction disturbances include the following:

1. Bundle branch block, right and left
2. Preexcitation (e.g., WPW-type preexcitation)
3. Intraventricular block

In bundle branch blocks (and ventricular rhythms), the prolongation is in the terminal portion of the QRS complex (i.e., "terminal slurring"). In preexcitation, the prolongation is in the initial portion of the QRS complex (i.e., "initial slurring"), producing "delta" waves. In intraventricular block, the prolongation is throughout the duration of the QRS complex (Fig. 3–19). Normal QRS duration varies with age; it is shorter in infants than in older children or adults (see Table 3–3). In adults, a QRS duration greater than 0.10 second is required for diagnosis of bundle branch block or ventricular conduction disturbance. In infants, a QRS duration of 0.08 second meets the requirement for bundle branch block.

By far the most commonly encountered form of ventricular conduction disturbance is RBBB. Although uncommon, WPW preexcitation is a well-defined entity that deserves a brief description. LBBB is extremely rare in children, although it is common in adults with ischemic and hypertensive heart disease. Intraventricular block is associated with metabolic disorders and diffuse myocardial diseases.

RIGHT BUNDLE BRANCH BLOCK

In RBBB, delayed conduction through the right bundle branch prolongs the time required for a depolarization of the RV. When the LV is completely depolarized, RV depolarization is still in progress. This produces prolongation of the QRS duration, involving the terminal portion of the QRS complex, called terminal slurring (see Fig. 3–19B) and the slurring is directed to the *right* and *anteriorly* because the RV is located rightward and anteriorly in relation to the LV.

In a normal heart, synchronous depolarization of the opposing electromotive forces of the RV and LV cancels out the forces to some extent, with the resulting voltages that we call normal. In RBBB (and other ventricular conduction disturbances), asynchronous depolarization of the opposing electromotive forces may produce a lesser degree of cancellation of the opposing forces and thus result in greater manifest potentials for both ventricles. Consequently, abnormally large voltages for *both* RV and LV may result even in the absence of ventricular hypertrophy. Therefore, the diagnosis of ventricular hypertrophy in the presence of bundle branch block (or WPW preexcitation or intraventricular block) is insecure.

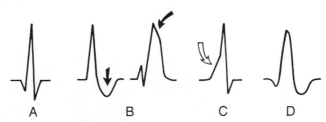

A   B   C   D

Figure 3–19. *Schematic diagram of three types of ventricular conduction disturbances.* **A,** *Normal QRS complex.* **B,** *QRS complex in right bundle branch block with prolongation of the QRS duration in the terminal portion (arrows, terminal slurring).* **C,** *Preexcitation with delta wave (arrow, initial slurring).* **D,** *Intraventricular block in which the prolongation of the QRS complex is throughout the duration of the QRS complex.*

Criteria for Right Bundle Branch Block

1. RAD, at least for the terminal portion of the QRS complex (the initial QRS force is normal)

2. QRS duration longer than the upper limit of normal for the patient's age (see Table 3–3)

3. Terminal slurring of the QRS complex that is directed to the right and usually, but not always, anteriorly:

   a. Wide and slurred S waves in leads I, V5, and V6

   b. Terminal, slurred R' in aVR and the right precordial leads (V4R, V1, and V2)

4. ST-segment shift and T-wave inversion are common in adults but not in children

Figure 3–20 is an example of RBBB. The QRS duration is increased (0.11 second), indicating a ventricular conduction disturbance. There is slurring of the terminal portion of the QRS complex, indicating a bundle branch block, and the slurring is directed to the right (slurred S waves in leads I and V6 and slurred R waves in aVR) and anteriorly (slurred R waves in V4R and V1), satisfying the criteria for RBBB. Although the S waves in leads I, V5, and V6 are abnormally deep and the R/S ratio in V1 is abnormally large, it cannot be interpreted as RVH in the presence of RBBB.

Two pediatric conditions commonly associated with RBBB are ASD and conduction disturbances after open heart surgery involving right ventriculotomy. Other congenital heart defects often associated with RBBB include Ebstein's anomaly, COA in infants younger than 6 months, ECD, and PAPVR; it is also occasionally seen in normal children. Rarely, RBBB is seen in myocardial diseases (cardiomyopathy, myocarditis), muscle diseases (Duchenne's muscular dystrophy, myotonic dystrophy), and Brugada syndrome.

The significance of RBBB in children is different from that in adults. In several pediatric examples of RBBB, the right bundle is intact. In ASD, the prolonged QRS duration is the result of a longer pathway through a dilated RV rather than an actual block in the right bundle. Right ventriculotomy for repair of VSD or tetralogy of Fallot disrupts the RV subendocardial Purkinje network and causes prolongation of the QRS duration without necessarily injuring the main right bundle, although the latter may occasionally be disrupted.

Some pediatricians are concerned with the rsR' pattern in V1. Although it is unusual to see this in adults, the rsR' pattern in V1 not only is normal but is expected to be present in infants and small children, provided that the QRS duration is not prolonged and the voltage of the primary or secondary R waves is not abnormally large. This is because the terminal QRS vector is normally more rightward and anterior in infants and children than adults.

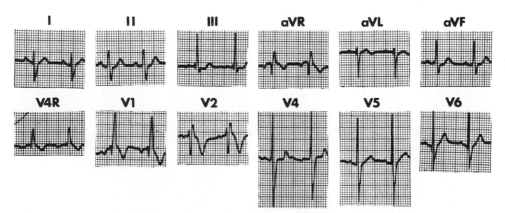

Figure 3–20. Tracing from a 6-year-old boy who had corrective surgery for tetralogy of Fallot that involved right ventriculotomy for repair of a ventricular septal defect and resection of infundibular narrowing.

LEFT BUNDLE BRANCH BLOCK

LBBB is extremely rare in children. In LBBB, the duration of the QRS complex is prolonged for age and the slurred portion of the QRS complex is directed leftward and posteriorly. A Q wave is absent in V6. A prominent QS pattern is seen in V1 and a tall R wave is seen in V6.

LBBB in children is associated with cardiac disease or surgery in the LV outflow tract, septal myomectomy, and replacement of the aortic valve. Other conditions rarely associated with LBBB include LVH, progressive conduction system disease, myocarditis, cardiomyopathy, myocardial infarction, and aortic valve endocarditis.

LBBB alone may rarely progress to complete heart block and sudden death, but the prognosis is more dependent on associated disease than on the LBBB itself.

INTRAVENTRICULAR BLOCK

In intraventricular block, the prolongation is throughout the duration of the QRS complex (see Fig. 3–19D). This usually suggests serious conditions such as metabolic disorders (e.g., hyperkalemia), diffuse myocardial diseases (e.g., myocardial fibrosis, systemic diseases with myocardial involvement), severe hypoxia, myocardial ischemia, or drug toxicity (quinidine or procainamide).

WOLFF-PARKINSON-WHITE PREEXCITATION

WPW preexcitation results from an anomalous conduction pathway (i.e., bundle of Kent) between the atrium and the ventricle, bypassing the normal delay of conduction in the AV node. The premature depolarization of a ventricle produces a delta wave and results in prolongation of the QRS duration (see Fig. 3–19C).

Criteria for Wolff-Parkinson-White Syndrome

1. Short PR interval, less than the lower limit of normal for the patient's age. The lower limits of normal of the PR interval according to age are as follows:

Younger than 12 months	0.075 second
1 to 3 years	0.080 second
3 to 5 years	0.085 second
5 to 12 years	0.090 second
12 to 16 years	0.095 second
Adults	0.120 second

2. Delta wave (initial slurring of the QRS complex)

3. Wide QRS duration beyond the upper limit of normal

Patients with WPW preexcitation are susceptible to attacks of paroxysmal supraventricular tachycardia (SVT) (see Chapter 24). When there is a history of SVT, the diagnosis of WPW syndrome is justified. WPW preexcitation may mimic other ECG abnormalities such as ventricular hypertrophy, RBBB, or myocardial disorders. In the presence of preexcitation, the diagnosis of ventricular hypertrophy cannot be safely made. Large QRS deflections are often seen in this condition because of an asynchronous depolarization of the ventricles rather than ventricular hypertrophy.

Figure 3–21 is an example of WPW preexcitation. The most striking abnormalities are a short PR interval (0.08 second) and a wide QRS duration (0.11 second). There are delta waves in most of the leads. Some delta waves are negative, as seen in leads III, aVR, V4R, and V1. The ST segments and T waves are shifted in the opposite direction of the QRS vector, resulting in a wide QRS-T angle. The leftward voltages are abnormally large, but the diagnosis of LVH cannot safely be made in the presence of WPW preexcitation.

Two other forms of preexcitation can also result in extreme tachycardia.

1. Lown-Ganong-Levine syndrome is characterized by a short PR interval and normal QRS duration. In this condition, James fibers (which connect the atrium and the bundle of His) bypass the upper AV node and produce a short PR interval, but the ventricles are depolarized normally through the His-Purkinje system. When there is

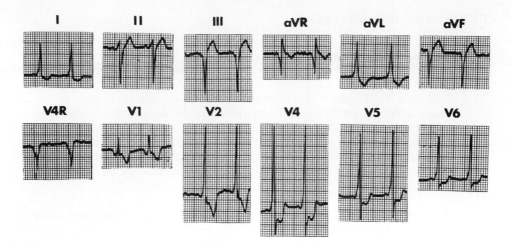

Figure 3–21. *Tracing from an asymptomatic 2-year-old boy whose ventricular septal defect underwent spontaneous closure. The tracing shows the Wolff-Parkinson-White preexcitation (see text for interpretation).*

no history of SVT, the ECG tracing should simply be read as showing a short PR interval rather than Lown-Ganong-Levine syndrome.

2. Mahaim-type preexcitation syndrome is characterized by a normal PR interval and long QRS duration with a delta wave. There is an abnormal Mahaim fiber that connects the AV node and one of the ventricles, bypassing the bundle of His, and "short-circuits" into the ventricle.

VENTRICULAR HYPERTROPHY VERSUS VENTRICULAR CONDUCTION DISTURBANCES

Two common ECG abnormalities in children, ventricular hypertrophy and ventricular conduction disturbances, are not always easy to distinguish; both arise with increased QRS amplitudes. The following approach may aid in the correct diagnosis of these conditions (Fig. 3–22). An accurate measurement of the QRS duration is essential.

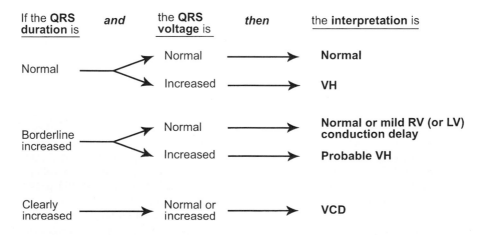

Figure 3–22. *Algorithm for differentiating between ventricular hypertrophy (VH) and ventricular conduction disturbances (VCDs). LV, left ventricle; RV, right ventricle.*

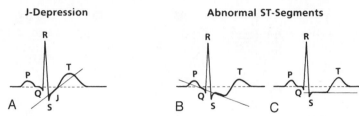

Figure 3–23. Nonpathologic (nonischemic) and pathologic (ischemic) ST-segment and T-wave changes. A, Characteristic nonischemic ST-segment change called J-depression; note that the ST slope is upward. B and C, Examples of pathologic ST-segment changes; note that the downward slope of the ST segment (B) or the horizontal segment is sustained (C). (From Park MK, Guntheroth WG: How to Read Pediatric ECGs, 4th ed. Philadelphia, Mosby, 2006.)

1. When the QRS duration is normal, normal QRS voltages indicate a normal ECG. Increased QRS voltages indicate ventricular hypertrophy.

2. When the QRS duration is clearly prolonged, a ventricular conduction disturbance is present whether the QRS voltages are normal or increased. Additional diagnosis of ventricular hypertrophy should not be made.

3. When the QRS duration is borderline prolonged, distinguishing these two conditions is difficult. Normal QRS voltages favor a normal ECG or a mild (right or left ventricular) conduction disturbance. An increased QRS voltage favors ventricular hypertrophy.

ST-Segment and T-Wave Changes

ECG changes involving the ST segment and the T wave are common in adults but relatively rare in children. This is because of a high incidence of ischemic heart disease, bundle branch block, myocardial infarction, and other myocardial disorders in adults. Some ST-segment changes are normal (nonpathologic) and others are abnormal (pathologic).

NONPATHOLOGIC ST-SEGMENT SHIFT

Not all ST-segment shifts are abnormal. Slight shift of the ST segment is common in normal children. Elevation or depression of up to 1 mm in the limb leads and up to 2 mm in the precordial leads is within normal limits. Two common types of nonpathologic ST-segment shifts are J-depression and early repolarization. The T vector remains normal in these conditions.

J-Depression. J-depression is a shift of the junction between the QRS complex and the ST segment (J-point) without sustained ST segment depression (Fig. 3–23A). The J-depression is seen more often in the precordial leads than in the limb leads (Fig. 3–24).

Early Repolarization. In early repolarization, all leads with upright T waves have elevated ST segments, and leads with inverted T waves have depressed ST segments (see Fig. 3–24). The T vector remains normal. This condition, seen in healthy adolescents and young adults, resembles the ST-segment shift seen in acute pericarditis; in the former, the ST segment is stable, and in the latter, the ST segment returns to the isoelectric line.

PATHOLOGIC ST-SEGMENT SHIFT

Abnormal shifts of the ST segment are often accompanied by T-wave inversion. A pathologic ST-segment shift assumes one of the following forms:

1. Downward slant followed by a diphasic or inverted T wave (see Fig. 3–23B)

2. Horizontal elevation or depression sustained for more than 0.08 second (see Fig. 3–23C)

Pathologic ST-segment shifts are seen in left or right ventricular hypertrophy with strain (discussed under ventricular hypertrophy); digitalis effect; pericarditis, including postoperative state; myocarditis (see under myocarditis, Chapter 19); myocardial infarction; and some electrolyte disturbances (hypokalemia and hyperkalemia).

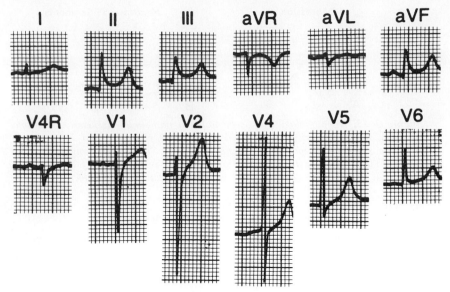

Figure 3–24. Tracing from a healthy 16-year-old boy that exhibits early repolarization and J-depression. The ST segment is shifted toward the direction of the T wave and is most marked in II, III, and aVF. J-depression is seen in most of the precordial leads.

T-WAVE CHANGES

T-wave changes are usually associated with the conditions manifesting with pathologic ST-segment shift. T-wave changes with or without ST-segment shift are also seen with bundle branch block and ventricular arrhythmias.

Pericarditis. The ECG changes seen in pericarditis are the result of subepicardial myocardial damage or pericardial effusion and consist of the following:

1. Pericardial effusion may produce low QRS voltages (QRS voltages <5 mm in every one of the limb leads).

2. Subepicardial myocardial damage produces the following time-dependent changes in the ST segment and T wave (Fig. 3–25):

   a. ST-segment elevation occurs in the leads representing the left ventricle.
   b. The ST-segment shift returns to normal within 2 to 3 days.
   c. T-wave inversion (with isoelectric ST segment) occurs 2 to 4 weeks after the onset of pericarditis.

Myocardial Infarction. Myocardial infarction is rare in infants and children, but correctly diagnosing the condition is important for proper care. All conditions that have

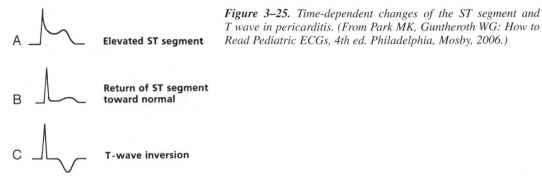

A — Elevated ST segment

B — Return of ST segment toward normal

C — T-wave inversion

Figure 3–25. Time-dependent changes of the ST segment and T wave in pericarditis. (From Park MK, Guntheroth WG: How to Read Pediatric ECGs, 4th ed. Philadelphia, Mosby, 2006.)

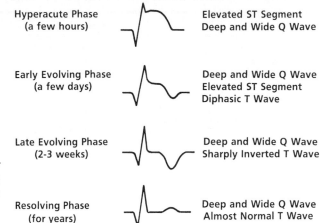

Hyperacute Phase (a few hours)		Elevated ST Segment Deep and Wide Q Wave
Early Evolving Phase (a few days)		Deep and Wide Q Wave Elevated ST Segment Diphasic T Wave
Late Evolving Phase (2-3 weeks)		Deep and Wide Q Wave Sharply Inverted T Wave
Resolving Phase (for years)		Deep and Wide Q Wave Almost Normal T Wave

Figure 3–26. Sequential changes of the ST segment and T wave in myocardial infarction. (From Park MK, Guntheroth WG: How to Read Pediatric ECGs, 4th ed. Philadelphia, Mosby, 2006.)

been associated with myocardial infarction in adults have been described as causing myocardial infarction in children, such as atherosclerosis, inflammatory disease of the myocardium, lupus erythematosus, syphilis, polyarteritis nodosa, hypertension, and diabetes mellitus. Uncommon causes of myocardial infarction in pediatric patients include anomalous origin of the left coronary artery from the pulmonary artery, endocardial fibroelastosis, coronary artery embolization resulting from infective endocarditis or from diagnostic procedures performed on the left side of the heart, and inadvertent surgical interruption of the coronary artery during cardiac surgery. Early and late sequelae of Kawasaki disease, surgical complications of the arterial switch operation for transposition of the great arteries, and dilated cardiomyopathy have emerged as important causes of myocardial infarction in the pediatric population.

The ECG findings of adult myocardial infarction are time dependent and are illustrated in Figure 3–26. Changes seen during the hyperacute phase are short lived. The more common ECG findings are those of the early evolving phase. These consist of pathologic Q waves (abnormally wide and deep), ST-segment elevation, and T-wave inversion. The duration of the Q wave is 0.04 second or greater in adults, and it should be at least 0.03 second in children. Over the next few weeks, the elevated ST segment gradually returns toward the baseline, but inverted T waves persist (late evolving phase). The pathologic Q waves persist for years after myocardial infarction (see Fig. 3–26). Leads that show these abnormalities vary with the location of the infarction and are summarized in Table 3–7.

In most pediatric patients with myocardial infarction, the time of onset is not clearly known, and the evolution of the different phases is difficult to document. Frequent ECG findings in children with acute myocardial infarction include the following (Towbin et al, 1992):

1. Wide Q waves (>0.035 second) with or without Q-wave notching

2. ST segment elevation (>2 mm)

3. Prolongation of QTc interval (>0.44 second) with accompanying abnormal Q waves

The width of the Q wave is more important than the depth; the depth of the Q wave varies widely in normal children (see Table 3–6).

Figure 3–27 is an ECG of myocardial infarction in an infant with anomalous origin of the left coronary artery from the pulmonary artery. The most important abnormality is the presence of a deep and wide Q wave (0.04 second) in leads I, aVL, and V6. A QS pattern appears in V2 through V5, indicating anterolateral myocardial infarction (see Table 3–7).

Table 3–7. **Leads Showing Abnormal ECG Findings in Myocardial Infarction**

	Limb Leads	Precordial Leads
Lateral	I, aVL	V5, V6
Anterior		V1, V2, V3
Anterolateral	I, aVL	V2–V6
Diaphragmatic	II, III, aVF	
Posterior		V1–V3*

*None of the leads is oriented toward the posterior surface of the heart. Therefore, in posterior infarction, changes that would have been present in the posterior surface leads will be seen in the anterior leads as a mirror image (e.g., tall and slightly wide R waves in V1 and V2, comparable with abnormal Q waves, and tall and wide, symmetrical T waves in V1 and V2).

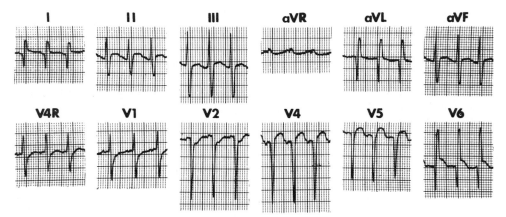

Figure 3–27. Tracing from a 2-month-old infant with anomalous origin of the left coronary artery from the pulmonary artery. An abnormally deep and wide Q wave (0.04 second) seen in I, aVL, and V6 and a QS pattern seen in V2 through V6 are characteristic of anterolateral myocardial infarction.

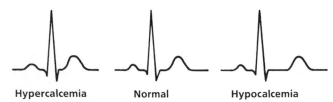

Figure 3–28. Electrocardiographic findings of hypercalcemia and hypocalcemia. Hypercalcemia shortens and hypocalcemia lengthens the ST segment. (From Park MK, Guntheroth WG: How to Read Pediatric ECGs, 4th ed. Philadelphia, Mosby, 2006.)

SERUM K

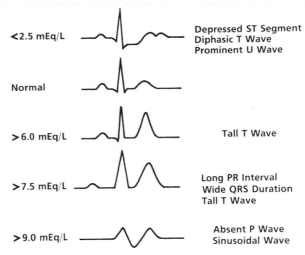

Figure 3–29. *Electrocardiographic findings of hypokalemia and hyperkalemia. (From Park MK, Guntheroth WG: How to Read Pediatric ECGs, 4th ed. Philadelphia, Mosby, 2006.)*

ELECTROLYTE DISTURBANCES

Two important serum electrolytes that produce ECG changes are calcium and potassium.

Calcium. Calcium ion affects the duration of the ST segment and thus changes the relative position of the T wave. Hypercalcemia or hypocalcemia does not produce ST-segment shift or T-wave changes. Hypocalcemia prolongs the ST segment and, as a result, prolongs the QTc interval (Fig. 3–28). Hypercalcemia shortens the ST segment, resulting in shortening of the QTc interval (see Fig. 3–28).

Potassium. Hypokalemia produces one of the least specific ECG changes. When the serum potassium level is below 2.5 mEq/L, ECG changes consist of a prominent U wave with apparent prolongation of the QTc, flat or diphasic T waves, and ST-segment depression (Fig. 3–29). With further lowering of serum potassium levels, the PR interval becomes prolonged, and sinoatrial block may occur.

The earliest ECG abnormality seen in hyperkalemia is tall, peaked, symmetrical T waves with a narrow base—the so-called tented T wave. In hyperkalemia, sinoatrial block, second-degree AV block (either Mobitz I or II), and passive or accelerated junctional or ventricular escape rhythm may occur. Severe hyperkalemia may result in either ventricular fibrillation or arrest. The following ECG sequence is associated with a progressive increase in the serum potassium level (see Fig. 3–29):

1. Tall, tented T waves

2. Prolongation of the QRS duration (intraventricular block)

3. Prolongation of the PR interval (first-degree AV block)

4. Disappearance of the P wave

5. Wide, bizarre diphasic QRS complex ("sine wave")

6. Eventual asystole

These ECG changes are usually seen best in leads II and II and the left precordial leads.

Chapter 4

Chest Roentgenography

The chest roentgenogram is an essential part of cardiac evaluation. The following information can be gained from x-ray films: heart size and silhouette; enlargement of specific cardiac chambers; pulmonary blood flow or pulmonary vascular markings; and other information regarding lung parenchyma, spine, bony thorax, abdominal situs, and so on. Posteroanterior and lateral views are routinely obtained.

Heart Size and Silhouette

HEART SIZE

Measurement of the cardiothoracic (CT) ratio is by far the simplest way to estimate the heart size in older children (Fig. 4–1). The CT ratio is obtained by relating the largest transverse diameter of the heart to the widest internal diameter of the chest:

$$CT \text{ ratio} = (A + B) \div C$$

where A and B are maximal cardiac dimensions to the right and left of the midline, respectively, and C is the widest internal diameter of the chest. A CT ratio of more than 0.5 indicates cardiomegaly. However, the CT ratio cannot be used with accuracy in newborns and small infants, in whom a good inspiratory chest film is rarely obtained. In this situation, the degree of inadequate inspiration should be taken into consideration. Also, an estimation of the cardiac volume should be made by inspecting the posteroanterior and lateral views instead of the CT ratio.

To determine the presence or absence of cardiomegaly, the lateral view of the heart should also be inspected. For example, isolated right ventricular enlargement may not be obvious on a posteroanterior film but is obvious on a lateral film. In a patient with

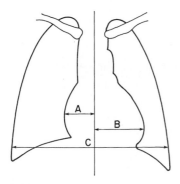

Figure 4–1. *Diagram showing how to measure the cardiothoracic (CT) ratio from the posteroanterior view of a chest x-ray film. The CT ratio is obtained by dividing the largest horizontal diameter of the heart (A + B) by the longest internal diameter of the chest (C).*

a flat chest (or narrow anteroposterior diameter of the chest), a posteroanterior film may erroneously show cardiomegaly.

An enlarged heart on chest x-ray films more reliably reflects a volume overload than a pressure overload. Electrocardiograms (ECGs) better represent a pressure overload.

NORMAL CARDIAC SILHOUETTE

The structures that form the cardiac borders in the posteroanterior projection of a chest roentgenogram are shown in Figure 4–2. The right cardiac silhouette is formed superiorly by the superior vena cava (SVC) and inferiorly by the right atrium (RA). The left cardiac border is formed from the top to the bottom by the aortic knob, the main pulmonary artery (PA), and the left ventricle (LV). The left atrial appendage is located between the main PA and the LV and is not prominent in a normal heart. The right ventricle (RV) does not form the cardiac border in the posteroanterior view. The lateral projection of the cardiac silhouette is formed anteriorly by the RV and posteriorly by the left atrium (LA) above and the LV below. In a normal heart, the lower posterior cardiac border (i.e., LV) crosses the inferior vena cava (IVC) line above the diaphragm (see Fig. 4–2).

However, in the newborn, a typical, normal cardiac silhouette is rarely seen because of the presence of a large thymus and because the films are often exposed during expiration. The thymus is situated in the superoanterior mediastinum. Therefore, the base of the heart may be widened, with resulting alteration in the normal silhouette in the posteroanterior view. In the lateral view, the retrosternal space, which is normally clear in older children, may be obliterated by the large thymus.

ABNORMAL CARDIAC SILHOUETTE

Although discerning individual chamber enlargement often helps diagnose an acyanotic heart defect, the overall shape of the heart sometimes provides important clues to the type of defect, particularly in dealing with cyanotic infants and children. A few examples follow, indicating the status of pulmonary blood flow or pulmonary vascular markings.

1. A "boot-shaped" heart with decreased pulmonary blood flow is typical in infants with cyanotic tetralogy of Fallot (TOF). This is also seen in some infants with tricuspid atresia. Typical of both conditions is the presence of a hypoplastic main

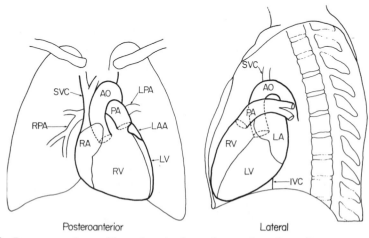

Posteroanterior   Lateral

Figure 4–2. *Posteroanterior and lateral projections of normal cardiac silhouette. Note that in the lateral projection, the right ventricle (RV) is contiguous with the lower third of the sternum and that the left ventricle (LV) normally crosses the posterior margin of the inferior vena cava (IVC) above the diaphragm. AO, aorta; LA, left atrium; LAA, left atrial appendage; LPA, left pulmonary artery; PA, pulmonary artery; RA, right atrium; RPA, right pulmonary artery; SVC, superior vena cava.*

PA segment (Fig. 4–3A). ECGs are helpful in differentiating these two conditions. The ECG shows right axis deviation (RAD), right ventricular hypertrophy (RVH), and occasional right atrial hypertrophy (RAH) in TOF, whereas it shows a "superior" QRS axis (i.e., left anterior hemiblock), RAH, and left ventricular hypertrophy (LVH) in tricuspid atresia.

2. A narrow-waisted and "egg-shaped" heart with increased pulmonary blood flow in a cyanotic infant strongly suggests transposition of the great arteries (TGA). The narrow waist results from the absence of a large thymus and the abnormal relationship of the great arteries (see Fig. 4–3B).

3. The "snowman" sign with increased pulmonary blood flow is seen in infants with the supracardiac type of total anomalous pulmonary venous return (TAPVR). The left vertical vein, left innominate vein, and dilated SVC make up the snowman's head (see Fig. 4–3C).

Evaluation of Cardiac Chambers and Great Arteries

INDIVIDUAL CHAMBER ENLARGEMENT

Identification of individual chamber enlargement is important in diagnosing a specific lesion, particularly when dealing with acyanotic heart defects. Although enlargement of a single chamber is discussed here, more than one chamber is usually involved.

Left Atrial Enlargement. An enlarged LA causes alterations not only of the cardiac silhouette but also of the various adjacent structures (Fig. 4–4). Mild left atrial enlargement is best appreciated in the lateral projection by the posterior protrusion of the left atrial border. Enlargement of the LA may produce "double density" on the posteroanterior view. With further enlargement, the left atrial appendage becomes prominent on the left cardiac border. The left main stem bronchus is elevated. The barium-filled esophagus is indented to the right.

Left Ventricular Enlargement. In the posteroanterior view, the apex of the heart is not only farther to the left but also downward. In the lateral view of left ventricular enlargement, the lower posterior cardiac border is displaced farther posteriorly and meets the IVC line below the diaphragm level (Fig. 4–5).

Right Atrial Enlargement. Right atrial enlargement is most obvious in the posteroanterior projection as an increased prominence of the lower right cardiac silhouette (Fig. 4–6). However, this is not an absolute finding because both false-positive and false-negative results are possible.

Right Ventricular Enlargement. Isolated right ventricular enlargement may not be obvious in the posteroanterior projection, and the normal CT ratio may be maintained because the RV does not make up the cardiac silhouette in the posteroanterior projection. Right ventricular enlargement is best recognized in the lateral view, in which it is manifest by filling of the retrosternal space (see Fig. 4–6, lateral view).

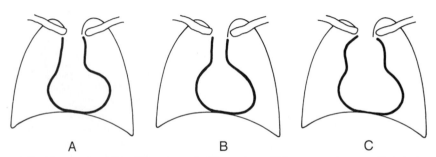

A   B   C

*Figure 4–3. Abnormal cardiac silhouettes. **A**, "Boot-shaped" heart seen in cyanotic tetralogy of Fallot or tricuspid atresia. **B**, "Egg-shaped" heart seen in transposition of the great arteries. **C**, "Snowman" sign seen in total anomalous pulmonary venous return (supracardiac type).*

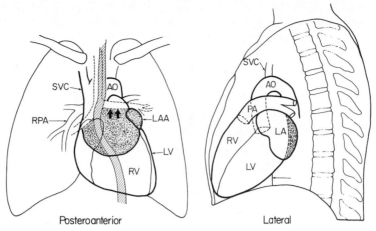

Figure 4–4. *Schematic diagram showing roentgenographic findings of enlargement of the left atrium (LA) in the posteroanterior and lateral projections. Arrows show left main stem bronchus elevation. In the posteroanterior view, double density and prominence of the left atrial appendage (LAA) are also illustrated. The barium-filled esophagus (crosshatched, vertical structure) is indented to the right. In the lateral view, posterior protrusion of the LA border is illustrated. The isolated enlargement of the LA shown here is only hypothetical because it usually accompanies other changes. Other abbreviations are the same as those in Figure 4–2.*

SIZE OF THE GREAT ARTERIES

As in the enlargement of specific cardiac chambers, the size of the great arteries often helps make a specific diagnosis.

Prominent Main Pulmonary Artery Segment. The prominence of a normally placed PA in the posteroanterior view (Fig. 4–7A) results from one of the following:

1. Poststenotic dilatation (e.g., pulmonary valve stenosis)

2. Increased blood flow through the PA (e.g., atrial septal defect [ASD], ventricular septal defect [VSD])

3. Increased pressure in the PA (e.g., pulmonary hypertension)

4. Occasional normal finding in adolescents, especially girls

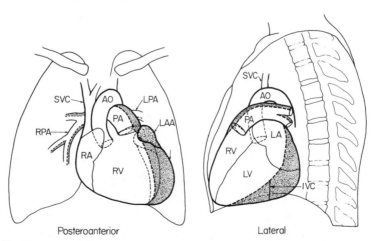

Figure 4–5. *Diagrammatic representation of changes seen in ventricular septal defect. Left ventricle (LV) enlargement in addition to enlargement of the left atrium (LA) and a prominent pulmonary artery (PA) segment. Other abbreviations are the same as those in Figure 4–2.*

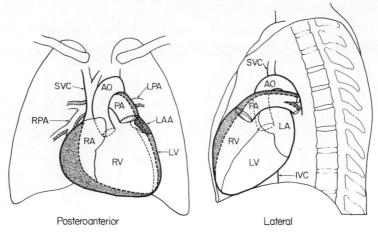

Posteroanterior   Lateral

Figure 4–6. *Schematic diagrams of posteroanterior and lateral chest roentgenograms of atrial septal defect. There is enlargement of the right atrium (RA) and right ventricle (RV) and increased pulmonary vascularity. Other abbreviations are the same as those in Figure 4–2.*

Hypoplasia of the Pulmonary Artery. A concave main PA segment with a resulting boot-shaped heart is seen in TOF and tricuspid atresia (Fig. 4–7B); obviously, malposition of the PA must be ruled out.

Dilatation of the Aorta. An enlarged ascending aorta may be observed in the frontal projection as a rightward bulge of the right upper mediastinum, but a mild degree of enlargement may easily escape detection. Aortic enlargement is seen in TOF and aortic stenosis (as poststenotic dilatation) and less often in patent ductus arteriosus (PDA), coarctation of the aorta (COA), Marfan syndrome, or systemic hypertension. When the ascending aorta and aortic arch are enlarged, the aortic knob may become prominent on the posteroanterior view (Fig. 4–7C).

Pulmonary Vascular Markings

One of the major goral of radiologic examination is assessment of the pulmonary vasculature. Although many textbooks explain how to detect increased pulmonary blood flow, this is one of the more difficult aspects of interpreting chest x-ray films of cardiac patients. There is no substitute for the experience gained by looking at many chest x-ray films with normal and abnormal pulmonary blood flow.

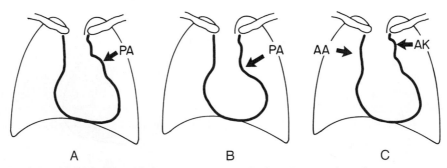

A   B   C

Figure 4–7. *cAbnormalities of the great arteries. **A,** Prominent main pulmonary artery (PA) segment. **B,** Concave PA segment resulting from hypoplasia. **C,** Dilatation of the aorta may be seen as a bulge on the right upper mediastinum by a dilated ascending aorta (AA) or as a prominence of the aortic knob (AK) on the left upper cardiac border.*

INCREASED PULMONARY BLOOD FLOW

Increased pulmonary vascularity is present when the right and left PAs appear enlarged and extend into the lateral third of the lung field, where they are not usually present; there is increased vascularity to the lung apices where the vessels are normally collapsed; and the external diameter of the right PA visible in the right hilus is wider than the internal diameter of the trachea.

Increased pulmonary blood flow in an acyanotic child represents ASD, VSD, PDA, ECD, partial anomalous pulmonary venous return (PAPVR), or any combination of these. In a cyanotic infant, increased pulmonary vascular markings may indicate TGA, TAPVR, HLHS, persistent truncus arteriosus, or a single ventricle.

DECREASED PULMONARY BLOOD FLOW

Decreased pulmonary blood flow is suspected when the hilum appears small, the remaining lung fields appear black, and the vessels appear small and thin. Ischemic lung fields are seen in cyanotic heart diseases with decreased pulmonary blood flow such as critical stenosis or atresia of the pulmonary or tricuspid valves, including TOF.

PULMONARY VENOUS CONGESTION

Pulmonary venous congestion is characterized by a hazy and indistinct margin of the pulmonary vasculature. This is caused by pulmonary venous hypertension secondary to left ventricular failure or obstruction to pulmonary venous drainage (e.g., mitral stenosis, TAPVR, cor triatriatum). Kerley's B lines are short, transverse strips of increased density best seen in the costophrenic sulci. This is caused by engorged lymphatics and interstitial edema of the interlobular septa secondary to pulmonary venous congestion.

NORMAL PULMONARY VASCULATURE

Pulmonary vascularity is normal in patients with obstructive lesions such as pulmonary stenosis or aortic stenosis. Unless the stenosis is extremely severe, pulmonary vascularity remains normal in pulmonary stenosis. Patients with small left-to-right shunt lesions also show normal pulmonary vascular markings.

Systematic Approach

The interpretation of chest x-ray films should include a systematic routine to avoid overlooking important anatomic changes relevant to cardiac diagnosis.

LOCATION OF THE LIVER AND STOMACH GAS BUBBLE

The cardiac apex should be on the same side as the stomach or opposite the hepatic shadow. When there is heterotaxia, with the apex on the right and the stomach on the left (or vice versa), the likelihood of a serious heart defect is great. An even more ominous situation exists with a "midline" liver, associated with asplenia (Ivemark's) syndrome or polysplenia syndrome (Fig. 4–8). These infants usually have complex cyanotic heart defects that are difficult to correct.

SKELETAL ASPECT OF CHEST X-RAY FILM

Pectus excavatum may flatten the heart in the anteroposterior dimension and cause a compensatory increase in its transverse diameter, creating the false impression of cardiomegaly. Thoracic scoliosis and vertebral abnormalities are frequent in cardiac patients. Rib notching is a specific finding of COA in an older child (usually older than 5 years) and is usually found between the fourth and eighth ribs (Fig. 4–9).

IDENTIFICATION OF THE AORTA

1. Identification of the descending aorta along the left margin of the spine usually indicates a left aortic arch; identification along the right margin of the spine indicates a right aortic arch. Right aortic arch is frequently associated with TOF or persistent truncus arteriosus.

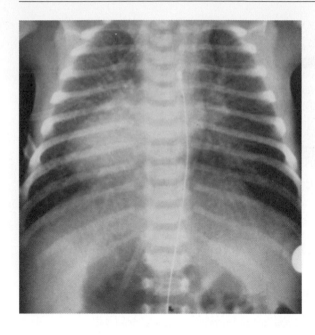

Figure 4–8. An x-ray film of the chest and upper abdomen of a newborn infant with polysplenia syndrome. Note a symmetrical liver ("midline liver"), a stomach bubble in the midline, dextrocardia, and increased pulmonary vascularity.

2. When the descending aorta is not directly visible, the position of the trachea and esophagus may help locate the descending aorta. If the trachea and esophagus are located slightly to the right of the midline, the aorta usually descends normally on the left (i.e., left aortic arch). In the right aortic arch, the trachea and esophagus are shifted to the left.

3. In a heavily exposed film, the precoarctation and postcoarctation dilatation of the aorta may be seen as a "figure of 3." This may be confirmed by a barium esophagogram with E-shaped indentation (Fig. 4–10).

UPPER MEDIASTINUM

1. The thymus is prominent in healthy infants and may give a false impression of cardiomegaly. It may give the classic "sail sign" (Fig. 4–11). The thymus often has

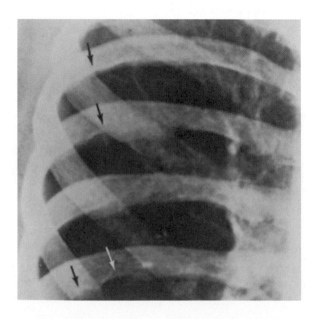

Figure 4–9. Rib notching (arrows) in an 11-year-old girl with coarctation of the aorta. (From Caffey J: Pediatric X-ray Diagnosis, 7th ed. Chicago, Mosby, 1978.)

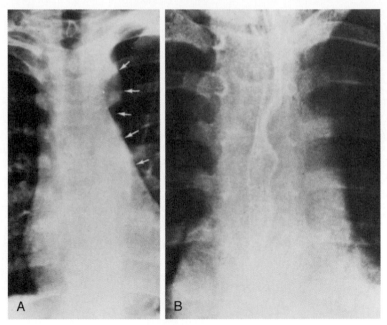

Figure 4–10. A, *The figure-of-3 configuration indicates the site of coarctation with the large proximal segment of aorta and/or prominent left subclavian artery above and the poststenotic dilatation of the descending aorta below it.* **B,** *Barium esophagogram reveals the E-shaped indentation or reversed figure-of-3 configuration. (From Caffey J: Pediatric X-ray Diagnosis, 7th ed. Chicago, Mosby, 1978.)*

a wavy border because this structure becomes indented by the ribs. On the lateral view, the thymus occupies the superoanterior mediastinum, obscuring the upper retrosternal space.

2. The thymus shrinks in cyanotic infants or infants under severe stress from congestive heart failure. In TGA, the mediastinal shadow is narrow ("narrow waist"), partly because of the shrinkage of the thymus gland. Infants with DiGeorge syndrome have an absent thymic shadow and a high incidence of aortic arch anomalies.

3. A snowman figure (or figure-of-8 configuration) is seen in infants, who are usually older than 4 months, with anomalous pulmonary venous return draining into the SVC through the left SVC (vertical vein) and the left innominate vein (see Fig. 4–3C).

Figure 4–11. *Roentgenogram showing the typical "sail sign" on the right mediastinal border.*

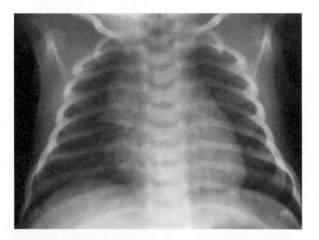

PULMONARY PARENCHYMA

1. Pneumonia is a common complication in patients with high pulmonary venous pressure, such as those with a large PDA or VSD.

2. A long-standing density, particularly in the lower left lung field, suggests pulmonary sequestration. In this condition, there is aberrant, nonfunctioning pulmonary tissue, which does not connect with the bronchial tree and derives its blood supply from the descending aorta. The venous drainage is usually to the pulmonary venous system.

3. A vertical vascular shadow along the lower right cardiac border may suggest PAPVR from the lower lobe and sometimes the middle lobe of the right lung, called scimitar syndrome. Its pulmonary venous drainage is usually to the IVC either just above or below the diaphragm. This syndrome is often associated with other anomalies including hypoplasia of the right lung and right pulmonary artery, sequestration of right lung tissue receiving arterial supply from the aorta, and other congenital heart diseases such as VSD, PDA, COA, or TOF.

Chapter 5

Flow Diagrams

Flow diagrams that help arrive at a diagnosis of congenital heart disease (CHD) are shown in Figures 5–1 and 5–2. They are based on the presence or absence of cyanosis and on the status of pulmonary blood flow—whether normal, increased, or decreased. The presence of right ventricular hypertrophy (RVH), left ventricular hypertrophy (LVH), or both further narrows the possibilities. Only common entities are listed in the flow diagrams.

In using these flow diagrams, certain adjustments are often necessary. For example, in some instances in which pulmonary vascularity on chest x-ray films may be interpreted as normal or at the upper limit of normal, the list may need to be checked under both normal and increased pulmonary blood flow. Likewise, an electrocardiogram (ECG) may show right ventricular dominance yet not meet strict criteria for RVH. Such a case may need to be treated as RVH. It should also be remembered that a normal ECG and normal pulmonary vascular markings on chest x-ray films do not rule out CHD. In fact,

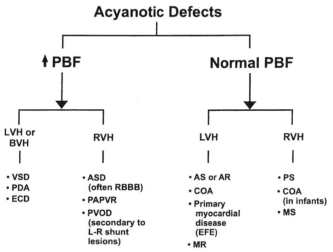

Figure 5–1. *Flow diagram of acyanotic congenital heart defects. AR, aortic regurgitation; AS, aortic stenosis; ASD, atrial septal defect; BVH, biventricular hypertrophy; COA, coarctation of the aorta; ECD, endocardial cushion defect; EFE, endocardial fibroelastosis; L-R, left-to-right; LVH, left ventricular hypertrophy; MR, mitral regurgitation; MS, mitral stenosis; PAPVR, partial anomalous pulmonary venous return; PBF, pulmonary blood flow; PDA, patent ductus arteriosus; PS, pulmonary stenosis; PVOD, pulmonary vascular obstructive disease (or Eisenmenger's syndrome); RBBB, right bundle branch block; RVH, right ventricular hypertrophy; VSD, ventricular septal defect.*

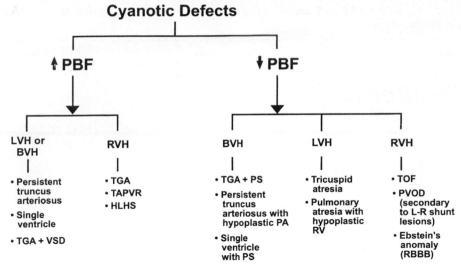

Figure 5–2. *Flow diagram of cyanotic congenital heart defects. BVH, biventricular hypertrophy; HLHS, hypoplastic left heart syndrome; L-R, left-to-right; LVH, left ventricular hypertrophy; PA, pulmonary artery; PBF, pulmonary blood flow; PS, pulmonary stenosis; PVOD, pulmonary vascular obstructive disease (or Eisenmenger's syndrome); RBBB, right bundle branch block; RV, right ventricle; RVH, right ventricular hypertrophy; TAPVR, total anomalous pulmonary venous return; TGA, transposition of the great arteries; TOF, tetralogy of Fallot; VSD, ventricular septal defect.*

many mild, acyanotic heart defects do not show abnormalities on the ECG or chest x-ray films. Diagnosis of these defects rests primarily on findings from the physical examination, particularly on auscultation.

In addition to ventricular hypertrophy seen on ECGs, other ECG findings are occasionally helpful in making the diagnosis. For example, a superiorly oriented QRS axis (i.e., left anterior hemiblock) in an acyanotic infant suggests endocardial cushion defect, whereas in a cyanotic infant it suggests tricuspid atresia, asplenia syndrome, or polysplenia syndrome. ECG findings of myocardial infarction may be seen in anomalous origin of the left coronary artery from the pulmonary artery, coronary aneurysms associated with Kawasaki's disease, or endocardial fibroelastosis. Common ECG manifestations of some CHDs are summarized in Table 5–1.

Table 5–1. **Common Electrocardiographic Manifestations of Congenital Heart Defects**

Congenital Defect	ECG Findings
Anomalous origin of the left coronary artery from the PA	Myocardial infarction, anterolateral
Anomalous pulmonary venous return	
Total	RAD, RVH, and RAH
Partial	Mild RVH or RBBB
AS	
Mild to moderate	Normal or LVH
Severe	LVH with or without "strain"
ASD	
Primum type	Superior QRS axis
	rsR′ pattern in V1 and aVR (RBBB or RVH)
	First-degree AV block (>50%)
	Counterclockwise QRS loop in the frontal plane of vectorcardiogram
Secundum type	RAD, RVH, or RBBB (rsR′ in V1 and aVR)
	First-degree AV block (10%)
COA	
Infants younger than 6 mo	RBBB or RVH
Older children	LVH, normal, or RBBB

Table 5–1. **Common Electrocardiographic Manifestations of Congenital Heart Defects**
(Continued)

Congenital Defect	ECG Findings
Common ventricle or single ventricle	Abnormal Q waves:
	Q in V1 and no Q in V6
	No Q in any precordial leads
	Q in all precordial leads
	Stereotype RS complex in most or all precordial leads
	WPW preexcitation or SVT
	First- or second-degree AV block
Cor triatriatum	Same as for MS
Ebstein's anomaly	RAH, RBBB
	First-degree AV block
	WPW preexcitation
	No RVH
ECD	
Complete	Superior QRS axis
	RVH or BVH, RAH
	First-degree AV block, RBBB
Partial	See ASD, primum type
Endocardial fibroelastosis	LVH
	Abnormal T waves
	Myocardial infarction patterns
HLHS (aortic and/or mitral atresia)	RVH
MS, congenital or acquired	RAD, RVH, RAH, LAH (±)
PDA	
Small shunt	Normal
Moderate shunt	LVH, LAH (±)
Large shunt	BVH, LAH
Eisenmenger's syndrome (PVOD)	RVH or BVH
Persistent truncus arteriosus	LVH or BVH
Pulmonary atresia (with hypoplastic RV)	LVH
PS	
Mild	Normal or mild RVH
Moderate	RVH
Severe	RVH with strain, RAH
PVOD (Eisenmenger's syndrome)	RVH or BVH
TOF	RAD
	RVH, with or without strain
	RAH (±)
D-TGA (complete transposition)	
Intact ventricular septum	RVH, RAH
VSD and/or PS	BVH, RAH, or BAH
L-TGA (congenitally corrected transposition)	AV block, first to third degree
	Atrial arrhythmias (SVT, atrial fibrillation)
	WPW preexcitation
	Absent Q in V5 and V6 and qR pattern in V1
	LAH or BAH
Tricuspid atresia	Superior QRS axis
	LVH, RAH
VSD	
Small shunt	Normal
Moderate shunt	LVH, LAH (±)
Large shunt	BVH, LAH
PVOD (Eisenmenger's syndrome)	RVH

AS, aortic stenosis; ASD, atrial septal defect; AV, atrioventricular; BAH, biatrial hypertrophy; BVH, biventricular hypertrophy; COA, coarctation of the aorta; ECD, endocardial cushion defect; HLHS, hypoplastic left heart syndrome; LAH, left atrial hypertrophy; LVH, left ventricular hypertrophy; MS, mitral stenosis; PA, pulmonary artery; PDA, patent ductus arteriosus; PS, pulmonary stenosis; PVOD, pulmonary vascular obstructive disease; RAD, right axis deviation; RAH, right atrial hypertrophy; RBBB, right bundle branch block; RV, right ventricle; RVH, right ventricular hypertrophy; SVT, supraventricular tachycardia; TGA, transposition of the great arteries; TOF, tetralogy of Fallot; VSD, ventricular septal defect; WPW, Wolff-Parkinson-White; ±, may or may not be present.

Chest x-ray findings other than pulmonary vascular markings also help detect a specific CHD. A few examples follow (see Chapter 4):

1. Heart size
   a. A large heart indicates large shunt lesions, myocardial failure, or pericardial effusion. An extremely large cardiac silhouette may be seen in Ebstein's anomaly.
   b. A large heart usually rules out tetralogy of Fallot.

2. Cardiac silhouette
   a. A "boot-shaped" heart suggests tetralogy of Fallot or tricuspid atresia.
   b. An "egg-shaped" heart with increased pulmonary vascularity suggests transposition of the great arteries.
   c. A "snowman" sign suggests anomalous pulmonary venous return.

3. Right aortic arch is commonly seen in tetralogy of Fallot or persistent truncus arteriosus.

4. A midline liver strongly suggests complex cardiac defects associated with asplenia or polysplenia syndrome.

Part II

SPECIAL TOOLS IN EVALUATION OF CARDIAC PATIENTS

Some readers may want to skip this part for now and return to it later as the need arises. The tools discussed in this section may be considered too specialized. Omission of this section will not affect one's understanding of the pathophysiology and most clinical aspects of pediatric cardiac problems.

A number of special tools are available to the cardiologist in the evaluation of cardiac patients. Some tools are readily available and frequently used in tertiary centers, whereas others are more specialized and are used less frequently. This part discusses only tests to which noncardiologists are exposed. Echocardiography (e.g., M-mode, two-dimensional, and Doppler), exercise stress test, and ambulatory electrocardiography (e.g., Holter monitor) are noninvasive tests; cardiac catheterization and angiocardiography are invasive tests. Although catheter intervention procedures are not diagnostic, this part discusses them because they are usually performed with cardiac catheterization.

Several other tests are not discussed because they are rarely performed or are too specialized. These tests include vectorcardiography, electrophysiologic study, nuclear cardiology (e.g., radionuclide cineangiography, myocardial scintigraphy), and magnetic resonance imaging.

Chapter 6

Noninvasive Techniques

Echocardiography

Echocardiography (echo) is an extremely useful, safe, and noninvasive test used for the diagnosis and management of heart disease. Echo studies, which use ultrasound, provide anatomic diagnosis as well as functional information. This is especially true with the incorporation of Doppler echo and color flow mapping.

The M-mode echo provides an "ice-pick" view of the heart. It has limited capability in demonstrating the spatial relationship of structures but remains an important tool in the evaluation of certain cardiac conditions and functions, particularly by measurements of dimensions and timing. It is usually performed as part of two-dimensional echo studies. The two-dimensional echo has an enhanced ability to demonstrate the spatial relationship of structures. This capability allows a more accurate anatomic diagnosis of abnormalities of the heart and great vessels. The Doppler and color mapping study has added the ability to detect easily valve regurgitation and cardiac shunts during the echo examination. It also provides some quantitative information such as pressure gradients across cardiac valves and estimation of pressures in the great arteries and ventricles. Echo examination can be applied in calculation of cardiac output and the magnitude of cardiac shunts. Discussion of instruments and techniques is beyond the scope of this book. Normal echo images and their role in the diagnosis of common cardiac problems in pediatric patients are briefly presented.

M-MODE ECHOCARDIOGRAPHY

An M-mode echo is obtained with the ultrasonic transducer placed along the left sternal border and directed toward the part of the heart to be examined. In Figure 6–1 the ultrasound is shown passing through three important structures of the left side of the heart. Line 1 passes through the aorta (AO) and left atrium (LA), where the dimensions of these structures are measured. Line 2 traverses the mitral valve. Line 3 goes through the main body of the right ventricle (RV) and left ventricle (LV). Along line 3 the dimensions of the RV and LV and the thickness of the interventricular septum and posterior LV wall are measured. Pericardial effusion is best detected at this level. An M-mode echo of the pulmonary valve is useful in the evaluation of pulmonary hypertension (see Chapter 29).

Although the two-dimensional echo has largely replaced the M-mode echo in the diagnosis of cardiac diseases, the M-mode echo retains many important applications, including the following:

1. Measurement of the dimensions of cardiac chambers and vessels, thickness of the ventricular septum, and free walls

2. Left ventricular systolic function

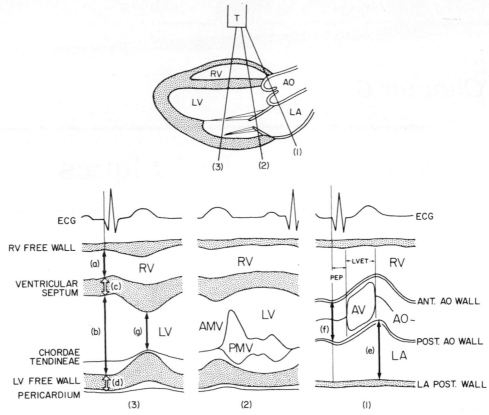

Figure 6–1. *A cross-sectional view of the left side of the heart along the long axis (top) through which "ice-pick" views of the M-mode echo recordings are made (bottom). Many other M-mode views are possible, but only three are shown in this figure. The dimension of the aorta (AO) and left atrium (LA) is measured along line (1). Systolic time intervals for the left side are also measured at the level of the aortic valve (AV). Line (2) passes through the mitral valve. Measurements made at this level are not very useful in pediatric patients. Measurement of chamber dimensions and wall thickness of right and left ventricles is made along line (3). The following measurements are shown in this figure. (a), Right ventricular (RV) dimension; (b), left ventricular (LV) diastolic dimension; (c), interventricular septal thickness; (d), LV posterior wall thickness; (e), LA dimension; (f), aortic dimension; (g), LV systolic dimension. AMV, anterior mitral valve; ECG, electrocardiogram; LVET, left ventricular ejection time; PEP, pre-ejection period; PMV, posterior mitral valve; T, transducer.*

   3. Study of the motion of the cardiac valves (e.g., mitral valve prolapse, mitral stenosis, pulmonary hypertension) and the interventricular septum
   4. Detection of pericardial fluid

Normal M-mode Echo Values

The dimensions of the cardiac chambers and the aorta increase with increasing age. Most dimensions are measured during diastole, coincident with the onset of the QRS complex; the LA dimension and LV systolic dimension are exceptions (see Fig. 6–1). Table 6–1 shows the mean values and ranges of common M-mode echo measurements of cardiac chamber size and wall thickness according to the patient's weight. In Appendix D, more detailed normal values of the chamber size, valve annulus size, and wall thickness are presented according to body surface area, age, weight, or height; for example, Table D–1 shows dimensions of LA, RV, and LV and the LV wall thickness by body surface area; Table D–2 the aortic annulus, LA, and LV dimensions by age; and Table D–3 the LA and LV dimensions by height.

Table 6–1. **Normal M-Mode Echo Values (mm) by Weight (lb): Mean (Range)**

	0–25 lb	26–50 lb	51–75 lb	76–100 lb	101–125 lb	126–200 lb
RV dimension	9 (3–15)	10 (4–15)	11 (7–18)	12 (7–16)	13 (8–17)	13 (12–17)
LV dimension	24 (13–32)	34 (24–38)	38 (33–45)	41 (35–47)	43 (37–49)	49 (44–52)
LV free wall (or septum)	5 (4–6)	6 (5–7)	7 (6–7)	7 (7–8)	7 (7–8)	8 (7–8)
LA dimension	17 (7–23)	22 (17–27)	23 (19–28)	24 (20–30)	27 (21–30)	28 (21–37)
Aortic root	13 (7–17)	17(13–22)	20 (17–23)	22 (19–27)	23 (17–27)	24 (22–28)

LA, left atrium; LV, left ventricle; RV, right ventricle.
Modified from Feigenbaum H: Echocardiography, 5th ed. Philadelphia, Lea & Febiger, 1995.

Left Ventricular Systolic Function

LV systolic function is evaluated by the fractional shortening (or shortening fraction), ejection fraction, and systolic time intervals. The ejection fraction is a derivative of the fractional shortening and offers no advantages over the fractional shortening. Serial determinations of these measurements are important in the management of conditions in which LV function may change (e.g., in patients with chronic or acute myocardial disease).

Fractional Shortening. Fractional shortening (or shortening fraction) is derived by the following:

$$FS(\%) = Dd - Ds/Dd \times 100$$

where FS is fractional shortening, Dd is end-diastolic dimension of the LV, and Ds is end-systolic dimension of the LV. This is a reliable and reproducible index of LV function, provided there is no regional wall-motion abnormality and there is concentric contractility of the LV. If the interventricular septal motion is flat or paradoxical, the shortening fraction will not accurately reflect ventricular ejection.

Mean normal value is 36%, with 95% prediction limits of 28% to 44%. Fractional shortening is decreased in a poorly compensated LV regardless of cause (e.g., pressure overload, volume overload, primary myocardial disorders, doxorubicin cardiotoxicity). It is increased in volume-overloaded ventricle (e.g., ventricular septal defect [VSD], patent ductus arteriosus [PDA], aortic regurgitation [AR], mitral regurgitation [MR]) and pressure overload lesions (e.g., moderately severe aortic valve stenosis, hypertrophic obstructive cardiomyopathy).

Ejection Fraction. Ejection fraction is related to the change in volume of the LV with cardiac contraction. It is obtained with the following formula:

$$EF(\%) = (Dd)^3 - (Ds)^3/(Dd)^3 \times 100$$

where EF is ejection fraction and Dd and Ds are end-diastolic and end-systolic dimensions, respectively, of the LV. The volume of the LV is derived from a single measurement of the dimension of the minor axis of the LV. In the preceding formula, the minor axis is assumed to be half of the major axis of the LV; this assumption is incorrect in children. Normal mean ejection fraction is 66% with a range of 56% to 78%.

Systolic Time Intervals. Since the introduction of two-dimensional and Doppler echo, this measurement is no longer routinely used. The systolic time interval of a ventricle includes the preejection period (measured from the onset of the Q wave of the electrocardiogram [ECG] to the opening of the semilunar valve), and the ventricular ejection time is measured from the cusp opening of the semilunar valve to the cusp closing (see Fig. 6–1). The former usually reflects the rate of pressure rise in the ventricle during isovolumic systole (i.e., dp/dt). The preejection period and ventricular ejection time are affected by the heart rate, but the ratio of preejection period to ventricular ejection time for both right and left sides is little affected by changes in the heart rate. The method of measuring left preejection period (LPEP) and left ventricular ejection time (LVET) is shown in the lower right panel of Figure 6–1.

The LPEP is prolonged and the LV ejection time is shortened in patients with LV failure with an increase in LPEP/LVET. In patients with aortic stenosis, the LPEP is shortened and the LVET is prolonged, and, thus, the ratio is decreased. Normal LPEP/LVET (with range) is 0.35 (0.30 to 0.39).

Measurement of the right preejection period (RPEP) and right ventricular ejection time (RVET) is sometimes difficult because only the posterior part of the pulmonary valve is normally recorded on the M-mode echo. The ratio increases in patients with pulmonary hypertension (large-shunt VSD, persistent pulmonary hypertension of the newborn) and those with increased pulmonary vascular resistance, but the correlation between the ratio and the conditions is relatively poor and the ratio alone should not be used in evaluation of patients with pulmonary hypertension. Normal RPRP/RVET (with range) is 0.24 (0.16 to 0.30).

TWO-DIMENSIONAL ECHOCARDIOGRAPHY

Two-dimensional echo examinations are performed by directing the plane of the transducer beam along a number of cross-sectional planes through the heart and great vessels. A routine two-dimensional echo is obtained from four transducer locations: parasternal, apical, subcostal, and suprasternal notch positions. Figures 6–2 through 6–10 illustrate some standard images of the heart and great vessels. Modified transducer positions and different angulations make many other views possible. Important cardiac structures can be measured on the freeze frame of two-dimensional echo studies. Normal values of the dimension of the great arteries and various valve annuli are shown in several tables in Appendix D (see Tables D–4 through D–7).

The Parasternal Views

For parasternal views, the transducer is applied to the left parasternal border in the second, third, or fourth space with the patient in the left lateral decubitus position.

Parasternal Long-Axis Views

The plane of sound is oriented along the major axis of the heart, usually from the patient's left hip to the right shoulder. There are three major views: standard long axis, long axis of the RV inflow, and long axis of the RV outflow (Fig. 6–2).

1. The *standard long-axis view* is the most basic view, which shows the LA, mitral valve, and the left ventricular inflow and outflow tracts (see Fig. 6–2A). This view is important in evaluating abnormalities in or near the mitral valve, LA, LV, left ventricular outflow tract, aortic valve, aortic root, ascending aorta, and ventricular septum. In normal heart, the anterior leaflet of the mitral valve is continuous with the posterior wall of the aorta (i.e., aortic-mitral continuity). The trabecular septum (apical ward) and infracristal outlet septum (near the aortic valve) constitute the interventricular septum in this view. Therefore, VSDs of tetralogy of Fallot (TOF) and persistent truncus arteriosus are best shown in this view. Detailed discussion of localizing the VSD is presented in Chapter 12. Pericardial effusion is readily imaged in this view. This is the view to evaluate mitral valve prolapse. Frequently, the coronary sinus can be seen as a small circle in the atrioventricular (AV) groove (see Fig. 6–2A). An enlarged coronary sinus may be seen with left superior vena cava, total anomalous pulmonary venous return to coronary sinus, coronary AV fistula, and rarely with elevated RA pressure.

2. In the *RV inflow view*, abnormalities in the tricuspid valve (TR, prolapse) and inflow portion of the RV are evaluated (see Fig. 6–2B). Ventricular septum in this view consists of the inlet muscular septum (near the AV valve) and trabecular septum (apicalward). The right atrial appendage (RAA) can also be seen in this view.

3. In the *RV outflow view*, the RV outflow tract, pulmonary valve, and proximal main PA are visualized (see Fig. 6–2C). The supracristal infundibular (outlet) septum is seen in this view.

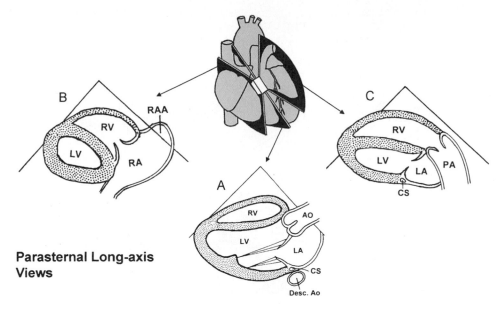

Parasternal Long-axis Views

Figure 6–2. *Diagram of important two-dimensional echo views obtained from the, parasternal long-axis transducer position. Standard long-axis view (A), RV inflow view (B), and RV outflow view (C). AO, aorta; CS, coronary sinus; Desc. Ao, descending aorta; LA, left atrium; LV, left ventricle; PA, pulmonary artery; RA, right atrium; RAA, right atrial appendage; RV, right ventricle.*

Parasternal Short-Axis Views

By rotating the transducer used for the long-axis views clockwise, one obtains a family of important short-axis views (Fig. 6–3). This projection provides cross-sectional images of the heart and the great arteries at different levels. The parasternal short-axis views are important in the evaluation of the aortic valve (i.e., bicuspid or tricuspid), pulmonary valve, PA and its branches, right ventricular outflow tract, coronary arteries (e.g., absence, aneurysm), LA, LV, ventricular septum, AV valves, LV, and right side of the heart.

1. *Aortic valve.* The aortic valve is seen in the center of the image with the right ventricular outflow tract anterior to the aortic valve and the main PA to the right of the aorta ("circle and sausage" view) (see Fig. 6–3A). The right, left, and non-coronary cusps of the aortic valve are best examined from this view. Stenosis and regurgitation of the pulmonary valve are also best examined in this plane. Stenosis of the pulmonary artery branches can be evaluated and Doppler interrogation of the ductal shunt is performed in this plane. Color flow studies show the membranous VSD just distal to the tricuspid valve (at the 10-o'clock direction) and both the infracristal and supracristal outlet VSDs (at the 12- to 2-o'clock direction) anterior to the aortic valve near the pulmonary valve.

2. *Coronary arteries.* With a slight manipulation of the transducer from the above plane, the ostia and the proximal portions of the coronary arteries are visualized. The right coronary artery arises from the anterior coronary cusp near the tricuspid valve, which should be confirmed to connect to the aorta; there are some venous structures (cardiac veins) that run in front of the aorta but do not connect to the aorta. The left main coronary artery arises in the left coronary cusp near the main pulmonary artery. Its bifurcation into the left anterior descending and circumflex coronary artery can usually be clearly seen. The proximal coronary arteries can also be seen in other long-axis views.

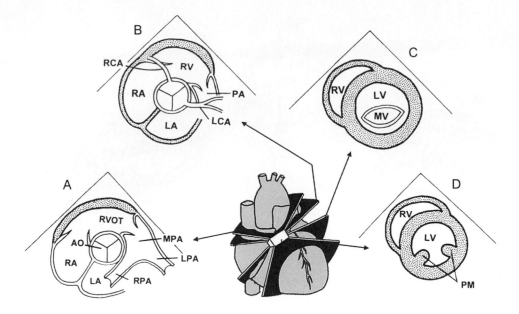

Parasternal Short-axis Views

Figure 6–3. Diagram of a family of parasternal short-axis views. Semilunar valves and great artery level *(A)*, coronary arteries *(B)*, mitral valve level *(C)*, and papillary muscle level *(D)*. AO, aorta; LA, 1eft atrium; LCA, left coronary artery; LPA, left pulmonary artery; LV, left ventricle; MPA, main pulmonary artery; MV, mitral valve; PM, papillary muscle; RA, right atrium; RCA, right coronary artery; RPA, right pulmonary artery; RV, right ventricle; RVOT, right ventricular outflow tract.

3. *Mitral valve.* The mitral valve is seen as a "fish mouth." The fibrous continuity of the anterior mitral valve and the aortic valve is present.

4. *Papillary muscles.* Two papillary muscles are normally seen at 4-o'clock (anterolateral) and 8-o'clock (posteromedial) directions. The trabecular septum is seen at this level.

The Apical Views

For apical views, the transducer is positioned over the cardiac apex with the patient in the left lateral decubitus position.

Apical Four-Chamber View. The plane of sound is oriented in a nearly coronal body plane and is tilted from posterior to anterior to obtain a family of apical four-chamber views (Fig. 6–4). This is the best view to image the left ventricular apex, where an apical VSD is commonly seen.

1. *Coronary sinus.* In the most posterior plane, the coronary sinus is seen to drain into the right atrium (see Fig. 6–4A). The ventricular septum seen in this view is the posterior trabecular septum.

2. The *apical four-chamber view* (see Fig. 6–4B) evaluates the atrial and ventricular septa, size and contractility of atrial and ventricular chambers, AV valves, and some pulmonary veins as well as identifying the anatomic RV and LV and detecting pericardial effusion. Normally, the tricuspid valve insertion to the septum is more apicalward than the mitral valve, with a small portion of the septum (called atrioventricular septum) separating the two AV valves. A defect in this portion of the septum may result in an LV-RA shunt. The inlet ventricular septum (where an endocardial cushion defect occurs) is well imaged in this

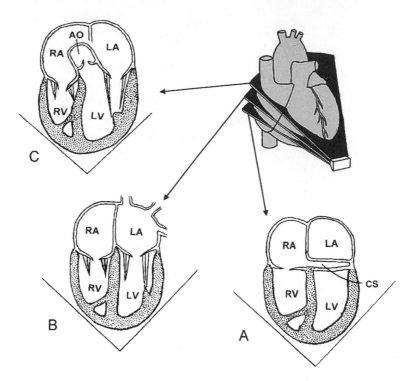

Apical Four-chamber Views

Figure 6–4. Diagram of two-dimensional echo views obtained with the transducer at the apical position. **A,** A posterior plane view showing the coronary sinus. **B,** The standard apical four-chamber view. **C,** The apical "five-chamber" view is obtained with further anterior angulation of the transducer. AO, aorta; CS, coronary sinus; LA, left atrium; LV, left ventricle; RA, right atrium; RV right ventricle.

view just under the AV valves. VSDs in the entire length of the trabecular septum are well imaged, including apical VSD. The membranous septum is *not* imaged in this view. The anatomic characteristics of each ventricle are also noted; with the heavily trabeculated RV showing the moderator band. The relative size of the ventricles is examined in this view. Abnormal chordal attachment of the AV valve (straddling) and overriding of the valve are also noted in this view.

3. *Apical "five-chamber" view.* Further anterior angulation of the transducer demonstrates the so-called apical five-chamber view. This view shows the LV outflow tract, aortic valve, subaortic area, and the proximal ascending aorta. The membranous VSD is visualized just under the aortic valve and the infracristal outlet VSD is also imaged in this plane.

Apical Long-Axis Views. The apical long-axis view (or apical three-chamber view) shows structures similar to those shown in the parasternal long-axis view (Fig. 6–5A). In the apical two-chamber view, the LA, mitral valve, and LV are imaged. The left atrial appendage can also be imaged (see Fig. 6–5B).

The Subcostal Views

Subcostal long-axis (coronal) and short-axis (sagittal) views are obtained from the subxiphoid transducer position with the patient in the supine position.

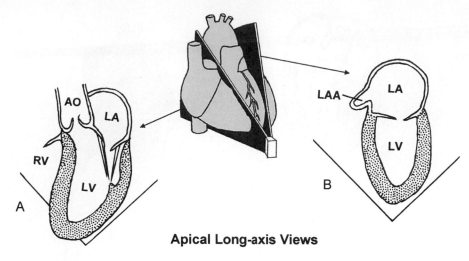

Apical Long-axis Views

Figure 6–5. *Apical long-axis views.* **A,** *Apical three-chamber view.* **B,** *Apical two-chamber view. AO, aorta; LA, left atrium; LAA, left atrial appendage; LV, left ventricle; RV right ventricle.*

Subcostal long-axis (coronal) views are obtained by tilting the coronal plane of sound from posterior to anterior (Fig. 6–6). They show posteriorly the coronary sinus draining into the right atrium, similar to that shown for the apical view (see Fig. 6–6A). Anterior angulation of the transducer shows the atrial and ventricular septa, and this is the best view for evaluating the atrial septum (see Fig. 6–6B). Further anterior angulation of the transducer shows the LV outflow tract, aortic valve, and ascending aorta (see Fig. 6–6C). The parts of the ventricular septum visualized in this view (apicalward) are membranous, subaortic outlet, and trabecular septa. The junction of the superior vena cava and the RA is seen to the right of the ascending aorta (see Fig. 6–6C). Further anterior angulation shows the entire RV including the inlet, trabecular and infundibular portions, the pulmonary valve, and the main pulmonary artery (see Fig. 6–6D). The ventricular septum seen in this view includes (apicalward) supracristal outlet, infracristal outlet, and anterior trabecular and posterior trabecular septa.

Subcostal short-axis (or sagittal) views (Fig. 6–7) are obtained by rotating the long-axis transducer 90 degrees to the sagittal plane.

To the right of the patient, both the superior and inferior venae cavae are seen to enter the right atrium (see Fig. 6–7A). A small azygos vein can be seen to enter the SVC, and the right PA can also be seen on end beneath this vein (see Fig. 6–7A).

A leftward angulation of the transducer shows the right ventricular outflow tract, pulmonary valve, and pulmonary artery and the tricuspid valve on end (see Fig. 6–7B). This view is orthogonal to the standard subcostal four-chamber view, and both views combined are good for evaluation of the size of a VSD.

Additional leftward angulation of the transducer shows the mitral valve (not shown) and papillary muscle (see Fig. 6–7C), a view similar to those seen in the parasternal short-axis views.

Subcostal Views of the Abdomen. Abdominal short- and long-axis views (Fig. 6–8) are obtained from the subxiphoid transducer position, with the patient in the supine position.

1. *Abdominal short-axis view* is obtained by placing the transducer in a transverse body plane (see Fig. 6–8, left). It demonstrates the descending aorta on the left and the inferior vena cava on the right of the spine as two round structures. The aorta should pulsate. Both hemidiaphragms, which move symmetrically with

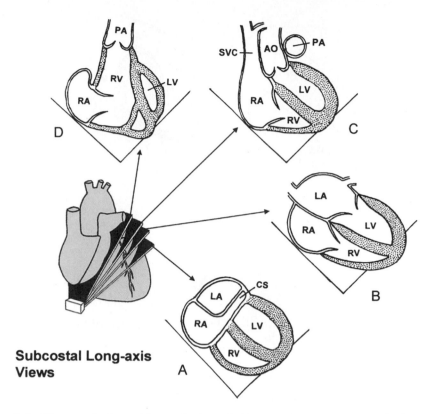

Subcostal Long-axis Views

Figure 6–6. Diagram of subcostal long-axis views. **A,** Coronary sinus view posteriorly. **B,** Standard subcostal four-chamber view. **C,** View showing the left ventricular outflow tract and the proximal aorta. **D,** View showing the right ventricular outflow tract (RVOT) and the proximal main pulmonary artery. AO, aorta; CS, coronary sinus; LA, left atrium; LV left ventricle; PA, pulmonary artery; RA, right atrium; RV right ventricle, SVS, superior vena cava.

respiration, are imaged. Asymmetric or paradoxical movement of the diaphragm is seen with paralysis of the hemidiaphragm.

2. *Abdominal long-axis views* are obtained by placing the transducer in a sagittal body plane. The inferior vena cava is imaged to the right (see Fig. 6–8, right, A) and the descending aorta is imaged to the left of the spine (see Fig. 6–8, right, B). The IVC collects the hepatic vein before draining into the right atrium. The eustachian valve may be seen at the junction of the IVC and the RA. Failure of the IVC to join the RA indicates interruption of the IVC (with azygos continuation, which is frequently seen with polysplenia syndrome). Major branches of the descending aorta, celiac artery, and superior mesenteric artery are easily visualized.

The Suprasternal Views

The transducer is positioned in the suprasternal notch to obtain suprasternal long-axis (Fig. 6–9, upper panel) and short-axis (see Fig. 6–9, lower panel) views, which are important in the evaluation of anomalies in the ascending and descending aortas (e.g., coarctation of the aorta), aortic arch (e.g., interruption), size of the PAs, and anomalies of systemic veins and pulmonary veins. In infants, the transducer can be sometimes placed in a high right subclavicular position.

A *suprasternal long-axis view* (see upper panel of Fig. 6–9) is obtained by 45-degree clockwise rotation from the sagittal plane in the suprasternal notch to visualize the entire

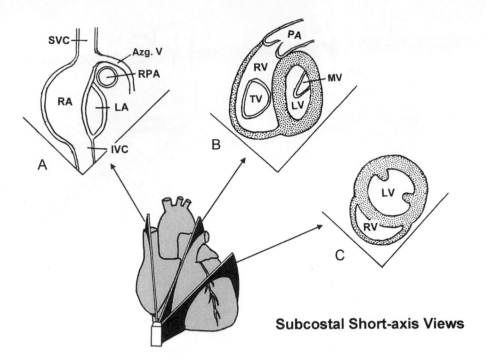

Subcostal Short-axis Views

Figure 6–7. Subcostal short-axis (sagittal) views. **A,** Entry of venae cavae with drainage of the azygos vein. **B,** View showing the RV, RVOT, and pulmonary artery. **C,** Short-axis view of the ventricles. Azg. V, azygos vein; LA, left atrium; LV, left ventricle; MV, mitral valve; PA, pulmonary artery; RA, right atrium; RPA, right pulmonary vein; RV right ventricle, SVC, superior vena cava, TV, tricuspid valve.

(left) aortic arch. Failure to visualize the aortic arch in this manner may suggest the presence of a right aortic arch. Three arteries arising from the aortic arch (the innominate, left carotid, and left subclavian arteries in that order) are seen. The innominate vein is seen in cross section in front of the ascending aorta and the right pulmonary artery behind the ascending aorta. Manipulation of the transducer further posteriorly and leftward emphasizes the isthmus and upper descending aorta, a very important segment to study for the coarctation of the aorta.

A *suprasternal short-axis view* (see lower panel of Fig. 6–9) is obtained by rotating the ultrasound plane parallel to the sternum. Superior to the circular transverse aorta, the innominate vein is seen, which is connected to the (right) superior vena cava and runs vertically to the right of the aorta. The right pulmonary artery is visualized in its length under the aorta. The LA is seen beneath the RPA. With a slight posterior angulation of the transducer, four pulmonary veins are seen to enter the LA.

The Subclavicular Views

The *right subclavicular view* (Fig. 6–10A) is obtained in the right second intercostal space in a sagittal projection. This view is useful in the assessment of the SVC and right atrial junction as well as the ascending aorta. The right upper pulmonary vein and the azygos vein can also be examined in this view.

The *left subclavicular view* (see Fig. 6–10B) is useful for examination of the branch pulmonary arteries. The transducer is positioned in a transverse plane in the second left intercostal space and a little tilted inferiorly. The main PA is seen left of the ascending aorta (circle), and it bifurcates into the right and left PA branches.

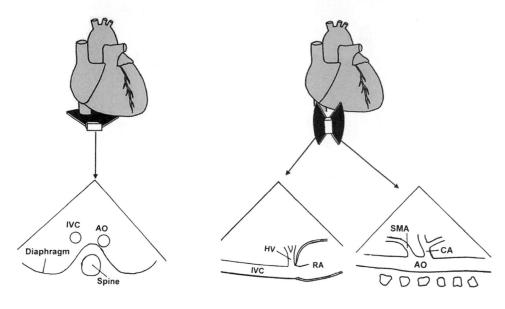

Abdominal Short-axis View   **Abdominal Long-axis Views**

Figure 6–8. Abdominal views. Left, abdominal short-axis view. Right, abdominal long-axis views. AO, aorta; CA, celiac axis; HV, hepatic vein; IVC, inferior vena cava; RA, right atrium; SMA, superior mesenteric artery.

Quantitative Values Derived from Two-Dimensional Echocardiography

1. Dimensions of cardiovascular structures

Several tables of normal values of cardiovascular structures that were measured from still frames of two-dimensional echocardiography are shown in Appendix D. These tables are frequently useful in the practice of pediatric cardiology. They include the aorta and pulmonary artery dimensions (see Table D–4), aortic root measurements (see Table D–5), valve annuli of neonates (see Table D–6), and mitral and tricuspid valve dimensions (see Table D–7), all indexed to body surface area.

2. Other measurements

Left Ventricular Mass. LV mass is derived from two-dimensional echo measurements of the LV and is indexed to body surface area. The normal value of LV mass for children (ages 2 to 17 years) is 60.8 ± 12 g/m^2.

Left ventricular hypertrophy (LVH) is considered present in children (6 to 23 years) when the LV mass is greater than 103 g/m^2 in males and greater than 84.2 g/m^2 in females. For adults, the value is greater than 134 g/m^2 for men and greater than 110 g/m^2 for women.

Indications

Indications for two-dimensional echo studies are expanding with their increasing diagnostic accuracy. The following are some selected indications for two-dimensional echo examinations.

1. To screen routinely newborns and small infants who appear to have cardiac defects or dysfunction
2. To rule out cyanotic congenital heart disease (CHD) in newborns with clinical findings of persistent pulmonary hypertension of the newborn (PPHN)

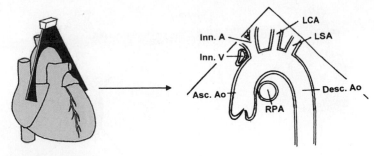

Suprasternal Long-axis View

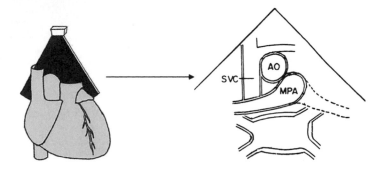

Suprasternal Short-axis View

Figure 6–9. *Diagram of suprasternal notch two-dimensional echo views. Top, Long-axis view. Bottom, Short-axis view. AO, aorta; Asc. Ao, ascending aorta; Desc. Ao, descending aorta; Inn. A, innominate artery; Inn. V, innominate vein; LA, left atrium; LCA, left carotid artery; LSA, left sub-clavian artery; MPA, main pulmonary artery; PA, pulmonary artery; RPA, right pulmonary artery; SVC, superior vena cava.*

3. To diagnose PDA, other heart defects, or ventricular dysfunction in a premature infant who is on a ventilator for pulmonary disease

4. To confirm the diagnosis in infants and children with findings atypical of certain defects

5. To rule in or rule out important cardiac conditions that are suspected on the basis of routine evaluation (e.g., cardiac examination, chest x-ray films, ECG)

6. To follow up on conditions that may change with time or treatment (e.g., before and after indomethacin treatment for PDA in premature infants, evaluation of drug therapy for CHF or LV dysfunction, follow-up examination for certain congenital or acquired heart diseases)

7. Before cardiac catheterization and angiocardiography, to obtain certain information that can reduce the amount of time spent in the cardiac catheterization laboratory and the amount of the radiopaque dye injected and to gain some information that angiography cannot provide. (Two-dimensional echo is superior to angiocardiography in demonstrating small, thin structures, such as subaortic membrane, straddling AV valve, or Ebstein's anomaly, that can easily be missed by angiocardiography.)

8. To replace cardiac catheterization and angiography in certain situations, such as uncomplicated VSD, PDA, or ASD

9. To evaluate the patient after surgery

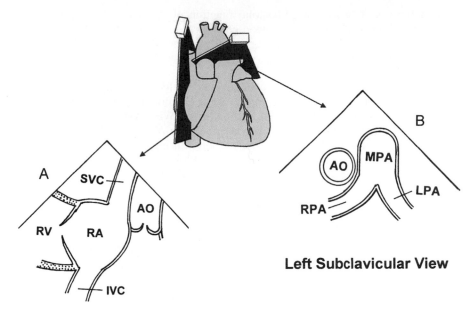

A / SVC / AO / RV / RA / IVC

Right Subclavicular View

B / AO / MPA / RPA / LPA

Left Subclavicular View

Figure 6–10. Diagram of subclavicular views. **A,** Right subclavicular view. **B,** left subclavicular view. *AO, aorta; IVC, inferior vena cava; LPA, left pulmonary artery; MPA, main pulmonary artery; RA, right atrium; RPA, right pulmonary artery; RV, right ventricle; SVC, superior vena cava.*

DOPPLER ECHOCARDIOGRAPHY

A Doppler echo combines the study of cardiac structure and blood flow profiles. The Doppler effect is a change in the observed frequency of sound that results from motion of the source or target. When the moving object or column of blood moves toward the ultrasonic transducer, the frequency of the reflected sound wave increases (i.e., a positive Doppler shift). Conversely, when blood moves away from the transducer, the frequency decreases (i.e., a negative Doppler shift). Doppler ultrasound equipment detects a frequency shift and determines the direction and velocity of red blood cell flow with respect to the ultrasound beam.

The two commonly used Doppler techniques are continuous wave and pulsed wave. The pulsed wave emits a short burst of ultrasound, and the Doppler echo receiver "listens" for returning information. The continuous wave emits a constant ultrasound beam with one crystal, and another crystal continuously receives returning information. Both techniques have their advantages and disadvantages. The pulsed-wave Doppler can control the site at which the Doppler signals are sampled, but the maximal detectable velocity is limited, making it unusable for quantification of severe obstruction. In contrast, continuous-wave Doppler can measure extremely high velocities (e.g., for the estimation of severe stenosis), but it cannot localize the site of the sampling; rather, it picks up the signal anywhere along the Doppler beam. When these two techniques are used in combination, clinical application expands.

The Doppler echo technique is useful in studying the direction of blood flow; in detecting the presence and direction of cardiac shunts; in studying stenosis or regurgitation of cardiac valves, including prosthetic valves; in assessing stenosis of blood vessels; in assessing the hemodynamic severity of a lesion, including pressures in various compartments of the cardiovascular system; in estimating the cardiac output or blood flow; and in assessing diastolic function of the ventricle (see later discussion). By convention, velocities of red blood cells moving toward the transducer are displayed above a zero baseline; those moving away from the transducer are displayed below the baseline. The Doppler echo is usually used with color flow mapping (see later) to enhance the technique's usefulness.

Normal Doppler velocities in children and adults are shown in Table 6–2. Normal Doppler velocity is less than 1 m/sec for the pulmonary valves and may be up to 1.8 m/sec for the ascending and descending aortas. With stenosis of the semilunar valves, the flow velocity of these valves increases. For the AV valve, the E wave is taller than the A wave except for the first 3 weeks of life, during which the A wave may be taller than the E wave. In normal subjects 11 to 40 years of age, mitral Doppler indexes are as follows (mean ± SD). The average peak E velocity is 0.73 ± 0.09 m/sec, the average peak A velocity is 0.38 ± 0.089 m/sec, and the average E/A velocity ratio is 2.0 ± 0.5.

Measurement of Pressure Gradients

The simplified Bernoulli equation can be used to estimate the pressure gradient across a stenotic lesion, regurgitant lesion, or shunt lesion. One may use one of the following equations.

$$P_1 - P_2 \text{ (mm Hg)} = 4(V_2^2 - V_1^2)$$

$$P_1 - P_2 \text{ (mm Hg)} = 4(V \max)^2$$

where $P_1 - P_2$ is the pressure difference across an obstruction, V_1 is the velocity (m/sec) proximal to the obstruction, and V_2 is the velocity (m/sec) distal to the obstruction in the first equation. When V_1 is less than 1 m/sec, it can be ignored, as in the second equation. However, when V_1 is more than 1.5 m/sec, it should be incorporated in the equation to obtain a more accurate estimation of pressure gradients. This is important in the study of the ascending and descending aortas, where flow velocities are often more than 1.5 m/sec. Ignoring V_1 may significantly overestimate pressure gradient in patients with aortic stenosis or coarctation of the aorta.

To obtain the most accurate prediction of the peak pressure gradient, the Doppler beam should be aligned parallel to the jet flow, the peak velocity of the jet should be recorded from several different transducer positions, and the highest velocity should be taken. An example of a Doppler study in a patient with moderate pulmonary stenosis is shown in Figure 6–11. The pressure gradient calculated from the Bernoulli equation is the peak instantaneous pressure gradient, *not* the peak-to-peak pressure gradient measured during cardiac catheterization. The peak instantaneous pressure gradient is larger than the peak-to-peak pressure gradient. The difference between the two is more noticeable in patients with mild to moderate obstruction and less apparent in patients with severe obstruction.

Prediction of Intracardiac or Intravascular Pressures

The Doppler echo allows estimation of pressures in the RV, PA, and LV using the flow velocity of certain valvular or shunt jets. Estimation of PA pressure is particularly important in pediatric patients.

Table 6–2. **Normal Doppler Velocities in Children and Adults: Mean (Range) (m/sec)**

	Children	Adults
Mitral flow	1.0 (0.8–1.3)	0.9 (0.6–1.3)
Tricuspid flow	0.6 (0.5–0.8)	0.6 (0.3–0.7)
Pulmonary artery	0.9 (0.7–1.1)	0.75 (0.6–0.9)
Left ventricle	1.0 (0.7–1.2)	0.9 (0.7–1.1)
Aorta	1.5 (1.2–1.8)	1.35 (1.0–1.7)

From Hatle L, Angelsen B: Doppler Ultrasound in Cardiology, 2nd ed. Philadelphia, Lea & Febiger, 1985.

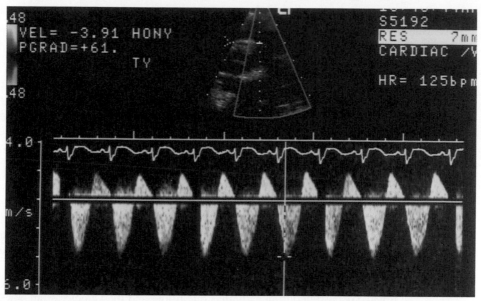

Figure 6–11. *Doppler echocardiographic study in a child with a moderate pulmonary valve stenosis. The Doppler cursor is placed in the main pulmonary artery near the pulmonary valve in the parasternal short-axis view. The maximum forward flow velocity (negative flow) is 3.91 m/second (with an estimated pressure gradient of 61 mm Hg). A small regurgitant (positive) flow is seen during diastole.*

The following are some examples of such applications

1. RV (or PA) systolic pressure (SP) can be estimated from the velocity of the tricuspid regurgitation (TR) jet, if present, by the following equation:

$$\text{RVSP (or PASP)} = 4(V)^2 + \text{RA pressure}$$

where V is the TR jet velocity.

For example, if the TR velocity is 2.5 m/sec, the instantaneous pressure gradient is $4 \times (2.5)^2 = 4 \times 6.25 = 25$ mm Hg. Using an assumed RA pressure of 10 mm Hg, the RV systolic pressure (or PA systolic pressure in the absence of PS) is 35 mm Hg.

2. RV (or PA) systolic pressure can also be estimated from the velocity of the VSD jet by the following equation:

$$\text{RVSP (or PASP)} = \text{systemic SP (or arm SP)} - 4(V)^2$$

where V is the VSD jet.

For example, if the VSD jet flow velocity is 3 m/sec, the instantaneous pressure drop between the LV and RV is $4 \times 3^2 = 36$ mm Hg. That is, the RV systolic pressure is 36 mm Hg lower than the LV systolic pressure. If the systemic systolic pressure is 90 mm Hg, which is close to (but usually 5 to 10 mm Hg higher than) the LV systolic pressure (see peripheral systolic amplification in Chapter 2), the RV pressure is estimated to be $90 - 36 = 54$ (or approximately 49) mm Hg. In the absence of PS, the PA systolic pressure is between 49 and 54 mm Hg.

3. LVSP can be estimated from the velocity of flow through the aortic valve by the following equation:

$$\text{LVSP} = 4(V)^2 + \text{systemic SP (or arm SP)}$$

where V is the aortic flow velocity. The same precaution applies as before in that the arm systolic pressure is slightly higher than the LV systolic pressure.

Measurement of Cardiac Output or Blood Flow

Both systemic blood flow and pulmonary blood flow can be calculated by multiplying the mean velocity of flow and the cross-sectional area as shown in the following equation:

$$\text{Cardiac output (L/min)} = V \times CSA \times 60 \text{ (sec/min)} \div 1000 \text{ cc/L}$$

where V is the mean velocity (cm/sec) obtained either by using a computer program or by manually integrating the area under the curve. CSA is the cross-sectional area of flow (cm^2) measured or computed from the two-dimensional echo. Usually, the PA flow velocity and diameter are used to calculate pulmonary blood flow; the mean velocity and diameter of the ascending aorta are used to calculate systemic blood flow, or cardiac output.

Diastolic Function

Signs of diastolic dysfunction may precede those of systolic dysfunction. LV diastolic function can be evaluated by mitral inflow velocities obtained in the apical four-chamber view. The following simple measurements are useful in evaluating diastolic function of the ventricle (Fig. 6–12):

1. The early (E) and second (A) peak velocities and their ratio: the velocity of an E wave occurring during early diastolic filling and the velocity of an A wave occurring during atrial contraction, as well as the ratio of the two

2. Deceleration time (DT): the interval from the early peak velocity to the zero intercept of the extrapolated deceleration slope

3. Atrial filling fraction: the integral of the A velocity divided by the integral of the total mitral inflow velocities

4. Isovolumic relaxation time (IVRT): the interval between the end of the LV outflow velocity and the onset of mitral inflow; this is easily obtained by pulsed-wave Doppler with the cursor placed in the LV outflow near the anterior leaflet of the mitral valve and is measured from the end of the LV ejection to the onset of the mitral inflow

Abnormalities of diastolic function are easy to find but are usually nonspecific and do not provide independent diagnostic information. In addition, they can be affected by loading conditions (i.e., increase or decrease in preload), heart rate, and the presence of atrial arrhythmias. Two well-known patterns of abnormal diastolic function are a decreased relaxation pattern and a "restrictive" pattern (see Fig. 18–6). The decreased relaxation

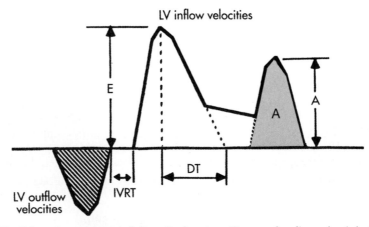

Figure 6–12. Selected parameters of diastolic function. (See text for discussion.) A, Second peak velocity; DT, deceleration time; E, early peak velocity; IVRT, isovolumic relaxation time; LV, left ventricle.

pattern is seen with hypertrophic and dilated cardiomyopathies, LVH of various causes, ischemic heart disease, other forms of myocardial disease, reduced preload (e.g., dehydration), and increased afterload (e.g., during infusion of arterial vasoconstrictors). The restrictive pattern is usually seen in restrictive cardiomyopathy but is also seen with increased preload (e.g., seen with MR) and a variety of heart diseases with heart failure.

COLOR FLOW MAPPING

A color-coded Doppler study provides images of the direction and disturbances of blood flow superimposed on the echo structural image. Although systematic Doppler interrogation can obtain similar information, this technique is more accurate and time saving. In general, red is used to indicate flow toward the transducer, and blue is used to indicate flow away from the transducer. Color may not appear when the direction of flow is perpendicular to the ultrasound beam. The turbulent flow is color coded as either green or yellow.

CONTRAST ECHOCARDIOGRAPHY

Injection of indocyanine green, dextrose in water, saline, or the patient's blood into a peripheral or central vein produces microcavitations and creates a cloud of echoes on the echocardiogram. Structures of interest are visualized or recorded, or both, by M-mode or two-dimensional echo at the time of the injection. This technique has successfully detected an intracardiac shunt, validated structures, and identified flow patterns within the heart. For example, an injection of any liquid into an intravenous line may confirm the presence of a right-to-left shunt at the atrial or ventricular level. This technique can be used in the diagnosis of cyanosis resulting from a right-to-left shunt at the atrial level (e.g., PPHN) or in postoperative patients with persistent arterial desaturation. To a large extent, this technique has been replaced by color flow mapping and Doppler studies.

OTHER ECHOCARDIOGRAPHIC TECHNIQUES

Fetal Echocardiography

Improvement in image resolution makes visualization of the fetal cardiovascular structure possible, thereby permitting in utero diagnosis of cardiovascular anomalies. Doppler examination and color mapping are performed at the same time. To obtain a complete examination, the transducer is placed at various positions on the maternal abdominal wall.

Fetal echo continues to teach physicians more about human fetal cardiac physiology. It also enables physicians to study the effects of cardiovascular abnormalities and abnormal cardiac rhythms in utero and then assess the need for therapeutic intervention. Indications for fetal echo include the following and are expanding:

1. A parent with a history of CHD

2. A history of previous children with CHD

3. The presence of fetal cardiac arrhythmias

4. The presence of certain maternal diseases (e.g., diabetes mellitus, collagen vascular disease)

5. The presence of chromosomal anomalies

6. The presence of extracardiac anomalies (e.g., diaphragmatic hernia, omphalocele, hydrops)

7. The presence of polyhydramnios or oligohydramnios

8. A history of maternal exposure to certain medications (e.g., lithium, amphetamine, anticonvulsants, addictive drugs, progesterone)

Transesophageal Echocardiography

By placing a two-dimensional or multiplane transducer at the end of a flexible endoscope, it is possible to obtain high-quality, two-dimensional images by way of the esophagus. Color flow mapping and Doppler examination are usually incorporated in this approach.

If satisfactory images of the heart or blood vessels are not possible from the usual transducer position on the surface of the patient's chest (e.g., in patients with obesity or chronic obstructive pulmonary disease), physicians may use a transesophageal echocardiography (TEE). This approach is especially helpful in assessing thrombus in native or prosthetic valves, endocarditis vegetations, thrombi in the left atrial chamber and appendage, and aortic dissections. TEE is often used for patients who are undergoing cardiac surgery. The TEE can monitor LV function throughout the surgical procedure as well as assess cardiac morphology and function before and after surgical repair of valvular or congenital heart defects. TEE requires general anesthesia or sedation and the presence of an anesthesiologist because lack of cooperation by the patient can result in serious complications. Use of this technique in pediatric patients is somewhat limited to intraoperative use and use in some obese adolescents and adolescents with complicated heart defects for whom the risk of general anesthesia or sedation is worth taking for the expected benefit. Schematic drawings of biplane images of TEE are shown in Appendix D (see Fig. D–1).

Intravascular Echocardiography

To provide an intravascular echo, the ultrasonic transducer is placed in a small catheter so that vessels can be imaged by means of the lumen. These devices can evaluate atherosclerotic arteries in adults and coronary artery stenosis or aneurysm in children with Kawasaki's disease.

Stress Testing

The cardiovascular system can be stressed either by exercise or by pharmacologic agents. Stress testing plays an important role in the evaluation of cardiac symptoms by quantifying the severity of the cardiac abnormality, assessing the effectiveness of management, and providing important indications of the need for new or further intervention.

The maximum oxygen uptake (Vo_2 max) that can be achieved during exercise is probably the best index for describing fitness or exercise capacity (also called maximum aerobic power). Vo_2 max is defined by the plateau of oxygen uptake (Vo_2) that occurs despite continued work. Beyond this level of Vo_2 max, the work can be performed using an anaerobic mechanism of energy production but the amount of work that can be performed using anaerobic means is quite limited. There is a linear relationship between the heart rate and progressive workload or Vo_2 max.

CARDIOVASCULAR RESPONSE IN NORMAL SUBJECTS

During upright dynamic exercise in normal subjects, the heart rate, cardiac index, and mean arterial pressure increase. In addition, the systemic vascular resistance drops, and blood flow to the exercising leg muscles greatly increases. Heart rate increase is the major determinant of the increased cardiac output seen during exercise. The heart rate reaches a maximum plateau just before the level of total exhaustion. For subjects between 5 and 20 years of age, the maximal heart rate is about 195 to 215 beats/minute. For subjects older than 20 years, the maximal heart rate is $210 - 0.65 \times$ age.

Blood pressure (BP) response varies depending on the type of exercise. During *dynamic exercise*, systolic BP increases but diastolic and mean arterial pressures remain nearly identical, varying within a few mm Hg from their levels at rest. The BP response to *isometric exercise* is quite different from that to dynamic exercise. With isometric exercise, both systolic and diastolic pressures increase.

Although changes that occur in the pulmonary circulation are similar to those seen in the systemic circulation, the increase in the mean PA pressure (100% increase) is more than twice that of systemic mean arterial pressure and the drop in pulmonary vascular resistance (17% decrease) is much less than that in systemic vascular resistance (49%). Because of this, children with RV dysfunction (after Fontan operation or surgery for TOF) or those with pulmonary hypertension may respond abnormally to exercise and demonstrate a decreased exercise capacity.

CARDIOVASCULAR RESPONSE IN CARDIAC PATIENTS

1. Congenital heart defects
   a. Patients with minor CHD (e.g., small left-to-right shunt lesions or mild obstructive lesions) experience little or no effect on exercise capacity.
   b. Large left-to-right shunt lesions decrease exercise capacity because a ventricle that has a much increased stroke volume at rest has a limited ability to increase the stroke volume further.
   c. In patients with severe obstructive lesions, the ventricle may not be able to maintain an adequate cardiac output, so that with exercise the systemic BP may not increase appropriately and decreased blood flow to exercising muscles may lead to premature fatigue.
   d. In cyanotic lesions, the arterial hypoxemia tends to increase cardiac output and decrease mixed venous oxygen saturation, thereby limiting the usual increment in stroke volume and oxygen extraction that occurs with exercise. Furthermore, these patients have an increased minute ventilation at rest and with exercise. In this way, ventilatory as well as cardiac mechanisms may limit exercise capacity.

2. Postsurgical patients
   a. For many patients with CHDs, normal or near-normal exercise tolerance is expected after surgery unless there are significant residual lesions or myocardial damage.
   b. After a successful Fontan operation for functional single ventricle, exercise capacity improves but it remains significantly less than normal. This results from both a subnormal heart rate response to exercise and an abnormal stroke volume (resulting from reduced systemic ventricular function). Cardiac arrhythmias are also common in patients both before and after the Fontan operation and may contribute to the decreased exercise capacity.
   c. After arterial switch operation for TGA, more than 95% of the children have normal exercise capacity. However, up to 30% of patients have chronotropic impairment with a peak heart rate of less than 180 beats/minute. Up to 10% of the patients develop significant ST-segment depression with exercise.

EXERCISE STRESS TESTING

Some exercise laboratories have developed bicycle ergometer protocols, but the equipment is not widely used. The treadmill protocols are well standardized and widely used because most hospitals have treadmills. In this chapter, exercise testing, in particular that using the Bruce protocol, is presented. In the Bruce protocol, the level of exercise is increased by increasing the speed and grade of the treadmill for each 3-minute stage.

During exercise stress testing, the patient is continually monitored for symptoms such as chest pain or faintness, ischemic changes or arrhythmias on the ECG, oxygen saturation, and responses in heart rate and BP. In the Bruce protocol, children are not allowed to hold on to the guardrails, except to maintain their balance at change of stage, because this can decrease the metabolic cost of work and therefore increase the exercise time.

Monitoring during Exercise Stress Testing

1. Endurance time
   Oxygen uptake is difficult to measure in children. However, there is a high correlation between maximal Vo_2 and endurance time, and thus endurance time is the best predictor of exercise capacity in children.

   The endurance data reported by Cummings and colleagues in 1978 have served as the reference for several decades. However, two reports from the United States (Chatrath et al, 2002; Ahmed et al, 2001) indicate that the endurance time has been reduced significantly since the 1970s. It is concerning that endurance times reported from two other countries (Italy in 1994; Turkey in 1998) are similar to those published by Cummings and colleagues and are significantly longer than those reported in the two U.S. reports. This may be an indication that U.S. youth are less physically fit than the youth from other countries, which may lead to increased risk of coronary artery disease and stroke in the U.S. population. A new set of endurance data from a U.S. study is presented in Table 6–3. The endurance times of boys and girls are close until early adolescence, at which time the endurance time of girls diminishes and that of boys' increases.

2. Heart rate

Heart rate is measured from the ECG signal. A heart rate of 180 to 200 beats/minute correlates with maximal oxygen consumption in both boys and girls. Therefore, an effort is made to encourage all children to exercise to attain this heart rate. The mean maximal heart rates for all subjects were virtually identical, 198 ± 11 for boys and 200 ± 9 for girls. Heart rate declined abruptly during the first minute of recovery to 146 ± 19 for boys and 157 ± 19 for girls.

Inadequate increments in heart rate may be seen with sinus node dysfunction, in congenital heart block, and after cardiac surgery. Sinus node dysfunction is common after surgery involving extensive atrial suture lines, such as a Senning operation or Fontan operation. It is also common after repair of TOF. Marked chronotropic impairment significantly decreases aerobic capacity. Trained athletes tend to have lower heart rate at each exercise level. An extremely high heart rate at low levels of work may indicate physical deconditioning or marginal circulatory compensation.

3. Blood pressure

BP can be measured with a cuff, a sphygmomanometer, and a stethoscope. Numerous commercially available electronic units are also available to measure BP during exercise. However, one must be concerned with the accuracy of these devices. Accurate measurement of BP, especially diastolic pressure, is probably not possible during exercise.

Systolic pressure increases linearly with progressive exercise. Systolic pressure usually rises as high as 180 mm Hg (Table 6–4) with little change in diastolic pressure. Maximal systolic pressure in children rarely exceeds 200 mm Hg. During recovery, it returns to baseline in about 10 minutes. The diastolic pressure ranges between 51 and 76 mm Hg at maximum systolic BP. Diastolic pressure also returns to the resting level by 8 to 10 minutes of recovery.

High systolic pressure in the arm, to the level of what is considered a hypertensive emergency, probably does not reflect the central aortic pressure, and the usefulness of arm BP in assessing cardiovascular function during upright exercise is questionable

Table 6–3. Percentiles of Endurance Time (min) by Bruce Treadmill Protocol

	Percentile					
Age Group	*10*	*25*	*50*	*75*	*90*	**Mean ± SD**
Boys						
4–5	6.8	7.0	8.2	10.0	12.7	8.9 ± 2.4
6–7	6.6	7.7	9.6	10.4	13.1	9.6 ± 2.3
8–9	7.0	9.1	9.9	11.1	15.0	10.2 ± 2.5
10–12	8.1	9.2	10.7	12.3	13.2	10.7 ± 2.1
13–15	9.6	10.3	12.0	13.5	15.0	12.0 ± 2.0
16–18	9.6	11.1	12.5	13.5	14.6	12.2 ± 2.2
Girls						
4–5	6.8	7.2	7.4	9.1	10.0	8.0 ± 1.1
6–7	6.5	7.3	9.0	9.2	12.4	8.7 ± 2.0
8–9	8.0	9.2	9.8	10.6	10.8	9.8 ± 1.6
10–12	7.3	9.3	10.4	10.8	12.7	10.2 ± 1.9
13–15	6.9	8.1	9.6	10.6	12.4	9.6 ± 2.1
16–18	7.4	8.5	9.5	10.1	12.0	9.5 ± 2.0

From Chatrath R, Shenoy R, Serratto M, Thoele DG: Physical fitness of urban American children. Pediatr Cardiol 23:608–612, 2002.

Table 6–4. **Systolic Blood Pressure Response to Bruce Treadmill Protocol**

Age Group	Rest	Maximal	Recovery (min)		
			6	8	10
Boys					
5, 6, 7	105 ± 10	141 ± 13	111 ± 14	108 ± 9	106 ± 12
8, 9	107 ± 10	149 ± 15	111 ± 10	107 ± 9	105 ± 6
10, 11	108 ± 7	153 ± 13	112 ± 8	107 ± 9	106 ± 8
12, 13	111 ± 12	165 ± 19	118 ± 12	113 ± 15	110 ± 9
14, 15	120 ± 12	179 ± 23	124 ± 15	118 ± 16	115 ± 12
16, 17, 18	122 ± 14	182 ± 17	136 ± 16	125 ± 13	125 ± 14
Girls					
5, 6, 7	106 ± 9	143 ± 15	103 ± 4	104 ± 8	98 ± 6
8, 9	108 ± 9	149 ± 11	114 ± 14	108 ± 11	108 ± 11
10, 11	106 ± 11	145 ± 12	106 ± 10	104 ± 8	102 ± 7
12, 13	112 ± 12	163 ± 16	120 ± 14	113 ± 10	108 ± 6
14, 15	111 ± 10	166 ± 16	117 ± 13	112 ± 12	111 ± 10
16, 17, 18	118 ± 14	170 ± 17	125 ± 14	119 ± 13	117 ± 14

From Ahmad F, Kavey R-E, Kveselis DA, Gaum WE: Response of non-obese white children to treadmill exercise. J Pediatr 139:284–290, 2001.

except in the case of failure to rise. The major portion of the rise in arm systolic pressure during treadmill exercise probably reflects peripheral amplification related to vasoconstriction in the nonexercising arms (associated with increased blood flow to vasodilated exercising legs); central aortic pressure would probably be much lower than the systolic pressure in the arm in most cases. Figure 6–13 is a dramatic illustration of a relationship between the central and peripheral arterial pressures measured directly with arterial cannulas inserted in the ascending aorta and radial artery during upright exercise in young adults. Note that when the radial artery systolic pressure is over 230 mm Hg, the aortic pressure is only 160 mm Hg, and that there is very little increase in diastolic pressure.

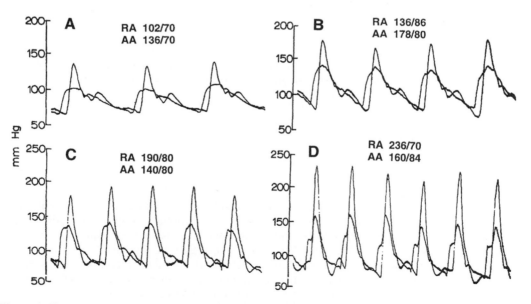

Figure 6–13. *Simultaneous recording of aortic and radial arterial pressure waves in a young adult during rest (**A**) and at 28.2% (**B**), 47.2% (**C**), and 70.2% (**D**) of maximal oxygen uptake during treadmill exercise. (From Rowell LB, Brengelmann GL, Blackmon JR, et al: Disparities between aortic and peripheral pulse pressure induced by upright exercise and vasomotor changes in man. Circulation 37:954–964, 1968.)*

An excessive rise in the peripheral BP has been reported in patients who have had surgical repair of coarctation of the aorta, patients with hypertension and those with the potential to develop hypertension, hypercholesterolemic patients, and patients with aortic regurgitation, but information on the central aortic pressure is lacking in these reports.

Failure of BP to rise to the expected level may be much more significant than the level of the rise in arm BP. The failure reflects an inadequate increase in cardiac output. This is commonly seen with cardiomyopathy, left ventricular outflow tract obstruction, coronary artery diseases, or the onset of ventricular or atrial arrhythmias.

4. ECG monitoring

The major reasons for monitoring ECG during exercise testing are to detect exercise-induced arrhythmias and ischemic changes. A complete ECG should be recorded at rest, at least once during each workload, and for several intervals after exercise.

  a. Exercise-induced arrhythmias. Arrhythmias that increase in frequency or begin with exercise are usually significant and require thorough evaluation. Type and frequency before and after the exercise and occurrence of new or more advanced arrhythmias should be noted. Occurrence of serious ventricular arrhythmias may be an indication to terminate the test. Changes in the QTc duration, including the recovery period, should be evaluated.

  b. Changes suggestive of myocardial ischemia. ST-segment depression is the most common manifestation of exercise-induced myocardial ischemia. For children, downsloping of the ST segment or sustained horizontal depression of the ST segment of 2 mm or greater when measured at 80 msec after the J point is considered abnormal (see Fig. 3–23). Most guidelines for adult exercise testing, however, recommend an ST-segment depression of 1 mm or greater as an abnormal response. With progressive exercise, the depth of ST-segment depression may increase, involving more ECG leads, and the patient may develop anginal pain. Five to 10 minutes after the termination of the exercise, the ST changes (and T-wave inversion) may return to the baseline. Occasionally, the ischemic ST-segment response may appear only in the recovery phase.

  The following lists evaluation of ST-segment shift in some special situations.

  1). If the ST segment is depressed at rest (which occurs occasionally), the J point and ST segment measured at 60 to 80 msec should be depressed an additional 1 mm or greater to be considered abnormal.

  2). Specificity of the exercise ECG is poor in the presence of ST-T abnormalities on a resting ECG or with digoxin use.

  3). When there is an abnormal depolarization, such as bundle branch block, ventricular pacemaker, or Wolff-Parkinson-White preexcitation, interpretation of ST-segment displacement is impossible.

  4). In patients with early repolarization and resting ST-segment elevation, return to the PQ junction is normal. In such cases, ST depression should be determined from the PQ point, not from the elevated J point.

  5). There is a poor correlation between ST-segment changes and nuclear perfusion imaging in such conditions as anomalous origin of the coronary artery from the pulmonary artery, Kawasaki disease, and postoperative arterial switch operation.

5. Oximetry

Ear or finger oximetry measurement of blood oxygen saturation is useful during exercise testing of children who have CHD. Normal children maintain oxygen saturation greater than 90% during maximal exercise when monitored by pulse oximetry. Desaturation (less than 90%) during exercise is considered an abnormal response and may reflect pulmonary, cardiac, or circulatory compromise. Children who received lateral tunnel Fontan operation with fenestration may desaturate during exercise due to a right-to-left shunt through the fenestration.

SAFETY OF EXERCISE TESTING

A properly supervised exercise study is safe. Exercise testing should be performed under the supervision of a physician who has been trained to conduct the test with patients' safety in mind. The examiner should pay close attention to the subject during the treadmill exercise testing and be alert to stopping the treadmill when the patient can no longer exercise or appears to be in jeopardy. At these times, an observer should be positioned to assist the subject. A well-stocked crash cart should be available in the laboratory. A defibrillator should be present. Additional equipment should include a delivery system for oxygen as well as ventilation and suction apparatus.

Indications

Indications for stress testing vary with institutions and cardiologists. However, some of the more common indications for exercise testing in children are as follows:

1. Evaluate specific signs or symptoms that are induced or exacerbated by exercise.
2. Assess or identify abnormal responses to exercise in children with cardiac, pulmonary, or other organ disorders, including the presence of myocardial ischemia and arrhythmias.
3. Assess efficacy of specific medical or surgical treatments.
4. Assess functional capacity for recreational, athletic, and vocational activities.
5. Evaluate prognosis, including both baseline and serial testing measurements.
6. Establish baseline data for institution of cardiac, pulmonary, or musculoskeletal rehabilitation.

Contraindications

Good clinical judgment should be foremost in deciding contraindications for exercise testing. Absolute contraindications include patients with acute myocardial or pericardial inflammatory diseases or patients with severe obstructive lesions for whom surgical intervention is clearly indicated (Paridon et al, 2006).

Patients with following diagnoses are considered a high-risk group.

1. Acute myocarditis or pericarditis
2. Severe aortic or pulmonary stenosis
3. Pulmonary hypertension
4. Documented long QT syndrome
5. Uncontrolled resting hypertension
6. Unstable arrhythmias
7. Routine testing in Marfan syndrome
8. Routine testing after heart transplantation

Termination of Exercise Testing

Three general indications for terminating an exercise test are that (1) diagnostic findings have been established and further testing would not yield any additional information, (2) monitoring equipment fails, and (3) signs or symptoms indicate that further testing may compromise the patient's well-being. The following indications for termination of exercise testing have been recommended by the American Heart Association (2006):

1. Failure of heart rate to increase or a decrease in ventricular rate with increasing workload associated with symptoms (such as extreme fatigue, dizziness)
2. Progressive fall in systolic pressure with increasing workload
3. Severe hypertension, greater than 250 mm Hg systolic or 125 mm Hg diastolic, or BP higher than can be measured by the laboratory equipment
4. Dyspnea that the patient finds intolerable
5. Symptomatic tachycardia that the patient finds intolerable
6. Progressive fall in oxygen saturation to less than 90% or a 10-point drop from resting saturation in a patient who is symptomatic

   7. Presence of 3-mm or greater flat or downward-sloping ST-segment depression

   8. Increasing ventricular ectopy with increasing workload

   9. Patient's request for termination of the study

ALTERNATIVE STRESS TESTING PROTOCOLS

Besides treadmill exercise, there are other types of stress testing that can be performed, including the 6-minute walk test, pharmacologic stress tests, and exercise-induced bronchospasm provocation tests (see later in this section).

Six-Minute Walk Test. This test may be more appropriate for assessing exercise tolerance in children with moderate to severe exercise limitation for traditional exercise testing.

The patient is encouraged to try to cover as much distance or as many laps on a measured course (often 30 m) as possible in 6 minutes. Patients using supplemental oxygen should perform the test with oxygen. Portable oximeters may be used if available to the patient. If monitoring equipment is not available, oxygen saturation and heart rate are monitored before, during, and after the test. The total distance walked is the primary outcome. At least two practice tests performed on a separate day are advisable. At this time, reference values for healthy children and adolescents are not available. However, the test is useful for following disease progression or measuring the response to medical interventions.

Pharmacologic Stress Protocol. This protocol is used when conventional exercise testing is unsuitable or impractical, such as for patients who are too young or those who are unable to perform an exercise test. Following pharmacologic stimulations, either echocardiography or nuclear imaging is performed. Two types of pharmacologic agents are used.

   1. Agents that increase myocardial oxygen consumption (dobutamine, isoproterenol), which simulate the effects of exercise.

   2. Agents that cause coronary dilatation (adenosine, dipyridamole). Adenosine causes dilatation of normal coronary artery segments, resulting in a shunting of myocardial blood flow away from diseased segments. Dipyridamole inhibits adenosine reuptake, resulting in the same physiologic response.

Dobutamine is administered in gradually increasing doses from a starting dose of 10 μg/kg/min to a maximal dose of 50 μg/kg/min in 3- to 5-minute stages to achieve the target heart rate. Atropine (0.01 mg/kg up to 0.25 mg every 1 to 2 minutes to a maximum of 1 mg) can be administered to augment heart rate, usually given at 40 to 50 μg/kg/min dobutamine. Esmolol (10 mg/mL dilution at a dose of 0.5 mg/kg) should be available to reverse the effects of dobutamine rapidly in the event of an adverse reaction or development of ischemia. If echo is used, the imaging should be performed at rest and at each dosing stage. A radioisotope for a nuclear myocardial perfusion scan should be injected 1 minute before the infusion of dobutamine at maximal dosage is stopped.

Adenosine is infused at 140 μg/kg/min for 6 minutes. If echo imaging is used, it should be continuous. Nuclear isotope is given at 3 minutes into the infusion. Dipyridamole is infused over the same time period at a dose of 0.6 mg/kg/min. Radioisotope delivery and echo imaging should be performed at the peak physiologic effect of the dipyridamole, usually 3 to 4 minutes after completion of the infusion. Administration of aminophylline is routinely used in many centers after termination of the dipyridamole infusion.

Exercise-Induced Bronchospasm Provocation. Bronchial reactivity is measured while a subject exercises for 5 to 8 minutes on a treadmill at an intensity of 80% of maximum capacity. The exercise room should be as cool (temperature 20°C to 25°C) and dry as possible.

The exercise protocol should be to increase the intensity to 80% of maximum capacity within 2 minutes (using predicted heart rate maximum as a surrogate). If the intensity is not reached quickly, the patient may develop refractoriness to bronchospasm. Incremental work used in many exercise tests, such as the Bruce protocol, is less likely to be effective in evaluating exercise-induced bronchospasm (EIB) because of its short duration of high ventilation and thus should be avoided in the evaluation of EIB.

Exercise is preceded by baseline spirometry. Spirometry is repeated immediately after exercise and again at minutes 5, 10, and 15 of recovery. Most pulmonary function test nadirs occur within 5 to 10 minutes after exercise. Accepted criteria for a significant decline in forced expiratory volume in 1 second (FEV_1) after exercise are variable. Declines of 12% to 15% in FEV_1 are typically diagnostic.

Long-term ECG Recording

Long-term ECG recording is the most useful method to document and quantitate the frequency of arrhythmias, correlate the arrhythmia with the patient's symptoms, and evaluate the effect of antiarrhythmic therapy. There are several different types of long-term ECG recorders, which detect arrhythmias for a varying length of time. The Holter monitor is used to record events occurring in 24 (or up to 72) hours; event recorders record arrhythmic episodes for up to 30 days, and implantable loop recorders record rhythm up to 14 months.

HOLTER RECORDING

The Holter monitor, invented by Dr. Norman Holter, is a device that records the heart rhythm continuously for 24 (to 72) hours, using ECG electrodes attached on the chest. The heart rhythm is recorded with cassette tape or flash card technology and then processed at a heart center. Two simultaneous channels are usually recorded, which helps to distinguish artifacts from arrhythmias. This recorder is useful when the child has symptoms almost daily. This type of monitoring is not helpful in the detection of episodes that occur infrequently (e.g., once a week or once a month). Patients are given a diary so that they can record symptoms and activities. The monitor has a built-in timer that is used with the patient's diary to allow subsequent correlation of symptoms and activities with arrhythmias. The importance of keeping an accurate and complete diary must be impressed on patients and parents. Events of interest can be picked out and printed for review. A wide variety of information can be obtained from the recording, including heart rates, abnormal heartbeats, and rhythm during any symptoms.

Indications

Ambulatory ECG monitoring is obtained for the following reasons:
1. To determine whether symptoms such as chest pain, palpitation, or syncope are caused by cardiac arrhythmias
2. To evaluate the adequacy of medical therapy for an arrhythmia
3. To screen high-risk cardiac patients such as those with hypertrophic cardiomyopathy or those who have had operations known to predispose to arrhythmias (e.g., Mustard, Senning, or Fontan-type operation)
4. To evaluate possible intermittent pacemaker failure in patients who have an implanted pacemaker
5. To determine the effect of sleep on potentially life-threatening arrhythmias

The Holter recordings should reveal the frequency, duration, and types of arrhythmias as well as their precipitating or terminating events. Significant arrhythmias rarely cause symptoms such as palpitation, chest pain, and syncope (<10% of cases). Marked bradycardia (<50 beats/minute in infants, <40 beats/minute in older children), supraventricular tachycardia with a rate greater than 200 beats/minute, and ventricular tachycardia are potentially life threatening. These arrhythmias do occur and may worsen during sleep.

Interpretations

Interpretation of the results usually includes the following:
1. A description of the basic rhythm and the range of the heart rate
2. A description of the characteristics, duration, and frequency of the arrhythmias identified

3. Correlation of the arrhythmias with the patient's activities and symptoms

4. Correlation of ST-segment changes with activities and symptoms if the patient complained of anginal pain.

Holter Findings in Normal Children

Meaningful interpretation of the Holter recordings of patients with organic heart disease or significant systemic illness requires knowledge of the range of heart rate and rhythm variations in normal subjects of comparable age. Holter ECG recordings of healthy pediatric populations have demonstrated that variations in rate and rhythm, which were previously thought to be abnormal, occur quite frequently.

1. *Premature or low-birth-weight infants.* The minimum heart rate of premature or low-birth-weight infants can be as low as 73 beats/minute; the maximum heart rate can be as high as 211 beats/minute. Junctional rhythm may be observed in 18% to 70%, premature atrial contractions (PACs) in 2% to 33%, and premature ventricular contractions (PVCs) in 6% to 17%. First-degree AV block or Wenckebach's second-degree AV block occurs in 4% to 6%. Sudden sinus bradycardia and sinus pause occur especially frequently.

2. *Full-term neonates.* In full-term neonates, the heart rate can be as low as 75 beats/minute and as high as 230 beats/minute. Junctional rhythm may be present in 28%, PACs in 10% to 35%, and PVCs in 1% to 13%. First-degree AV block or Wenckebach's second-degree AV block may be recorded in 25% of neonates. Sinus pause is quite frequent.

3. *Children between 7 and 16 years of age.* During sleep, the heart rate can become as low as 23 beats/minute and the maximum rate as high as 110 beats/minute in older children. While the children are awake, minimum and maximum heart rates are 45 and 200 beats/minute, respectively. First-degree AV block and Wenckebach's second-degree AV block are also common during sleep (occurring in 3% to 12%). PVCs (occurring in 26% to 57%), which include multiform PVCs; PACs (occurring in 13% to 20%); and junctional rhythm (occurring in 5% to 15%) are also observed.

EVENT RECORDERS

Event monitors are devices that are used by patients over a longer period (weeks to months, typically 1 month). The monitor is used when symptoms suggestive of an arrhythmia occur infrequently. A drawback of this device is that the patient must be able to press the event button to begin recording. The information collected by the event monitor can be sent over the telephone to a doctor's office, clinic, or hospital. Two general types of cardiac event monitors are available:

1. *Looping memory (presymptom) event monitor.* Two electrodes are attached on the chest. The monitor is always on but stores the patient's rhythm only when the patient or caregiver pushes the button. Most monitors save the rhythm for 30 seconds before the device is activated. This feature is especially useful for people who pass out when their heart problems occur and can press the button only after they wake up.

2. *Postsymptom event monitor.* This monitor does not have electrodes that are attached to the chest. One type is worn on the wrist like a watch. When symptoms occur, a button is pressed to start the recording. The other type is a small device that has small metal disks that function as the electrodes. When symptoms occur, the device is pressed against the chest to start the recording.

IMPLANTABLE LOOP RECORDER

For patients with very infrequent symptoms, such as once every 6 months, neither Holter recorders nor 30-day event recorders may yield diagnostic information. In such patients, implantable loop recorders, about the size of a pack of chewing gum, are implanted beneath the skin in the upper left chest. The patient uses a handheld activator to record and permanently store the cardiac rhythm when symptoms occur. The device can be "interrogated" through the skin to determine what the heart was doing when the symptoms occurred. This device was shown to be instrumental in establishing the diagnosis in patients with infrequent syncope, in whom other recording devices failed to document the cause of syncope.

Ambulatory Blood Pressure Monitoring

BP is not a static variable; it changes not only from daytime to nighttime but also from minute to minute. Casual BP measurement provides only a snapshot of the daytime BP pattern, which is higher than nighttime readings. In some patients, there is a transient elevation of systolic, diastolic, or mean BP when BP is measured in a health care facility (i.e., "white coat hypertension"). This could lead to an overdiagnosis of hypertension and to unnecessarily aggressive and costly diagnostic studies and treatment. Ambulatory BP monitoring (ABPM) has emerged as a technology that addresses some of the limitations of casual BP measurements.

With ABPM, BP is measured multiple times during a predefined period in the patient's normal living environment during both awake and sleep periods, thus helping to identify those with white coat hypertension. In addition, ABPM may be better at identifying early markers of hypertensive end-organ injury, such as left ventricular mass. It also allows evaluation of the need for and the effectiveness of pharmacologic therapy for hypertension. Some researchers advocate the use of ABPM in all patients with casual BP elevation.

Multiple BP measurements are obtained with a preapplied BP cuff, using either the auscultatory method (with or without the ECG's R-wave gating) or the oscillometric method for a 24-hour period while children participate in their normal daily activities. Typically, BP measurements are programmed to occur every 20 minutes during awake periods and every 30 to 60 minutes during expected sleep periods. Sleep periods can be identified by either diary or actigraphy. The most common complaint is sleep disruption. Successful recording has been reported in more than 70% of children younger than 6 years.

There are three basic calculations of ABPM.

1. The *mean BP value* can be determined for the entire 24-hour period or for awake and sleep periods separately. Soergel and colleagues (1997) have published mean normative ambulatory BP levels for gender- and height-specific 95th percentile values from mid-European white children.

2. Alternatively, the *BP load* can be calculated. BP load is the percentage of BP readings for a given period that exceeds the 95th percentile of normal for the individual patient. This may be a better measure of the hemodynamic stress placed on end organs susceptible to hypertensive injury.

3. The *percent sleep decline* in BP (nocturnal dipping) is calculated by subtracting the mean sleep BP from the mean awake BP and dividing this value by the mean awake BP. Normal nocturnal dipping is at least 10% of mean awake BP. Nondipping (defined as a decline of <10%) has been associated with hypertensive end-organ injury, end-stage renal disease, renal transplantation, or insulin-dependent diabetes mellitus. Black children have higher sleep BP levels and less significant decreases in BP during sleep than age-matched white counterparts.

Although the advantages of ABPM are clear, there are still some technical difficulties and problems with normative ambulatory BP levels in children. With the auscultatory method, it is difficult to keep a microphone under the BP cuff over the brachial artery, and ambient noise levels interfere with accurate detection of Korotkoff sounds. Thus, oscillometric devices are more popular. In addition, there have not been published normative oscillometric BP standards until recently, and they have been shown to be higher than the auscultatory BP levels (see Blood Pressure Measurement in Chapter 2). The significance of each of the three calculations needs to be further defined. Another problem is that this technology is not always available, and the cost of the study may be prohibitive.

Chapter 7

Invasive Procedures

Two kinds of invasive procedures are used in the practice of pediatric cardiology. The first is cardiac catheterization and angiocardiography, which are used for diagnostic purposes (diagnostic catheterization). The second, used to treat certain structural heart defects nonsurgically, employs specially designed catheters and implantable devices that are delivered through cardiac catheters (therapeutic cardiac catheterization).

Cardiac Catheterization and Angiocardiography

Cardiac catheterization and angiocardiography usually constitute the final definitive diagnostic tests for most cardiac patients. They are carried out under general sedation using various sedatives discussed later. For newborns, cyanotic infants, and hemodynamically unstable children, general anesthesia with intubation may be used.

Under local anesthesia and with strict aseptic preparation of the skin, catheters are placed in peripheral (most commonly the femoral) vessels and advanced to the heart and central vessels under fluoroscopy with image intensification to reduce radiation exposure. At each position in the heart and blood vessels, values of pressure and oxygen saturation of blood are obtained. The oxygen saturation data provide information on the site and magnitude of the left-to-right or right-to-left shunt, if any. The pressure data provide information on the site and severity of obstruction. Cardiac output may be obtained from oxygen saturation data (e.g., the Fick principle) or by the indicator dilution (e.g., indocyanine green dye) or thermodilution (e.g., cold saline injection) technique. Selective angiocardiography is usually performed as part of the catheterization procedure (described later).

NORMAL HEMODYNAMIC VALUES

Normal oxygen saturation in the right side of the heart is usually 70% but it may vary between 65% and 80%, depending on cardiac output. Left-sided saturations are usually 95% to 98% in room air. In newborns and heavily sedated children, the oxygen saturation may be lower. Pressures are lower in the right side than in the left side of the heart, with systolic pressures in the right ventricle (RV) and pulmonary artery (PA) about 20% to 30% of those in the left side of the heart (Fig. 7–1).

ROUTINE HEMODYNAMIC CALCULATIONS

The following calculations are routinely obtained: flow and resistance for systemic and pulmonary circuits and left-to-right or right-to-left shunt.

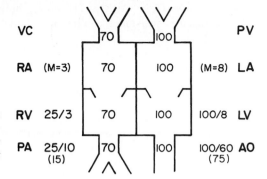

Figure 7–1. Average values of pressure and oxygen saturation in normal children. AO, aorta; LA, left atrium; LV, left ventricle; M, mean pressure; PA, pulmonary artery; PV, pulmonary vein; RA, right atrium; RV, right ventricle; VC, vena cava.

Flows (Cardiac Output) and Shunts. Flow is calculated by use of the Fick formula:

$$\text{Pulmonary flow } (\dot{Q}p) = \frac{Vo_2}{C_{PV} - C_{PA}}$$

$$\text{Systemic flow } (\dot{Q}s) = \frac{Vo_2}{C_{AO} - C_{MV}}$$

where flows are in L/minute, Vo_2 is oxygen consumption (mL/minute), C is oxygen content (mL/L) at various positions, PV is pulmonary vein, PA is pulmonary artery, AO is aorta, and MV is mixed systemic venous blood (superior vena cava or right atrium). Normal systemic flow or pulmonary flow in the absence of a shunt is 3.1 ± 0.4 L/minute/m^2 (i.e., cardiac index).

Oxygen consumption is either directly measured during the procedure or estimated from a table for children 3 years and older (see Appendix A, Table A–5). An assumed oxygen consumption of 150 to 160 mL/min/m^2 is used for older infants and children. For infants younger than 2 to 3 weeks, 120 to 130 mL/min/m^2 may be used. *Oxygen capacity* is the maximum quantity of oxygen that can be bound to each gram of hemoglobin (i.e., 1.36 mL × Hb level; each gram of hemoglobin [Hb] combines maximally with 1.36 mL of oxygen). *Oxygen saturation* is the amount of oxygen bound to hemoglobin compared with the oxygen capacity, and it is expressed as a percentage.

When there is a pure left-to-right or right-to-left shunt, the magnitude of the shunt is calculated as follows:

$$\text{Left-to-right shunt} = \dot{Q}p - \dot{Q}s$$

$$\text{Right-to-left shunt} = \dot{Q}s - \dot{Q}p$$

The flow data are subject to much error because of difficulties in measuring accurate oxygen consumption or because of the frequent use of assumed oxygen consumption in pediatric patients. Therefore, the ratio of pulmonary to systemic flow is frequently used because it does not require an oxygen consumption value. The ratio provides information on the magnitude of the shunt. A ratio of 1:1 would indicate no shunting in either direction or bidirectional shunting of equal magnitude. A ratio of 2:1 implies that there is a left-to-right shunt equal to systemic blood flow. A ratio of 0.8:1 signifies that the pulmonary blood flow is 20% less than the systemic blood flow (e.g., the flow ratio seen in a cyanotic patient). Patients with a flow ratio greater than 2:1 are usually surgical candidates.

Resistance. Hydraulic resistance (R) is defined by analogy to Ohm's law as the ratio of the mean pressure drop (ΔP) to flow (Q) between two points in a liquid flowing in a tube (R = ΔP/Q). Therefore, pulmonary vascular resistance (PVR) and systemic vascular resistance (SVR) are calculated using the following formulas:

$$PVR = \frac{\text{Mean PA pressure} - \text{Mean left atrium (LA) pressure}}{\dot{Q}p}$$

$$SVR = \frac{\text{Mean arotic pressure} - \text{Mean right atrium (RA) pressure}}{\dot{Q}s}$$

The normal SVR is about 20 units/m² in children, but it varies markedly between 15 and 30 units/m². In newborn infants, the SVR is lower (about 10 to units/m²), and it rises gradually to about 20 units/m² by 12 to 18 months of age. The normal PVR is high at birth but approaches adult values by about 6 to 8 weeks after birth. Normal values in children and adults are 1 to 3 units/m². Obviously, the ratios of PVR to SVR range from 1:10 to 1:20. High PVR values increase the risk associated with corrective surgery for many congenital cardiac defects.

SELECTIVE ANGIOCARDIOGRAPHY

Information derived from echocardiography and oxygen saturation and pressure data from catheterization help determine the number and sites of selective angiocardiograms required to delineate cardiovascular structures. A radiopaque dye is rapidly injected into a certain site, and angiograms are recorded, often on biplane views. Depending on the cardiovascular anomaly under study, special views are obtained by moving the fluoroscopic camera (or by positioning the patient at desired angles). Multiple injection sites are often necessary to obtain a complete anatomic diagnosis (Fig. 7–2A).

Contrast agents used in angiocardiography are water-soluble, complex organic compounds with three iodine atoms bound to a benzene ring. Old contrast agents (e.g., Renografin 76, Renovist, Hypaque M-75, Vascoray) are ionic agents with high osmolality (i.e., osmolality of 1690 to 2150 mOsm/kg, much [five to eight times] higher than the serum osmolality of 275 to 300 mOsm). Nonionic contrast agents (e.g., Isovue, Omnipaque) are low-osmolality agents (i.e., osmolality of 200 to 300 mOsm/kg), and some are hypotonic to the serum. After the injection of a high-osmolality contrast medium, there is a rapid shift of fluid from the interstitial and intracellular spaces into the intravascular space. This shift causes volume expansion, a slight drop in hematocrit, and a change in electrolyte concentration. These changes adversely affect newborns and

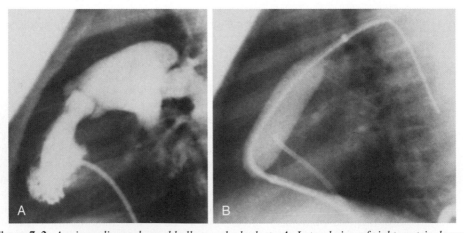

Figure 7–2. Angiocardiography and balloon valvuloplasty. **A,** *Lateral view of right ventriculogram showing a thick, dome-shaped pulmonary valve and a marked poststenotic dilatation of the pulmonary artery.* **B,** *A maximally inflated sausage-shaped valvuloplasty balloon is seen, which suggests that the stenotic pulmonary valve has been widened. The balloon catheter was introduced over a guide wire, which was positioned in the left pulmonary artery.*

infants with congestive heart failure (CHF). Low-osmolality agents cause less volume shift and are safer. Other toxic effects of high-osmolality agents include decreased red cell pliability, increased viscosity, osmolar diuresis, proteinuria, hematuria, and renal failure (occasionally).

RISKS

Cardiac catheterization and angiocardiography can lead to serious complications and occasionally death. Complications related to catheter insertion and manipulation include serious arrhythmias, heart block, cardiac perforation, hypoxic spells, arterial obstruction, hemorrhage, and infection. Complications related to contrast injection include reactions to the contrast material, intramyocardial injection, and renal complications (e.g., hematuria, proteinuria, oliguria, anuria). Complications related to exposure, sedation, and medications include hypothermia, acidemia, hypoglycemia, convulsions, hypotension, and respiratory depression, which are more likely to occur in newborns.

The risk of cardiac catheterization and angiocardiography varies with the patient's age and illness, the type of lesion, and the experience of the physician doing the procedure. The reported rate of fatal complications varies from lower than 1% to as high as 5% in the newborn period. In one study, the incidence of significant but nonfatal complications requiring treatment (e.g., arrhythmias and arterial complications) was 12% in infants younger than 4 months. In comparison, the incidence of such complications was 1.5% in older infants. Major complications (e.g., ventricular arrhythmias, hypotension, arterial complications, perforation of the heart, breakage or knotting of catheters, allergic reactions, hypoxic spells) occurred 1.4% of the time, and minor complications occurred 6.8% of the time. With better preparation and monitoring, as well as the use of prostaglandin infusion in critically ill newborns, the mortality and morbidity rates can be minimized.

INDICATIONS

Indications for these invasive studies vary from institution to institution and from cardiologist to cardiologist. With improved capability of noninvasive techniques (e.g., two-dimensional echo and color flow Doppler studies), many cardiac problems are adequately diagnosed and managed without the invasive studies. The following are considered indications by most cardiologists:

1. Selected newborns with cyanotic congenital heart disease (CHD) who may require palliative surgery or balloon atrial septostomy during the procedure
2. Selected children with CHD when the lesion is severe enough to require surgical intervention
3. Children who appear to have had unsatisfactory results from cardiac surgery
4. Infants and children with lesions amenable to balloon angioplasty or valvuloplasty
5. Children with hypoplastic or stenotic pulmonary arteries, especially those associated with pulmonary atresia and TOF, with extensive collateral arteries require angiography to delineate the extent of the abnormalities (echocardiography is not useful in studying blood vessels within the lung parenchyma)

SEDATION

A number of sedatives have been used by different institutions with equal success rates. Smaller doses of sedatives are usually used in cyanotic infants. When an interventional procedure is planned, general anesthesia is usually employed.

1. No sedation is used in newborns.
2. For small infants weighing less than 10 kg, a combination of chloral hydrate (75 mg/kg, maximum of 2 g) and diphenhydramine (2 mg/kg, maximum of 100 mg) by mouth has been used with good results.
3. For older children, Demerol compound (i.e., a solution containing 25 mg/mL of meperidine [Demerol], 12.5 mg/mL of promethazine [Phenergan], and 12.5 mg/ mL of chlorpromazine [Thorazine]) is a popular sedative mixture. The dosage

of the Demerol compound is 0.11 mL/kg intramuscularly. Some centers exclude chlorpromazine from the sedative mixture. In cyanotic children, the dosage of the Demerol compound is reduced by a third. For children in severe CHF, the dose is reduced by half.

4. Some cardiologists use a combination of meperidine (1 mg/kg) and hydroxyzine (Vistaril) (1 mg/kg) intramuscularly; others use a combination of fentanyl (1.25 µg/kg, maximum of 50 µg) and droperidol (62.5 µg/kg, maximum of 2500 µg) with equal success.

5. Ketamine (3 mg/kg intramuscularly or 1 to 2 mg/kg intravenously) may be used, but it can change the hemodynamic data because it increases the systemic vascular resistance and blood pressure.

6. Morphine (0.1 to 0.2 mg/kg) administered subcutaneously can be used to prevent or treat hypoxic spells.

7. If more sedation is required during the study, intravenous diazepam (Valium) (0.1 mg/kg) or morphine (0.1 mg/kg) is used.

PREPARATION AND MONITORING

Adequate preparation of the patient before the procedure and careful monitoring during the procedure can minimize complications and fatality from invasive studies.

Every child undergoing cardiac catheterization should have the following studies.

1. A 12-lead ECG, chest radiographs (both PA and lateral), two-dimensional echo, urinalysis, and a complete blood count within days or weeks in advance of the study

2. Baseline coagulation studies and a platelet count for deeply cyanotic child

3. Blood type and cross-match for infants less than 5 kg of body weight

The following areas of preparation and monitoring are particularly important for the safety of the patient.

1. Increasing the temperature in the cardiac catheterization laboratory when an infant is being studied

2. Using a warming blanket and a rectal thermistor to monitor rectal temperature to avoid hypothermia

3. Checking arterial blood gases and pH in addition to correcting acidemia and hypoxemia

4. Correcting hypoglycemia or hypocalcemia before and during the procedure.

5. Monitoring oxygen saturation and administering oxygen (if indicated) during the procedure

6. Having a reliable intravenous line (for sedation, resuscitation, or volume replacement) for all patients undergoing catheterization

7. Giving overnight intravenous fluid to reduce the risk of dehydration, thrombosis, and hypotension to children with a high hemoglobin level

8. Holding digitalis beginning the night prior to catheterization in order to reduce the risks of catheterization-induced arrhythmias

9. Having emergency medications (e.g., atropine, epinephrine, bicarbonate) drawn up and ready

10. Initiating prostaglandin infusion in cyanotic infants who seem to be ductus dependent

11. Intubating or readiness for intubating infants with respiratory difficulties

12. Whenever possible, having another physician (preferably an anesthesiologist) available to monitor the noncardiac aspects of the patient so that the operator can concentrate on the procedure

Catheter Intervention Procedures

Recent advances have allowed the development of a variety of therapeutic procedures using specially modified catheters and catheter-delivered devices. The lives of critically ill neonates may be saved by these procedures. They may also eliminate or delay the need for elective surgical procedures in children with certain CHDs. These procedures can open things that are closed, widen things that are too small, or close things that are open. More specifically, blood vessels and heart valves that are too small can be enlarged using balloon catheters or implantable devices known as stents, or both. Too small an opening in the atrial septum can be enlarged by using a balloon or blade catheter. An opening can be created in an intact atrial septum for left-to-right or right-to-left shunt to occur. Abnormal connections within the heart (atrial and ventricular septal defects) can be closed using innovative devices. Abnormal blood vessels (PDAs or collaterals) can also be closed using coils or plugging devices.

BALLOON AND BLADE ATRIAL SEPTOSTOMY

In balloon atrial septostomy (Rashkind's procedure), a special balloon-tipped catheter is placed in the LA from the RA through a patent foramen ovale (PFO) or an existing atrial septal defect (ASD). The balloon is inflated with diluted contrast material, and the catheter is rapidly pulled back to the RA through the interatrial communication, thereby creating a large opening in the atrial septum. This procedure is indicated in patients with an intact or nearly intact atrial septum in whom a better mixing of systemic and pulmonary venous blood would benefit their oxygenation, cardiac output, or both. Infants who have transposition of the great arteries (TGA), with or without associated ASD, are candidates for the procedure unless an arterial switch operation is to be performed immediately. It is also indicated in infants with total anomalous pulmonary venous return (TAPVR) with restrictive ASD if surgery is delayed for some reason. The procedure may be appropriate in selected patients with pulmonary atresia, mitral atresia, and tricuspid atresia.

In infants older than 6 to 8 weeks, the atrial septum may be too thick to allow an effective balloon septostomy. In such cases, the atrial septum can be opened with a blade catheter (i.e., Park blade). The blade catheter uses a small blade that unfolds from the tip of the catheter to incise the atrial septum as the catheter tip is withdrawn from the LA to the RA. The opening can be torn further with a balloon catheter. Conditions for which the procedure is necessary are the same as those listed for balloon atrial septostomy.

BALLOON VALVULOPLASTY

The balloons used in these interventional procedures are made of special plastic polymers and retain their predetermined diameters. A long guide wire is advanced far beyond the valve of interest, and the balloon catheter is placed over the wire. The middle of the elongated, sausage-shaped balloon is placed in the valve position. The balloon is then inflated with diluted contrast material to relieve obstruction at the valve.

Pulmonary Valve Stenosis. This technique is the treatment of choice for valvular pulmonary stenosis (PS) in children and, to a large extent, has replaced the surgical pulmonary valvotomy (see Fig. 7–2B). Balloon valvuloplasty may be indicated in patients with a Doppler peak gradient of 40 mm Hg or greater. The results of this technique are excellent, and it does not have significant complications. This technique can be used in neonates with critical PS, although the complication rate is higher. The effectiveness of balloon valvuloplasty for a severe dysplastic pulmonary valve is questionable, but it may be attempted. The procedure is not useful for the treatment of infundibular PS that is not associated with valvular PS.

Aortic Valve Stenosis. This procedure is more difficult and carries a higher complication rate than pulmonary valve balloon dilatation, especially for infants. The gradient reduction is less effective than for the pulmonary valve. Indications for balloon valvotomy include peak systolic pressure gradients greater than 50 to 60 mm Hg without significant aortic regurgitation (AR) in children and adolescents. Newborns or small infants with critical valve obstruction are also candidates for the procedure, regardless of the measured pressure gradient value. Complications include production or worsening of AR, iliofemoral artery injury and occlusion, ventricular fibrillation, and even death in small infants. Although the effectiveness of the procedure has been questioned, it may be tried in discrete membranous subaortic stenosis but not in fibromuscular subaortic (or "tunnel") stenosis.

Mitral Stenosis. Balloon dilatation valvuloplasty has been effective for rheumatic mitral stenosis (MS) but less effective for congenital MS. Passage of the balloon catheter across the atrial septum is necessary. Complications include perforation of the left ventricle, transient complete atrioventricular block, tearing of the anterior leaflet of the mitral valve, and severe mitral regurgitation.

Stenosis of Prosthetic Conduits and Valves within Conduits. The balloon dilatation procedure may reduce the transconduit gradient across stenotic areas of prosthetic conduits and across valves contained within conduits.

BALLOON ANGIOPLASTY

Balloon catheters similar to those used in balloon valvuloplasties are used for the relief of stenosis of blood vessels. Appropriate guide wires are placed beyond the point of narrowing, and the balloon catheter is placed over the guide wires. The midportion of the balloon is positioned at the point of narrowing, and the balloon is inflated with diluted contrast material to relieve the narrowing of vascular structures. This procedure has been used for coarctation of the aorta (COA), PA branch stenosis, and stenosis of the systemic veins. Following the balloon procedure, some blood vessels recoil and do not maintain the dilated caliber of the vessel.

Endovascular stents are sometimes used to maintain vessel patency after balloon angioplasty of any vascular structure. The stent prevents recoil of the vessel, providing better acute results and a considerably reduced rate of restenosis than with balloon angioplasty alone. The stent is positioned over an angioplasty balloon and the balloon is inflated after positioning it at an appropriate site. After stent placement, the vascular endothelium grows over the struts of the stent over several months, functionally incorporating the stent into the vessel wall. Occasionally, however, the endothelialization may go awry, resulting in a thick neointimal layer causing a functional stenosis. There is also active work in the development of biodegradable stents, which would eliminate some concerns about repeated dilatation in a growing child.

Recoarctation of the Aorta. Balloon angioplasty is an extremely useful tool in the management of postoperative residual obstruction of COA. It has become the procedure of choice for patients with this condition because reoperation carries a significant risk of morbidity and mortality. The procedure's success rate is close to 80%, and late development of an aortic aneurysm rarely occurs. Some centers use a stent to prevent restenosis.

Native (or Unoperated) Coarctation of the Aorta. Balloon angioplasty for native unoperated coarctation is controversial. The benefit is incomplete and inferior to the benefit resulting from surgery. The rate of recoarctation following the balloon procedure appears higher than that following surgery in infants. The complication rate is 17%, with aortic aneurysm formation (both acute and late) occurring in 6% of patients. The long-term effects of the procedure for native coarctation, which produces tearing of the intima and media of the coarctation segment, are unknown with regard to the development of an aortic aneurysm. Therefore, surgery may be a better choice than the balloon procedure for native coarctation. However, the use of stents may reduce the incidence of aneurysm formation and other complications.

Branch Pulmonary Artery Stenosis. The most frequent use of stents in pediatric patients is to treat peripheral PA stenosis. The peripheral PA stenosis may be seen as an isolated lesion but more commonly as a component of complex cyanotic heart defects. Hypoplastic and stenotic branch PAs are seen with postoperative tetralogy of Fallot (TOF), pulmonary atresia, and hypoplastic left heart syndrome. The immediate success rate of the balloon procedure is about 60%, but restenosis occurs in a significant number of patients and aneurysm formation occurs in approximately 3% of patients. Modification of the balloon technique, using an intravascular stent, has improved immediate results and may improve the long-term success rate. Because operative treatment of peripheral PA stenosis is often not possible, attempting the balloon procedure with a stent for this condition is well accepted.

Systemic Venous Stenosis. For obstructed venous baffles after the Mustard or Senning operation for TGA, the balloon procedure is an attractive alternative. The procedure is inappropriate for stenosis of the pulmonary vein because stenosis recurs in each case.

CLOSURE TECHNIQUES

Various devices have been used for nonsurgical closure of ASD, patent ductus arteriosus (PDA), and muscular ventricular septal defect (VSD) in the cardiac catheterization laboratory. All closure devices are delivered through a catheter that goes through long, large sheaths. The sheaths are inserted into the femoral vein, the femoral artery, or both. These nonsurgical devices have the advantages of a short hospital stay, rapid recovery, and no residual thoracic scar. In many centers, these devices and techniques are considered the procedures of choice for ASD, PDA, and collateral arteries.

Atrial Septal Defect. In the past, a double-umbrella device was used to close secundum ASD, but because of fractures of its arms, it has been taken off the market in this country. Currently, there are several devices available; some are approved by the U.S. Food and Drug Administration (FDA) and others are in clinical trial stages. They include the Sideris buttoned device, Angel Wings ASD device, CardioSEAL device (approved by the FDA), ASDOS (Atrial Septal Defect Occluder System), Amplatzer ASD occlusion device (approved by the FDA), and modified Clamshell double-umbrella device.

The Amplatzer device has been used worldwide and is most popular. The device is available in a range of sizes from 4 to 32 mm. The ASD must be less than or equal to 32 mm in diameter, and there must be at least a 4-mm rim of atrial septal tissue around the defect. The appropriate size of the device allows the connecting stalk to fill the ASD, self-centering the device for a better result. The procedure is performed under general anesthesia under the guidance of transesophageal echo. The patient is observed overnight and discharged the next morning. Patients take a baby aspirin daily for 6 months until endothelialization of the device is complete. Follow-up consists of an echo study and a chest radiograph at 6 months and 1 year. Rare possible complications include infection, arrhythmia, stroke, cardiac perforation, device embolization, and incomplete closure.

Successful closure of a muscular VSD, which is remote from cardiac valves, has been reported in selected patients by using the double-umbrella, Clamshell device.

Patent Ductus Arteriosus. A double-umbrella plug has been used outside the United States to close PDA in infants and young children, with a closure rate better than 85%. More recently, less costly coils have become popular in this country. Most transcatheter PDA closures are now performed using Gianturco vascular occlusion coils. They are small, coiled wires coated with thrombogenic Dacron strands that open like a small "pigtail" when placed in the vessel. When delivered to the aortic ampulla, blood clot is formed around the coil, obstructing blood flow with ultimate endothelialization. Good candidates for the coil occlusion are children weighing 6 kg and larger with the ductus 4 mm and smaller. The incidence of minor complications is low (less than 5%), and they include coil embolization, incomplete closure, mild LPA stenosis, and very rarely hemolysis. For a larger ductus, the Amplatzer PDA occluder may be used. Very large ducti in small infants are still probably best treated surgically.

Occlusion of Collaterals and Other Vessels. This technique is used for closing aortopulmonary collaterals (often seen with TOF), systemic arteriovenous fistulas, pulmonary arteriovenous fistulas, or surgically placed shunts that are no longer needed. The Gianturco coil and the White balloon are examples. When delivered, the coil occludes the vessel by creating a thrombus around the coil. Alternatively, a balloon is placed in a selected spot with an elaborate harpoon-like hydraulic delivery system on a thin catheter. Both devices need a discrete area of stenosis within a tubular vessel for fixation. The vessel should not be larger than 6 to 7 mm in diameter. Peripheral embolization of the coil or balloon into the PAs or the aorta is a major risk.

Part III

PATHOPHYSIOLOGY

In this section, discussion of fetal and perinatal circulation and the circulatory changes that take place after birth is followed by discussion of the pathophysiology of some representative congenital and acquired heart diseases.

Knowledge of fetal and perinatal circulation is extremely helpful in understanding the clinical manifestations and natural history of congenital heart diseases. A few examples of clinical importance in relation to fetal and perinatal circulation are examined. In discussing the pathophysiology of congenital and acquired heart diseases, attempts are made to explain why particular ECG, chest x-ray, and physical findings are associated with each defect, based on hemodynamic abnormalities. This necessitates a simplistic approach and the avoidance of controversies. Careful study of the pathophysiology section will enable readers to not only explain but also recall and predict the physical findings and abnormalities of the ECG and chest x-ray films of many cardiac anomalies.

Chapter 8

Fetal and Perinatal Circulation

Knowledge of fetal and perinatal circulation is an integral part of understanding the pathophysiology, clinical manifestations, and natural history of congenital heart disease (CHD). Only a brief discussion of clinically important aspects of fetal and perinatal circulation is presented.

Fetal Circulation

Fetal circulation differs from adult circulation in several ways. Almost all differences are attributable to the fundamental difference in the site of gas exchange. In the adult, gas exchange occurs in the lungs. In the fetus, the placenta provides the exchange of gases and nutrients.

COURSE OF FETAL CIRCULATION

There are four shunts in fetal circulation: placenta, ductus venosus, foramen ovale, and ductus arteriosus (Fig. 8–1). The following summarizes some important aspects of fetal circulation:

1. The placenta receives the largest amount of combined (i.e., right and left) ventricular output (55%) and has the lowest vascular resistance in the fetus.

2. The superior vena cava (SVC) drains the upper part of the body, including the brain (15% of combined ventricular output), whereas the inferior vena cava (IVC) drains the lower part of the body and the placenta (70% of combined ventricular output). Because the blood is oxygenated in the placenta, the oxygen saturation in the IVC (70%) is higher than that in the SVC (40%). The highest partial pressure of oxygen (Po_2) is found in the umbilical vein (32 mm Hg) (see Fig. 8–1).

3. Most of the SVC blood goes to the right ventricle (RV). About one third of the IVC blood with higher oxygen saturation is directed by the crista dividens to the left atrium (LA) through the foramen ovale, whereas the remaining two thirds enters the RV and pulmonary artery (PA). The result is that the brain and coronary circulation receive blood with higher oxygen saturation (Po_2 of 28 mm Hg) than the lower half of the body (Po_2 of 24 mm Hg) (see Fig. 8–1).

4. Less oxygenated blood in the PA flows through the widely open ductus arteriosus to the descending aorta and then to the placenta for oxygenation.

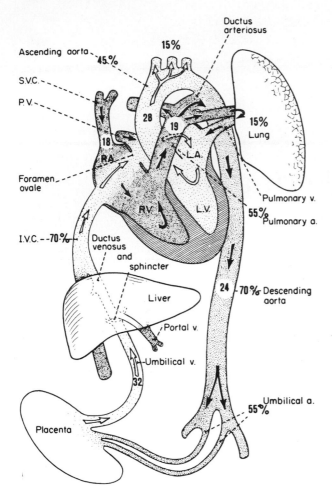

Figure 8–1. *Diagram of the fetal circulation showing the four sites of shunt: placenta, ductus venosus, foramen ovale, and ductus arteriosus. Intravascular shading is in proportion to oxygen saturation, with the lightest shading representing the highest P_{O_2}. The numerical value inside the chamber or vessel is the P_{O_2} for that site in mm Hg. The percentages outside the vascular structures represent the relative flows in major tributaries and outlets for the two ventricles. The combined output of the two ventricles represents 100%. a, artery; IVC, inferior vena cava; LA, left atrium; LV, left ventricle; PV, pulmonary vein; RA, right atrium; RV, right ventricle; SVC, superior vena cava; v, vein. (From Guntheroth WG, Kawabori I, Stevenson JG: Physiology of the circulation: Fetus, neonate and child. In Kelley VC [ed]: Practice of Pediatrics, vol 8. Philadelphia, Harper & Row, 1982–1983.)*

DIMENSIONS OF CARDIAC CHAMBERS

The proportions of the combined ventricular output traversing the heart chambers and the major blood vessels are reflected in the relative dimensions of these chambers and vessels (see Fig. 8–1).

Because the lungs receive only 15% of combined ventricular output, the branches of the PA are small. This is important in the genesis of the pulmonary flow murmur of the newborn (see Chapter 2).

Also, the RV is larger and more dominant than the left ventricle (LV). The RV handles 55% of the combined ventricular output, whereas the LV handles 45% of the combined ventricular output. In addition, the pressure in the RV is identical to that in the LV (unlike that in the adult). This fact is reflected in the ECG of the newborn, which shows more RV force than the adult ECG.

FETAL CARDIAC OUTPUT

Unlike the adult heart, which increases its stroke volume when the heart rate decreases, the fetal heart is unable to increase stroke volume when the heart rate falls because it has a low compliance. Therefore, the fetal cardiac output depends on the heart rate; when the heart rate drops, as in fetal distress, a serious fall in cardiac output results.

Changes in Circulation after Birth

The primary change in circulation after birth is a shift of blood flow for gas exchange from the placenta to the lungs. The placental circulation disappears, and the pulmonary circulation is established.

1. The removal of the placenta results in the following:

    a. An increase in systemic vascular resistance (because the placenta had the lowest vascular resistance in the fetus)

    b. Cessation of blood flow in the umbilical vein resulting in closure of the ductus venosus

2. Lung expansion results in the following:

    a. A reduction of the pulmonary vascular resistance (PVR), an increase in pulmonary blood flow, and a fall in PA pressure (Fig. 8–2)

    b. Functional closure of the foramen ovale as a result of increased pressure in the LA in excess of the pressure in the right atrium (RA). The LA pressure increases as a result of the increased pulmonary blood flow and increased pulmonary venous return to the LA. The RA pressure falls as a result of closure of the ductus venosus.

    c. Closure of patent ductus arteriosus (PDA) as a result of increased arterial oxygen saturation

Changes in the PVR and closure of the PDA are so important in understanding many CHDs that further discussion is necessary.

PULMONARY VASCULAR RESISTANCE

The PVR is as high as the systemic vascular resistance near or at term. The high PVR is maintained by an increased amount of smooth muscle in the walls of the pulmonary arterioles and alveolar hypoxia resulting from collapsed lungs.

With expansion of the lungs and the resulting increase in the alveolar oxygen tension, there is an initial, rapid fall in the PVR (Fig. 8–3). This rapid fall is secondary to the vasodilating effect of oxygen on the pulmonary vasculature. Between 6 and 8 weeks after birth, there is a slower fall in the PVR and the PA pressure. This fall is associated with thinning of the medial layer of the pulmonary arterioles. A further decline in the PVR occurs after the first 2 years. This may be related to the increase in the number of alveolar units and their associated vessels.

Many neonatal conditions causing inadequate oxygenation may interfere with the normal maturation (i.e., thinning) of the pulmonary arterioles, resulting in persistent

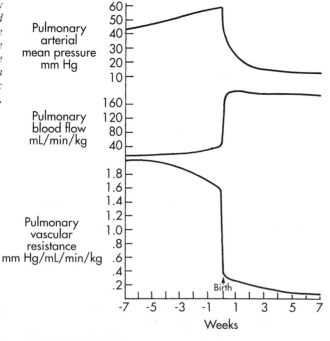

Figure 8–2. Changes in pulmonary artery pressure, pulmonary blood flow, and pulmonary vascular resistance, during the 7 weeks preceding birth, at birth, and in the 7 weeks after birth. The prenatal data were derived from lambs and the postnatal data from other species. (From Rudolph AM: Congenital Diseases of the Heart. Chicago, Mosby, 1974.)

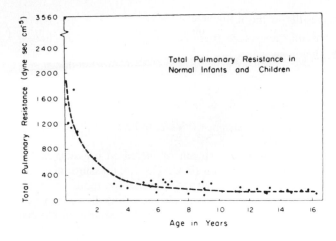

Figure 8–3. Postnatal changes in pulmonary vascular resistance. (From Moller JH, Amplatz K, and Edwards JE: Congenital Heart Disease. Kalamazoo, Mich, Upjohn Company, 1974.)

pulmonary hypertension or delay in the fall of PVR (Box 8–1). A few examples of clinical importance follow:

1. Infants with a large ventricular septal defect (VSD) may not develop congestive heart failure (CHF) while living at a high altitude, but they may develop CHF if they move to sea level. This is because of the delayed fall in the PVR associated with altitude.

2. Premature infants with severe hyaline membrane disease usually do not develop CHF because of their high PVR, which restricts the left-to-right shunt. Acidosis, which is often present in these infants, may contribute to maintaining a high PVR. CHF may develop as their hyaline membrane disease improves because the resulting increase in arterial Po_2 dilates pulmonary vasculature.

3. In infants with a large VSD, a high PA pressure, resulting from a direct transmission of the LV pressure to the PA through the defect, delays the fall in the PVR. As a result, CHF does not develop until 6 to 8 weeks of age or older. In contrast, the PVR falls normally in infants with a small VSD because direct transmission of the LV pressure to the PA does not occur in this situation.

CLOSURE OF THE DUCTUS ARTERIOSUS

Functional closure of the ductus arteriosus occurs within 10 to 15 hours after birth by constriction of the medial smooth muscle in the ductus. Anatomic closure is completed by 2 to 3 weeks of age by permanent changes in the endothelium and subintimal layers of the ductus. Oxygen, prostaglandin E_2 (PGE_2) levels, and maturity of the newborn are important factors in closure of the ductus. Acetylcholine and bradykinin also constrict the ductus.

BOX 8–1	NEONATAL CONDITIONS THAT MAY INTERFERE WITH THE NORMAL MATURATION OF PULMONARY ARTERIOLES

Hypoxia and/or altitude
Lung disease (e.g., hyaline membrane disease)
Acidemia
Increased pulmonary artery pressure secondary to large ventricular septal defect or patent ductus arteriosus
Increased pressure in the left atrium or pulmonary vein

Oxygen and the Ductus. A postnatal increase in oxygen saturation of the systemic circulation (from Po_2 of 25 mm Hg in utero to 50 mm Hg after lung expansion) is the strongest stimulus for constriction of the ductal smooth muscle, which leads to closure of the ductus. The responsiveness of the ductal smooth muscle to oxygen is related to the gestational age of the newborn; the ductal tissue of a premature infant responds less intensely to oxygen than that of a full-term infant. This decreased responsiveness of the immature ductus to oxygen is due to its decreased sensitivity to oxygen-induced contraction; it is not the result of a lack of smooth muscle development, as the immature ductus constricts well in response to acetylcholine. It may also be due to persistently high levels of PGE_2 in preterm infants (see later section).

Prostaglandin E and the Ductus. A few clinical situations are worth mentioning to show the importance of the prostaglandin E series in maintaining the patency of the ductus arteriosus in the fetus.

1. A decrease in PGE_2 levels after birth results in constriction of the ductus. This decrease results from removal of the placental source of PGE_2 production at birth and from the marked increase in pulmonary blood flow, which allows effective removal of circulating PGE_2 by the lungs.

2. Constricting effects of indomethacin and the dilator effects of PGE_2 and prostaglandin I_2 are greater in the ductal tissues of an immature fetus than of a near-term fetus.

3. Prolonged patency of the ductus can be maintained by intravenous infusion of a synthetic PGE_1, in infants such as those with pulmonary atresia, whose survival depends on patency of the ductus.

4. Indomethacin, a prostaglandin synthetase inhibitor, can be used to close a significant PDA in premature infants (see Chapter 12).

5. Maternal ingestion of a large amount of aspirin, an inhibitor of prostaglandin synthetase, may harm the fetus because the aspirin may constrict the ductus during fetal life and may result in persistent pulmonary hypertension of the newborn (PPHN). It has been suggested that some cases of PPHN (or persistent fetal circulation syndrome) may be caused by a premature constriction of the ductus arteriosus.

Reopening of a Constricted Ductus. Before true anatomic closure occurs, the functionally closed ductus may be dilated by a reduced arterial Po_2 or an increased PGE_2 concentration. The reopening of the constricted ductus may occur in asphyxia and various pulmonary diseases (as hypoxia and acidosis relax ductal tissues). Ductal closure is delayed at high altitude. There is a much higher incidence of PDA at high altitudes than at sea level. In some newborn infants (such as those with coarctation of the aorta), intravenous infusion of PGE_1 can open a partially or completely constricted ductus.

Responses of Pulmonary Artery and Ductus Arteriosus to Various Stimuli. The PA responds to oxygen and acidosis in the opposite manner from the ductus arteriosus. Hypoxia and acidosis relax the ductus arteriosus but constrict the pulmonary arterioles. Oxygen constricts the ductus but relaxes the pulmonary arterioles. The PAs are also constricted by sympathetic stimulation and α-adrenergic stimulation (e.g., epinephrine, norepinephrine). Vagal stimulation, β-adrenergic stimulation (e.g., isoproterenol), and bradykinin dilate the PAs.

Premature Newborns

Two important problems that premature infants may face are related to the rate at which PVR falls and the responsiveness of the ductus arteriosus to oxygen.

The ductus arteriosus is more likely to remain open in preterm infants after birth because the premature infant's ductal smooth muscle does not have a fully developed constrictor response to oxygen. In addition, premature infants have persistently high circulating levels of PGE_2 (possibly caused by increased production or decreased degradation in the lungs), and the premature ductal tissue exhibits an increased dilatory response to PGE_2.

In premature infants, the pulmonary vascular smooth muscle is not as well developed as in full-term infants. Therefore, the fall in PVR occurs more rapidly than in mature infants. This accounts for the early onset of a large left-to-right shunt and CHF.

Chapter 9

Pathophysiology of Left-to-Right Shunt Lesions

Before discussing the hemodynamic abnormalities of left-to-right shunt lesions, knowledge of the model that is used throughout this section will be helpful. Figure 9–1 is a block diagram of a normal heart, in which one arrow represents a "unit" of normal cardiac output. It is assumed that the cardiac chambers and great arteries and veins indicated by one arrow are normal in size. If a cardiac chamber or great artery has more than one arrow in it, that chamber or blood vessel is dilated. A diagram of a normal cardiac roentgenogram was presented in an earlier chapter (see Fig. 4–2). Modifications in the appearance of chest roentgenograms secondary to enlargement or reduction of cardiac chambers or great vessels are presented in diagrammatic drawings to aid in the interpretation of chest x-ray films.

Atrial Septal Defect

In acyanotic patients with atrial septal defect (ASD), the direction of the shunt is from left to right and the magnitude of the left-to-right shunt is determined by the size of the defect and the relative compliance of the right ventricle (RV) and left ventricle (LV). Because the compliance of the RV is greater than that of the LV, a left-to-right shunt is present. The magnitude of the shunt is reflected in the degree of cardiac enlargement. Let it be assumed that there is a left-to-right shunt of one arrow at the atrial level. As seen in Figure 9–2, the right atrium (RA), RV, and main pulmonary artery (PA) and its

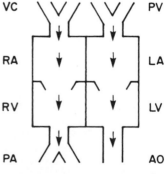

Figure 9–1. *Block diagram of a normal heart. One arrow represents a unit of normal cardiac output. AO, aorta; LA, left atrium; LV, left ventricle; PA, pulmonary artery; PV, pulmonary vein; RA, right atrium; RV, right ventricle; VC, vena cava.*

125

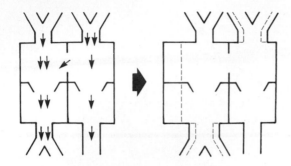

Figure 9–2. *Block diagram of an atrial septal defect. The number of arrows in each chamber represents the amount of blood to be handled by that particular chamber. When one redraws the chambers with two arrows larger than normal, one can predict which chambers will be enlarged.*

branches have two arrows and are therefore dilated. These findings are translated into the chest x-ray films (Fig. 9–3), which reveal enlargement of the RA, RV, and PA as well as an increase in pulmonary vascular markings. Note that the left atrium (LA) is not enlarged (see Figs. 9–2 and 9–3). This is because the increased pulmonary venous return to the LA does not stay in that chamber; rather, it is shunted immediately to the RA. The absence of left atrial enlargement is one of the helpful x-ray signs for differentiating an ASD from a ventricular septal defect (VSD).

The dilated RV cavity prolongs the time required for depolarization of the RV because of its longer pathway, producing a right bundle branch block (RBBB) pattern (with rsR′ in V1) in the ECG. The RBBB pattern in children with ASDs is not the result of actual block in the right bundle. If the duration of the QRS complex is not abnormally prolonged, the ECG may be read as mild right ventricular hypertrophy (RVH). Therefore, either RBBB or mild RVH is seen on the ECG of children with ASD.

The heart murmur in ASD is not caused by the shunt at the atrial level. Because the pressure gradient between the atria is so small and the shunt occurs throughout the cardiac cycle, in both systole and diastole, the left-to-right shunt is silent. The heart murmur in ASD originates from the pulmonary valve because of the increased blood flow (denoted by two arrows) passing through this normal-sized valve, producing a relative stenosis of the pulmonary valve (see Fig. 9–2). Therefore, the murmur is systolic in timing and is maximal at the pulmonary valve area (i.e., at the upper

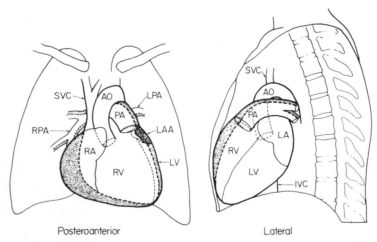

Posteroanterior   Lateral

Figure 9–3. *Posteroanterior and lateral view diagrams of chest roentgenograms. Enlargement of the right atrium (RA) and pulmonary artery (PA) segment and increased pulmonary vascular markings are present in the posteroanterior view. The right ventricular enlargement is best seen in the lateral view. AO, aorta; IVC, inferior vena cava; LA, left atrium; LAA, left atrial appendage; LPA, left pulmonary artery; LV, left ventricle; RPA, right pulmonary artery; RV, right ventricle; SVC, superior vena cava.*

left sternal border). When the shunt is large, increased blood flow through the tricuspid valve (denoted by two arrows) results in a relative stenosis of this valve, producing a diastolic murmur at the tricuspid valve area (i.e., lower left sternal border). The widely split S2 that is a characteristic finding in ASD results partially from RBBB. The RBBB delays both the electrical depolarization of the RV and the ventricular contraction, resulting in delayed closure of the pulmonary valve. In addition, the large atrial shunt tends to abolish respiration-related variations in systemic venous return to the right side of the heart, resulting in a fixed S2.

It should be noted that infants and small children rarely manifest with the clinical findings just described even in the presence of a moderately large ASD (proved by echo studies) until they are 3 to 4 years of age. It is because the compliance of the RV improves slowly so that any significant shunt does not occur until that age.

Children with ASD rarely experience congestive heart failure (CHF), even in the presence of a large left-to-right shunt. The PAs can handle an increased amount of blood flow for a long time without developing CHF because there is no direct transmission of the systemic pressure to the PA, and PA pressure remains normal. However, CHF and pulmonary hypertension eventually develop in the third and fourth decades of life.

Ventricular Septal Defect

The direction of the shunt in acyanotic VSD is left to right. The magnitude of the shunt is determined by the size, not the location, of the defect and the level of pulmonary vascular resistance (PVR). With a small defect, a large resistance to the left-to-right shunt occurs at the defect, and the shunt does not depend on the level of PVR. Decrease in the PVR occurs normally in this situation. With a large VSD, the resistance offered by the defect is minimal, and the left-to-right shunt depends largely on the level of PVR. The lower the PVR, the greater the magnitude of the left-to-right shunt. This type of left-to-right shunt is called a dependent shunt. Even in the presence of a large VSD in a newborn, the PVR remains elevated and therefore a large shunt does not occur until the infant reaches 6 to 8 weeks of age, when the shunt increases and CHF may develop.

In a VSD of moderate size, the cardiac chambers or vessels with two arrows enlarge, resulting in enlargement of the main PA, LA, and LV as well as an increase in pulmonary vascular markings (Fig. 9–4). In VSD, it is the LV that does volume overwork, not the RV. This results in LV enlargement; the RV does not enlarge. Because the shunt of VSD occurs mainly during systole when the RV also contracts, the shunted blood goes directly to the PA rather than remaining in the RV cavity. Therefore, there is no significant volume overload to the RV, and the RV remains relatively normal in size (Fig. 9–5; see Fig. 9–4). It should be noted that LA enlargement is present only with VSD but not with ASD. It should also be noted that both VSD and patent ductus arteriosus (PDA) produce an enlargement of the LA and LV.

Figure 9–6 summarizes the hemodynamics of VSDs of varying sizes and helps in the understanding of clinical manifestations. The size of a cardiac chamber directly relates to the amount of blood (or the number of arrows) handled by the chamber. The total number of arrows in the heart diagram also determines the overall size of the heart.

Figure 9–4. Block diagram of ventricular septal defect that shows the chambers and vessels that will be enlarged. There is an enlargement of the left atrium and left ventricle. The pulmonary artery is prominent, and the pulmonary vascularity is increased. Note the absence of right ventricular enlargement (see text for explanation).

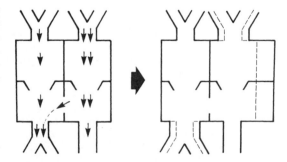

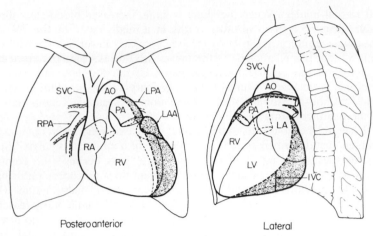

Figure 9–5. Posteroanterior and lateral view diagrams of chest roentgenograms of a moderate ventricular septal defect. Enlargement of the left atrium (LA), left ventricle (LV), and pulmonary artery (PA) and increased pulmonary vascular markings are present. Note the presence of left atrial enlargement, which is absent in atrial septal defect. Other abbreviations are the same as those in Figure 9–3.

With a small VSD, there is only half an arrow coming from the LV to the main PA. In addition, the degree of pulmonary vascular congestion and chamber enlargement is either minimal or too small to result in a significant change in the chest x-ray films (see Fig. 9–6). The degree of volume work imposed on the LV is also too small to produce left ventricular hypertrophy (LVH) on the ECG. The shunt itself produces a heart murmur (regurgitant systolic), and the intensity of the P2 is normal because the PA pressure is normal.

With a VSD of moderate size, one arrow shunts from the LV to the RV, and all the chambers that are enlarged handle two arrows. Therefore, the degree of cardiomegaly on the x-ray film is significant. The volume overwork done by the LV is significant, so that the ECG shows LVH of the volume overload type. Although the shunt is large,

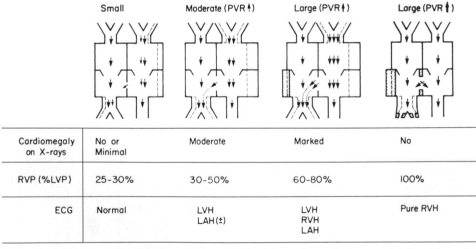

	Small	Moderate (PVR↑)	Large (PVR↑)	Large (PVR↑)
Cardiomegaly on X-rays	No or Minimal	Moderate	Marked	No
RVP (%LVP)	25-30%	30-50%	60-80%	100%
ECG	Normal	LVH LAH(±)	LVH RVH LAH	Pure RVH

Figure 9–6. Diagrammatic summary of the pathophysiology of ventricular septal defect. Most of the x-ray and ECG findings can be deduced from this diagram (see text for full description). LAH, left atrial hypertrophy; LVH, left ventricular hypertrophy; LVP, left ventricular pressure; PVR, pulmonary vascular resistance; RVH, right ventricular hypertrophy; RVP, right ventricular pressure.

the RV is not significantly dilated, and the pressure in this chamber is elevated only slightly (see Fig. 9–6). In other words, in a moderate VSD, the RV is not under significant volume or pressure overload; therefore, ECG signs of RVH are absent. As in a small VSD, a heart murmur (regurgitant systolic type) is produced by the left-to-right shunt. The normal-sized mitral valve handles two arrows. This relative mitral stenosis produces a mid-diastolic rumble at the apex. The PA pressure is mildly elevated; therefore, the intensity of the P2 may increase slightly.

With a large VSD, the overall heart size is larger than that seen with a moderate VSD because there is a much greater shunt. Because there is direct transmission of the LV pressure through the large defect to the RV in addition to a much greater shunt, the RV becomes enlarged and hypertrophied. Therefore, the x-ray film shows biventricular enlargement, left atrial enlargement, and greatly increased pulmonary vascularity (see Fig. 9–6). The ECG shows biventricular hypertrophy (BVH) and sometimes left atrial hypertrophy (LAH). A large VSD usually results in CHF in early infancy.

When a large VSD is left untreated, irreversible changes take place in the pulmonary arterioles, producing pulmonary vascular obstructive disease (or Eisenmenger's syndrome). It may take years to develop this condition. When Eisenmenger's syndrome occurs, striking changes take place in the heart size, ECG, and clinical findings. Because the PVR is notably elevated at this stage, approaching the systemic level, the magnitude of the left-to-right shunt decreases. This results in removal of the volume overload placed on the LV as well as the LA. Therefore, the size of the LV and the overall heart size decrease, and the ECG evidence of LVH disappears, leaving only RVH because of the persistence of pulmonary hypertension. Although the heart size becomes small, the PA segment remains enlarged because of persistent pulmonary hypertension. In other words, with the development of pulmonary vascular obstructive disease (PVOD), the heart size returns to normal except for a prominent PA segment, and a pure RVH on the ECG results. A bidirectional shunt causes cyanosis. Because the shunt is small, the loudness of the murmur decreases, or it may even disappear. The S2 is loud and single owing to pulmonary hypertension.

Patent Ductus Arteriosus

The hemodynamics of PDA are similar to those of VSD. The magnitude of the left-to-right shunt is determined by the resistance offered by the ductus (i.e., diameter, length, and tortuosity) when the ductus is small and by the level of PVR when the ductus is large (i.e., dependent shunt). Therefore, the onset of CHF with PDA is similar to that with VSD.

The chambers and vessels that enlarge are the same as those in VSD, except for an enlarged aorta to the level of the PDA (i.e., enlarged ascending aorta and transverse arch), which also handles an increased amount of blood flow (Fig. 9–7). Therefore, in PDA, chest x-ray films show enlargement of the LA and LV, a large ascending aorta and PA, and an increase in pulmonary vascular markings (Fig. 9–8). Although the aorta is enlarged, it usually does not produce an abnormal cardiac silhouette because

Figure 9–7. Block diagram of the heart in patent ductus arteriosus (PDA). Note the similarities between PDA and ventricular septal defect as to chamber enlargement. There is enlargement of the aorta to the level of the ductus arteriosus.

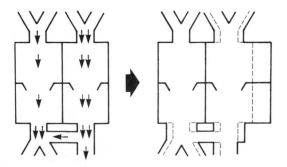

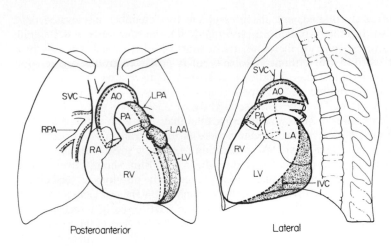

Figure 9–8. Diagrams of the posteroanterior and lateral chest x-ray films of patent ductus arteriosus (PDA). Note the similarities between PDA and ventricular septal defect. Abbreviations are the same as those in Figure 9–3.

the aorta does not form the cardiac silhouette. Therefore, chest x-ray films of PDA are indistinguishable from those of VSD.

Hemodynamic consequences of PDA are similar to those of VSD. In PDA with a small shunt, the left ventricular enlargement is minimal; therefore, the ECG and chest x-ray findings are close to normal. Because there is a significant pressure gradient between the aorta and the PA in both systole and diastole, the left-to-right shunt occurs in both phases of the cardiac cycle, producing the characteristic continuous murmur of this condition. With a small shunt, the intensity of the P2 is normal because the PA pressure is normal.

In PDA with a moderately large shunt, the heart size is moderately enlarged with increased pulmonary blood flow. The chambers enlarged are the LA, LV, and PA segment. The ECG shows LVH as in moderate VSD. In addition to the characteristic continuous murmur, there may be an apical diastolic flow rumble as a result of relative stenosis of the mitral valve. The P2 slightly increases in intensity if it can be separated from the loud heart murmur.

In a large PDA, marked cardiomegaly and increased pulmonary vascular markings are present. The volume overload is on the LV and LA, which produces LVH and occasional LAH on the ECG. The free transmission of the aortic pressure to the PA produces pulmonary hypertension and RV hypertension, with resulting RVH on the ECG. Therefore, the ECG shows BVH and LAH, as in a large VSD. The continuous murmur is present, with a loud apical diastolic rumble owing to relative mitral stenosis. The P2 is accentuated in intensity because of pulmonary hypertension.

An untreated large PDA can also produce pulmonary vascular obstructive disease, with a resulting bidirectional (i.e., right-to-left and left-to-right) shunt at the ductus level. The bidirectional shunt may produce cyanosis only in the lower half of the body (i.e., differential cyanosis). As in VSD with Eisenmenger's syndrome, the heart size returns to normal because of the reduced magnitude of the shunt. The peripheral pulmonary vascularity decreases, but the central hilar vessels and the main PA segment are greatly dilated owing to severe pulmonary hypertension. The ECG shows pure RVH because the LV is no longer under volume overload. Auscultation no longer reveals the continuous murmur or the apical rumble as a result of the shunt reduction. The S2 is single and loud because of pulmonary hypertension.

Endocardial Cushion Defect

During fetal life, the endocardial cushion tissue contributes to the closure of both the lower part of the atrial septum (i.e., ostium primum) and the upper part of the ventricular septum, in addition to the formation of the mitral and tricuspid valves. The failure of this tissue to develop may be complete or partial. A simple way of understanding the complete form of endocardial cushion defect (ECD) is that the tissue in the center of the heart is missing, with resulting VSD, the primum type of ASD, and clefts in the mitral and tricuspid valves. In the partial form of the defect, only an ASD is present in the ostium primum septum (primum type of ASD), often associated with a cleft in the mitral valve.

Hemodynamic abnormalities of primum-type ASD are similar to those of secundum-type ASD, in which the RA and RV are dilated with increased pulmonary blood flow (Fig. 9–9). These changes are expressed in the chest x-ray films (see Fig. 9–3). The cleft mitral valve is usually insignificant from a hemodynamic point of view because blood regurgitated into the LA is immediately shunted to the RA, thereby decompressing the LA. The physical findings are also similar to those of secundum ASD: a widely split and fixed S2, a systolic ejection murmur at the upper left sternal border, and a mid-diastolic rumble of relative tricuspid stenosis at the lower left sternal border. In addition, a systolic murmur of mitral regurgitation (MR) is occasionally present. The ECG findings are also similar: RBBB (with rsR' in V1) or mild RVH. One exception, which is important in differentiating between the two types of ASDs, is the presence of a "superior" QRS axis or left anterior hemiblock (with the QRS axis in the range of −20 to −150 degrees) in primum-type ASD. The abnormal QRS axis seen in ECD

Endocardial Cushion Defect

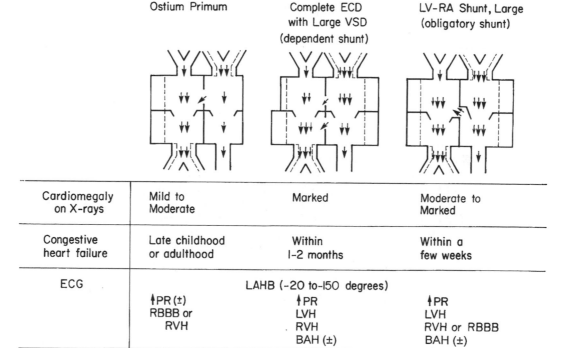

	Ostium Primum	Complete ECD with Large VSD (dependent shunt)	LV-RA Shunt, Large (obligatory shunt)
Cardiomegaly on X-rays	Mild to Moderate	Marked	Moderate to Marked
Congestive heart failure	Late childhood or adulthood	Within 1-2 months	Within a few weeks
ECG	↕PR (±) RBBB or RVH	LAHB (-20 to-150 degrees) ↕PR LVH RVH BAH (±)	↕PR LVH RVH or RBBB BAH (±)

Figure 9–9. Hemodynamic changes in different types of endocardial cushion defect (ECD). Hemodynamics of the ostium primum type of atrial septal defect (ASD) are identical to those of the secundum type of ASD. The cleft mitral valve is usually not significant from a hemodynamic point of view, and its effect is not shown here. In complete ECD, the hemodynamic changes are the sum of those of ventricular septal defect (VSD) and ASD, resulting in enlargement of all four cardiac chambers and increased pulmonary blood flow. The shunt depends on the level of the pulmonary vascular resistance (PVR; dependent shunt). In the left ventricular–to–right atrial (LV-RA) shunt, the shunt depends not on the level of PVR but on the size of the defect (obligatory shunt). Therefore, congestive heart failure may occur within the first weeks of life. BAH, biatrial hypertrophy; LAHB, left anterior hemiblock; LVH, left ventricular hypertrophy; ↑ PR, prolongation of the PR interval on ECG; RBBB, right bundle branch block; RVH, right ventricular hypertrophy.

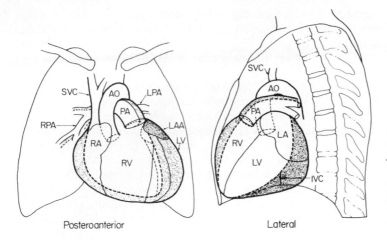

Figure 9–10. *Diagrams of chest roentgenograms in the complete form of endocardial cushion defect. All four cardiac chambers are enlarged, with increased pulmonary vascular markings. Abbreviations are the same as those in Figure 9–3.*

(both partial and complete forms) is not the result of axis deviation or any of the hemo-dynamic abnormalities mentioned; rather, the abnormal QRS axis occurs as a result of the primary abnormality in the development of the bundle of His and the bundle branches.

Hemodynamic changes seen with complete ECD are the sum of the changes of ASD and VSD. The magnitude of the left-to-right shunt in both ASD and VSD is determined by the level of PVR (i.e., dependent shunt). It has volume overload of the LA and LV as in VSD and partially due to MR. In addition, it has volume overload of the RA and RV as in ASD (see Fig. 9–9). This is translated to the chest x-ray films as biatrial and biventricular enlargement (Fig. 9–10). The ECG also reflects these changes as BVH and occasional biatrial hypertrophy. "Superior" QRS axis is also characteristic of ECD as discussed earlier. Physical examination is characterized by a hyperactive precordium and regurgitant systolic murmurs of VSD and MR, loud and narrowly split S2 (because of pulmonary hypertension), apical and/or tricuspid diastolic rumble, and signs of CHF. Those who survive infancy may develop pulmonary vascular obstructive disease, as already discussed for large VSD and large PDA.

A direct communication between the LV and RA may occur as part of ECD or as an isolated defect unrelated to ECD. The direction of the shunt is from the high-pressure LV to the low-pressure RA. The magnitude of the shunt is determined by the size of the defect, regardless of the state of PVR; blood shunted to the RA must go forward through the lungs even if the PVR is high. This type of shunt, which is inde-pendent of the status of PVR, is called an obligatory shunt (see Fig. 9–9). CHF occurs within a few weeks, which is earlier than in the usual VSD. The enlarged chambers are identical to those of the complete form of ECD. Therefore, the chest x-ray films and ECG findings are similar to those seen in complete ECD. Physical findings also resemble those of complete ECD, although the holosystolic murmur (resulting from the LV-RA shunt) may be more prominent at the mid-right sternal border.

Chapter 10

Pathophysiology of Obstructive and Valvular Regurgitation Lesions

This chapter discusses hemodynamic abnormalities of obstructive and valvular regurgitant lesions of congenital and acquired causes. For convenience, they are divided into the following three groups on the basis of their hemodynamic similarities:

1. Ventricular outflow obstructive lesions (e.g., aortic stenosis [AS], pulmonary stenosis [PS], coarctation of the aorta [COA])

2. Stenosis of atrioventricular (AV) valves (e.g., mitral stenosis [MS], tricuspid stenosis [TS])

3. Valvular regurgitant lesions (e.g., mitral regurgitation [MR], tricuspid regurgitation [TR], aortic regurgitation [AR], pulmonary regurgitation [PR])

Obstruction to Ventricular Output

Common congenital obstructive lesions to ventricular output are AS, PS, and COA. All these obstructive lesions produce the following three pathophysiologic changes (Fig. 10–1):

1. An ejection systolic murmur (as heard on auscultation)

2. Hypertrophy of the respective ventricle (as seen in the ECG)

3. Poststenotic dilatation (as seen in chest-x ray films). (This is not seen with subvalvular stenosis.)

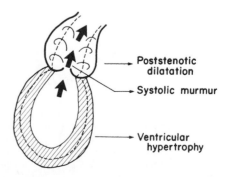

Figure 10–1. Three secondary changes are seen in aortic valve and pulmonary valve stenosis: an ejection systolic murmur, hypertrophy of the responsible ventricle, and poststenotic dilatation of a great artery. A normal-sized ventricle and a great artery are shown by broken lines. The end results of a semilunar valve stenosis are illustrated by solid lines. A similar change occurs with coarctation of the aorta.

Poststenotic dilatation

Systolic murmur

Ventricular hypertrophy

AORTIC AND PULMONARY VALVE STENOSES

An ejection type of systolic murmur can best be heard when the stethoscope is placed over the area distal to the obstruction. Therefore, the murmur of AS is usually loudest over the ascending aorta (i.e., aortic valve area or upper right sternal border), and the murmur of PS is loudest over the pulmonary artery (i.e., pulmonary valve area or upper left sternal border). However, the actual location of the aortic valve is under the sternum at the level of the third left intercostal space; therefore, the murmur of AS may be quite loud at the third left intercostal space.

In isolated stenosis of the pulmonary or aortic valve, the intensity and duration of the ejection systolic murmur are directly proportional to the severity of the stenosis. In mild stenosis of a semilunar valve, the murmur is of low intensity (grade 1 to 2/6) and occurs early in systole, with the apex of the "diamond" in the first half of systole. With increasing severity of the stenosis, the murmur becomes longer and louder (often with a thrill) with the apex of the murmur moving toward the S2. With mild pulmonary valve stenosis, the S2 is normal or split widely because of prolonged "hangout time" (see Chapter 2). With severe PS, the murmur is long and may continue beyond the A2, the S2 splits widely, but the intensity of the P2 decreases (Fig. 10–2A). With severe AS, the S2 becomes single or splits paradoxically because of the delayed closure of the aortic valve (A2) in relation to the P2 (see Fig. 10–2B). In semilunar valve stenosis, an ejection click may be audible. The click is produced by a sudden checking of the valve motion or possibly by the sudden distention of the dilated great arteries.

If the obstruction is severe, the ventricle that has to pump blood against the obstruction hypertrophies. The left ventricle (LV) hypertrophies in AS and the right ventricle (RV) in PS, which results in left ventricular hypertrophy (LVH) and right ventricular hypertrophy (RVH), respectively, on the ECG. Cardiac output is maintained unless myocardial failure occurs in severe cases; therefore, the heart size remains normal.

Poststenotic dilatation is the hallmark of an obstruction at the valvular level. The artery distal to the stenotic semilunar valve dilates circumferentially. Poststenotic dilatation is not seen with subvalvular stenosis; it is only mild or not seen at all with supravalvular stenosis. It was believed that the jet of blood resulting from the stenosis strikes a localized area of the great artery with weakening of that area causing the dilatation. However, there is also circumferential dilatation of the great artery where the jet does not strike. Sustained vibration of the vessel distal to the narrowing causes generalized fatigue of collagen fibers with resulting dilatation, which may add circumferential dilatation. In pulmonary valve stenosis, a prominent PA segment is visible on chest x-ray film (see Fig. 4–7A). In aortic valve stenosis, the dilated aorta may look like a bulge on the right upper mediastinum or a prominence of the aortic knob on the left upper mediastinum (see Fig. 4–7C). Mild dilatation of the ascending aorta secondary to aortic valve stenosis is usually not visible on plain chest x-ray films because the ascending aorta does not form the cardiac border.

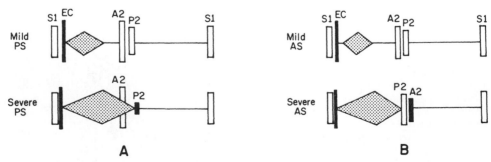

A   **B**

Figure 10–2. Systolic murmurs of pulmonary valve stenosis (**A**) and aortic valve stenosis (**B**). The duration and intensity of the murmur increase with increasing severity of the stenosis. Note the changes in the splitting of S2 (see text). An ejection click (EC) is present in both conditions. Abnormal heart sounds are shown as black bars. AS, aortic stenosis; PS, pulmonary stenosis.

COARCTATION OF THE AORTA

In older children with COA, an ejection-type systolic murmur is present over the descending aorta, distal to the site of coarctation (i.e., in the left interscapular area). Because many of these patients also have abnormal aortic valves (most commonly bicuspid aortic valves), a soft AS murmur, ejection click, and occasional AR murmur may be heard. Depending on the severity of the obstruction, the femoral pulses are either weak and delayed or absent. The weak pulse results primarily from a slow upstroke of the arterial pulse in the lower extremity sites. On chest x-ray films, poststenotic dilatation of the descending aorta (distal to the coarctation) often produces the figure-of-3 sign on the plain film or an E-shaped indentation on the barium esophagogram (see Fig. 4–9). The ECG shows LVH because of a pressure overload on the LV. In newborns and small infants, RVH or right bundle branch block (RBBB) is commonly seen, but LVH is not (see later section for the reasons).

Previously, terms such as *preductal* and *infantile coarctation* were used to describe symptomatic infants. Terms such as *postductal* and *adult-type coarctation* described asymptomatic children. Neither terminology is correct (see Chapter 13). The coarctation is almost always juxtaductal (i.e., located opposite the entry of the ductus arteriosus). Major differences in pathology between symptomatic infants and asymptomatic children often occur and contribute significantly to hemodynamic abnormalities (Fig. 10–3).

1. Many patients who become symptomatic early in life have associated defects such as ventricular septal defect (VSD) or left-sided obstructive lesions, or both. The obstructive lesions may be in the left ventricular outflow tract, the aortic valve, or the proximal aorta (see Fig. 10–3A). These associated defects tend to decrease blood flow to the ascending aorta and to the aortic isthmus (i.e., the segment between the left subclavian artery and the ductus arteriosus) during fetal life. As a result, these structures become relatively hypoplastic.

2. These associated anomalies result in more volume work delegated to the RV, which supplies blood to the descending aorta through a large ductus arteriosus. The RV, which is normally dominant, becomes more dilated and hypertrophied, whereas the LV becomes smaller than normal. This may explain why infants with COA show RVH rather than LVH on the ECG (see later).

3. Decreased flow in the proximal aorta does not produce a pressure gradient between the aortic segments proximal and distal to the coarctation. The absence of pressure gradient does not stimulate the development of collateral circulation

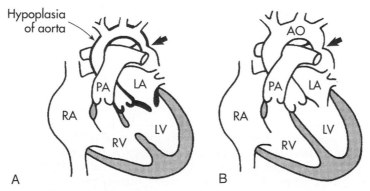

Figure 10–3. Diagrammatic comparison of the heart and aorta in symptomatic infants and asymptomatic children with coarctation of the aorta. *A,* In symptomatic infants, associated defects are frequently found, which include ventricular septal defect, aortic and mitral valve abnormalities, and hypoplasia of the ascending and transverse aortas. These abnormalities are shown in heavy lines. *B,* In asymptomatic children, the coarctation is usually an isolated lesion, except for bicuspid aortic valve (not shown). AO, aorta; LA, left atrium; LV, left ventricle; PA, pulmonary artery; RA, right atrium; RV, right ventricle.

between the ascending and descending aortas. When the ductus closes after birth, the pressure work imposed on the relatively small LV suddenly increases. This results in a noticeable decrease in the perfusion of the descending aorta (with resulting circulatory shock), renal failure, and signs of left heart failure (i.e., dyspnea and pulmonary venous congestion).

4. On the contrary, in the absence of the associated defects, normal amounts of blood reaching the isthmus area produce a pressure gradient between the aortic segments above and below the coarctation, and it stimulates the development of collateral circulation between them. Most of these infants, who do not have associated defects, tolerate the postnatal closure of the ductus well and remain asymptomatic (see Fig. 10–3B), although some infants develop LV failure.

The changes in fetal circulation just described account for the presence of RVH (or RBBB), rather than LVH, on the ECG. During fetal life, the RV normally performs 55% of the combined ventricular volume work and the LV performs 45%, for an RV/LV volume work ratio of 55:45. This is the reason why normal newborn infants have RV dominance on the ECG. An associated VSD or obstructive lesion described previously, or both, delegates more volume work to the RV; for example, if the RV/LV volume work ratio is 70:30, the RV dominance is greater than normal, with resulting RVH on the ECG. Thus, RVH in symptomatic infants usually results from an increased volume overload placed on the RV during fetal life. The RVH is gradually replaced by LVH by 2 years of age.

Stenosis of Atrioventricular Valves

Stenosis of the AV valves produces obstruction to pulmonary or systemic venous return. Passive congestion in the pulmonary or systemic venous system causes the clinical manifestations associated with these conditions.

MITRAL STENOSIS

Stenosis of the mitral valve is more often rheumatic than congenital in origin. It produces a pressure gradient in diastole between the left atrium (LA) and the LV, which in turn produces a series of changes in the structures proximal to the mitral valve (e.g., the LA, pulmonary veins, PAs, and RV). When a significant MS is present, the LA becomes dilated and hypertrophied. The pressure in the LA is raised, which in turn raises pressures in the pulmonary veins and capillaries (Fig. 10–4). Pulmonary edema may result if the hydrostatic pressure in the capillaries exceeds the osmotic pressure of the blood. Therefore, chest x-ray films may reveal pulmonary venous congestion or pulmonary edema and enlargement of the LA. Dyspnea with or without exertion and orthopnea may manifest. The high pulmonary capillary pressure results in reflex arteriolar constriction, which in turn causes pulmonary arterial hypertension and eventually hypertrophy of the RV. These changes are seen as RVH on the ECG and as prominence of the PA segment on chest x-ray films. Right heart failure may eventually develop (with cardiomegaly seen on x-ray films).

The pressure gradient during diastole produces a mid-diastolic rumble that is best heard at the apex on auscultation. When the mitral valve is mobile (not severely stenotic), an opening snap precedes the murmur (see Fig. 21–1). During the last part of diastole, if the pressure gradient persists, the LA contracts to push blood forward, producing a presystolic murmur. At the time of the onset of ventricular contraction, the mitral valve leaflets are relatively wide apart because of the prolonged atrial contraction, producing a loud S1. If the cardiac output decreases significantly, thready pulses result. The dilated LA contributes to the frequent occurrence of atrial fibrillation, which may result in loss of the presystolic murmur.

The following conditions all have in common an elevated pulmonary venous pressure, with similar pathophysiology, and must be differentiated from mitral stenosis:

1. Total anomalous pulmonary venous return with obstruction (see Chapter 14)

2. Cor triatriatum (see Chapter 17)

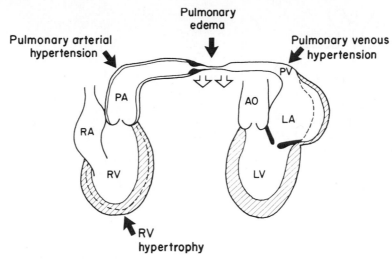

Figure 10–4. *Hemodynamic. changes in severe mitral stenosis. Enlargement and hypertrophy of the left atrium (LA), pulmonary venous hypertension, and possible pulmonary edema result. Reflex vasoconstriction of pulmonary arterioles leads to pulmonary arterial hypertension and right ventricular hypertrophy. AO, aorta; LV, left ventricle; PA, pulmonary artery; PV, pulmonary vein; RA, right atrium; RV, right ventricle.*

3. Stenosis of individual pulmonary vein
4. Hypoplastic left heart syndrome (see Chapter 14)
5. Left atrial myxoma (see Chapter 22)

TRICUSPID STENOSIS

Stenosis of the tricuspid valve is rare and usually congenital. It produces dilatation and hypertrophy of the right atrium (RA) for obvious reasons. Therefore, chest x-ray films reveal right atrial enlargement, and the ECG may show right atrial hypertrophy (RAH).

Increased pressure in the systemic veins produces hepatomegaly and distended neck veins. A pressure gradient across this valve during diastole produces a mid-diastolic murmur. A prolonged contraction of the RA to push blood through the narrow valve may produce a presystolic murmur. It is occasionally associated with congenital hypoplasia of the RV, which worsens the obstructed blood flow into the RV.

Valvular Regurgitant Lesions

Important valvular regurgitant lesions are AR and MR. Severe pulmonary valve regurgitation is relatively rare except in a postoperative state, such as those seen following surgery for TOF and other conditions that require conduit placement between the RV and the PA. Significant tricuspid valve regurgitation is also rare.

In general, when regurgitation is severe, the chambers both proximal and distal to a regurgitant valve become dilated, with volume overload of these chambers. With MR, both the LV and LA dilate, whereas with AR, the LV enlarges and the aorta enlarges or increases its pulsation. If the regurgitation is minimal, only auscultatory abnormalities indicate its presence.

MITRAL REGURGITATION

The major problem in MR is volume overload of both the LA and LV, with resulting enlargement of these chambers (Fig. 10–5). Therefore, chest x-ray films reveal enlargement of the LA and LV, and the ECG may show LVH and left atrial hypertrophy.

Regurgitation of blood from the LV to the LA produces a regurgitant systolic murmur that is best heard near the apex. Because of an increased amount of blood flows

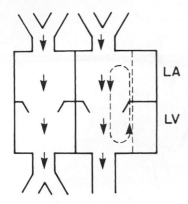

Figure 10–5. *Diagrammatic representation of hemodynamic changes in mitral regurgitation. Note that the chambers with two arrows (left atrium [LA] and left ventricle [LV]) are enlarged.*

across the mitral orifice during the rapid filling phase of diastole, the S3 is usually loud. When the regurgitation is severe, a mid-diastolic rumble may be present because of "relative" MS that results from handling an excessive amount of left atrial blood through the normal-sized mitral orifice. The dilated LA chamber tends to dampen the transmission of the pressure from the LV, and the pressure in the LA is usually not notably elevated. Therefore, unlike the situation with mitral stenosis, marked pulmonary hypertension occurs only occasionally with MR.

TRICUSPID REGURGITATION

In TR, hemodynamic changes similar to those described for MR result. The RA and RV enlarge for obvious reasons. The ECG may show RAH and RVH (or RBBB).

A systolic regurgitant murmur, a loud S3, and a diastolic rumble develop, as in MR, but they are audible at the tricuspid area (both sides of the lower sternal border) rather than at the apex. With severe regurgitation, pulsation of the liver and neck veins may occur, reflecting a phasic increase in right atrial pressure by the regurgitation.

AORTIC REGURGITATION

There is volume overload of the LV because this chamber must handle normal cardiac output in addition to the amount that leaks back to the LV (Fig. 10–6). This is represented as left ventricular enlargement on x-ray films and LVH on the ECG. Because of the increase in stroke volume received by the aorta, the aorta pulsates more than normal and becomes somewhat dilated, although the aorta does not retain all the increased stroke volume.

An increase in systolic pressure results from an increase in stroke volume. The diastolic pressure is lower because of a continuous leak back to the LV during diastole. This results in a wide pulse pressure and bounding peripheral pulse. The regurgitation

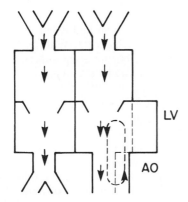

Figure 10–6. *Diagrammatic representation of hemodynamic changes in aortic regurgitation. Note that the left ventricle (LV) and aorta (AO), with two arrows, are enlarged.*

during diastole produces a high-pitched, decrescendo diastolic murmur immediately after the S2 (see Fig. 21–4). The regurgitant flow is directed toward the apex; therefore, the diastolic decrescendo murmur is well audible at the apex as well as in the third left intercostal space. The AR flow, which coincides with the forward flow of left atrial blood, produces a flutter motion of the mitral valve, producing an Austin Flint murmur in diastole. With severe AR, a high left ventricular end-diastolic pressure approximates the mitral valve leaflets at the onset of ventricular systole, resulting in reduced intensity of the S1.

PULMONARY REGURGITATION

The pathophysiology of PR is similar to that of AR. The RV dilates, and the PA may enlarge. This is represented in x-ray films as right ventricular enlargement and prominence of the PA segment. The ECG may show RVH or RBBB.

Because of the low diastolic pressure of the PA, the murmur of PR is low pitched, and the gap between the S2 and the onset of the decrescendo diastolic murmur is wider than that seen in AR. In the presence of pulmonary hypertension, however, the murmur of PR resembles that of AR. The direction of the regurgitation is to the body of the RV; therefore, the PR murmur is audible along the left sternal border rather than at the apex (where the AR murmur is loud). The different direction of the radiation of the diastolic murmur is helpful in differentiating PR from AR.

Chapter 11

Pathophysiology of Cyanotic Congenital Heart Defects

Clinical Cyanosis

DETECTION OF CYANOSIS

Cyanosis is a bluish discoloration of the skin and mucous membranes resulting from an increased concentration of reduced hemoglobin to about 5 g/100 mL in the cutaneous veins. This level of reduced hemoglobin in the cutaneous vein may result from either desaturation of arterial blood or increased extraction of oxygen by peripheral tissue in the presence of normal arterial saturation (e.g., circulatory shock, hypovolemia, vasoconstriction from cold). Cyanosis associated with desaturation of arterial blood is called central cyanosis; cyanosis with normal arterial oxygen saturation is called peripheral cyanosis.

Cyanosis is more difficult to detect in children with dark pigmentation. Although cyanosis may be detected on many parts of the body, including the lips, fingernails, oral mucous membranes, and conjunctivae, the tip of the tongue is a good place to look for cyanosis; the color of the tongue is not affected by race or ethnic background, and the circulation is not sluggish in the tongue. In a newborn, acrocyanosis may cause confusion. In addition, some newborns are polycythemic, which may contribute to the appearance of cyanosis without arterial desaturation (see later). In older infants and children, chronic subclinical cyanosis produces clubbing.

When in doubt, arterial oxygen saturation should be obtained by a pulse oximeter or arterial partial pressure of oxygen (Po_2) by blood gas determination. Normal Po_2 in a 1-day-old infant may be as low as 60 mm Hg. In certain cyanotic congenital heart defects with increased pulmonary blood flow, the Po_2 may be greater than 60 mm Hg, but the Po_2 usually does not show a large increase with a hyperoxitest (see later). An arterial oxygen saturation of 90% or above does not completely rule out a cyanotic heart defect in a newborn infant. An arterial oxygen saturation of 90% can be seen with a Po_2 of 45 to 50 mm Hg in newborns because of the normally leftward oxygen hemoglobin dissociation curve (see later). In older children and adults, a Po_2 of 60 to 65 mm Hg is needed to have 90% oxygen saturation.

INFLUENCE OF HEMOGLOBIN LEVEL ON CYANOSIS

The level of hemoglobin greatly influences the occurrence of cyanosis. This effect is graphically illustrated in Figure 11–1. As stated earlier, about 5 g/100 mL of

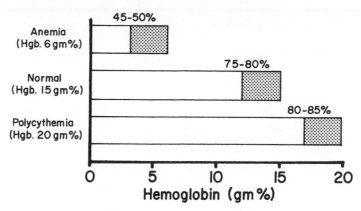

Figure 11–1. Influence of hemoglobin levels on clinical recognition of cyanosis. Cyanosis is recognizable at a higher arterial oxygen saturation in patients with polycythemia and at a lower arterial oxygen saturation in patients with anemia. See text for explanation.

reduced hemoglobin in cutaneous veins is required for the appearance of cyanosis. Normally, about 2 g/100 mL of reduced hemoglobin is present in the venules, so that an additional 3 g/100 mL of reduced hemoglobin in arterial blood produces clinical cyanosis. For a normal person with hemoglobin of 15 g/100 mL, 3 g of reduced hemoglobin results from 20% desaturation (because 3 is 20% of 15). Thus, cyanosis appears when the oxygen saturation is reduced to about 80%. Cyanosis is recognized at a higher level of oxygen saturation in patients with polycythemia and at a lower level of oxygen saturation in patients with anemia (see Fig. 11–1). For example, in a person with polycythemia with hemoglobin of 20 g/100 mL, 3 g of reduced hemoglobin results from only 15% desaturation (or at 85% arterial saturation). On the other hand, in a patient with a marked anemia (hemoglobin of 6 g/100 mL, for example), cyanosis does not appear until arterial oxygen saturation is reduced to 50% (3 g of reduced hemoglobin results from 50% desaturation).

CAUSES OF CYANOSIS

Cyanosis may have a number of causes (Box 11–1). Central cyanosis with reduced arterial oxygen saturation is significant and may be due to cyanotic congenital heart defects, lung disease, or central nervous system depression. Cyanosis of cardiac origin must be diagnosed early for proper management, but the detection of mild cyanosis is not always easy.

Rarely, cyanosis is due to methemoglobinemia. Methemoglobinemia may occur as a hereditary disorder or may be caused by toxic substances. Toxic methemoglobinemia (such as seen with ingestion of water high in nitrate or exposure to aniline teething gels) is more common than hereditary methemoglobinemia (absence of reductive pathways—NADH cytochrome b_5 reductase deficiency). When methemoglobin levels are greater than 15% of normal hemoglobin, cyanosis is visible, and a level of 70% methemoglobin is lethal. Compensatory polycythemia may occur in this condition. In methemoglobinemia, the color of the blood may remain brown, even after a full oxygenation or a long exposure to room air.

Acrocyanosis, a bluish color of fingers seen in neonates and infants, is a form of peripheral cyanosis and reflects sluggish blood flow in the fingers. It has no clinical significance unless associated with circulatory shock. Circumoral cyanosis refers to a bluish skin color around the mouth. This is a form of peripheral cyanosis seen in a healthy child with fair skin because of sluggish capillary blood flow in association with vasoconstriction. Isolated circumoral cyanosis is of no concern unless it occurs as a result of a low cardiac output.

CYANOSIS OF CARDIAC VERSUS PULMONARY ORIGIN

Differentiation of cardiac cyanosis from cyanosis caused by pulmonary diseases is crucially important for proper management of cyanotic infants. The hyperoxitest helps

BOX 11–1	CAUSES OF CYANOSIS

REDUCED ARTERIAL OXYGEN SATURATION (I.E., CENTRAL CYANOSIS)

Inadequate alveolar ventilation

Central nervous system depression

Inadequate ventilatory drive (e.g., obesity, pickwickian syndrome)

Obstruction of the airway, congenital or acquired

Structural changes in the lungs and/or ventilation-perfusion mismatch (e.g., pneumonia, cystic fibrosis, hyaline membrane disease, pulmonary edema, congestive heart failure)

Weakness of the respiratory muscles.

Desaturated blood bypassing effective alveolar units

Intracardiac right-to-left shunt (i.e., cyanotic congenital heart defect)

Intrapulmonary shunt (e.g., pulmonary atrioventricular fistula, chronic hepatic disease resulting in multiple microvascular fistulas in the lungs)

Pulmonary hypertension with the resulting right-to-left shunt at the atrial, ventricular, or ductal levels (e.g., Eisenmenger's syndrome, persistent pulmonary hypertension of the newborn)

NORMAL ARTERIAL OXYGEN SATURATION (I.E., PERIPHERAL CYANOSIS)

Increased deoxygenation in the capillaries

Circulatory shock

Congestive heart failure

Acrocyanosis of newborns

METHEMOGLOBINEMIA

Congenital methemoglobinemia

Toxic substances

Ingestion of water high in nitrates

Exposure to aniline dye teething gels

differentiate cyanosis caused by cardiac disease from that caused by pulmonary disease. In the hyperoxitest, one tests the response of arterial P_{O_2} to 100% oxygen inhalation. With pulmonary disease, arterial P_{O_2} usually rises to a level greater than 100 mm Hg. When there is a significant intracardiac right-to-left shunt, the arterial P_{O_2} does not exceed 100 mm Hg and the rise is usually not more than 10 to 30 mm Hg, although some exceptions exist. See Chapter 14 for exceptions and further discussion.

Figure 11–2 explains why breathing 100% oxygen does not significantly increase P_{O_2} in the presence of a right-to-left intracardiac shunt. Figure 11–2A is a schematic illustration of the effect of a right-to-left shunt on the P_{O_2} while breathing in room air. Assuming a cardiac output of 2 L/minute, 1 L of venous blood is distributed to ventilated alveoli, and 1 L is shunted right to left through a cardiac defect. Mixing 1 L of venous blood with an oxygen content of 19.4 mL/100 mL (P_{O_2} of 30 mm Hg) with 1 L of pulmonary venous blood containing 26.3 mL/100 mL (P_{O_2} of 100 mm Hg) results in an oxygen content of 22.8 mL/100 mL. The corresponding P_{O_2} from the dissociation curve is 41 mm Hg. Therefore, mixing 1 L of blood with a P_{O_2} of 100 mm Hg with 1 L of blood with a P_{O_2} of 30 mm Hg results in a P_{O_2} of 41 mm Hg (see Fig. 11–2A), not an arithmetic average of 65 mm Hg. With the patient breathing 100% oxygen (see Fig. 11–2B), the alveolar P_{O_2} becomes 600 mm Hg (with a corresponding oxygen content of 28.6 mL/100 mL, assuming a hemoglobin level of 20 g/100 mL; this figure is derived from 26.8 mg/100 mL of oxygen bound to hemoglobin plus 1.8 mL of oxygen dissolved in plasma [0.003×600]). When 1 L of blood with a P_{O_2} of 600 mm Hg (oxygen content 28.6 mg/100 mL) is mixed with 1 L of venous blood with a P_{O_2} of 30 mm Hg (oxygen content of 19.4 mL/100 mL), the resulting oxygen content is 24 mg/100 mL ([$28.6 + 19.4$]/2), with a corresponding P_{O_2} of 46 mm Hg (see Fig. 11–2B). Thus, breathing 100% oxygen does not significantly alter the P_{O_2} (an increase from 41 to 46 mm Hg), even though the alveolar P_{O_2} increases from 100 to 600 mm Hg.

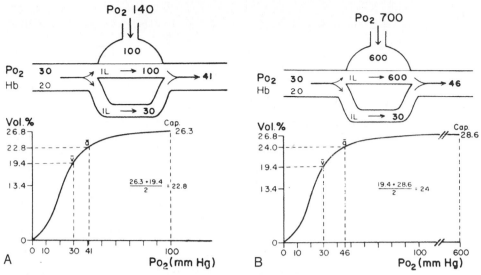

Figure 11–2. Result of hyperoxitest in cyanotic heart defects. **A,** Effect of a right-to-left shunt on the arterial Po_2 in room air. The mixing of 1 L of blood coming from normal ventilated alveoli (Po_2 of 100 mm Hg) with 1 L of venous blood flowing through the cardiac defect (Po_2 of 30 mm Hg) results in a significant decrease in arterial Po_2 (41 mm Hg). **B,** Effect of a right-to-left shunt on the arterial Po_2 in 100% oxygen. The mixing of 1 L of blood coming from normal ventilated alveoli (Po_2 of 600 mm Hg) with 1 L of venous blood flowing through the shunt (Po_2 of 30 mm Hg) results in an arterial Po_2 of 46 mm Hg. Breathing 100% oxygen does not significantly influence the hypoxemia, as the arterial Po_2 increases only from 41 to 46 mm Hg. Note that the oxygen content was calculated using an old number of 1.34 mL (rather than 1.36 mL), which can be bound to 1 g of hemoglobin. See text for a detailed description. (From Duc G: Assessment of hypoxia in the newborn: Suggestions for a practical approach. Pediatrics 48:469–481, 1971.)

HEMOGLOBIN DISSOCIATION CURVE

A full understanding of the hyperoxitest and the unique behavior of fetal hemoglobin requires knowledge of the hemoglobin dissociation curve. The relationship between the Po_2 and the amount of oxygen bound to hemoglobin and the relationship between the Po_2 and the oxygen dissolved in plasma are different. The relationship is S shaped (sigmoid) for hemoglobin; the relationship is linear for plasma. For dissolved oxygen in plasma, the solubility coefficient is 0.003 mL/100 mL at a Po_2 of 1 mm Hg at 37°C (or 0.3 mL of oxygen/100 mL plasma at a Po_2 of 100 mm Hg).

The sigmoid relationship between the Po_2 and the amount of oxygen bound to hemoglobin is expressed by the oxygen-hemoglobin dissociation curve (Fig. 11–3). The Po_2 at which 50% of hemoglobin is saturated has been chosen as the reference point, called P50. The P50 averages 27 mm Hg in the adult and 22 mm Hg in the fetus and newborn. The position of the dissociation curve is an expression of the affinity of hemoglobin for oxygen. The newborn's curve (curve A), with high oxygen affinity, favors the extraction of oxygen from the maternal circulation and suits the conditions of the intrauterine environment, but fetal hemoglobin is "stingy" hemoglobin; it does not allow easy release of oxygen to tissues as in adults. The adult curve (curve B), with a decreased affinity for oxygen, allows the release of more oxygen to tissues. The adult curve is reached by 3 months of age.

The pH, Pco_2, and erythrocyte concentrations of 2,3-diphosphoglycerate (2,3-DPG), adenosine triphosphate (ATP), methemoglobin, and carboxyhemoglobin influence the position of the dissociation curve (see Fig. 11–3).

1. A decrease in hydrogen ion concentration (or increased pH), Pco_2, temperature, 2,3-DPG, and ATP concentrations shifts the curve to the left (curve A).

2. An increase in these parameters shifts the curve to the right (curve C).

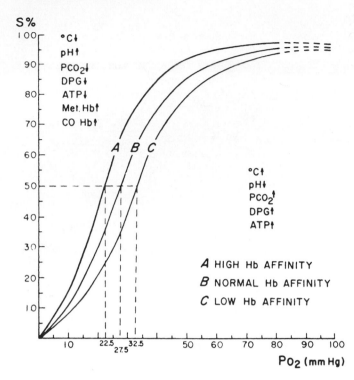

Figure 11–3. Factors that influence the position of the oxygen-hemoglobin dissociation curve. Curve B is from a normal adult at 38°C, pH 7.40, and Pco_2 35.0 mm Hg. Curves A and C illustrate the effect on the affinity for oxygen (P50) of variations in temperature (°C), pH, Pco_2, 2,3-diphosphoglycerate, adenosine triphosphate, methemoglobin, and carboxyhemoglobin. Curve A is of the newborn. (From Duc G: Assessment of hypoxia in the newborn: Suggestions for a practical approach. Pediatrics 48:469–481, 1971.)

3. Fetal hemoglobin has considerably less affinity for 2,3-DPG (40%) than adult hemoglobin. This makes fetal hemoglobin behave as if 2,3-DPG levels are low, thus shifting the curve to the left.

4. The curve shifts to the right in compensation for high altitude, cyanosis, or anemia, as a result of an increase in the red cell concentration of 2,3-DPG.

CONSEQUENCES AND COMPLICATIONS

Polycythemia. Low arterial oxygen content stimulates bone marrow through erythropoietin release from the kidneys and produces an increased number of red blood cells. Polycythemia, with a resulting increase in oxygen-carrying capacity, benefits cyanotic children. However, when the hematocrit reaches 65% or higher, a sharp increase in the viscosity of blood occurs, and the polycythemic response becomes disadvantageous, particularly if there is congestive heart failure (CHF). Some cyanotic infants have a relative iron deficiency state, with normal or lower than normal hemoglobin and hypochromia on blood smear. A normal hemoglobin in a cyanotic patient represents a relative anemic state. Although less cyanotic, these infants are usually more symptomatic and improve when iron therapy raises the hemoglobin.

Clubbing. Clubbing is caused by soft tissue growth under the nail bed as a consequence of central cyanosis. The mechanism for soft tissue growth is unclear. One hypothesis is that megakaryocytes present in the systemic venous blood may be responsible for the change. In normal persons, platelets are formed from the cytoplasm of the megakaryocytes by fragmentation during their passage through the pulmonary circulation. The cytoplasm of megakaryocytes contains growth factors (e.g., platelet-derived growth factor and transforming growth factor β). In patients with right-to-left shunts, megakaryocytes with their cytoplasm may enter the systemic circulation, become trapped in the capillaries of the digits, and release growth factors, which in turn cause clubbing. Clubbing usually does not occur until a child is 6 months or older, and it is seen first and is most pronounced in the thumb. In the early stage, it appears as shininess and redness of the fingertips. When it is fully developed, the fingers and toes become thick and wide and have convex nail beds (see Fig. 2–1). Clubbing is also seen in patients with liver disease or subacute bacterial endocarditis and on a hereditary basis without cyanosis.

Central Nervous System Complications. Either very high hematocrit levels or iron-deficient red blood cells place individuals with cyanotic congenital heart defects at risk for disorders of the central nervous system, such as brain abscess and vascular stroke. In the past, cyanotic CHDs accounted for 5% to 10% of all cases of brain abscesses. The predisposition for brain abscesses may partially result from the fact that right-to-left intracardiac shunts may bypass the normally effective phagocytic filtering actions of the pulmonary capillary bed. This predisposition may also result from the fact that polycythemia and the consequent high viscosity of blood lead to tissue hypoxia and microinfarction of the brain, which are later complicated by bacterial colonization. The triad of symptoms of brain abscesses are fever, headache, and focal neurologic deficit.

Vascular stroke caused by embolization arising from thrombus in the cardiac chamber or in the systemic veins may be associated with surgery or cardiac catheterization. Cerebral venous thrombosis may occur, often in infants younger than 2 years who have cyanosis and relative iron deficiency anemia. A possible explanation for these findings is that microcytosis further exacerbates hyperviscosity resulting from polycythemia.

Bleeding Disorders. Disturbances of hemostasis are frequently present in children with severe cyanosis and polycythemia. Most frequently noted are thrombocytopenia and defective platelet aggregation. Other abnormalities include prolonged prothrombin time and partial thromboplastin time and lower levels of fibrinogen and factors V and VIII. Clinical manifestations may include easy bruising, petechiae of the skin and mucous membranes, epistaxis, and gingival bleeding. Red cell withdrawal and replacement with an equal volume of plasma tend to correct the hemorrhagic tendency and lower blood viscosity.

Hypoxic Spells and Squatting. Although most frequently seen in infants with tetralogy of Fallot (TOF), hypoxic spells may occur in infants with other congenital heart defects (see later section on TOF for further discussion).

Depressed Intelligent Quotient. Children with chronic hypoxia and cyanosis have a lower than expected intelligence quotient as well as poorer perceptual and gross motor functions than children with acyanotic congenital heart defects, even after surgical repair of cyanotic heart defects.

Scoliosis. Children with chronic cyanosis, particularly girls and patients with TOF, often have scoliosis.

Hyperuricemia and Gout. Hyperuricemia and gout tend to occur in older patients with uncorrected or inadequately repaired cyanotic heart defects.

The pathophysiology of individual cyanotic heart defects is discussed in the following section.

Common Cyanotic Heart Defects

COMPLETE TRANSPOSITION OF THE GREAT ARTERIES

Complete transposition of the great arteries (D-TGA) is the most common cyanotic congenital heart defect in newborns, at least in Western countries. In this condition, the aorta arises from the right ventricle (RV) and the pulmonary artery (PA) arises from the left ventricle (LV). As the result, the normal anteroposterior relationship of the great arteries is reversed, so that the aorta is anterior to the PA (transposition), but the aorta remains to the right of the PA; thus, the prefix D is used for dextroposition. In levo-transposition of the great arteries (L-TGA, or congenitally corrected TGA), the aorta is anterior to and to the left of the PA; therefore, the prefix L is used (see Chapter 14). The atria and ventricles are in normal relationship. The coronary arteries arise from the aorta, as in a normal heart. Desaturated blood returning from the body to the right atrium (RA) flows out of the aorta without being oxygenated in the lungs and then returns to the RA. Therefore, tissues, including vital organs such as the brain and heart, are

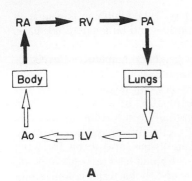

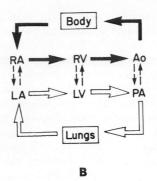

Figure 11–4. Circulation pathways of normal "in series" circulation (**A**) and the "in parallel" circulation of transposition of the great arteries (**B**). Open arrows denote oxygenated blood; closed arrows, desaturated blood. AO, aorta; LA, left atrium; LV, left ventricle; PA, pulmonary artery; RA, right atrium; RV, right ventricle.

perfused by blood with a low oxygen saturation. Conversely, well-oxygenated blood returning to the left atrium (LA) flows out of the PA and returns to the LA. This results in a complete separation of the two circuits. The two circuits are said to be in parallel rather than in series, as in normal circulation (Fig. 11–4). This defect is incompatible with life unless communication between the two circuits occurs to provide the necessary oxygen to the body. This communication can occur at the atrial, ventricular, or ductal level or at any combination of these levels.

In the most frequently encountered form of D-TGA, only a small communication exists between the atria, usually a patent foramen ovale (PFO) (Fig. 11–5A). The newborn is notably cyanotic from birth and has an arterial oxygen saturation of 30% to 50%. The low arterial Po_2, which ranges from 20 to 30 mm Hg, causes an anaerobic glycolysis, with resulting metabolic acidosis. Hypoxia and acidosis are detrimental to myocardial function. The normal postnatal decrease in pulmonary vascular resistance (PVR) results in increased pulmonary blood flow (PBF) and volume overload to the LA and LV. Severe hypoxia and acidosis (with a resulting decrease in myocardial function) and volume overload to the left side of the heart cause CHF during the first week of life. Therefore, chest x-ray films show cardiomegaly and increased pulmonary vascularity. Unless hypoxia and acidosis are corrected, the condition of these infants deteriorates rapidly. Hypoxia and acidosis stimulate the carotid and cerebral chemoreceptors, causing hyperventilation and a low Pco_2 in the pulmonary circulation. Other metabolic problems encountered are hypoglycemia, which is probably secondary to pancreatic islet hypertrophy and hyperinsulinism, and a tendency toward hypothermia. The ECG shows

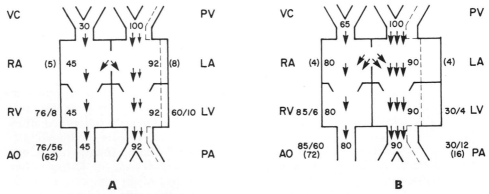

Figure 11–5. Diagrammatic representation of the hemodynamics of transposition of the great arteries with inadequate mixing (**A**) and with good mixing at the atrial level (**B**). Numbers within the diagram denote oxygen saturation values, and those outside the diagram denote pressure values. AO, aorta; LA, left atrium; LV, left ventricle; PA, pulmonary artery; PV, pulmonary vein; RA, right atrium; RV, right ventricle; VC, vena cava.

right ventricular hypertrophy (RVH), but RVH may be difficult to diagnose in the first days of life because of the normal dominance of the RV at this age. Usually no heart murmur is noted in a neonate with D-TGA, although a murmur is commonly found in other forms of cyanotic heart defects. The S2 is single, mainly because the pulmonary valve is farther from the chest wall, causing the P2 to be inaudible. A deeply cyanotic newborn with increased pulmonary vascular markings and cardiomegaly without heart murmur can be considered to have TGA until proved otherwise.

The presence of a large atrial septal defect (ASD) is most desirable in infants with TGA. When a large ASD is present, infants have good arterial oxygen saturation (as high as 80% to 90%) because of good mixing (see Fig. 11–5B). Therefore, hypoxia and metabolic acidosis are not the problems in these children. In fact, the idea of the balloon atrial septostomy (Rashkind procedure) was derived from the natural history of infants with TGA and large ASDs. However, the frequency of a large ASD occurring naturally in TGA is low. Infants who have had successful balloon atrial septostomies behave like those with naturally occurring ASDs. As the PVR falls after birth, PBF increases, with an increase in the size of the LA and LV. Although these infants are not hypoxic or acidotic, CHF develops because of volume overload to the left side of the heart. Because the RV is the systemic ventricle, RVH becomes evident on the ECG.

When associated with a large ventricular septal defect (VSD), only minimal arterial desaturation is present, and cyanosis may be missed (Fig. 11–6A). Therefore, metabolic acidosis does not develop, but left-sided heart failure results within the first few weeks of life as the PBF increases with decreasing PVR. Chest x-ray films reflect this, showing cardiomegaly with increased pulmonary vascularity. The ECG may show biventricular hypertrophy (BVH) when the VSD is large: RVH because of the systemic RV, and left ventricular hypertrophy (LVH) because of volume overload of the left side of the heart. A heart murmur of VSD is present, and the S2 is single because the P2 is inaudible or pulmonary hypertension is present.

When the VSD is associated with pulmonary stenosis (PS) in infants with TGA, although the VSD helps good mixing, the volume of fully saturated blood returning from the lungs is inadequate (see Fig. 11–6B). Likewise, even after a well-performed Rashkind procedure, the arterial oxygen saturation does not increase much because of the decreased PBF. These infants have severe hypoxia and acidosis and may succumb early in life. This is a good illustration of how the magnitude of PBF affects the arterial oxygen saturation in a given cyanotic congenital heart defect. Because PBF is not increased, the left cardiac chambers are not under increased volume work; therefore, cardiac enlargement and CHF do not develop. X-ray films, therefore, show normal heart size and normal or decreased pulmonary vascularity. The ECG shows evidence of BVH; LVH is

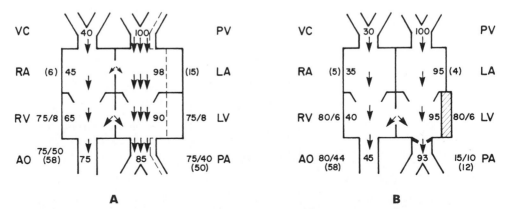

Figure 11–6. *Diagrammatic representation of the hemodynamic abnormalities in transposition of the great arteries with a large ventricular septal defect (VSD) (**A**) and with VSD and pulmonary stenosis (**B**). Numbers within the diagram denote oxygen saturation values, and those outside the diagram denote pressure values. Abbreviations are the same as those in Figure 11–5.*

present because of PS, and RVH is present because of the nature of TGA. Physical examination reveals a PS murmur and a single S2, in addition to cyanosis.

PERSISTENT TRUNCUS ARTERIOSUS AND SINGLE VENTRICLE

In persistent truncus arteriosus (Fig. 11–7A), a single arterial blood vessel (truncus arteriosus) arises from the heart. The PA or its branches arise from the truncus arteriosus, and the truncus continues as the aorta. A large VSD is always present in this condition. In single ventricle (also called double-inlet ventricle) (see Fig. 11–7B), two atrioventricular (AV) valves empty into a single ventricular chamber from which a great artery (either the aorta or PA) arises. The other great artery arises from a rudimentary ventricular chamber attached to the main ventricle. The opening between the single ventricle and the rudimentary chamber is called the bulboventricular foramen. No ventricular septum of significance is present (see Fig. 14–61).

The following similarities exist between persistent truncus arteriosus and single ventricle from a hemodynamic point of view:

1. There is almost complete mixing of systemic and pulmonary venous blood in the ventricle, and the oxygen saturation of blood in the two great arteries is similar.

2. Pressures in both ventricles are identical.

3. The level of oxygen saturation in the systemic circulation is proportional to the magnitude of PBF.

In addition to the level of PVR, the magnitude of PBF is determined by the caliber of the PA in the case of persistent truncus arteriosus and by the presence or absence of PS and the size of the VSD (i.e., the bulboventricular foramen) in the case of single ventricle. When the PBF is large, the patient is minimally cyanotic but may develop CHF because of an excessive volume overload placed on the ventricle. In contrast, when the PBF is small, the patient is severely cyanotic and does not develop CHF because there is no volume overload. The latter group of patients and those with TOF share similar clinical pictures.

Physical examination reveals varying degrees of cyanosis, depending on the magnitude of PBF. A heart murmur of the VSD is rarely audible because of the presence of a huge defect. There may be an ejection systolic murmur caused by the stenosis of the pulmonary valve or of the PA branches. An early diastolic murmur of truncal valve regurgitation may be heard. The ECG usually shows BVH in both conditions. In single ventricle, the QRS complexes of all precordial leads (i.e., V1 through V6) are recorded over one ventricle, and therefore they are similar (with poor R/S progression), suggestive of BVH. Chest x-ray findings are determined by the magnitude of PBF—if the magnitude of the PBF is large, the heart size is large and the pulmonary vascularity increases; if the magnitude is small, the heart size is small and the pulmonary vascularity decreases.

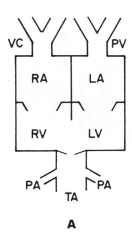
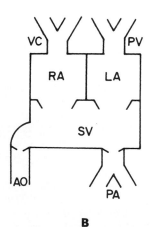

A   **B**

Figure 11–7. *Diagrammatic representation of persistent truncus arteriosus (**A**) and a common form of single ventricle (**B**). AO, aorta; LA, left atrium; LV, left ventricle; PA, pulmonary artery; PV, pulmonary vein; RA, right atrium; RV, right ventricle; SV, single ventricle; TA, truncus arteriosus; VC, vena cava.*

With increased PBF and resulting pulmonary hypertension, CHF and later pulmonary vascular obstructive disease (i.e., Eisenmenger's syndrome) may develop.

TETRALOGY OF FALLOT

The classic description of TOF includes the following four abnormalities: VSD, pulmonary stenosis (PS), RVH, and overriding of the aorta. From a physiologic point of view, TOF requires only two abnormalities—a VSD large enough to equalize systolic pressures in both ventricles and a stenosis of the right ventricular outflow tract (RVOT) in the form of infundibular stenosis, valvular stenosis, or both. RVH is secondary to PS, and the degree of overriding of the aorta varies widely and it is not always present. The severity of the RVOT obstruction determines the direction and the magnitude of the shunt through the VSD. With mild stenosis, the shunt is left to right, and the clinical picture resembles that of a VSD. This is called acyanotic or pink TOF (Fig. 11–8A). With a more severe stenosis, the shunt is right to left, resulting in "cyanotic" TOF (see Fig. 11–8B). In the extreme form of TOF, the pulmonary valve is atretic, with right-to-left shunting of the entire systemic venous return through the VSD. In this case, the PBF is provided through a patent ductus arteriosus (PDA) or multiple collateral arteries arising from the aorta, or both. In TOF, regardless of the direction of the ventricular shunt, the systolic pressure in the RV equals that of the LV and the aorta (see Fig. 11–8A and B). The mere combination of a small VSD and a PS is not TOF; the size of the VSD must be nearly as large as the annulus of the aortic valve to equalize the pressure in the RV and LV.

In acyanotic TOF, a small to moderate left-to-right ventricular shunt is present, and the systolic pressures are equal in the RV, LV, and aorta (see Fig. 11–8A). There is a mild to moderate pressure gradient between the RV and PA, and the PA pressure may be slightly elevated (because of a less severe stenosis of the RVOT). Because the presence of the PS minimizes the magnitude of the left-to-right shunt, the heart size and the pulmonary vascularity increase only slightly to moderately. These increases are indistinguishable from those of a small to moderate VSD. However, unlike the finding with VSDs, the ECG always shows RVH because the RV pressure is always high. Occasionally, LVH is also present. The heart murmurs are caused by the PS and the VSD. Therefore, the murmur is a superimposition of an ejection systolic murmur of PS and a regurgitant systolic murmur of a VSD. The murmur is best audible along the lower left and mid-left sternal borders, and it sometimes extends to the upper left sternal border. Therefore, in a child who has physical and x-ray findings similar to those of a small VSD,

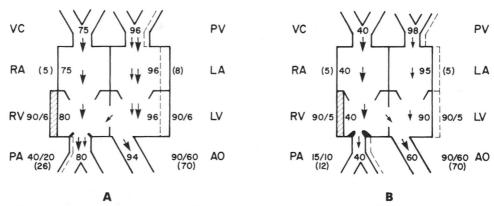

*Figure 11–8. Hemodynamics of acyanotic (**A**) and cyanotic (**B**) tetralogy of Fallot. Numbers within the diagram denote oxygen saturation values, and those outside the diagram denote pressure values. In both conditions, the systolic pressure in the right ventricle (RV) is identical to that in the left ventricle (LV) and the aorta (AO) and there is a significant pressure gradient between the RV and the pulmonary artery (PA). In the acyanotic form (**A**), pulmonary blood flow is slightly to moderately increased, whereas in the cyanotic form (**B**), pulmonary blood flow is decreased. Other abbreviations are the same as those in Figure 11–5.*

the presence of RVH or BVH on the ECG should raise the possibility of acyanotic TOF. (A small VSD is associated with LVH or a normal ECG rather than with RVH or BVH.) Right aortic arch, if present, confirms the diagnosis. Infants with acyanotic TOF become cyanotic over time, usually by 1 or 2 years of age, and have clinical pictures of cyanotic TOF, including exertional dyspnea and squatting.

In infants with classic cyanotic TOF, the presence of severe PS produces a right-to-left shunt at the ventricular level (i.e., cyanosis), with decreased PBF (see Fig. 11–8B). The PAs are small, and the LA and LV may be slightly smaller than normal because of a reduction in the pulmonary venous return to the left side of the heart. Therefore, chest x-ray films show a normal heart size with decreased pulmonary vascularity. The systolic pressures are identical in the RV, LV, and aorta. The ECG demonstrates RVH because of the high pressure in the RV. The right-to-left ventricular shunt is silent, and the heart murmur audible in this condition originates in the PS (ejection-type murmur). The ejection systolic murmur is best audible at the mid-left sternal border (over the infundibular stenosis) or occasionally at the upper left sternal border (in patients with pulmonary valve stenosis). The intensity and the duration of the heart murmur are proportional to the amount of blood flow through the stenotic valve. When the PS is mild, a relatively large amount of blood goes through the stenotic valve (with a relatively small right-to-left ventricular shunt), producing a loud, long systolic murmur (Fig 11–9A). However, with severe PS, there is a relatively large right-to-left ventricular shunt that is silent, and only a small amount of blood goes through the PS, producing a short, faint systolic murmur (see Fig 11–9A). In other words, the intensity and duration of the systolic murmur are inversely related to the severity of the PS. These findings are in contrast to those seen in isolated PS (see Fig. 11–9A and B). Because of low pressure in the PA, the P2 is soft and often inaudible, resulting in a single S2. The heart size on x-ray films is normal in TOF because none of the heart chambers handle an increased amount of blood. If a cyanotic infant has a large heart on the chest x-ray examination, especially with an increase in pulmonary vascularity, TOF is extremely unlikely unless the child has undergone a large systemic-to-PA shunt operation. Another important point is that an infant with TOF does not develop CHF. This is because no cardiac chamber is under volume overload and the pressure overload placed on the RV (not higher than the aortic pressure, which is under baroreceptor control) is well tolerated.

The extreme form of TOF is that associated with pulmonary atresia, in which the only source of PBF is through a constricting PDA or through multiple aortic collateral arteries. All systemic venous return is shunted right to left at the ventricular level, resulting in a marked systemic arterial desaturation. Probably the more important reason for such severe cyanosis is the markedly reduced PBF, with resulting reduction of pulmonary venous return to the left side of the heart. Unless the patency of the ductus is maintained, the infant may die. Infusion of prostaglandin E$_1$ has been successful in keeping the ductus open in this and other forms of cyanotic congenital heart defects that

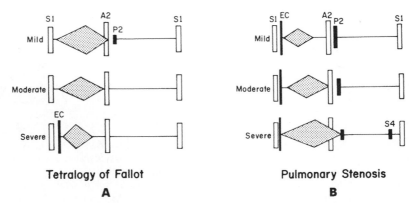

Tetralogy of Fallot

A

Pulmonary Stenosis

B

*Figure 11–9. Comparison of ejection systolic murmurs in tetralogy of Fallot (**A**) and isolated pulmonary valve stenosis (**B**) (see text). EC, ejection click.*

rely on the patency of the ductus arteriosus for PBF. Heart murmur is absent, or a faint murmur of PDA is present. RVH is present on the ECG as in other forms of TOF. Chest x-ray films show a small heart and a markedly reduced PBF.

It is important to understand what controls the degree of cyanosis and the amount of PBF in patients with TOF because this concept relates to the mechanism and treatment of the "hypoxic" spell of TOF. Because the VSD of TOF is large enough to equalize systolic pressures in both ventricles, the RV and LV may be viewed as a single chamber that ejects blood to the systemic and pulmonary circuits (Fig. 11–10). The ratio of flows to the pulmonary and systemic circuits ($\dot{Q}p/\dot{Q}s$) is related to the ratio of resistance offered by the right ventricular outflow obstruction (shown as pulmonary resistance in Fig. 11–10) and the systemic vascular resistance (SVR). Either an increase in the pulmonary resistance or a decrease in the SVR increases the degree of the right-to-left shunt, producing more severe arterial desaturation. On the contrary, more blood passes through the right ventricular outflow obstruction when the SVR increases or when the pulmonary resistance decreases. Although controversies exist over the role of the spasm of the RVOT as an initiating event for the hypoxic spell, there is no evidence that the spasm actually occurs as a primary event. Pulmonary valve stenosis has a fixed resistance and does not produce spasm. The infundibular stenosis, which consists of disorganized muscle fibers intermingled with fibrous tissue, is almost nonreactive to sympathetic stimulation or catecholamines. The hypoxic spell also occurs in patients with TOF with pulmonary atresia in which the presence or absence of spasm would have no role in the spell. Therefore, it is more likely that changes in the SVR play a primary role in controlling the degree of the right-to-left shunt and the amount of PBF. A decrease in the SVR increases the right-to-left shunt and decreases the PBF with a resulting increase in cyanosis. In this case, the RVOT dimension may decrease, but it is probably secondary to the decreased amount of blood flowing through it rather than primary spasm. Conversely, an increase in SVR decreases the right-to-left shunt and forces more blood through the stenotic RVOT. This results in an improvement in the arterial oxygen saturation. Therefore, the likelihood of the RVOT spasm initiating the right-to-left shunt is remote. Also, excessive tachycardia or hypovolemia can increase the right-to-left shunt through the VSD, resulting in a fall in the systemic arterial oxygen saturation. The resulting hypoxia can initiate the hypoxic spell. Tachycardia or hypovolemia may narrow down the RV outflow tract, and a reduction of blood pressure related to hypovolemia can initiate hypoxic spell by increasing right-to-left ventricular shunt. Slowing of the heart rate by β-adrenergic blockers, volume expansion, and interventions that increase the SVR have all been used to terminate the hypoxic spell.

The hypoxic spell, also called the cyanotic spell, tet spell, or hypercyanotic spell, occurs in young infants with TOF. It consists of hyperpnea (i.e., rapid and deep respiration), worsening cyanosis, and disappearance of the heart murmur. This occasionally results in complications of the central nervous system and even death. Any event such as crying, defecation, or increased physical activity that suddenly lowers the SVR or produces a large right-to-left ventricular shunt may initiate the spell and, if not corrected, establishes a vicious circle of hypoxic spells (Fig. 11–11). The sudden onset of tachycardia or hypovolemia can also cause the spell as discussed earlier. The resulting

Figure 11–10. Simplified concept of tetralogy of Fallot that demonstrates how a change in the systemic vascular resistance (SVR) or right ventricular outflow tract (RVOT) obstruction (pulmonary resistance [PR]) affects the direction and the magnitude of the ventricular shunt. AO, aorta; LV, left ventricle; PA, pulmonary artery; RV, right ventricle.

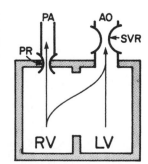

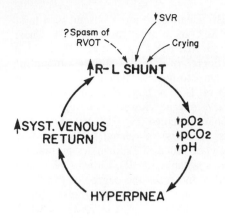

Figure 11–11. *Mechanism of hypoxic spell. A decrease in the arterial PO$_2$ stimulates the respiratory center, and hyperventilation results. Hyperpnea increases systemic venous return. In the presence of a fixed right ventricular outflow tract (RVOT), the increased systemic venous return results in increased right-to-left (R-L) shunt, worsening cyanosis. A vicious circle is established. SVR, systemic vascular resistance.*

fall in arterial Po$_2$, in addition to an increase in Pco$_2$ and a fall in pH, stimulates the respiratory center and produces hyperpnea. The hyperpnea, in turn, makes the negative thoracic pump more efficient and results in an increase in the systemic venous return to the RV. In the presence of fixed resistance at the RVOT (i.e., pulmonary resistance) or decreased SVR, the increased systemic venous return to the RV must go out the aorta. This leads to a further decrease in the arterial oxygen saturation, which establishes a vicious circle of hypoxic spells (see Fig. 11–11).

Treatment of hypoxic spells is aimed at breaking this circle by using one or more of the following maneuvers:

1. Picking up the infant in such a way that it assumes the knee-chest position and traps systemic venous blood in the legs, thereby temporarily decreasing systemic venous return and helping to calm the baby. The knee-chest position may also increase SVR by reducing arterial blood flow to the lower extremities.

2. Morphine sulfate suppresses the respiratory center and abolishes hyperpnea.

3. Sodium bicarbonate (NaHCO$_3$) corrects acidosis and eliminates the respiratory center–stimulating effect of acidosis.

4. Administration of oxygen may improve arterial oxygen saturation a little.

5. Vasoconstrictors such as phenylephrine raise SVR and improve arterial oxygen saturation.

6. Ketamine is a good drug to use because it simultaneously increases SVR and sedates the patient. Both effects are known to help terminate the spell.

7. Propranolol has been used successfully in some cases of hypoxic spell, both acute and chronic. Its mechanism of action is not entirely clear. When administered for acute cases, propranolol may slow the heart rate and perhaps reduce the spasm of the RVOT (although this is not likely as discussed previously) More important, propranolol may increase SVR by antagonizing the vasodilating effects of β-adrenergic stimulation. The successful use of propranolol in the prevention of hypoxic spell is more likely the result of the drug's peripheral action. The drug may stabilize vascular reactivity of the systemic arteries, thereby preventing a sudden decrease in SVR (see Chapter 14).

Infants and toddlers with mildly cyanotic TOF often assume a squatting position after having played hard. During the play, these infants become tachypneic and dusky. When they assume a squatting position and rest a little while, these symptoms disappear and they resume playing. What is the mechanism of recovery from these symptoms during squatting? The squatting position is the same as the knee-chest position (which is used to treat hypoxic spells). The squatting or knee-chest position increases systemic arterial oxygen saturation as shown in an experimental study (Fig. 11–12). Three mechanisms

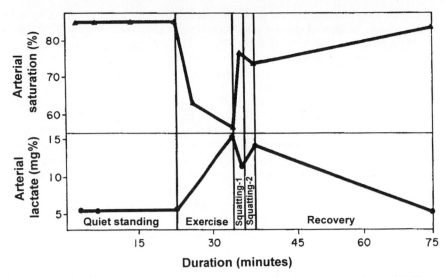

Figure 11–12. *Hemodynamic changes with squatting. An adult patient with tetralogy of Fallot was studied during cardiac catheterization with determinations of arterial oxygen saturation and arterial lactate levels. The latter was used as an indicator of the change in the systemic venous return. With exercise, there is an immediate drop in the arterial saturation and an increase in systemic venous return. With squatting (a knee-chest position), there is an immediate rise in arterial oxygen saturation and a drop in systemic venous return. (From Guntheroth WG, Morgan BC, Mullins GL, Baum D: Venous return with knee-chest position and squatting in tetralogy of Fallot. Am Heart J 75:313–318, 1968.)*

may be involved. First, reduction of the systemic venous return by trapping venous blood in the lower extremities reduces right-to-left shunt at the ventricular level (evidenced by reduced arterial lactate levels in Fig. 11–12). Second, reduced arterial blood flow to the legs reduces venous washout from leg muscles. Third, squatting may also increase SVR, a known mechanism to reduce right-to-left ventricular shunt.

TRICUSPID ATRESIA

In tricuspid atresia, the tricuspid valve and a portion of the RV do not exist (Fig. 11–13). Because no direct communication exists between the RA and RV, systemic venous return to the RA must be shunted first to the LA through an ASD or PFO. There is usually a VSD (or PDA) for the pulmonary arteries to receive some blood for survival. In order

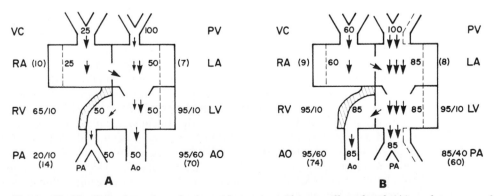

Figure 11–13. *Hemodynamics of tricuspid atresia with normally related (A) and transposed (B) great arteries. Numbers within the diagram denote oxygen saturations, and those outside the diagram denote pressure values. Abbreviations are the same as those in Figure 11–5.*

for the right-to-left shunt to occur, the RA pressure is elevated in excess of the LA pressure, and enlargement of the RA results (i.e., right atrial hypertrophy [RAH] on the ECG and right atrial enlargement on x-ray films). The LA and LV receive both systemic and pulmonary venous returns and thereby dilate (i.e., enlargement of the LA and LV on x-ray films). The volume overload placed on the LV is unopposed by the hypoplastic RV, with resulting LVH on the ECG. Therefore, the ECG shows RAH and LVH, and the x-ray films show an enlargement of the RA, LA, and LV. In addition, a "superior" QRS axis is a characteristic ECG finding in tricuspid atresia, as in endocardial cushion defect. Embryologically, there is a similarity between these two defects; tricuspid atresia results from an abnormal development of the endocardial cushion tissue, that is, an incomplete shift of the common AV canal to the right. Developmental abnormalities in the endocardial cushion tissue may explain the similar QRS axis in both conditions.

Oxygen saturation values are equal in the aorta and the PA because there is complete mixing of systemic and pulmonary venous blood in the LV, from which both the systemic and the pulmonary circulations receive blood. The level of arterial saturation directly relates to the magnitude of PBF. Anatomically, the great arteries are normally related in about 70% of cases and transposed in about 30% of cases (see Fig 11–13A and B). In patients with normally related great arteries (see Fig. 11–13A) the PBF is generally reduced because it comes through a small VSD, hypoplastic RV, and/or small PAs. Therefore, arterial oxygen saturation is low, and the infant is notably cyanotic. In infants with transposed great arteries (see Fig. 11–13B) the PBF is usually increased. Therefore, these infants are only mildly cyanotic; their heart size is large, and their pulmonary vascular markings are increased. However, because of an interplay of other factors such as the size of the VSD, the presence or absence of PS or pulmonary atresia, as well as the patency of the ductus arteriosus, some infants with normally related great arteries may have increased PBF, and some infants with TGA may have decreased PBF. The magnitude of PBF determines not only the level of arterial oxygen saturation but also the degree of enlargement of the cardiac chambers.

No physical findings are characteristic of tricuspid atresia. These infants have varying degrees of cyanosis, and most have a heart murmur of VSD. A PS murmur, if present, is characteristic. In patients with increased PBF, an increased amount of blood passing through the mitral valve may produce an apical diastolic rumble. The liver may be enlarged because of increased pressure in the RA, which may result from an inadequate interatrial communication or heart failure.

In summary, tricuspid atresia is the most likely diagnosis if a cyanotic infant has an ECG that shows a superior QRS axis, RAH, and LVH and chest x-ray films that show enlargement of the RA (with or without left atrial enlargement), a concave PA segment, and decreased pulmonary vascularity.

PULMONARY ATRESIA

In pulmonary atresia, direct communication between the RV cavity and the PA does not exist; the PDA (or collateral arteries) is the major source of blood flow to the lungs. The systemic venous return to the RA must go to the LA through an ASD or a PFO. The RA enlarges and hypertrophies to maintain a right-to-left atrial shunt (resulting in right atrial enlargement on x-ray films and RAH on the ECG). The RV is usually hypoplastic with a thick ventricular wall, but occasionally the RV is normal in size; tricuspid regurgitation (TR) is usually present in the latter situation. Systemic and pulmonary venous returns mix in the LA and go to the LV to supply the body and lungs (Fig. 11–14). The volume load placed on the left side of the heart (i.e., LA and LV) is proportionally related to the magnitude of PBF. Because the PDA is the major source of PBF and it may close after birth, the PBF is usually decreased. When multiple collateral arteries are the only source of PBF, they are usually not adequate and PBF is reduced. Therefore, the infant is severely cyanotic, and the overall heart size is normal or only slightly increased. The hypoplasia of the RV and possible volume overload to the LV produce LVH on the ECG.

The infant is usually notably cyanotic, and the S2 is single because there is only one semilunar valve to close. A faint, continuous murmur of PDA may be present.

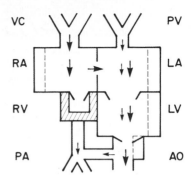

Figure 11–14. *Hemodynamics of pulmonary atresia. The chambers that enlarge are similar to those in tricuspid atresia; therefore, x-ray findings are similar in tricuspid atresia and pulmonary atresia. The ECG also shows left ventricular hypertrophy but without the characteristic "superior" QRS axis of tricuspid atresia. Because of the decreased pulmonary blood flow, the aortic saturation is low, and the infant is notably cyanotic. Abbreviations are the same as those in Figure 11–5.*

Closure of the ductus results in a rapid deterioration of the infant's condition unless there are enough collateral arteries supplying PBF. Reopening or maintaining the patency of the ductus arteriosus with infusion of prostaglandin E_1 increases the PBF, improves cyanosis, and stabilizes the infant's condition.

In summary, a severely cyanotic newborn with decreased pulmonary vascularity and normal or slightly enlarged heart size on chest x-ray films and RAH or biatrial hypertrophy and LVH on the ECG may have pulmonary atresia. The QRS axis is usually normal, in contrast to the superior QRS axis seen in tricuspid atresia. Either a faint, continuous murmur of PDA or a soft regurgitant systolic murmur of TR may be present.

TOTAL ANOMALOUS PULMONARY VENOUS RETURN

In total anomalous pulmonary venous return (TAPVR), the pulmonary veins drain abnormally to the RA, either directly or indirectly through its venous tributaries. An ASD is usually present to send blood from the RA to the LA and LV. Depending on the drainage site, TAPVR may be divided into the following three types (see Fig. 14–30):

1. Supracardiac: The common pulmonary vein drains to the superior vena cava through the vertical vein and the left innominate vein.

2. Cardiac: The pulmonary veins empty into the RA directly or indirectly through the coronary sinus.

3. Infracardiac (or subdiaphragmatic): The common pulmonary vein traverses the diaphragm and drains into the portal or hepatic vein or the inferior vena cava.

Physiologically, however, TAPVR may be divided into two types—obstructive and nonobstructive, depending on the presence or absence of an obstruction to the pulmonary venous return. The infracardiac type is usually obstructive, and the majority of the cardiac and supracardiac types are nonobstructive.

The hemodynamics of the nonobstructive types of TAPVR are similar to those of a large ASD. The amount of blood that goes to the LA through the ASD, rather than to the RV, is determined by the size of the interatrial communication and the relative compliance of the ventricles. Because right ventricular compliance normally increases after birth, with a rapid fall in PVR, and the ASD may be inadequate in size, more blood enters the RV than the LA. Thus, volume overload of the right side of the heart and the pulmonary circulation results, with enlargement of the RA, RV, PA, and pulmonary veins (Fig. 11–15A). Chest x-ray films show this as an enlargement of the RA and RV, a prominent PA segment, and increased pulmonary vascular markings. The pressures in the RA, RV, and PA are slightly elevated. The ECG shows RBBB or RVH, as in secundum ASD, and occasional RAH. Because there is complete mixing of systemic and pulmonary venous blood in the RA, oxygen saturation values are almost identical in the aorta and the PA. Cardiac examination reveals an ejection systolic murmur of PS (at the upper left sternal border) and a diastolic murmur of tricuspid stenosis because the pulmonary and tricuspid valves handle three arrows (see Fig. 11–15A). The S2 splits widely for the same reasons as it does for ASD. This contributes to the characteristic "quadruple" rhythm of TAPVR, which consists of an S1, a widely

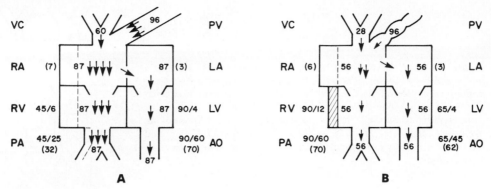

Figure 11–15. *Hemodynamics of total anomalous pulmonary venous return without (**A**) and with (**B**) obstruction to the pulmonary venous return. In the nonobstructive type (**A**), the hemodynamics are similar to those of a large atrial septal defect, with the exception of a mild systemic arterial desaturation. In the obstructive type (**B**), the hemodynamics are characterized by pulmonary venous hypertension, pulmonary edema, pulmonary arterial hypertension, and marked arterial desaturation. The heart size is not enlarged on chest x-ray films. Severe right ventricular hypertrophy is present on the ECG. Abbreviations are the same as those in Figure 11–5.*

split S2, and an S3 or S4. Children with large PBF are only minimally desaturated, and cyanosis is often missed because the arterial oxygen saturation ranges from 85% to 90% (see Fig. 11–15A).

If there is an obstruction to the pulmonary venous return, the hemodynamic consequences are notably different from those without pulmonary venous obstruction. The obstruction to the pulmonary venous return causes pulmonary venous hypertension and secondary PA and RV hypertension (Fig. 11–15B), a situation similar to that seen in mitral stenosis (see Fig. 10–4). Pulmonary edema results when the hydrostatic pressure in the capillaries exceeds the osmotic pressure of the blood. As long as a large ASD permits a right-to-left shunt, the RV cavity remains relatively small (i.e., smaller than one arrow). This is because the RV hypertension prevents the RV compliance from increasing, and the PVR remains elevated. Therefore, chest x-ray films show a relatively small heart and characteristic patterns of pulmonary venous congestion or pulmonary edema (i.e., "ground-glass" appearance). The ECG reflects the high pressure in the RV (i.e., RVH). The oxygen saturation values are equal in the aorta and the PA because of the complete mixing of systemic and pulmonary venous return at the RA level, and the arterial saturation is much lower than that found in patients without obstruction. The degree of arterial desaturation or cyanosis inversely relates to the amount of PBF. Infants with obstruction have severe cyanosis and respiratory distress. The latter results from pulmonary edema and may cause pulmonary crackles on auscultation. The pulmonary valve closure sound (P2) is loud because of pulmonary hypertension, which results in a single, loud S2. The heart murmur may be absent or soft because of normal or decreased flow through the pulmonary or tricuspid valve (i.e., smaller than one arrow) (see Fig. 11–15B).

Full comprehension of the relationship between the magnitude of PBF and the systemic arterial oxygen saturation helps in understanding and managing most cyanotic congenital heart defects. The two extreme examples of TAPVR shown in Figure 11–15 illustrate this relationship.

If the PBF is three times as great as the systemic blood flow (i.e., $\dot{Q}p/\dot{Q}s = 3:1$), as in most nonobstructive cases (see Fig. 11–15A), the arterial oxygen saturation is close to 90%, and cyanosis does not become obvious. This figure is derived as follows. An assumed pulmonary vein saturation of 96% and a vena caval saturation of 60% result in an average mixed venous saturation of 87%. Of course, the aortic saturation is 87% in this case.

$$\frac{(96\times3)+(60\times1)}{4}=87(\%)$$

The difference in the arterial and venous oxygen saturation is kept at 27% to indicate the absence of heart failure (see Fig. 11–15A).

If an obstruction to the pulmonary venous return exists and the PBF is small, a marked arterial desaturation results, based on the following calculation. It is assumed that the PBF is 70% of the systemic flow (i.e., $\dot{Q}p/\dot{Q}s$ = 0.7:1) and the pulmonary vein saturation is 96%. The RA saturation (and thus the aortic saturation) is 56%.

$$\frac{(96\times0.7)+(28\times1)}{1.7}=56(\%)$$

It is also assumed that the infant is not experiencing heart failure (i.e., the systemic AV difference is 28%) (see Fig. 11–15B).

This relationship holds true for other forms of cyanotic congenital heart defects. For a given defect, an increase in the magnitude of PBF results in a rise in the systemic arterial oxygen saturation; a decrease in PBF results in a decrease in the arterial oxygen saturation. An improvement in cyanosis after a systemic-to-PA shunt operation in an infant with decreased PBF is an example of this relationship. Conversely, infants with a single ventricle may be in CHF from a large PBF but not be cyanotic. CHF improves following a PA banding operation (which decreases PBF and lowers PA pressure), but the arterial oxygen saturation usually decreases, and cyanosis may appear.

Part IV

SPECIFIC CONGENITAL HEART DEFECTS

The next three chapters discuss common left-to-right shunt lesions, obstructive lesions, and cyanotic cardiac defects. Other chapters in this part discuss aortic arch anomalies, primarily "vascular ring" and cardiac malposition. Miscellaneous, rare anomalies that do not belong to these categories are briefly discussed in another chapter. These chapters are intended to be used as a quick reference; therefore, descriptions are brief.

Chapter 12

Left-to-Right Shunt Lesions

This chapter discusses common left-to-right shunt lesions such as atrial septal defect (ASD), ventricular septal defect (VSD), patent ductus arteriosus (PDA), endocardial cushion defect (ECD), and partial anomalous pulmonary venous return (PAPVR).

Atrial Septal Defect

PREVALENCE

ASD (ostium secundum defect) occurs as an isolated anomaly in 5% to 10% of all congenital heart defects. It is more common in females than in males (male/female ratio of 1:2). About 30% to 50% of children with congenital heart defects have an ASD as part of the cardiac defect.

PATHOLOGY

1. Three types of ASDs exist—secundum defect, primum defect, and sinus venosus defect. Another rare form of defect is coronary sinus ASD. Patent foramen ovale (PFO) does not ordinarily produce intracardiac shunts (see Chapter 17).

2. Ostium secundum defect is the most common type of ASD, accounting for 50% to 70% of all ASDs. This defect is present at the site of fossa ovalis, allowing left-to-right shunting of blood from the left atrium (LA) to the right atrium (RA) (Fig. 12–1). Anomalous pulmonary venous return is present in about 10% of cases.

Figure 12–1. *Anatomic types of atrial septal defects (ASDs) viewed with the right atrial wall removed. IVC, inferior vena cava; SVC, superior vena cava.*

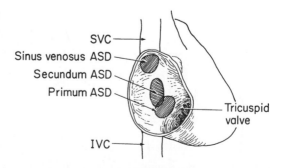

3. Ostium primum defects occur in about 30% of all ASDs, if those that occur as part of complete ECD are included (see Fig. 12–1). Isolated ostium primum ASD occurs in about 15% of all ASDs. This is discussed in greater detail in the section on partial ECD.

4. Sinus venosus defect occurs in about 10% of all ASDs. The defect is most commonly located at the entry of the superior vena cava (SVC) into the RA (superior vena caval type) and rarely at the entry of the inferior vena cava (IVC) into the RA (inferior vena caval type). The former is very commonly associated with anomalous drainage of the right upper pulmonary vein (into the RA), and the latter is often associated with anomalous drainage of the right lung into the IVC ("scimitar syndrome") (see Chapter 17).

5. In coronary sinus ASD, there is a defect in the roof of the coronary sinus and the LA blood shunts through the defect and the coronary sinus ostium into the RA, which produces clinical pictures similar to those in other types of ASD.

6. Mitral valve prolapse (MVP) occurs in 20% of patients with either ostium secundum or sinus venosus defects.

CLINICAL MANIFESTATIONS

History. Infants and children with ASDs are usually asymptomatic.

Physical Examination (Fig. 12–2)

1. A relatively slender body build is typical. (The body weight of many is less than the 10th percentile.)

2. A widely split and fixed S2 and a grade 2 to 3/6 systolic ejection murmur are characteristic findings of ASD in older infants and children. With a large left-to-right shunt, a mid-diastolic rumble resulting from relative tricuspid stenosis may be audible at the lower left sternal border.

3. Classic auscultatory findings (and ECG and chest x-ray findings) of ASD are not present unless the shunt is reasonably large (at least $\dot{Q}p/\dot{Q}s$ of 1.5 or greater). The typical auscultatory findings may be absent in infants and toddlers, even in those with a large defect, if the RV is poorly compliant.

Electrocardiography (Fig. 12–3). Right axis deviation of +90 to +180 degrees and mild right ventricular hypertrophy (RVH) or right bundle branch block (RBBB) with an rsR′ pattern in V1 are typical findings. In about 50% of the patients with sinus venosus ASD, the P axis is less than 30 degrees.

X-ray Studies (Fig. 12–4)

1. Cardiomegaly with enlargement of the RA and right ventricle (RV) may be present.

2. A prominent pulmonary artery (PA) segment and increased pulmonary vascular markings are seen when the shunt is significant.

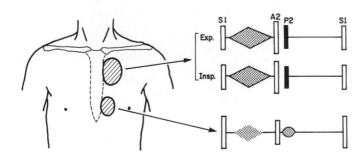

Figure 12–2. Cardiac findings of atrial septal defect. Throughout this book, heart murmurs with solid borders are the primary murmurs, and those without solid borders are transmitted murmurs or those occurring occasionally. Abnormalities in heart sounds are shown in black. Exp., expiration; Insp., inspiration.

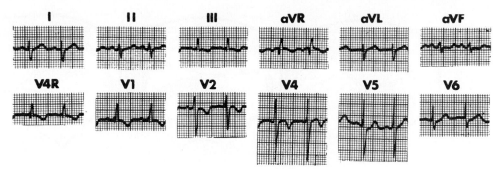

Figure 12–3. *Tracing from a 5-year-old girl with secundum-type atrial septal defect.*

Echocardiography

1. A two-dimensional echo study is diagnostic. The study shows the position as well as the size of the defect, which can best be seen in the subcostal four-chamber view (Fig. 12–5). In secundum ASD, a dropout can be seen in the midatrial septum. The primum type shows a defect in the lower atrial septum; the SVC type of sinus venosus defect shows a defect in the posterosuperior atrial septum.

2. Indirect signs of a significant left-to-right atrial shunt include RV enlargement and RA enlargement, as well as dilated PA, which often accompanies an increase in the flow velocity across the pulmonary valve. These findings indicate the functional significance of the defect.

3. Pulsed Doppler examination reveals a characteristic flow pattern with the maximum left-to-right shunt occurring in diastole. Color flow mapping enhances the evaluation of the hemodynamic status of the ASD.

4. M-mode echo may show increased RV dimension and paradoxical motion of the interventricular septum, which are signs of RV volume overload.

5. In older children and adolescents, especially in those who are overweight, adequate imaging of the atrial septum may not be possible with the ordinary transthoracic echo study. Transesophageal echocardiography (TEE) may be used as an alternative.

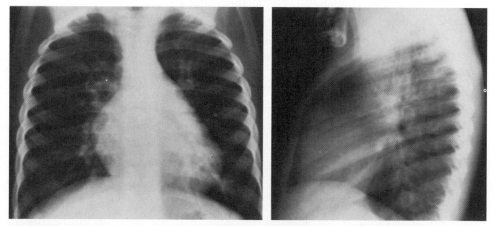

Figure 12–4. *Posteroanterior and lateral views of chest roentgenograms from a 10-year-old child with atrial septal defect. The heart is mildly enlarged, with involvement of the right atrium (best seen in the posteroanterior view) and the right ventricle (best seen in the lateral view with obliteration of the retrosternal space). Pulmonary vascularity is increased, and the main pulmonary artery segment is slightly prominent.*

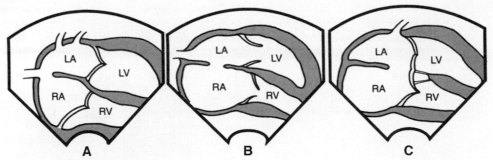

Figure 12–5. *Diagram of two-dimensional echocardiography of the three types of atrial septal defect (ASD). The subcostal transducer position provides the most diagnostic view. **A,** Sinus venosus defect. The defect is located in the posterosuperior atrial septum, usually just beneath the orifice of the superior vena cava. This defect is often associated with partial anomalous return of the right upper pulmonary vein. **B,** Secundum ASD. The defect is located in the middle portion of the atrial septum. **C,** Primum ASD. The defect is located in the anteroinferior atrial septum, just over the inflow portion of each atrioventricular valve. LA, left atrium; LV, left ventricle; RA, right atrium; RV, right ventricle.*

NATURAL HISTORY

1. Earlier reports have indicated that spontaneous closure of the secundum defect occurs in about 40% of patients in the first 4 years of life (reported rates vary between 14% and 55% of patients). The defect may decrease in size in some patients. However, a more recent report indicates the overall rate of spontaneous closure to be 87%. In patients with an ASD less than 3 mm in size diagnosed before 3 months of age, spontaneous closure occurs in 100% of patients at 1½ years of age. Spontaneous closure occurs more than 80% of the time in patients with defects between 3 and 8 mm before 1½ years of age. An ASD with a diameter greater than 8 mm rarely closes spontaneously.

   It may be that "small ASDs" detected by color Doppler studies are not true ASDs; they may simply be an incompetent foramen ovale that resolved to a competent PFO without shunt. (Spontaneous closure of VSD is associated with high velocities across the defect with resulting platelet adhesion to a jet lesion on the septal leaflet of the tricuspid valve. Such hemodynamic abnormalities do not exist with ASD.)

2. Most children with an ASD remain active and asymptomatic. Rarely, congestive heart failure (CHF) can develop in infancy.

3. If a large defect is untreated, CHF and pulmonary hypertension develop in adults who are in their 20s and 30s.

4. With or without surgery, atrial arrhythmias (flutter or fibrillation) may occur in adults.

5. Infective endocarditis does not occur in patients with isolated ASDs.

6. Cerebrovascular accident, resulting from paradoxical embolization through an ASD, is a rare complication.

MANAGEMENT

Medical

1. Exercise restriction is unnecessary.

2. Prophylaxis for infective endocarditis is not indicated unless the patient has associated MVP or other associated defects. Prophylaxis is indicated in patients with primum ASD.

3. In infants with CHF, medical management is recommended because of its high success rate and the possibility of spontaneous closure of the defect.

Nonsurgical Closure. Nonsurgical closure using a catheter-delivered closure device has become a preferred method, provided the indications are met. Several closure devices that can be delivered through cardiac catheters have been shown to be safe and efficacious for ASD closure. These devices are applicable only to secundum ASD with an adequate septal rim. Devices available for clinical use have included the Sideris buttoned device, the Angel Wings device, the CardioSEAL device, and the Amplatzer ASD Occlusion Device. Among these, the Amplatzer Septal Occluder appears to enjoy widespread use.

Use of the closure device may be indicated to close a secundum ASD, measuring 5 mm or more in diameter (but less than 32 mm), and a significant left-to-right shunt with clinical evidence of right ventricular volume overload (i.e., $\dot{Q}p/\dot{Q}s$ ratio of 1.5:1 or greater or RV enlargement). There must be enough rim (4 mm) of septal tissue around the defect for appropriate placement of the device. The timing of the device closure for secundum ASD is not entirely clear. Considering the possibility of spontaneous closure, it is wise not to use the device in infancy unless the patient is symptomatic with heart failure.

Advantages of nonsurgical closure include complete avoidance of cardiopulmonary bypass with its attendant risk, avoidance of pain and residual thoracotomy scars, a less than 24-hour hospital stay, and rapid recovery. All these devices are associated with a higher rate of small residual leak than is operative closure.

Post–device closure follow-up. The patients are administered aspirin 81 mg/day for 6 months. Postprocedure echo studies check for a residual atrial shunt and unobstructed flow of pulmonary veins, coronary sinus, and venae cavae and proper function of the mitral and tricuspid valves. Some cardiologists prescribe aspirin 81 mg for patients with residual shunt to prevent paradoxical embolization, but most cardiologists do not.

Surgical Closure

Indications and Timing

1. A left-to-right shunt with a pulmonary-to-systemic blood flow ratio ($\dot{Q}p/\dot{Q}s$) of ≥1.5:1 is a surgical indication only if device closure is not considered appropriate. Surgery is usually delayed until 2 to 4 years of age because the possibility of spontaneous closure exists and because children tolerate the defect well.

2. If CHF does not respond to medical management, surgery is performed during infancy, again if device closure is considered inappropriate.

3. If oxygen and other medical therapy are needed for infants with associated bronchopulmonary dysplasia and the device closure is not considered appropriate, surgery is performed during infancy.

4. High pulmonary vascular resistance (i.e., >10 units/m^2, >7 units/m^2 with vasodilators) may be a contraindication for surgery.

Procedure. For secundum ASD, the defect is traditionally repaired through a midsternal incision under cardiopulmonary bypass by either a simple suture or a pericardial or Teflon patch. Recently, so-called minimally invasive cardiac surgical techniques with smaller skin incisions have become popular, especially for female patients. For ASDs (including simple primum ASDs and sinus venosus defects), one of the following techniques can be used: midline short transxiphoid incision with minimal sternal split (preferred), transverse inframammary incision with vertical or transverse sternotomy, or small lower midline skin incision with either partial or full median sternotomy. The benefit of this technique appears to be an improved cosmetic result; it does not reduce pain, hospital stay, or surgical stress.

For sinus venosus defect without associated anomalous pulmonary venous return, the defect is closed using an autologous pericardial patch. When it is associated with a pulmonary venous anomaly, a tunnel is created between the anomalous pulmonary vein and the ASD by using a Teflon or pericardial patch. A plastic or pericardial gusset is placed in the SVC to prevent obstruction of the SVC. Alternatively, one may use the Warden procedure. In this procedure, the SVC is divided above the level of the pulmonary venous entry. The cardiac end of the SVC is oversewn, and a pericardial baffle is placed in such a way as to drain the pulmonary venous blood through the sinus venosus ASD into the LA. The proximal SVC is sewn to the right atrial appendage to drain the SVC blood to the RA.

For coronary sinus ASD, the ostium of the coronary sinus is closed with an autologous pericardium with care to avoid conduction tissues, provided it is not associated with persistent left SVC. This results in drainage of coronary sinus blood into the left atrium.

Mortality. Fewer than 0.5% of patients die; however, there is a greater risk for small infants and those with increased pulmonary vascular resistance.

Complications. Cerebrovascular accident and postoperative arrhythmias may develop in the immediate postoperative period.

Postoperative Follow-up

1. Cardiomegaly on x-ray film and enlarged RV dimension on echo as well as the wide splitting of the S2 may persist for 1 or 2 years postoperatively. The ECG typically demonstrates RBBB (or RV conduction disturbance).

2. Atrial or nodal arrhythmias occur in 7% to 20% of postoperative patients. Occasionally, sick sinus syndrome, which occurs especially after the repair of a sinus venosus defect, may require antiarrhythmic drugs, pacemaker therapy, or both.

3. Rarely, patients with residual shunt may be administered aspirin 81 mg to prevent paradoxical embolization.

Ventricular Septal Defect

PREVALENCE

VSD is the most common form of congenital heart defect and accounts for 15% to 20% of all such defects, not including those occurring as part of cyanotic congenital heart defects.

PATHOLOGY

1. The ventricular septum may be divided into a small membranous portion and a large muscular portion (Fig. 12–6A). The muscular septum has three components: the inlet septum, the trabecular septum, and the outlet (infundibular or conal) septum. The trabecular septum (also simply called muscular septum) is further divided into anterior, posterior, middle, and apical portions. Therefore, a VSD may be classified as a membranous, inlet, outlet (or infundibular), midtrabecular (or midmuscular), anterior trabecular (or anterior muscular), posterior trabecular (or posterior muscular), or apical muscular defect (see Fig. 12–6B).

   a. The membranous septum is a relatively small area immediately beneath the aortic valve. The membranous defect involves varying amounts of muscular tissue adjacent to the membranous septum (perimembranous VSD). According to the accompanying defect in the adjacent muscular septum, perimembranous VSDs have been called perimembranous inlet (atrioventricular [AV] canal type), perimembranous trabecular, or perimembranous outlet (tetralogy type) defects. Perimembranous defects are most common (70%).

   b. Outlet (infundibular or conal) defects account for 5% to 7% of all VSDs in the Western world and about 30% in Far Eastern countries. The defect is located within the outlet (conal) septum, and part of its rim is formed by the aortic and pulmonary annulus. An aortic leaflet can prolapse through the VSD and cause aortic insufficiency (see later for further discussion). It has been called a supracristal, conal, subpulmonary, or subarterial defect.

   c. Inlet (or AV canal) defects account for 5% to 8% of all VSDs. The defect is located posterior and inferior to the perimembranous defect, beneath the septal leaflet of the tricuspid valve (see Fig. 12–6B).

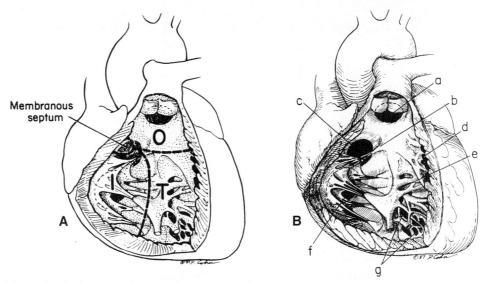

Figure 12–6. *Anatomy of ventricular septum and ventricular septal defect (VSD).* **A,** *Ventricular septum viewed from the right ventricular (RV) side. The membranous septum is small. The large muscular septum has three components: the inlet septum (I), the trabecular septum (T), and the outlet (or infundibular) septum (O).* **B,** *Anatomic locations of various VSDs and landmarks, viewed with the RV free wall removed. a, outlet (infundibular) defect; b, papillary muscle of the conus; c, perimembranous defect; d, marginal muscular defect; e, central muscular defect; f, inlet defect; g, apical muscular defect. (From Graham TP Jr, Bender HW, Spach MS: Ventricular septal defect. In Adams FH, Emmanouilides GC, Riemenschneider TA (eds): Moss' Heart Disease in Infants, Children and Adolescents, 4th ed. Baltimore, Williams and Wilkins, 1989.)*

    d. Trabecular (or muscular) defects account for 5% to 20% of all VSDs. They frequently appear to be multiple when viewed from the right side. A midmuscular defect is posterior to the septal band. An apical muscular defect is near the cardiac apex and is difficult to visualize and repair. The anterior (marginal) defects are usually multiple, small, and tortuous. The "Swiss cheese" type of multiple muscular defect (involving all components of the ventricular septum) is extremely difficult to close surgically.

2. The defects vary in size, ranging from tiny defects without hemodynamic significance to large defects with accompanying CHF and pulmonary hypertension.

3. The bundle of His is related to the posteroinferior quadrant of perimembranous defects and the superoanterior quadrant of inlet muscular defects. Defects in other parts of the septum are usually unrelated to the conduction tissue.

4. In an infundibular defect, the right coronary cusp of the aortic valve may herniate through the defect. This may result in an actual reduction of the VSD shunt but may produce aortic regurgitation (AR) and cause an obstruction in the right ventricular outflow tract. A similar herniation of the right and/or noncoronary cusp occasionally occurs through perimembranous defects.

CLINICAL MANIFESTATIONS

History

1. With a small VSD, the patient is asymptomatic with normal growth and development.

2. With a moderate to large VSD, delayed growth and development, decreased exercise tolerance, repeated pulmonary infections, and CHF are relatively common during infancy.

3. With long-standing pulmonary hypertension, a history of cyanosis and a decreased level of activity may be present.

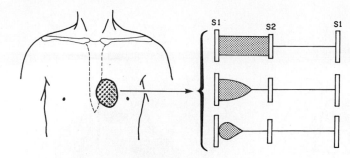

Figure 12–7. Cardiac findings of a small ventricular septal defect. A regurgitant systolic murmur is best audible at the lower left sternal border; it may be holosystolic or less than holosystolic. Occasionally, the heart murmur is in early systole. A systolic thrill (dots) may be palpable at the lower left sternal border. The S2 splits normally, and the P2 is of normal intensity.

Physical Examination (Figs. 12–7 and 12–8)

1. Infants with small VSDs are well developed and acyanotic. Before 2 or 3 months of age, infants with large VSDs may have poor weight gain or show signs of CHF. Cyanosis and clubbing may be present in patients with pulmonary vascular obstructive disease (Eisenmenger's syndrome).

2. A systolic thrill may be present at the lower left sternal border. Precordial bulge and hyperactivity are present with a large-shunt VSD.

3. The intensity of the P2 is normal with a small shunt and moderately increased with a large shunt. The S2 is loud and single in patients with pulmonary hypertension or pulmonary vascular obstructive disease. A grade 2 to 5/6 regurgitant systolic murmur is audible at the lower left sternal border (see Figs. 12–7 and 12–8). It may be holosystolic or early systolic. An apical diastolic rumble is present with a moderate to large shunt (because of increased flow through the mitral valve during diastole).

4. With infundibular VSD, a grade 1 to 3/6 early diastolic decrescendo murmur of AR may be audible. This murmur may be due to herniation of an aortic cusp.

Electrocardiography

1. With a small VSD, the ECG is normal.

2. With a moderate VSD, left ventricular hypertrophy (LVH) and occasional left atrial hypertrophy (LAH) may be seen.

3. With a large defect, the ECG shows biventricular hypertrophy (BVH) with or without LAH (Fig. 12–9).

4. If pulmonary vascular obstructive disease develops, the ECG shows RVH only.

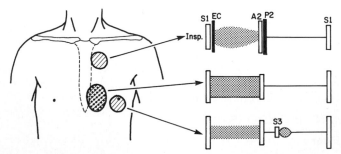

Figure 12–8. Cardiac findings of a large ventricular septal defect. A classic holosystolic regurgitant murmur is audible at the lower left sternal border. A systolic thrill is also palpable at the same area (dots). There is usually a mid-diastolic rumble, resulting from relative mitral stenosis, at the apex. The S2 is narrowly split, and the P2 is accentuated in intensity. Occasionally an ejection click (EC) may be audible in the upper left sternal border when associated with pulmonary hypertension. The heart murmurs shown without solid borders are transmitted from other areas and are not characteristic of the defect. Abnormal sounds are shown in black. Insp., inspiration.

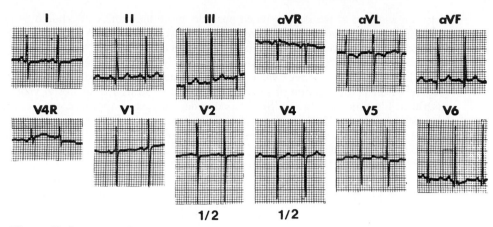

Figure 12–9. *Tracing from a 3-month-old infant with a large ventricular septal defect, patent ductus arteriosus, and pulmonary hypertension. The tracing shows biventricular hypertrophy with left dominance. Note that V2 and V4 are in ½ standardization.*

X-ray Studies (Fig. 12–10)

1. Cardiomegaly of varying degrees is present and involves the LA, left ventricle (LV), and sometimes RV. Pulmonary vascular markings increase. The degree of cardiomegaly and the increase in pulmonary vascular markings directly relate to the magnitude of the left-to-right shunt.

2. In pulmonary vascular obstructive disease (PVOD), the main PA and the hilar PAs enlarge noticeably, but the peripheral lung fields are ischemic. The heart size is usually normal.

Echocardiography. Two-dimensional and Doppler echo studies can identify the number, size, and exact location of the defect; estimate PA pressure by using the modified Bernoulli equation; identify other associated defects; and estimate the magnitude of the shunt. Because the ventricular septum is a large, complex structure, examination for a VSD should be carried out in a systematic manner to be able to specify the exact

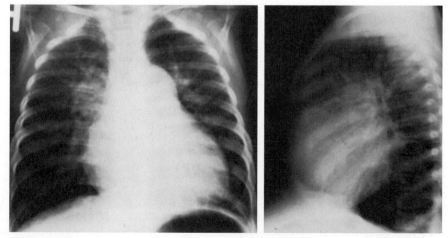

Figure 12–10. *Posteroanterior and lateral views of chest roentgenograms of a ventricular septal defect with a large shunt and pulmonary hypertension. The heart size is moderately increased, with enlargement on both sides. Pulmonary vascular markings are increased, with a prominent main pulmonary artery segment.*

location and size of the defect. When possible, more than one view should be obtained, preferably a combination of the long- and short-axis views.

The cardiac valves serve as markers of specific types of VSDs, except for the trabecular septum. The membranous VSD is closely related to the aortic valve, the inlet VSD to the tricuspid (or AV) valve, and the infundibular VSD to the semilunar valves. Figure 12–11 is a collection of selected parasternal, apical, and subcostal views that are useful in locating the site of VSDs. Good understanding of these views is necessary in the assessment of a VSD in terms of location and size of the defect.

The membranous septum is closely related to the aortic valve. In the apical and subcostal "five-chamber" views, it is seen in the LV outflow tract just under the aortic valve (see Fig. 12–11, C3). In the parasternal short-axis view at the level of aortic valve, it is seen adjacent to the tricuspid valve (see Fig. 12–11, B1). These are the best views to confirm the membranous VSD. The membranous VSD is not visible in the standard parasternal long-axis view, but by tilting the transducer slightly to the right, away from the aorta, the membranous VSD becomes visible. Figure 12–12 shows a membranous VSD imaged in the apical five-chamber view.

The inlet septum is best imaged in the apical or subcostal four-chamber view beneath the AV valves (see Fig. 12–11, C2 and D1). It can also be seen equally well in the parasternal short-axis view in the posterior interventricular septum at the levels between the mitral valve and the papillary muscle (see Fig. 12–11, B2). Simple inlet VSD (not that associated with AV canal defect) is seen beneath the AV valve, but a small amount of tissue remains under the valves. In the AV canal type of VSD, the AV valves are at the same level. There may be straddling or overriding.

The infundibular (or outlet) septum lies inferior to the semilunar valves. The subpulmonary, supracristal infundibular VSD lies under the pulmonary valve (see Fig. 12–11, A2 and D3), and the subaortic infracristal VSD (TOF type, also called conoventricular VSD) lies under the aortic valve (see Fig. 12–11, A2 and D2). From the RV side, if the outlet septum lies inferior to the pulmonary valve, it is supracristal. The infracristal VSD lies much closer to the aortic valve but away from the pulmonary valve (see Fig. 12–11, A1 and C3), and the supracristal is closer to the pulmonary valve (see Fig. 12–11, A2, D3, and E1).

Figure 12–11. *Selected two-dimensional echo views of the ventricular septum. These schematic drawings are helpful in determining the site of a VSD. Different shading has been used for easy recognition of different parts of the ventricular septum. In the standard parasternal long-axis view (**A1**), the ventricular septum consists of (from the aortic valve toward the apex) the infracristal outlet (Inf-C outlet) septum (the VSD of TOF is seen here) and the trabecular (middle and apical) septum. In the parasternal RVOT view (**A2**), the septum consists of the supracristal outlet (Sup-C outlet) septum and the trabecular septum. In the parasternal short-axis view showing the aortic valve (**B1**), the membranous septum is toward the 10 o'clock direction, the infracristal outlet septum at the 12 o'clock direction, and the supracristal outlet septum immediately adjacent to the pulmonary valve. The ventricular septum at the mitral valve (**B2**), the posterior muscular septum, is the inlet (INLET) septum. The ventricular septum at the papillary muscle (**B3**) is all trabecular septum, so that one can easily classify the defect into anterior (ANT), middle (MID), and posterior (POST) trabecular defects. In the apical four-chamber view showing the coronary sinus (**C1**), the ventricular septum is the posterior (POST) trabecular septum. In the apical four-chamber view showing both AV valves (**C2**), the septum immediately beneath the tricuspid valve is the inlet septum (INLET) and the remainder is the middle and apical septa. The thin septum between the insertion of the mitral and tricuspid valves is the atrioventricular septum (**C2**), a defect that can result in an LV-to-RA shunt. In the standard apical four-chamber view, the membranous septum is not visible. In the apical "five-chamber" view (**C3**), the membranous (MEMB) septum is seen beneath the aortic valve and below it is the infracristal outlet (Inf-C outlet) septum. The ventricular septum seen in the subcostal four-chamber view (**D1**) is similar to the apical four-chamber view (**C2**). With anterior angulation of the horizontal transducer, the LVOT is seen (**D2**) and the septum seen here is similar to the apical five-chamber view (**C3**). With further anterior angulation, the RVOT is seen (**D3**). The superior part is the supracristal outlet (Sup-C outlet) septum and the inferior part is the anterior (ANT) trabecular septum (**D3**).*

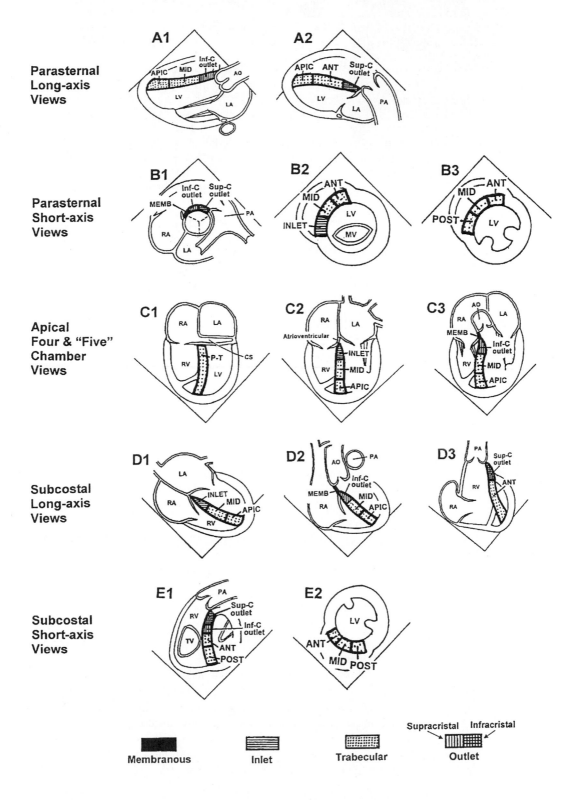

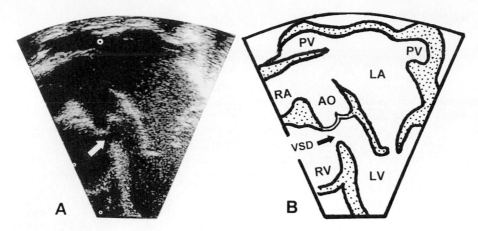

Figure 12–12. *Two-dimensional echocardiogram showing membranous ventricular septal defect (VSD). The membranous VSD is seen underneath the aortic valve in the left ventricular outflow tract (in the apical "five-chamber" view). This view is equivalent to Figure 12–11C3. AO, aorta; LA, left atrium; LV, left ventricle; RA, right atrium; RV, right ventricle; PV, pulmonary vein.*

The trabecular septum is the largest portion of the ventricular septum and extends from the membranous septum to the cardiac apex. Four types of trabecular VSD are (1) anterior, (2) midmuscular, (3) apical, and (4) posterior. Echo views that show the locations of different types of trabecular VSDs are shown in Figure 12–11. The apical VSD occurs near the cardiac apex (see Fig. 12–11, A1, A2, C2, C3, D1, and D2). The entire ventricular septum seen at the papillary muscle level is the trabecular septum (see Fig. 12–11, B3 and E2). For imaging of an apical muscular VSD, the transducer must be maximally angled toward the cardiac apex.

The subcostal short-axis view showing the RVOT (E1) is orthogonal to the standard subcostal four-chamber view and is an important view for evaluating the site and size of a VSD. In this view both supracristal outlet (Sup-C outlet) and infracristal outlet (Inf-C outlet) septa (in that order) are seen beneath the pulmonary valve and the trabecular septum (ANT and POST) is seen apical ward. The ventricular septum seen at the papillary muscle (E2) is all trabecular septum and is similar to the parasternal short-axis view (B3).

NATURAL HISTORY

Understanding the natural history of a VSD is important when planning its management.

1. Spontaneous closure occurs in 30% to 40% of patients with membranous VSDs and muscular VSDs during the first 6 months of life. It occurs more frequently in small defects. These VSDs do not become bigger with age; rather, they decrease in size. However, inlet defects and outlet (infundibular) defects do not become smaller or close spontaneously.

2. CHF develops in infants with large VSDs but usually not until 6 to 8 weeks of age.

3. Pulmonary vascular obstructive disease may begin to develop as early as 6 to 12 months of age in patients with large VSDs, but the resulting right-to-left shunt usually does not develop until the teenage years.

4. Infundibular stenosis may develop in some infants with large defects and result in a decrease in the magnitude of the left-to-right shunt (i.e., acyanotic TOF), with an occasional occurrence of a right-to-left shunt.

5. Infective endocarditis rarely occurs.

Management

Medical

1. Treatment of CHF, if it develops, is indicated with digoxin and diuretics (see Chapter 27) for 2 to 4 months to see if growth failure can be improved. Addition of spironolactone may be helpful to minimize potassium loss. Concomitant use of an afterload-reducing agent, such as captopril, has gained popularity. Angiotensin-converting enzyme inhibitors may raise the serum potassium level, and spironolactone or potassium supplementation should be discontinued. Frequent feedings of high-calorie formulas, by either nasogastric tube or oral feeding, may help. Anemia, if present, should be corrected by oral iron therapy. These measures often allow delay of surgical treatment and may promote spontaneous reduction or closure of the VSD.

2. No exercise restriction is required in the absence of pulmonary hypertension.

3. Maintenance of good dental hygiene and antibiotic prophylaxis against infective endocarditis are important (see Chapter 19).

4. Nonsurgical closure of selected muscular VSDs is possible using the "umbrella" device, but this is still in the experimental stage.

Surgical

Indications and Timing

1. Small infants who have large VSDs and develop CHF and growth retardation are managed first with digoxin, diuretics, and afterload-reducing agents. If growth failure cannot be improved by medical therapy, the VSD should be operated on within the first 6 months of life. Surgery should be delayed for infants who respond to medical therapy. However, if the PA pressure is greater than 50% of systemic pressure, surgical closure should be done by the end of the first year.

2. After 1 year of age, a significant left-to-right shunt with $\dot{Q}p/\dot{Q}s$ of at least 2:1 indicates that surgical closure is needed, regardless of PA pressure.

3. Infants with evidence of pulmonary hypertension but no CHF or growth failure should have a cardiac catheterization at 6 to 12 months of age. Surgery should follow soon after cardiac catheterization. Older infants with large VSDs and evidence of elevated pulmonary vascular resistance should be operated on as soon as possible.

4. Infants who have small VSDs and have reached the age of 6 months without CHF or evidence of pulmonary hypertension are usually not candidates for surgery. Surgery is not indicated for a small VSD with $\dot{Q}p/\dot{Q}s$ less than 1.5:1.

5. Some centers close VSD when there is evidence of aortic valve prolapse (even without AR), history of prior endocarditis, or evidence of LV dilatation, even if the $\dot{Q}p/\dot{Q}s$ is less then 2:1.

6. Surgery is contraindicated in patients with a pulmonary-to-systemic vascular resistance ratio of 0.5 or greater or with pulmonary vascular obstructive disease with a predominant right-to-left shunt.

Procedure

1. PA banding as a palliative procedure is no longer performed unless additional lesions make complete repair difficult.

2. Direct closure of the defect is carried out under hypothermic cardiopulmonary bypass, preferably without right ventriculotomy. Most perimembranous and inlet VSDs are repaired by a transatrial approach. Outlet (conal) defects are best approached through an incision in the main PA. Apical VSD may require apical right ventriculotomy.

As with the closure of ASDs, minimally invasive surgical techniques with smaller skin incisions are becoming popular for the closure of VSDs. The major benefit of this approach appears to be cosmetic.

Mortality. Surgical mortality is less than 1%. Mortality is higher for small infants younger than 2 months of age, infants with associated defects, or infants with multiple VSDs.

Complications

1. RBBB is frequent in patients repaired by right ventriculotomy. This is usually due to the disruption of the Purkinje fibers, but it can also be caused by direct injury to the right bundle itself.

2. RBBB and left anterior hemiblock, which occurs in less than 10% of patients, is a controversial cause of sudden death. Complete heart block requiring a pacemaker occurs in 1% to 2% of patients.

3. Residual shunt occurs in less than 5%. Intraoperative TEE has reduced the incidence of the residual shunt.

4. Injuries to the tricuspid valve (with resulting TR) and the aortic valve (with resulting AR) rarely occur.

5. The incidence of neurologic complications is directly related to the circulatory arrest time.

Surgical Approaches for Special Situations

1. *Ventricular septal defect and patent ductus arteriosus.* If the PDA is large, the ductus alone may be closed in the first 6 to 8 weeks in the hope that the VSD is restrictive. If the VSD is large and not restrictive, PDA should be ligated at the time of VSD repair, through the median sternotomy.

2. *Ventricular septal defect and coarctation of the aorta.* A VSD is present in 15% to 20% of patients with coarctation of the aorta (COA). Several options exist in this controversial situation.

    a. Initial repair of the COA alone, if the VSD appears relatively small. The VSD is closed later, if indicated.
    b. Coarctation repair and PA banding when the VSD appears unrestrictive.
    c. Repair of both defects at the same time using one or two incisions.

3. *Ventricular septal defect and aortic regurgitation syndrome.* The prolapsed aortic cusp, with resulting AR, is usually associated with outlet VSD and occasionally with perimembranous VSD. It occurs in about 5% of patients with VSD, but the prevalence is much higher in Far Eastern countries (15% to 20%). The adjacent (i.e.., right and/or noncoronary) aortic valve cusps prolapse through the defect into the right ventricular outflow tract, actually reducing the VSD shunt. Once AR appears, it gradually worsens. Surgery is usually performed promptly when AR is present, even if the $\dot{Q}p/\dot{Q}s$ is less than 2:1, so that progression of AR (by the Venturi effect through the open VSD) is either aborted or abolished. Some centers close the VSD even in the absence of AR if the aortic prolapse is demonstrated. When AR is trivial or mild, the VSD alone is closed. When AR is moderate or severe, the aortic valve is repaired or replaced. Not every case of VSD and AR results from the prolapsed aortic cusps; it may be the result of a VSD and bicuspid aortic valve.

4. *Development of subaortic stenosis.* A discrete fibrous or fibromuscular subaortic stenosis is occasionally associated with perimembranous VSD. It is also seen in patients with COA and VSD, after PA banding or repair of a VSD. The mechanism for the development is unclear. Because of its progressive nature and potential damage to the aortic valve, surgical resection is usually undertaken relatively early if a gradient greater than 30 mm Hg is present. Long-term follow-up of these stenoses is mandatory because they tend to recur (also see subaortic membrane in Chapter 13).

Postoperative Follow-up

1. An office examination should be scheduled every 1 to 2 years.

2. Activity should not be restricted unless complications have resulted from surgery.

3. The ECG shows RBBB in 50% to 90% of patients who had VSD repair through right ventriculotomy and up to 40% of the patients who had repair through a right atrial approach.

4. Although it is rare these days, patients who had VSD and mild pulmonary hypertension and repair of the VSD after 3 years of age should be checked for possible progressive pulmonary vascular disease.

5. Bacterial endocarditis prophylaxis may be discontinued 6 months after surgery. If a residual shunt is present, endocarditis prophylaxis should be continued indefinitely when the indications arise.

6. A patient with a postoperative history of transient heart block with or without pacemaker therapy requires long-term follow-up.

Patent Ductus Arteriosus

PREVALENCE

PDA occurs in 5% to 10% of all congenital heart defects, excluding premature infants. It is more common in females than in males (male/female ratio of 1:3). PDA is a common problem in premature infants, which is discussed under a separate heading in this chapter.

PATHOLOGY

1. There is a persistent patency of a normal fetal structure between the left PA and the descending aorta, that is, about 5 to 10 mm distal to the origin of the left subclavian artery.

2. The ductus is usually cone shaped with a small orifice to the PA, which is restrictive to blood flow. The ductus may be short or long, straight or tortuous.

CLINICAL MANIFESTATIONS

History

1. Patients are usually asymptomatic when the ductus is small.

2. A large-shunt PDA may cause a lower respiratory tract infection, atelectasis, and CHF (accompanied by tachypnea and poor weight gain).

3. Exertional dyspnea may be present in children with a large-shunt PDA

Physical Examination (Fig. 12–13)

1. Tachycardia and tachypnea may be present in infants with CHF.

2. Bounding peripheral pulses with wide pulse pressure (with elevated systolic pressure and lower diastolic pressure) are characteristic findings. With a small shunt, these findings do not occur.

3. The precordium is hyperactive. A systolic thrill may be present at the upper left sternal border. The P2 is usually normal, but its intensity may be accentuated if pulmonary hypertension is present. A grade 1 to 4/6 continuous ("machinery")

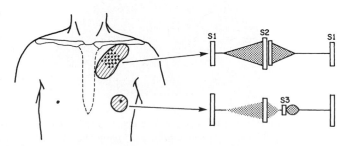

Figure 12–13. Cardiac findings of patent ductus arteriosus. A systolic thrill may be present in the area shown by dots.

murmur is best audible at the left infraclavicular area or upper left sternal border. The heart murmur may be crescendo systolic at the upper left sternal border in small infants or infants with pulmonary hypertension. An apical diastolic rumble may be heard when the PDA shunt is large. Patients with a small ductus do not have the preceding findings.

4. If pulmonary vascular obstructive disease develops, a right-to-left ductal shunt results in cyanosis only in the lower half of the body (i.e., differential cyanosis).

Electrocardiography. The ECG findings in PDA are similar to those in VSD. A normal ECG or LVH is seen with small to moderate PDA. BVH is seen with large PDA. If pulmonary vascular obstructive disease develops, RVH is present.

X-ray Studies. X-ray findings are also similar to those of VSD.

1. Chest x-ray films may be normal with a small-shunt PDA.

2. Cardiomegaly of varying degrees occurs in moderate- to large-shunt PDA with enlargement of the LA, LV, and ascending aorta. Pulmonary vascular markings are increased.

3. With pulmonary vascular obstructive disease, the heart size becomes normal, with a marked prominence of the PA segment and hilar vessels.

Echocardiography

1. The PDA can be imaged in most patients. Its size can be assessed by two-dimensional echo in a high parasternal view or in a suprasternal notch view (Fig. 12–14).

2. Doppler studies that are performed with the sample volume in the PA immediately proximal to the ductal opening provide important functional information (see discussion in "Patent Ductus Arteriosus in Preterm Neonates").

3. The dimensions of the LA and LV provide an indirect assessment of the magnitude of the left-to-right ductal shunt. The larger the shunt, the greater the dilatation of these chambers.

NATURAL HISTORY

1. Unlike that in premature infants, spontaneous closure of a PDA does not usually occur in full-term infants and children. This is because the PDA in term infants results from a structural abnormality of the ductal smooth muscle rather than decreased responsiveness of the premature ductus to oxygen.

2. CHF or recurrent pneumonia or both develop if the shunt is large.

3. Pulmonary vascular obstructive disease may develop if a large PDA with pulmonary hypertension is left untreated.

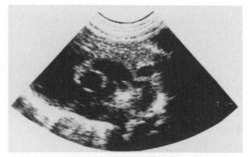 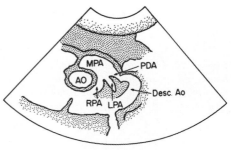

Figure 12–14. Parasternal short-axis view demonstrating patent ductus arteriosus (PDA) that connects the main pulmonary artery (MPA) and the descending aorta (Desc Ao). AO, aorta; LPA, left pulmonary artery; RPA, right pulmonary artery.

4. Infective endocarditis may occur.

5. Although rare, an aneurysm of PDA may develop and possibly rupture in adult life.

DIFFERENTIAL DIAGNOSIS

The following conditions occur with a heart murmur that is similar to the continuous murmur of PDA or with bounding pulses, or both, and they require differentiation from PDA:

1. *Coronary arteriovenous fistula*: A continuous murmur is usually maximally audible along the right sternal border, not at the left infraclavicular area or upper left sternal border.

2. *Systemic arteriovenous fistula*: A bounding pulse with a wide pulse pressure and signs of CHF may develop without continuous murmur over the precordium. A continuous murmur is present over the fistula (i.e., head or liver).

3. *Pulmonary arteriovenous fistula*: A continuous murmur is audible over the back. Cyanosis and clubbing are present in the absence of cardiomegaly.

4. *Venous hum*: A venous hum is maximally audible in the right or left infraclavicular and supraclavicular areas, or both, when the patient is examined in the sitting position. It usually disappears when the patient lies in a supine position.

5. *Collaterals in COA*: A continuous murmur is audible in the intercostal spaces, usually bilaterally.

6. *VSD with AR*: A to-and-fro murmur, rather than a continuous murmur, is audible at the mid-left sternal border or lower left sternal border.

7. *Absence of the pulmonary valve*: A to-and-fro murmur ("sawing wood" sound) is audible at the upper left sternal border. Large hilar PAs on x-ray films and RVH on the ECG are characteristic. These patients are frequently cyanotic because this defect is usually associated with TOF.

8. *Persistent truncus arteriosus*: A continuous murmur is occasionally audible at the second right intercostal space or at the back in a cyanotic infant, rather than in the upper left sternal border. The ECG may show BVH, and chest x-ray films show varying degrees of cardiomegaly and increased pulmonary vascularity. A right aortic arch is frequently found.

9. *Aortopulmonary septal defect (aortopulmonary window)*: This extremely rare condition produces a bounding pulse, but the murmur resembles that of a VSD. CHF develops in early infancy.

10. *Peripheral PA stenosis*: A continuous murmur is audible all over the thorax. The ECG may show RVH if the stenosis is severe. This often accompanies Williams' syndrome or rubella syndrome.

11. *Ruptured sinus of Valsalva aneurysm*: The sudden onset of chest pain and signs of severe heart failure with dyspnea develop. A continuous murmur or a to-and-fro murmur is present at the base. This condition is more commonly seen in patients with Marfan's syndrome.

12. *Total anomalous pulmonary venous return (TAPVR) draining into the RA*: A murmur that sounds similar to a venous hum may be heard along the right sternal border in a child with mild cyanosis. The ECG shows RVH in the presence of cardiomegaly and increased pulmonary vascular markings on chest x-ray films.

MANAGEMENT

Medical

1. Indomethacin is ineffective in term infants with PDA and should not be used.

2. Standard anticongestive measures with digoxin and diuretics are indicated when CHF develops.

3. No exercise restriction is needed in the absence of pulmonary hypertension.

4. Prophylaxis for subacute bacterial endocarditis (SBE) is indicated when indications arise.

Nonsurgical Closure. Catheter closure of the ductus using several different devices is having varying degrees of success. At many centers, small ductus less than 4 mm in diameter are closed by coils and larger ones by an Amplatzer PDA device.

1. Gianturco stainless coils, which were introduced by Gambier and coworkers, have become the standard device for closure of PDA for all children with ducts less than 4 mm in diameter in the United States. In optimal candidates for the device, the ductus is 2.5 mm in size but the use of multiple coils can close a ductus up to 5 mm. The residual shunt rate is 5% to 15% at 12 months' follow-up. According to the European experience, the immediate occlusion rate of 59% rose to 95% at 1 year.

2. Some centers use the Amplatzer device for PDAs ranging in size from 4 to 10 mm (with 100% closure rate).

The advantages of nonsurgical closure of the ductus include no need for general anesthesia, shorter hospital stay and convalescent period, and elimination of a thoracotomy scar. Disadvantages and potential complications include residual leaks, PA coil embolization, hemolysis, left PA stenosis, aortic occlusion with the Amplatzer device, and femoral vessel occlusion.

Surgical Closure

Indications and Timing. A hemodynamically significant ductus needs to be closed by either surgery or interventional techniques at any age. An interventional device rather than surgery is used to close small ducti with no hemodynamic significance by many centers. Surgical closure is reserved for patients in whom a nonsurgical closure technique is not considered applicable. The presence of pulmonary vascular obstructive disease is a contraindication to surgery. In infants with CHF, pulmonary hypertension, or recurrent pneumonia, surgery is performed on an urgent basis.

Procedure

1. Ligation and division through left posterolateral thoracotomy without cardiopulmonary bypass is the standard procedure.

2. The technique of video-assisted thoracoscopic clip ligation has become the standard of care for surgical management of a ductus with adequate length (to allow safe ligation), which is performed through three small ports in the fourth intercostal space.

Mortality. The surgical mortality rate is zero for both techniques.

Complications. Complications are rare. Injury to the recurrent laryngeal nerve (hoarseness), the left phrenic nerve (paralysis of the left hemidiaphragm), or the thoracic duct (chylothorax) is possible. Recanalization (reopening) of the ductus is possible, although rare, occurring after ligation alone (without division).

Postoperative Follow-up

1. Regular follow-up is unnecessary after PDA ligation unless surgical complications are present.

2. SBE prophylaxis is not needed beyond 6 months after surgery.

Patent Ductus Arteriosus in Preterm Neonates

PREVALENCE

Clinical evidence of PDA appears in 45% of infants with birth weight less than 1750 g and in about 80% of infants with birth weight less than 1200 g. Significant PDA with CHF occurs in 15% of premature infants with birth weight less than 1750 g and in 40% to 50% of those with birth weight less than 1500 g.

PATHOPHYSIOLOGY

1. PDA is a special problem in premature infants who are recovering from hyaline membrane disease. With improvement in oxygenation, the pulmonary vascular resistance falls rapidly, but the ductus remains patent because its responsiveness to oxygen is immature in premature newborns (see Chapter 8). The resulting large left-to-right shunt makes the lung stiff, and weaning the infant from the ventilator and oxygen therapy becomes difficult.

2. If the infant must remain on ventilator and oxygen therapy for a long time, bronchopulmonary dysplasia develops, with resulting pulmonary hypertension (cor pulmonale) and right-sided heart failure. Early recognition and appropriate management are keys to improving the prognosis of these infants.

CLINICAL MANIFESTATIONS

1. The history is important in suspecting a significant PDA in a premature neonate. Typically, a premature infant with hyaline membrane disease shows some improvement during the first few days after birth. This is followed by an inability to wean the infant from the ventilator or a need to increase ventilator settings or oxygen requirements in 4- to 7-day-old premature infants. Episodes of apnea or bradycardia may be the initial sign of PDA in infants who are not on ventilators.

2. The physical examination commonly reveals bounding peripheral pulses, a hyperactive precordium, and tachycardia with or without gallop rhythm. The classic continuous murmur at the left infraclavicular area or upper left sternal border is diagnostic, but the murmur may be only systolic and is difficult to hear in infants who are on ventilators. Premature infants who are fluid overloaded or retaining fluid may also present with findings of PDA as described earlier (hyperdynamic precordium, systolic ejection murmur, bounding pulses, and wide pulse pressures), requiring differentiation from PDA.

3. The ECG is not diagnostic. It is usually normal but occasionally shows LVH.

4. Chest x-ray films show cardiomegaly in larger premature infants who are not intubated. The infant may have evidence of pulmonary edema or increased pulmonary vascular markings, but these may be difficult to assess in the presence of hyaline membrane disease. In infants who are intubated and on high ventilator settings, chest x-ray films may show the heart to be either of normal size or only mildly enlarged.

5. Two-dimensional echo and color flow Doppler studies provide accurate anatomic and functional information.

    a. Two-dimensional echo provides anatomic information about the diameter, length, and shape of the ductus (see Fig. 12–14).

    b. Doppler studies of the ductus (with the sample volume placed at the pulmonary end of the ductus) provide important functional information, such as ductal shunt patterns (pure left-to-right, bidirectional, or predominant right-to-left shunt), pressures in the PA, and magnitude of the ductal shunt or pulmonary perfusion status:

      1). Ductal shunt pattern. A continuous positive flow indicates a pure left-to-right shunt with the PA pressure lower than the aortic pressure. In pure right-to-left shunts, flow is continuously negative away from the PA, indicating that the PA pressure is suprasystemic. A bidirectional shunting pattern (with an early negative flow in systole followed by a late positive flow in diastole) is found in infants with PDA and severe pulmonary hypertension.

      2). Estimation of PA pressures. A high ductal flow velocity indicates a low PA pressure, and a low flow velocity indicates a high PA pressure. The pressure drop may be underestimated in patients with a small pulmonary end of the ductus, tortuous PDAs, or tunnel-like PDAs with diameters less than 3 mm and lengths greater than 10 mm (because of viscous energy loss).

However, the easiest and most accurate estimate of the PA systolic pressure is obtained from the peak velocity of tricuspid regurgitation, when it is present.

3). Perfusion status. Increased flow velocity in the left PA suggests a large left-to-right shunt through the ductus. High PA pressure and a lower flow velocity (with a pressure drop of <5 mm Hg) indicate poor perfusion of the lungs, which is a bad prognostic sign during the first 24 to 36 hours.

MANAGEMENT

For symptomatic infants, either pharmacologic or surgical closure of the ductus is indicated. A small PDA that does not cause symptoms should be observed medically for 6 months without surgical ligation because of the possibility of spontaneous closure.

Medical

1. Fluid restriction to 120 mL/kg per day and a diuretic (e.g., furosemide, 1 mg/kg, two to three times a day) may be tried for 24 to 48 hours, but these regimens have a low success rate. Digoxin is not used because it has little hemodynamic benefit and a high incidence of digitalis toxicity.

2. Pharmacologic closure of the PDA can he achieved with indomethacin (a prostaglandin synthetase inhibitor). Indications and dosages vary from center to center (see later). One popular approach is to give indomethacin (Indocin) 0.2 mg/kg intravenously every 12 hours for up to three doses in selected cases. A second course of indomethacin treatment is occasionally necessary to achieve adequate ductal closure. Contraindications to the use of indomethacin include high blood urea nitrogen (>25 mg/dL) or creatinine (>1.8 mg/dL) levels, low platelet count (<80,000/mm^3), bleeding tendency (including intracranial hemorrhage), necrotizing enterocolitis, and hyperbilirubinemia.

   Many dosage regimens exist, and dose is dependent on the postnatal age of the infant at the time of the first dose; one example is as follows. The dose is given intravenously every 12 hours for a total of three doses. For infants less than 48 hours old, 0.2 mg/kg is followed by 0.1 mg/kg times 2. For those 2 to 7 days old, 0.2 mg/kg times 3, and for infants older than 7 days, 0.2 mg/kg followed by 0.25 mg/kg times 2.

3. A multicenter prospective study from Europe showed that intravenous ibuprofen (10 mg/kg, followed at 24-hour intervals by two doses of 5 mg/kg) starting on the third day of life was as effective as indomethacin in closing the ductus in preterm newborns. Ibuprofen was associated with a significantly lower incidence of oliguria, and it does not appear to have a deleterious effect on cerebral blood flow. Ibuprofen significantly reduces plasma concentrations of prostaglandin. An earlier study from Canada reported that intravenous ibuprofen 10 mg/kg given at 3 hours of age, followed by 5 mg/kg given at 24 and 48 hours of age, was effective in reducing the incidence of PDA without causing notable adverse drug reactions. Thus, ibuprofen appears to be a valuable alternative to indomethacin for both the treatment and the prophylaxis of PDA in preterm newborns. Ibuprofen may prove to be a better choice than indomethacin. A dose-finding study conducted in Europe confirmed the dosage of 10-5-5 mg/kg to be correct for ductal closure (Desfrere et al, 2005). Recent reports from Europe concluded that prophylactic use of ibuprofen in small preterm infants was not useful because, although it reduced the occurrence and the need for surgical ligation of the ductus, it did not reduce the frequency of intraventricular hemorrhage, mortality, or morbidity.

Surgical. If medical treatment is unsuccessful or if the use of indomethacin is contraindicated, surgical ligation of the ductus is indicated. The standard operative approach to PDA is through a posterolateral thoracotomy. The PDA is simply ligated or hemoclipped (without division). Many centers now perform PDA ligation in the neonatal intensive care unit at the bedside. The operative mortality is 0% to 3%.

Recently, the use of minimally invasive video-assisted thoracoscopic surgery has been reported for the management of PDA in low-birth-weight infants. This technique allows PDA interruption without the muscle cutting or rib spreading of a standard thoracotomy. Reduced compromise of respiratory mechanics and less chest wall deformity associated with a large thoracotomy incision may also be advantages.

Complete Endocardial Cushion Defect

PREVALENCE

Complete ECD (also called complete AV canal defect or AV communis) occurs in 2% of all congenital heart defects. Of patients with complete ECD, about 70% are children with Down syndrome. Of children with Down syndrome, about 40% have congenital heart defects and 50% of the defects are ECD. ECD is also a component of heart defects in asplenia and polysplenia syndromes (see Chapter 14).

PATHOLOGY

1. Abnormalities seen in complete ECD affect the structures normally derived from the endocardial cushion tissue. Ostium primum ASD, VSD in the inlet ventricular septum, and clefts in the anterior mitral valve and the septal leaflet of the tricuspid valve (forming the common AV valve) are all present in the complete form of ECD (Fig. 12–15). The combination of these defects may result in interatrial and interventricular shunts, LV-to-RA shunt, and AV valve regurgitation. Although rare, the entire atrial septum may be absent (common atrium). When two AV valve orifices are present without an interventricular shunt, the defect is called partial ECD or ostium primum ASD (which is presented under a separate heading in this chapter).

2. Both complete and partial forms of ECD are characterized by a deficiency of the inlet portion of the ventricular septum, with a "scooped-out" appearance of the muscular septum and an excessively long infundibular septum, as well as by an abnormal position of the aortic valve (i.e., anterosuperior to, rather than wedged between, the right and left AV valves). The latter results in lengthening and narrowing of the left ventricular outflow tract, producing the characteristic "goose-neck deformity" on angiocardiogram (see Fig. 12–20).

3. In complete ECD, a single valve orifice connects the atrial and ventricular chambers, whereas in the partial form, there are separate mitral and tricuspid orifices.

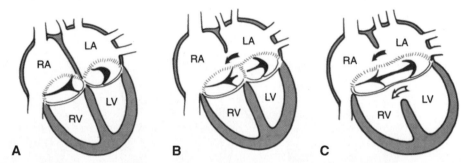

Figure 12–15. *Diagram of the atrioventricular (AV) valve and cardiac septa in partial and complete endocardial cushion defects (ECDs).* ***A,*** *Normal AV valve anatomy with no septal defect.* ***B,*** *Partial ECD with clefts in the mitral and tricuspid valves and an ostium primum atrial septal defect (ASD) (solid arrow).* ***C,*** *Complete ECD. There is a common AV valve with large anterior and posterior bridging leaflets. An ostium primum ASD (solid arrow) and an inlet ventricular septal defect (open arrow) are present. LA, left atrium; LV, left ventricle; RA, right atrium; RV, right ventricle.*

The common AV valve usually has five leaflets (see Fig. 12–15). The arrangement of the LV papillary muscles may be abnormal in that either they are closer together or only one papillary muscle is present in the LV, which makes surgical repair difficult.

4. In the majority of complete ECD cases, the AV orifices are equally committed to the RV and LV. In some patients, however, the orifices are committed primarily to one ventricle, with hypoplasia of the other ventricle (i.e., "unbalanced" AV canal with RV or LV dominance). Hypoplasia of one ventricle may necessitate one ventricular repair (Fontan operation).

5. A universally accepted classification for complete ECD does not exist. The Rastelli classification was based on the relationships of the anterior bridging leaflets to the crest of the ventricular septum or RV papillary muscles (Fig. 12–16). In type A, the anterior bridging leaflet is tightly tethered to the crest of the ventricular septum, occurring in 50% to 70%. This type is commonly associated with Down syndrome. In type B (3%), the anterior bridging leaflet is not attached to the ventricular septum; rather, it is attached to an anomalous RV papillary muscle and is almost always associated with unbalanced AV canal with right dominance. In type C (30%), a free-floating anterior leaflet is attached to the anterior papillary muscle. This type is often seen in visceral heterotaxia and conotruncal malformations.

6. Additional cardiac anomalies include TOF (called "canal tet," occurring in 6% of patients), double-outlet right ventricle with more than 50% overriding of the aorta (occurring in 6%), and TGA (occurring in 3%). Associated defects are rare in children with Down syndrome.

CLINICAL MANIFESTATIONS

History. Failure to thrive, repeated respiratory infections, and signs of CHF are common.

Physical Examination (Fig. 12–17)

1. Infants with ECD are usually undernourished and have tachycardia and tachypnea (signs of CHF). This defect is common in infants with Down syndrome.

2. Hyperactive precordium with a systolic thrill at the lower left sternal border is common (shown as the area with dots in Fig. 12–17).

3. The S1 is accentuated. The S2 narrowly splits, and the P2 increases in intensity. A grade 3 to 4/6 holosystolic murmur is usually audible along the lower left sternal border. The systolic murmur may transmit well to the left back and be heard well at the apex when mitral regurgitation (MR) is significant. A mid-diastolic

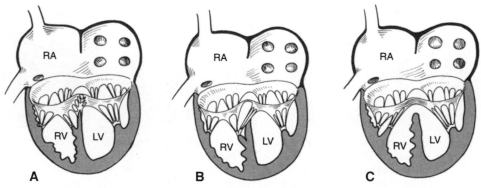

*Figure 12–16. Rastelli's classification of complete endocardial cushion defect. **A**, Type A. **B**, Type B. **C**, Type C. (See text for descriptions.) LV, left ventricle; RA, right atrium; RV, right ventricle.*

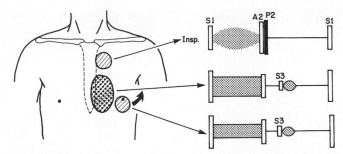

Figure 12–17. *Cardiac findings of complete endocardial cushion defect, which resemble those of a large ventricular septal defect. An apical holosystolic murmur (due to mitral regurgitation) may transmit toward the left axilla. A systolic thrill may be present at the lower left sternal border (dotted area), where the systolic murmur is loudest. Insp., inspiration.*

rumble may be present at the lower left sternal border or at the apex as a result of relative stenosis of the tricuspid or mitral valve.

4. Signs of CHF (e.g., hepatomegaly, gallop rhythm) may be present.

Electrocardiography

1. "Superior" QRS axis with the QRS axis between −40 and −150 degrees is characteristic of the defect (Fig. 12–18).

2. Most of the patients have a prolonged PR interval (first-degree AV block).

3. RVH or RBBB is present in all cases, and many patients have LVH, too.

X-ray Studies. Cardiomegaly is always present and involves all four cardiac chambers. Pulmonary vascular markings are increased, and the main PA segment is prominent.

Echocardiography. Two-dimensional and Doppler echo studies allow imaging of all components of complete ECD and an assessment of the severity of these components. The following surgically important information can be gained: size of the ASD and VSD, size of the AV valve orifices, anatomy of leaflets, chordal attachment, relative and absolute size of the RV and LV (balance of the canal), and papillary muscle architecture (one versus two) in the LV.

1. The apical and subcostal four-chamber views are most useful in evaluating the anatomy and the functional significance of the defect. These views show both an ostium primum ASD and an inlet muscular VSD (Fig. 12–19). Either the anterior

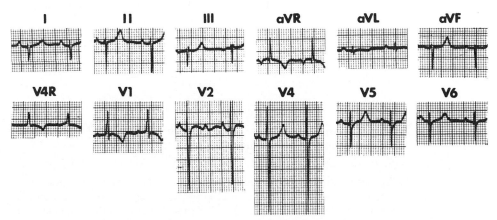

Figure 12–18. *Tracing from a 5-year-old boy with Down syndrome and complete atrioventricular canal. Note the "superior" QRS axis (−110 degrees) and right ventricular hypertrophy.*

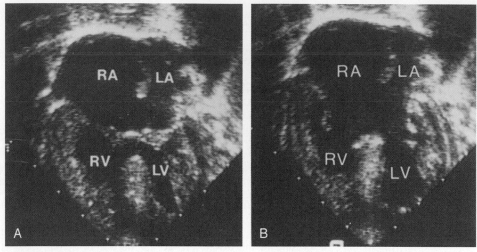

Figure 12–19. *Apical four-chamber views in systole (**A**) and diastole (**B**) from a patient with a complete endocardial cushion defect. In systole, an ostium primum defect and an inlet ventricular septal defect are imaged. The atrioventricular (AV) valve appears to be attached to the crest of the ventricular septum by chordae (type A). When the AV valve opens in diastole, a large deficiency in the center of the heart is visible. Note that there is a common AV valve instead of two separate AV valves. LA, left atrium; LV, left ventricle; RA, right atrium; RV, right ventricle. (From Snider AR, Serwer GA: Echocardiography in Pediatric Heart Disease. St Louis, Mosby, 1990.)*

bridging leaflet crosses the ventricular septum, or the right and left AV valve leaflets can be seen at the same level from the crest of the ventricular septum. The full extent of the ASD and VSD can be imaged during systole when the common anterior leaflet is closed.

2. A combined use of the subcostal transducer position (i.e., about 45 degrees clockwise from a standard four-chamber view) and the parasternal short-axis examination may show a cleft in the mitral valve, the presence of bridging leaflets, the number of AV valve orifices (e.g., double-orifice mitral valve), and the AV valve leaflets. These views may also image the abnormal position of the anterolateral papillary muscle, which is displaced posteriorly from its normal position, and the number (i.e., single or triple) of papillary muscles.

3. The subcostal five-chamber view may image a goose-neck deformity, which is characteristic of an angiocardiographic finding (Fig. 12–20).

4. In real time, the subcostal and apical four-chamber views can image the chordal attachment of the anterior bridging leaflet to the crest of the ventricular septum (type A), to the right side of the septum (type B), or to a papillary muscle at the apex of the RV or on its free wall (type C).

NATURAL HISTORY

1. For patients with complete ECD, heart failure occurs 1 to 2 months after birth and recurrent pneumonia is common.

2. Without surgical intervention, most patients die by the age of 2 to 3 years.

3. In the latter half of the first year of life, the survivors begin to develop pulmonary vascular obstructive disease. These survivors usually die in late childhood or as young adults. Infants with Down syndrome are particularly susceptible to the early development of pulmonary vascular obstructive disease during infancy. As a result, surgery should be performed during infancy.

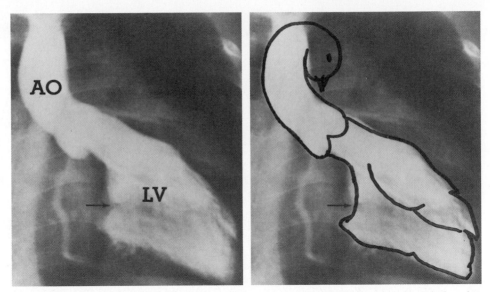

Figure 12–20. *Frontal view of a left ventriculogram of a patient with partial endocardial cushion defect showing a goose-neck deformity. The left ventricular outflow tract is elongated and narrowed. The arrows point to the mitral cleft. AO, aorta: LV, left ventricle.*

MANAGEMENT

Medical

1. In small infants with CHF, anticongestive management consisting of digoxin, diuretics, captopril, and so on should be started (see Chapter 27).

2. Antibiotics and other supportive measures are indicated for pneumonia and other infections.

3. Antibiotic prophylaxis against SBE is recommended.

Surgical

Indications. The presence of complete ECD indicates the need for surgery because an important hemodynamic derangement is usually present. Most of these infants have CHF that is unresponsive to medical therapy, and some have elevated pulmonary vascular resistance.

Timing. Although timing varies among institutions and with the hemodynamics of the defect, most centers perform the repair at 2 to 4 months of age. Early surgical repair is especially important for infants with Down syndrome and complete ECD because of their known tendency to develop early pulmonary vascular obstructive disease.

Procedures

Palliative. Banding of the PA in early infancy is no longer recommended unless other associated abnormalities make complete repair a high-risk procedure. The mortality rate for PA banding may be as high as 15%.

Corrective. Given two ventricles of suitable size and no additional defects, closure of the primum ASD and inlet VSD and construction of two separate and competent AV valves are carried out under cardiopulmonary bypass or deep hypothermia, or both. Some surgeons use a single patch to close the ASD and VSD and reconstruction of the left AV valve as a bileaflet valve, whereas others use a two-patch technique; one patch for the VSD and a second for the ASD. The left AV valve is allowed to persist as a trileaflet structure. A schematic drawing of the surgery is shown in Figure 12–21. This figure illustrates the complexity of anatomy of the AV canal. Mitral valve replacement may become necessary in a few patients.

Patients with an unbalanced AV canal (with hypoplasia of the right or left ventricle) may be treated by an earlier PA banding and later by a modified Fontan operation.

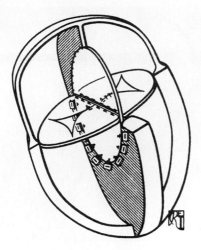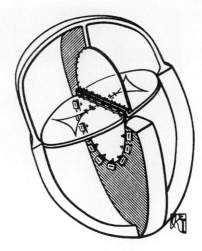

Figure 12–21. *Schematic three-dimensional reconstructive surgery for complete atrioventricular canal defect.* ***A,*** *Single-patch technique.* ***B,*** *Two-patch technique. (From Backer CL, Mavroudis C: Atrioventricular canal defect. In Mavroudis C, Backer CL [eds]: Pediatric Cardiac Surgery, 3rd ed. Philadelphia, Mosby, 2003, pp 321–338.)*

Mortality. The mortality rate has been 3% to 10%. The survival rate is the same for patients with and without Down syndrome. Factors that increase the surgical risk are young age, severe AV valve regurgitation, hypoplasia of the LV, increased and fixed pulmonary vascular resistance, and severe preoperative symptoms. Other defects (e.g., double-orifice mitral valve, single left-sided papillary muscle, additional muscular VSD) increase the surgical risk. The hospital mortality rate for complete ECD and TOF is around 10%.

Complications

1. MR becomes persistent or worsens 10% of the time.
2. Sinus node dysfunction resulting in bradyarrhythmias may occur.
3. Although complete heart block occurs rarely (in <5% of patients), it occurs more frequently when mitral valve replacement is required (up to 20% of patients).
4. Postoperative arrhythmias occur and are usually supraventricular.

Special Situations

1. Because of the early development of pulmonary vascular obstructive disease in patients with Down syndrome and complete ECD, a cardiac catheterization should be performed before 3 months of age, and elective surgery should follow shortly thereafter. Down syndrome itself is not a risk factor.
2. Patients with severe hypoplasia of the LV and low PA pressure may receive a combination of the Damus-Kaye-Stansel operation (see Fig. 14–11 or Fig. 14–62) and a Fontan-type operation. The proximal PA is anastomosed end to side to the ascending aorta and systemic venous return is channeled to the right PA, bypassing the RV.
3. In patients with TOF and complete ECD (i.e., canal tet) who are severely cyanotic, a systemic-to-PA shunt is carried out during infancy. A complete repair is done between 2 and 4 years of age.
4. Parachute deformity of the mitral valve may result in an obstructed mitral orifice. If there is a significant MR, valve replacement may be required.
5. Double-orifice mitral valve (found in 4%) is usually left alone. Incision of the valve may create more problems with MR.

Postoperative Follow-up

1. An office evaluation should be performed every 6 months to 1 year.

2. SBE prophylaxis should be continued as indicated, even after surgery.

3. Medications (e.g., digitalis, diuretics, captopril) may be required if residual hemodynamic abnormalities are present.

4. Some restriction of activities may be necessary if significant MR or other complications exist.

5. Rarely, subaortic stenosis may appear after surgical repair of complete ECD (although it is less frequent than in patients who had primum ASD repair), requiring surgical resection.

Partial Endocardial Cushion Defect

PREVALENCE

Partial ECD (partial AV canal defect or ostium primum ASD) occurs in 1% to 2% of all congenital heart defects, which is considerably less than the prevalence of secundum ASD.

PATHOLOGY

1. In partial ECD, there is a defect in the lower part of the atrial septum near the AV valves, without an interventricular communication (see Fig. 12–1). The anterior and posterior bridging leaflets are fused by a connecting tongue to form separate right and left AV orifices (see Fig. 12–15). There are clefts in the septal leaflets of the mitral and tricuspid valves. The conjoined leaflets are displaced into the ventricle and are usually firmly attached to the crest of the ventricular septum. The aortic valve and AV valves are distanced from one another, which accounts for the characteristic goose-neck deformity in angiocardiograms (see Fig. 12–20).

2. Less common forms of partial ECD include common atrium, VSD of the inlet septum (i.e., AV canal–type VSD), and isolated cleft of the mitral valve. A common atrium, in which the atrial septum is virtually absent, is either a characteristic lesion in patients with the Ellis-van Creveld syndrome or a component of complex cyanotic heart defects such as those associated with asplenia or polysplenia syndrome.

3. Occasional associated anomalies include secundum ASD and persistent left SVC that drains into the coronary sinus.

CLINICAL MANIFESTATIONS

History

1. Patients with ostium primum ASD are usually asymptomatic during childhood.

2. A history of symptoms such as dyspnea, easy fatigability, recurrent respiratory infections, and growth retardation may be present early in life if associated with major MR or common atrium.

Physical Examination

1. Cardiac findings are the same as those of secundum ASD (see Fig. 12–2), with the exception of a regurgitant systolic murmur of MR (owing to a cleft mitral valve), which may be present at the apex.

2. Mild cyanosis and clubbing may be present in patients with a common atrium.

Electrocardiography

1. "Superior" QRS axis with the QRS axis ranging from −30 to −150 degrees is characteristic of the condition (see Fig. 12–18).

2. RVH or RBBB (with rsR′ pattern in V1) is present, as in secundum ASD.

3. First-degree AV block (i.e., prolonged PR interval) is present in about 50% of cases.

X-ray Studies. The x-ray findings are the same as those of a secundum ASD (see Fig. 12–4), except for enlargement of the LA and LV when MR is significant. A characteristic goose-neck deformity is seen on a left ventriculogram (see Fig. 12–20).

Echocardiography

1. Two-dimensional and Doppler echo allow accurate diagnosis of primum ASD. The defect is in the lower atrial septum (see Fig. 12–5). No visible or Doppler-detectable VSD is present. The septal portions of the AV valves insert at the same level on the crest of the ventricular septum.

2. A cleft in the anterior leaflet of the mitral valve is commonly imaged. Less common abnormalities of the mitral valve include double-orifice mitral valve and parachute mitral valve.

3. The atrial septum may be completely absent (common atrium) in patients with Ellis-van Creveld syndrome.

4. Color flow and Doppler studies are useful in the detection of stenosis or regurgitation of the AV valve and in the assessment of the RV and PA pressures.

NATURAL HISTORY

1. Spontaneous closure of the defect does not occur.

2. CHF may develop in childhood earlier than with secundum ASD. CHF is related to major MR or other associated defects.

3. Pulmonary hypertension (i.e., pulmonary vascular obstructive disease) develops in adulthood.

4. SBE, usually of the AV valve, is a rare complication.

5. Arrhythmias occur in 20% of patients.

MANAGEMENT

Medical

1. No exercise restriction is indicated.

2. Precaution against SBE should be observed.

3. Anticongestive therapy with digoxin and diuretics may be indicated for some patients.

Surgical

Indications and Timing. The presence of a partial AV canal or primum ASD is an indication for surgical repair. Elective surgery can be performed in asymptomatic children between 2 and 4 years of age. Surgery can be performed earlier in infants with CHF, failure to thrive, MR, or a common atrium.

Procedure. Under cardiopulmonary bypass, the primum ASD is closed and the cleft mitral and tricuspid valves are reconstructed. Some surgeons leave the mitral valve as a trileaflet valve (without suturing the cleft) by performing various mitral annuloplasties. Minimally invasive cardiac surgical techniques with smaller skin incisions have become popular, especially for female patients (discussed under "Atrial Septal Defect").

Mortality. The surgical mortality rate is approximately 3%. Risk factors include the presence of CHF or cyanosis, failure to thrive, and moderate to severe MR.

Complications

1. Reoperation is needed in about 15% of the patients who have residual or worsening MR.

2. Atrial or nodal arrhythmias occasionally occur.

3. Complete heart block rarely results and requires a permanent cardiac pacemaker.

4. Although rare, subaortic stenosis can develop after surgery.

Postoperative Follow-up

1. Usually no restriction in activity is indicated.

2. Unlike the management of secundum ASD, continued SBE prophylaxis is indicated even after completing surgery for a residual AV valve regurgitation, which is likely to be present in most patients.

3. Sinus node dysfunction may require permanent pacemaker therapy.

4. Periodic echocardiographic evaluation for the development of subaortic stenosis and for worsening of MR should be performed. Subaortic stenosis develops more frequently after repair of partial ECD than complete ECD.

Partial Anomalous Pulmonary Venous Return

PREVALENCE

PAPVR occurs in less than 1% of all congenital heart defects.

PATHOLOGY

1. One or more (but not all) pulmonary veins drain into the RA or its venous tributaries such as the SVC, IVC, coronary sinus, and left innominate vein. The right pulmonary veins are involved twice as often as the left pulmonary veins.

2. The right pulmonary veins may drain into the SVC, which is often associated with sinus venosus defect (Fig. 12–22A), or drain into the IVC (see Fig. 12–22B) in association with an intact atrial septum and bronchopulmonary sequestration (see Chapter 17).

3. The left pulmonary veins either drain into the left innominate vein (see Fig. 12–22C) or drain into the coronary sinus (see Fig. 12–22D). ASD is usually present with anomalous drainage of the left pulmonary veins.

PATHOPHYSIOLOGY

1. Hemodynamic alterations are similar to those in ASD. Pulmonary blood flow increases as a result of recirculation through the lungs.

2. The magnitude of the pulmonary recirculation is determined by the number of anomalous pulmonary veins, the presence and size of the ASD, and the pulmonary vascular resistance.

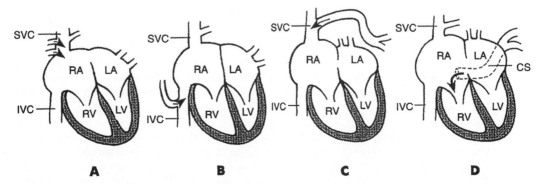

A   **B**   **C**   **D**

Figure 12–22. *Common types of partial anomalous pulmonary venous return.* *A,* *The right pulmonary veins drain anomalously to the superior vena cava (SVC). Sinus venosus atrial septal defect (ASD) is usually present.* *B,* *The right lower pulmonary vein drains anomalously into the inferior vena cava (IVC), usually without an associated ASD.* *C,* *The left pulmonary veins drain into the left innominate vein.* *D,* *The left pulmonary veins drain into the coronary sinus (CS). LA, left atrium; LV, left ventricle; RA, right atrium; RV, right ventricle.*

CLINICAL MANIFESTATIONS

History. Children with PAPVR are usually asymptomatic.

Physical Examination

1. Cardiac findings are similar to those of ASD (see Fig. 12–2).

2. When associated with ASD, the S2 is split widely and fixed. When the atrial septum is intact, the S2 is normal. A grade 2 to 3/6 midsystolic murmur is present at the upper left sternal border. A mid-diastolic rumble, resulting from relative tricuspid stenosis, may be present.

Electrocardiography. RVH, RBBB, or a normal ECG may be seen.

X-ray Studies. The findings are similar to those of secundum ASD (see Fig. 12–4).

1. Cardiomegaly involving the RA and RV, prominence of the PA segment, and increased pulmonary vascularity are all present.

2. Occasionally a dilated SVC, a crescent-shaped vertical shadow in the right lower lung (scimitar syndrome), or a distended vertical vein may suggest the site of anomalous drainage.

Echocardiography. The diagnosis of PAPVR requires a high index of suspicion. A systematic attempt to visualize each pulmonary vein should be made during any routine echo studies.

1. The inability to visualize all four pulmonary veins in the presence of mild dilatation of the RA and RV strongly suggests the diagnosis of PAPVR, especially in the presence of a demonstrable ASD.

2. PAPVR is frequently found in patients with ASD of any type and in those with persistent left SVC.

3. In sinus venosus defect, the chance of anomalous drainage of the right upper pulmonary vein is high.

NATURAL HISTORY

1. Cyanosis and exertional dyspnea may develop during the third and fourth decades of life. This results from pulmonary hypertension and pulmonary vascular obstructive disease.

2. Pulmonary infections are common in patients with anomalous drainage of the right pulmonary veins to the IVC.

MANAGEMENT

Medical

1. Exercise restriction is not required.

2. SBE prophylaxis is probably not indicated.

Surgical

Indications and Timing. Indications for surgery include a significant left-to-right shunt with a Qp/Qs greater than 2:1 and, if the anatomy is uncomplicated, a ratio greater than 1.5:1. Surgery is indicated in patients with scimitar syndrome with severe hypoplasia of the right lung even with a Qp/Qs less than 2:1. Surgery is carried out between the ages of 2 and 5 years. Isolated single lobe anomaly without an ASD is usually not corrected.

Procedures. Surgical correction is carried out under cardiopulmonary bypass. The procedure to be performed depends on the site of the anomalous drainage.

To the Right Atrium. The ASD is widened, and a patch is sewn in such a way that the anomalous pulmonary veins drain into the LA (similar to that shown in Fig. 14–33B).

To the Superior Vena Cava. A tunnel is created between the anomalous vein and the ASD through the SVC and the RA by using a Teflon or pericardial patch. A plastic or pericardial gusset is placed in the SVC to prevent obstruction to the SVC.

To the Inferior Vena Cava. In scimitar syndrome, the resection of the involved lobe or lobes may be indicated without connecting the anomalous vein to the heart. When the anomalous venous drainage is an isolated lesion, the vein is reimplanted to the RA, and an intra-atrial tunnel is created to drain into the LA.

To the Coronary Sinus. This defect is repaired in the same manner as for TAPVR to the coronary sinus (see Fig. 14-33C).

Mortality. Surgical mortality occurs less than 1% of the time.

Complications

1. SVC obstruction for patients with anomalous drainage into the SVC.

2. Postoperative arrhythmias (usually supraventricular) occur.

Postoperative Follow-up

1. An examination should be done every 1 to 2 years or at longer intervals.

2. No restriction in activities is indicated.

3. SBE prophylaxis is not indicated beyond 6 months after surgery.

Chapter 13

Obstructive Lesions

Lesions that produce obstruction to ventricular outflow such as pulmonary stenosis (PS), aortic stenosis (AS), and coarctation of the aorta (COA) are discussed in this chapter.

Pulmonary Stenosis

PREVALENCE

Isolated PS occurs in 8% to 12% of all congenital heart defects. PS is often associated with many other CHDs, such as tetralogy of Fallot and single ventricle.

PATHOLOGY

1. PS may be valvular, subvalvular (infundibular), or supravalvular. An obstruction may occur within the right ventricular (RV) cavity by an abnormal muscle bundle (i.e., "double-chambered RV").

2. In *valvular PS*, the pulmonary valve is thickened, with fused or absent commissures and a small orifice (Fig. 13–1A). Although the RV is usually normal in size, it is hypoplastic in infants with critical PS (with a nearly atretic valve). Dysplastic valves (consisting of thickened, irregular, immobile tissue and a variably small pulmonary valve annulus) are frequently seen with Noonan's syndrome.

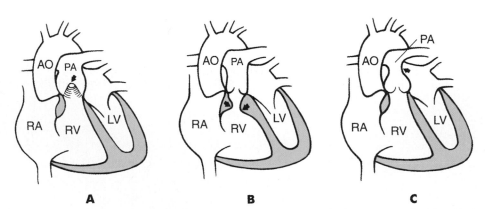

Figure 13–1. *Anatomic types of pulmonary stenosis (PS).* **A,** *Valvular stenosis.* **B,** *Infundibular stenosis.* **C,** *Supravalvular PS (or stenosis of the main pulmonary artery [PA]). Abnormalities are indicated by arrows. AO, aorta; LV, left ventricle; RA, right atrium; RV, right ventricle.*

3. Isolated *infundibular PS* is rare; it is usually associated with a large ventricular septal defect (VSD), as seen in tetralogy of Fallot (TOF) (see Fig. 13–1B).

4. Aberrant hypertrophied muscular bands (running between the ventricular septum and the anterior wall) divide the RV cavity into a proximal high-pressure chamber and a distal low-pressure chamber (double-chambered RV). A "dimple" in the ordinarily smooth RV surface is found at surgery (see Chapter 17).

5. Supravalvular PS (or stenosis of the pulmonary arteries), isolated or in association with other CHDs, occurs in 2% to 3% of all patients with CHD. The stenosis may be single, involving the main pulmonary artery (see Fig. 13–1) or either of its branches, or multiple, involving both the main and several smaller peripheral PA branches (not shown). Common associated defects are pulmonary valve stenosis, VSD, and TOF. Peripheral PA stenosis is often seen in association with congenital syndromes, such as congenital rubella syndrome, Williams' syndrome, Noonan's syndrome, Alagille's syndrome, Ehlers-Danlos syndrome, and Silver-Russell syndrome.

CLINICAL MANIFESTATIONS

History

1. Children with mild PS are completely asymptomatic. Exertional dyspnea and easy fatigability may be present in patients with moderately severe cases. Heart failure or exertional chest pain may develop in severe cases.

2. Newborns with critical PS may present with poor feeding, tachypnea, and cyanosis.

Physical Examination (Fig. 13–2)

1. Most patients are acyanotic and well developed. Newborns with critical PS are cyanotic and tachypneic.

2. An RV tap and a systolic thrill may be present at the upper left sternal border (and occasionally in the suprasternal notch).

3. A systolic ejection click is present at the upper left sternal border only with valvular stenosis. The S2 may split widely, and the P2 may be diminished in intensity. An ejection-type systolic murmur (grade 2 to 5/6) is best audible at the upper left sternal border, and it transmits well to the back, too. The louder and longer the murmur, the more severe the stenosis.

4. Hepatomegaly may be present if congestive heart failure (CHF) develops.

5. In newborns with critical PS, cyanosis may be present (due to a right-to-left atrial shunt), and signs of CHF with hepatomegaly and peripheral vasoconstriction may be found.

6. In patients with peripheral PA stenosis, a midsystolic murmur in the pulmonary valve area is well transmitted to the axillae and back. Occasionally, a continuous murmur is audible over the involved lung field.

Electrocardiography

1. The ECG is normal in mild cases.

2. Right axis deviation (RAD) and right ventricular hypertrophy (RVH) are present in moderate PS. The degree of RVH on the ECG correlates with the severity of PS

Figure 13–2. Cardiac findings of pulmonary valve stenosis. Abnormal sounds are shown in black. Dots represent areas with systolic thrill. EC, ejection click.

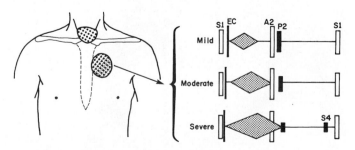

(i.e., the R wave in V1 >20 mm is usually associated with systemic pressure in the RV).

3. Right atrial hypertrophy (RAH) and RVH with "strain" may be seen in severe PS.

4. Neonates with critical PS may show left ventricular hypertrophy (LVH) because of a hypoplastic RV and relatively large left ventricle (LV).

X-ray Studies

1. Heart size is usually normal, but the main PA segment is prominent (because of poststenotic dilatation) (Fig. 13–3). Cardiomegaly is present if CHF develops.

2. Pulmonary vascular markings are usually normal but may decrease with severe PS.

3. In neonates with critical PS, lung fields are oligemic with a varying degree of cardiomegaly.

Echocardiography

1. Two-dimensional echo in the parasternal short-axis view shows thick pulmonary valve cusps with restricted systolic motion (doming). The size of the pulmonary valve annulus can be estimated. The main PA is often dilated (poststenotic dilatation).

2. Dysplastic valves are characterized by a noticeably thickened and immobile leaflet and hypoplasia of the pulmonary valve annulus.

3. The Doppler study can estimate the pressure gradient across the stenotic valve by the simplified Bernoulli equation (see Fig. 6–6). Multiple transducer positions should be used to obtain the maximum flow velocity. A pressure gradient less than 35 to 40 mm Hg (or RV systolic pressure <50% of the LV pressure) is considered mild. A valve pressure gradient of 40 to 70 mm Hg (or RV pressure 50% to 75% of the LV pressure) is considered moderate, and a pressure gradient greater than 70 mm Hg (or RV pressure = 75% LV pressure) is severe. The instantaneous pressure gradient estimated by Doppler echo is slightly greater than the peak-to-peak systolic pressure gradient obtained by cardiac catheterization.

4. In neonates, the severity of PS can be underestimated because their PA pressure may be higher than normal, especially in those with patent ductus arteriosus (PDA) with a left-to-right shunt.

NATURAL HISTORY

1. The severity of stenosis is usually not progressive in mild PS. For example, over 95% of patients who had an initial Doppler gradient less than 25 mm Hg were free of cardiac operation over a 25-year period. The severity tends to progress with age in moderate or severe PS.

2. CHF may develop in patients with severe stenosis.

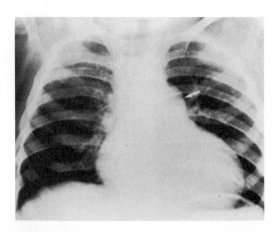

Figure 13–3. Posteroanterior view of chest film in pulmonary valve stenosis. Note a marked poststenotic dilatation (arrow) and normal pulmonary vascularity. (Courtesy Dr. Ewell Clarke, San Antonio, Texas.)

3. Infective endocarditis occasionally occurs.

4. Sudden death is possible in patients with severe stenosis during heavy physical activities.

5. Without appropriate management, most neonates with critical PS die (see "Management").

MANAGEMENT

Medical

1. Newborns with critical PS and cyanosis require emergency treatment to reduce mortality. These babies may temporarily improve with prostaglandin E_1 (PGE_1) infusion, which reopens the ductus arteriosus, and other supportive measures. Balloon valvuloplasty is the procedure of choice in critically ill neonates. Immediate reduction in pressure gradient can be achieved in more than 90% of these neonates but some of these infants are not able to maintain effective forward flow through the pulmonary valve because of noncompliant or hypoplastic RV, requiring surgical intervention. If ductal dependence persists, a shunt operation is indicated. In neonates, complications of the balloon procedure are more common than in older patients, with a mortality rate of up to 3%, a major complication rate of 3.5%, and a minor complication rate of 15%. Even dysplastic valves appear to mature after the procedure. Some patients require reintervention (either repeated valvuloplasty or surgery) at a later time.

2. Balloon valvuloplasty, which is performed at the time of cardiac catheterization, is the procedure of choice for the valvular stenosis; it is preferable to surgical repair for significant pulmonary valve stenosis.

    Indications for balloon valvuloplasty for pulmonary valve stenosis in adolescents are as follows, according to ACC/AHA 2006 Guidelines (American College of Cardiology, 2006). The same indications may apply for younger children.

    a. Symptomatic patients* with catheterization gradient greater than 30 mm Hg.
    b. Asymptomatic patients with catheterization gradient greater than 40 mm Hg.

    c. If the catheterization gradient is 30 to 39 mm Hg, a balloon procedure may be reasonable.

    Cardiac catheterization is recommended in patients with a borderline gradient, such as Doppler peak jet velocity greater than 3 mm (or peak gradient >36 mm Hg). The balloon dilatation can be performed in the same setting if indicated.

    A good outcome is achieved in 85% of patients with valvular stenosis. Mild to moderate PR may occur in less than 15% of the patients. The balloon procedure carries an extremely low risk, is painless, is less costly than surgery, and shortens hospital stay. This procedure is useful even for dysplastic pulmonary valves, although the success rate is lower (65%). If balloon valvuloplasty is unsuccessful, surgery is indicated.

3. Surgical treatment is not possible when the stenosis is within the lung parenchyma. Balloon angioplasty has a lower success rate (about 50%) because of recurrence. The stainless steel balloon-expandable intravascular stent has dramatically improved the effectiveness of balloon angioplasty (75% to 100%).

4. Restriction of activity is not necessary in children with this condition, except in cases of severe PS (Doppler gradient >70 mm Hg).

5. Antibiotic prophylaxis against subacute bacterial endocarditis (SBE) should be observed when indications arise.

---

*Symptoms may include angina, syncope or presyncope, and exertional dyspnea.

Surgical

Indications and Timing

1. Surgical valvotomy is indicated on an elective basis for patients with dysplastic pulmonary valves resistant to dilatation and occasional patients in whom balloon valvuloplasty is unsuccessful.

2. Other types of obstruction (e.g., infundibular stenosis, anomalous RV muscle bundle) with significant pressure gradients also require surgery on an elective basis.

3. If balloon valvuloplasty is unsuccessful or unavailable, infants with critical PS and CHF require surgery on an urgent basis.

Procedure

1. Through a midsternal incision, pulmonary valvotomy is performed for pulmonary valve stenosis under cardiopulmonary bypass. The approach is through the PA. Neonates with critical PS may require a transventricular valvotomy and/or the insertion of a transannular patch while receiving PGE_1 infusion. If severe infundibular hypoplasia is present, a systemic-to-PA shunt is also performed. Minimally invasive surgery through a right posterior thoracotomy has been reported for pulmonary valve stenosis.

2. Dysplastic valves often require complete excision of the valves. Simple valvotomy may be ineffective.

3. Infundibular stenosis requires resection of the infundibular muscle and patch widening of the RV outflow tract.

4. Stenosis at the main pulmonary artery level requires patch widening of the narrow portion.

5. Anomalous muscle bundles require surgical resection.

Mortality. Surgical mortality occurs in less than 1% of older children. The rate is about 10% in critically ill infants.

Postoperative Follow-up

1. Following relief of severe PS, hypertrophied dynamic infundibulum may cause a persistent pressure gradient, with rare occurrences of a fatal outcome ("suicidal" right ventricle). Propranolol may be given to reduce hyperdynamic infundibular obstruction. The reduction of this gradient occurs gradually over weeks.

2. SBE prophylaxis is needed even after relief of stenosis.

3. Periodic echo and Doppler studies are needed to reassess the pressure gradient.

Aortic Stenosis

PREVALENCE

Left ventricular outflow tract (LVOT) obstruction, which includes stenosis at, below, or above the aortic valve, represents up to 10% of all CHDs. Valvular AS is the most frequent (71%), followed by subvalvular stenosis (23%) and supravalvular stenosis (6%). Aortic valve stenosis occurs more often in males (male/female ratio of 4:1).

PATHOLOGY

1. Stenosis may be at the valvular, subvalvular, or supravalvular level (Fig. 13–4).

2. Valvular AS may be caused by a bicuspid aortic valve, a unicuspid aortic valve, or stenosis of the tricuspid aortic valve (see Fig. 13–4B). A bicuspid aortic valve with a fused commissure and an eccentric orifice accounts for the most common form of aortic valve stenosis (75%) (Fig. 13–5B). Less common is the unicuspid valve with one lateral attachment (see Fig. 13–5A). A valve that has three unseparated cusps with a stenotic central orifice is the least common form (see Fig. 13–5C). Many bicuspid aortic valve are nonobstructive during childhood and become stenotic in adult life because of calcification of the valve.

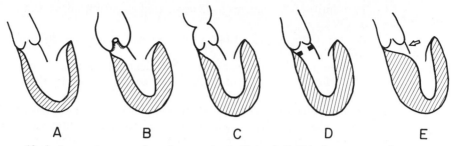

Figure 13–4. Anatomic types of aortic stenosis. **A,** Normal. **B,** Valvular stenosis. **C,** Supravalvular stenosis. **D,** Discrete subaortic stenosis. **E,** Idiopathic hypertrophic subaortic stenosis (this condition is discussed in Chapter 18).

3. Symptomatic neonates with so-called critical neonatal aortic valve stenosis have primitive, myxomatous valve tissue, with a pinhole opening. The aortic valve and ascending aorta are almost always hypoplastic. Hypoplasia of the mitral valve, LV cavity, or LV outflow tract and a VSD are also frequently found, often requiring one ventricular repair (Norwood and Fontan operations).

4. Supravalvular AS is an annular constriction at the upper margin of the sinus of Valsalva (see Fig. 13–4C). Occasionally, the ascending aorta is diffusely hypoplastic. This is often associated with Williams' syndrome (which includes mental retardation, characteristic facies, and multiple PA stenosis).

5. Subvalvular (subaortic) stenosis may be in the form of a simple diaphragm (discrete) (see Fig. 13–4D) or a long, tunnel-like fibromuscular narrowing (tunnel stenosis) of the left ventricular outflow tract.

   a. Discrete membranous subaortic stenosis accounts for about 10% of all AS cases, and it occurs more often than tunnel stenosis. It is believed to develop as the result of turbulence in an abnormally shaped LVOT, which causes endocardial injury and subsequent proliferation and fibrosis.

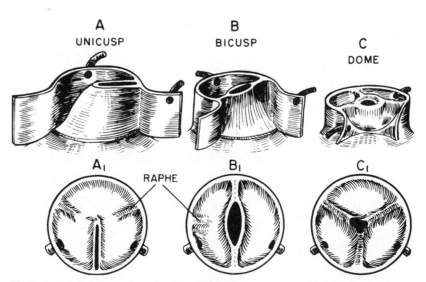

Figure 13–5. Anatomic types of aortic valve stenosis. Top row is the side view, and bottom row is the view as seen in surgery during aortotomy. **A,** Unicuspid aortic valve. **B,** Bicuspid aortic valve. **C,** Stenosis of a tricuspid aortic valve. (From Goor DA, Lillehei CW: Congenital Malformations of the Heart. New York, Grune & Stratton, 1975.)

1). Two thirds of the patients have associated cardiac lesions, such as VSD, PDA, or COA.

2). In one third of the patients, the stenosis is isolated; familial subaortic membrane has been reported.

3). In some patients, there is history of surgical intervention, such as membranous VSD closure or PA banding (9 months to 8 years before the development of the membrane).

b. Tunnel-like subaortic stenosis is often associated with hypoplasia of the ascending aorta and aortic valve ring, as well as thickened aortic valve leaflets. It is usually associated with other LV anomalies, including Shone's complex (comprising supramitral ring, parachute mitral valve, subaortic stenosis, and COA).

c. Another type of subvalvular stenosis is idiopathic hypertrophic subaortic stenosis (see Fig. 13–4E), a primary disorder of the heart muscle (see Chapter 18).

CLINICAL MANIFESTATIONS

History

1. Neonates with critical or severe stenosis of the aortic valve may develop signs of hypoperfusion or respiratory distress related to pulmonary edema within days to weeks after birth.

2. Most children with mild to moderate AS are asymptomatic. Occasionally, exercise intolerance may be present.

3. Exertional chest pain, easy fatigability, or syncope may occur in a child with a severe degree of obstruction.

Physical Examination (Fig. 13–6)

1. Infants and children with AS are acyanotic and are normally developed.

2. Except for neonates with critical AS, blood pressure is normal in most patients, but a narrow pulse pressure is present in severe AS. Patients with supravalvular AS may have a higher systolic pressure in the right arm than in the left (because of the jet of stenosis directed into the innominate artery, so-called Coanda effect).

3. A systolic thrill may be palpable at the upper right sternal border, in the suprasternal notch, or over the carotid arteries.

4. An ejection click may be heard with valvular AS. The S2 splits either normally or a bit narrowly. The S2 may split paradoxically in severe AS (see Fig. 13–6). A harsh, grade 2 to 4/6, midsystolic murmur is best heard at the second right or left intercostal space, with good transmission to the neck and apex. A high-pitched, early diastolic decrescendo murmur, which results from aortic regurgitation (AR), may be audible in patients with bicuspid aortic valve and in those with discrete subvalvular stenosis.

5. Peculiar "elfin facies," mental retardation, and friendly "cocktail party" personalities may be associated with supravalvular AS (e.g., Williams' syndrome).

6. Newborns with critical AS may develop signs of reduced peripheral perfusion (with weak and thready pulses, pale cool skin, and slow capillary refill) triggered by

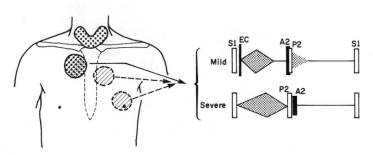

Figure 13–6. Cardiac findings of aortic valve stenosis. Abnormal sounds are indicated in black. Systolic thrill may be present in areas with dots. EC, ejection click.

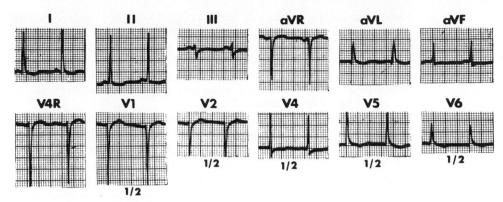

Figure 13–7. Tracing from a 7-year-old boy with severe aortic stenosis. It shows left ventricular hypertrophy, with probable "strain" pattern.

ductal constriction. The clinical picture may mimic overwhelming sepsis with low cardiac output. The heart murmur may be absent or faint but becomes louder when CHF improves.

Electrocardiography. In mild cases the ECG is normal. LVH with or without strain pattern may be present in severe cases (Fig. 13–7). Correlation of the severity of AS and the ECG abnormalities is relatively poor.

X-ray Studies

1. The heart size is usually normal in children, but a dilated ascending aorta or a prominent aortic knob may be seen occasionally in valvular AS, resulting from poststenotic dilatation.
2. Significant cardiomegaly does not develop unless CHF occurs later in life or if AR becomes substantial.
3. Newborns with critical AS show generalized cardiomegaly with pulmonary venous congestion.

Echocardiography

1. Valvular AS:

   a. The coaptation line of a normal aortic valve is seen in the center of the aortic root in an M-mode echo (Fig. 13–8A). In the M-mode echo of a bicuspid valve, an eccentric closure line or multiple closure lines of the aortic valve may be present during diastole (see Fig. 13–8B and C).

   b. In the parasternal short-axis view of the two-dimensional echo, normal aortic valves are tricuspid, with three cusps of approximately equal size. In diastole, the normal

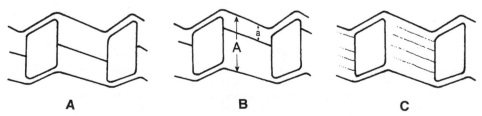

Figure 13–8. Diagram demonstrating M-mode echocardiography of a normal aortic valve (A) and of a bicuspid aortic valve (B and C). In the bicuspid aortic valve, an eccentric coaptation line is seen (B). The eccentricity index (0.5 × A/a) is usually greater than 1.5, where A is the aortic root diameter and a is the distance from the diastolic closure line to the nearest aortic wall. The normal eccentricity index is 1.0 to 1.2. Multiple lines may be present in diastole in a bicuspid aortic valve (C).

aortic cusp margins form a Y pattern (Fig. 13–9). In systole, a bicuspid aortic valve appears as a noncircular (i.e., football-shaped) orifice (see Fig. 13–9). Stenosis of the tricuspid aortic valve appears as a heavy Y pattern in diastole and as a small, centrally located orifice in systole, with three thickened commissures distinctly visible. A unicommissural aortic valve, which is seen often in infants with critical AS, is seen as a circular orifice positioned eccentrically within the aortic root and without visible distinct cusps.

  c. In the parasternal long-axis view of the two-dimensional echo, doming of the thick aortic valve with restriction to the opening is seen in systole. Reverse doming during diastole commonly occurs in the unicuspid valve, occurs less frequently in the bicuspid valve, and does not occur in the tricuspid aortic valve.

2. The parasternal long-axis view, apical long-axis view, and apical "five-chamber" view show the discrete subaortic membrane as a thin echo stretching across the LVOT just beneath the aortic valve. The fibromuscular type (i.e., tunnel stenosis) involves a more extensive area of the LVOT, as seen in the parasternal long-axis view or apical long-axis view.

3. Supravalvular AS is seen as a narrowing of the ascending aorta in the parasternal long-axis view and apical long-axis view. The suprasternal view best shows diffuse hypoplasia of the ascending aorta.

4. Doppler studies can estimate the severity of the stenosis by using the simplified Bernoulli equation (see Chapter 6). The Doppler-derived gradient (i.e., instantaneous gradient) is approximately 20% higher than the peak-to-peak systolic pressure gradient obtained during cardiac catheterization.

NATURAL HISTORY

1. Chest pain, syncope, and even sudden death (1% to 2% of cases) may occur in children with severe AS.

2. Heart failure occurs with severe AS during the newborn period or later in adult life.

3. Mild stenosis becomes more severe with time in a significant number of patients.

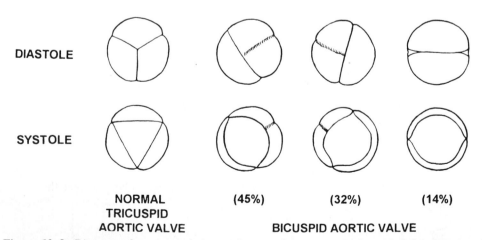

DIASTOLE

SYSTOLE

NORMAL TRICUSPID AORTIC VALVE   (45%)   (32%)   (14%)

BICUSPID AORTIC VALVE

Figure 13–9. Diagram of parasternal short-axis scan shows normal tricuspid (left column) and bicuspid aortic valves (three right columns) during diastole and systole. Three nearly equal-sized aortic cusps are imaged in a normal aortic valve, which opens widely during systole. The systolic opening pattern distinguishes a raphe from a commissure. With a bicuspid aortic valve, various commissural orientations are imaged. The most common pattern demonstrates commissures at the 4- or 5-o'clock and the 9- or 10-o'clock positions, with raphe at the 1- or 2-o'clock position (46%). (Modified from Brandenburg RO Jr, Tajik AJ, Edwards WD, et al: Accuracy of 2-dimensional echocardiographic diagnosis of congenitally bicuspid aortic valve: Echocardiographic-anatomic correlation in 115 patients. Am J Cardiol 51:1469–1473, 1983.)

4. The stenosis may worsen with aging as the result of calcification of the valve cusps, which may require valve replacement in many adult patients.

5. Progressive worsening of AR is possible in discrete subaortic stenosis. The jet of the subaortic stenosis damages the aortic valve with resulting AR.

6. SBE occurs in approximately 4% of patients with valvular AS.

MANAGEMENT

Medical

1. For critically ill newborns with CHF, the patients are stabilized before surgery or balloon valvuloplasty by the use of rapidly acting inotropic agents (usually dopamine) and diuretics to treat CHF and intravenous infusion of PGE_1 to reopen the ductus. Mechanical ventilation may be useful. Neonates and young infants with CHF from critical AS require balloon valvuloplasty (or surgery) on an urgent basis.

2. Serial echo-Doppler ultrasound evaluation is needed at approximately 1- to 2-year intervals in asymptomatic children with mild to moderate stenosis and more often in children with severe stenosis because AS of all severities tends to worsen with time.

3. An exercise stress test (EST) may be indicated in asymptomatic children with mean Doppler gradient greater than 30 mm Hg or peak gradient greater than 50 mm Hg who are interested in athletic participation or in becoming pregnant.

4. The following are indications for cardiac catheterization in adolescents and young adults, according to the ACC/AHA 2006 Guidelines (American College of Cardiology, 2006). The same guidelines may apply in children as well.

   a. In asymptomatic patients with moderate AS (mean gradient >30 mm Hg or peak gradient >50 mm Hg), when T-wave inversion develops over the left precordial leads at rest.

   b. In symptomatic patients* with mean Doppler gradient greater than 30 mm Hg (or peak gradient >50 mm Hg).

   c. In asymptomatic patients when Doppler echo results are equivocal or when there is a discrepancy between symptoms and gradients.

   d. Catheterization may be indicated in asymptomatic patients with moderate AS (mean gradient >30 mm Hg or peak gradient >50 mm Hg), if the patient is interested in athletic participation or becoming pregnant.

   e. Asymptomatic patients with severe AS (mean Doppler gradient >40 mm Hg) may benefit from cardiac catheterization.

5. Percutaneous balloon valvuloplasty is now regarded as the first step in the management of symptomatic neonates in many centers. It is also the first interventional method for children older than 1 year.

   Indications for the balloon procedure in adolescents are as follows according to the ACC/AHA 2006 Guidelines. The same guidelines may apply for younger children.

   a. In symptomatic patients* with catheterization pressure gradient (cath gradient) greater than 50 mm Hg.

   b. In asymptomatic patients with catheterization gradient greater than 60 mm Hg.

   c. In asymptomatic patients who develop ST or T changes on ECG at rest or EST and who have a catheterization gradient greater than 50 mm Hg.

   d. In asymptomatic patients with cath gradient greater than 50 mm Hg who want to play competitive sports. (Balloon angioplasty is not indicated when the cath gradient is <40 mm Hg.)

   Although the results of aortic balloon valvuloplasty are promising, they are not as good as those for PS. Serious complications (e.g., major hemorrhage, loss of the

---

*Symptoms may include angina, syncope, or dyspnea on exertion.

femoral artery pulse, avulsion of part of the aortic valve leaflet, perforation of the mitral valve or left ventricle) can occur.

6. For subaortic stenosis, the balloon procedure is not effective.

7. Maintenance of good oral hygiene and antibiotic prophylaxis against bacterial endocarditis are especially important for patients with AS, regardless of the type or severity of the stenosis (see Chapter 19).

8. Activity restrictions. No limitation in activity is required for mild AS (with peak Doppler gradient < 40 mm Hg). Moderate AS (peak Doppler gradient 40 to 70 mm Hg) requires restriction from high dynamic or static competitive athletics (allowing only golf, baseball, doubles tennis, and so forth). With severe AS (peak Doppler gradient >70 mm Hg), no competitive sports are allowed (see Table 34–1).

Surgical

Indications and Timing

1. Valvular AS: Surgery is indicated if the balloon valvuloplasty has failed to relieve the pressure gradient or if severe AR results following the balloon procedure.

2. Subvalvular AS: An earlier elective operation may be considered for discrete membranous subvalvular AS of moderate degree (i.e., gradient >30 mm Hg) because of the progressive nature of AR. Most centers accept the onset of AR as an indication for surgical removal of the membrane, and some centers consider the mere presence of a significant membrane to be an indication for surgery. The risk of recurrence after surgical removal is higher in children younger than 10 years, and therefore some centers recommend deferring surgery until after 10 years of age. A gradient of 50 mm Hg or greater is considered an indication for surgery for tunnel-type subaortic stenosis.

3. Supravalvular AS: Surgery is advisable for patients with supravalvular AS when there is a peak pressure gradient across the stenosis greater than 50 to 60 mm Hg, severe LVH, or appearance of new AR. The operation is performed whenever the patient meets the criteria for surgery.

Procedures

1. Closed aortic valvotomy, using calibrated dilators or balloon catheters without cardiopulmonary bypass, may be performed in sick infants if balloon valvuloplasty has been unsuccessful or if it is not available. This procedure is associated with low surgical mortality.

2. Newborns with "critical AS" (with hypoplasia of the aortic annulus, ascending aorta, and mitral annulus, small LV cavity, and MR from papillary muscle infarction) have a poor prognosis. The Norwood procedure (see Chapter 14) may be preferable (for future Fontan operation) to aortic valvotomy.

3. Valvular AS. The following procedures are performed for aortic valve stenosis: aortic valve commissurotomy, aortic valve replacement, or the Ross procedure.

    a. Aortic valve commissurotomy is usually tried if stenosis is the predominant lesion. Fused commissures are divided with a knife to within 1 mm of the aortic wall. Only commissures with adequate leaflet attachments to the aortic wall are opened because division of rudimentary commissures produces severe AR.

    b. Aortic valve replacement may be necessary if AR is the predominant lesion. Valve replacement is done by using a mechanical prosthetic valve or homografts. The advantage of the mechanical valve is durability, but there is a tendency for thrombus formation on the valve with a potential embolization. Because of this tendency, patients require warfarin with its attendant risks of bleeding as well as aspirin. Homografts have the advantage of a lower incidence of thromboembolism, but deterioration of the homograft (related to degeneration and calcification) is likely to occur within a decade or two. Current recommendations for adolescents and young adults who need valve replacement are for mechanical valves using the St. Jude valve (with two tilting disks).

Because of accelerated degeneration of homograft or bioprosthetic valves, a mechanical valve is usually used in adolescents. For adolescent girls or women in whom pregnancy is desired, homografts may be a good alternative until childbearing years are completed because of the known teratogenic effects of warfarin. A study in an adult population has revealed that an increased serum cholesterol level (>200 mg/dL) may be a risk factor for bioprosthetic valve calcification. Therefore, monitoring serum cholesterol levels is important for patients who have received a bioprosthesis (Farivar et al, 2003).

   c. In pulmonary root autografts (i.e., the Ross procedure), the autologous pulmonary valve replaces the aortic valve, and an aortic or a pulmonary allograft replaces the pulmonary valve. The Ross procedure is more complex than simple aortic valve replacement because it requires coronary artery implantation, but it can be carried out with a low mortality rate in selected patients (Fig. 13–10). The pulmonary valve autograft has the advantage of documented long-term durability; it does not require anticoagulation, and remains uncompromised by host reactions. There is evidence of the autograft's growth, making it an attractive option for aortic valve replacement in infants and children. Mild regurgitation of the neoaortic valve occurs frequently and may result from preexisting pulmonary valve regurgitation. The patient's own aortic valve may be used for a pulmonary position after aortic valvotomy ("double" Ross procedure).

3. Subvalvular AS. Excision of the membrane is done for discrete subvalvular AS. A tendency for recurrence exists after surgical excision. The recurrence rate is as high as 25% to 30%. Excision combined with myectomy or myotomy of the septal muscle tends to improve the result. Occasionally, it may be necessary to perform the Konno procedure, which enlarges the LV outflow tract anteriorly by incision of the aortic annulus and the interventricular septum of the outflow tract.

   For complex LVOT obstruction (such as AS combined with a diffuse subaortic stenosis or hypoplastic annulus), the Ross procedure can be combined with Konno operation (the Ross-Konno procedure) (Fig. 13–11).

4. Supravalvular AS. With the most common hourglass type of supravalvular AS, a reconstructive surgery is done using a Y-shaped patch. For the diffuse form of obstruction, the patch is extended superiorly into the transverse arch to relieve all obstruction.

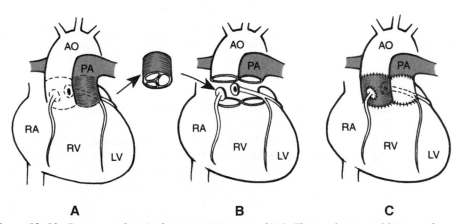

A   **B**   **C**

Figure 13–10. *Ross procedure (pulmonary root autograft).* ***A,*** *The two horizontal lines on the aorta (AO) and pulmonary artery (PA) and two broken circles around the coronary artery ostia are lines of proposed incision. The pulmonary valve, with a small rim of right ventricle (RV) muscle, and the adjacent PA are removed.* ***B,*** *The aortic valve and the adjacent aorta have been removed, leaving buttons of aortic tissue around the coronary arteries.* ***C,*** *The pulmonary autograft is sutured to the aortic annulus and to the distal aorta, and the coronary arteries are sutured to openings made in the PA. The pulmonary valve is replaced with either an aortic or a pulmonary allograft. LV, left ventricle; RA, right atrium.*

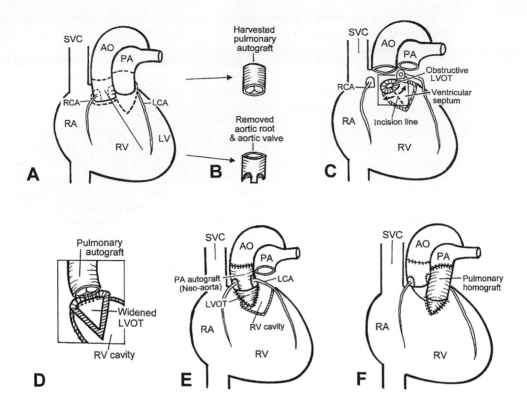

Figure 13–11. *The Ross-Konno procedure.* ***A.*** *Intended incision in the ascending aorta and around the aortic annulus and excision boundaries for the pulmonary artery and right ventricle (RV) are shown. Intended incisions to harvest buttons of aortic wall around the coronary artery ostia are also shown.* ***B.*** *The pulmonary artery autograft has been harvested (with an extra portion of the RV, not shown) for the Ross procedure. The aortic root and aortic valve are completely excised.* ***C.*** *Small obstructed left ventricular outflow tract (LVOT) is shown. Intended incision in the LVOT and the interventricular septum is noted by the dotted line, which will result in a V-shaped widening of the LVOT.* ***D.*** *The posterior portion of the pulmonary autograft is sutured to the original LVOT.* ***E.*** *The LVOT is reconstructed by suturing the extra portion of the RV to the widened V-shaped LVOT. The coronary arteries have been reimplanted.* ***F.*** *The RVOT is reconstructed by inserting a pulmonary homograft between the RV body and the distal end of the pulmonary artery. LCA, left coronary artery; RCA, right coronary artery; SVC, superior vena cava. Other abbreviations used are the same as in Figure 13–10.*

Mortality. The mortality rate for sick neonates with critical AS has decreased to around 10%, although it was much higher in the past, up to 40% to 50%. The hospital mortality in older children with valvular AS is 1% to 2%. The early mortality rate for Ross and Ross-Konno procedures is less than 5%. The mortality for subaortic membrane is near zero and that for tunnel subaortic stenosis is less than 5%. Death occurs in supravalvular stenosis in less than 1% of cases, although diffuse narrowing of the ascending aorta is a risk factor.

Postballoon and Postoperative Follow-up

1. An annual follow-up examination is necessary for all patients who have the aortic valve balloon procedure or surgery in order to detect development of stenosis or regurgitation. In 10% to 30% of patients, significant AR develops after valvotomy or the balloon procedure.

2. Recurrence of discrete subaortic stenosis occurs in 25% to 30% after surgical resection of the membrane and as long as 17 years after the initial procedure,

requiring long, periodic follow-up. Some of these patients require reoperation at a later age.

3. Anticoagulation is needed after a prosthetic mechanical valve replacement. The International Normalized Ratio (INR) should be maintained between 2.5 and 3.5 for the first 3 months and 2.0 to 3.0 beyond that time. Low-dose aspirin (75 to 100 mg/day for adolescents) is indicated in addition to warfarin (American College of Cardiology, 2006).

4. After aortic valve replacement with a bioprosthesis and no risk factors, aspirin (75 to 100 mg), but not warfarin, is indicated. When there are risk factors (which include atrial fibrillation, previous thromboembolism, LV dysfunction, and hypercoagulable state), warfarin is indicated to achieve an INR of 2.0 to 3.0 (American College of Cardiology, 2006).

5. Restriction from competitive, strenuous sports may be necessary for children with moderate residual AS or AR, or both (see Table 34-1).

6. SBE prophylaxis should be used for all types of aortic valve abnormalities. The incidence of SBE does not decrease with valve surgery or a balloon procedure.

Coarctation of the Aorta

PREVALENCE

COA occurs in 8% to 10% of all cases of congenital heart defect. It is more common in males than in females (male/female ratio of 2:1). Among patients with Turner's syndrome, 30% have COA.

PATHOLOGY

1. The terms used in the past such as *preductal* and *postductal* as well as *infantile* or *adult-type* COA are misleading. COA is almost always in a juxtaductal position (i.e., neither preductal nor postductal).

2. In *symptomatic infants* with COA, during fetal life (and at birth), the descending aorta is supplied mostly by right-to-left ductal flow and by a reduced amount of antegrade aortic flow through the aortic isthmus. Other associated cardiac defects such as aortic hypoplasia, abnormal aortic valve, VSD, and mitral valve anomalies are often present. All these cardiac defects tend to decrease antegrade aortic blood flow in utero (see Fig. 10–3). With ductal closure, a reduced antegrade aortic flow to the descending aorta produces symptoms early in life. Good collateral circulation has not developed in these infants (see Chapter 10). Occasionally, infants without associated defects may become symptomatic because of LV failure, which results from a sudden increase in pressure work in early postnatal life. COA also occurs as part of other CHDs, such as transposition of the great arteries and double-outlet right ventricle (e.g., Taussig-Bing abnormality).

3. In *asymptomatic infants and children* with COA, during fetal life, the descending aorta is supplied by both a normal amount of antegrade aortic flow through the aortic isthmus and normal ductal flow because associated cardiac defects are rare in these children, except for bicuspid aortic valve. Good collateral circulation gradually develops between the proximal aorta and the distal aorta during fetal life.

4. Major collateral circulations between the aortic segments proximal and distal to the coarctation comprise (1) the internal mammary artery anteriorly, (2) arteries arising from the subclavian artery by way of the intercostal arteries, and (3) the anterior spinal artery (Fig. 13–12).

5. As many as 85% of patients with COA have a bicuspid aortic valve.

The presentation of patients with COA occurs in a bimodal distribution. There is a group that presents in the first weeks of life with circulatory symptoms requiring timely diagnosis and correct management. The other group consists of infants and children with

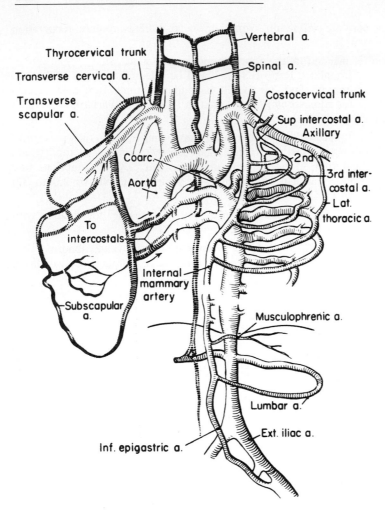

Figure 13–12. Collateral circulation in coarctation of the aorta. Anteriorly, the internal mammary artery leads to the epigastric arteries for the supply to the lower extremity. The arteries arising from the subclavian artery and supplying the scapula communicate, by way of intercostal arteries, with the descending aorta, thereby supplying blood to the abdominal organs. The anterior spinal artery is also enlarged. (From Moller JH, Amplatz K, Edwards JE: Congenital Heart Disease. Kalamazoo, MI, Upjohn, 1971.)

COA who are essentially asymptomatic. Clinical manifestation and management are quite different in these two groups, and therefore they are discussed under separate headings.

SYMPTOMATIC INFANTS

Clinical Manifestations

History. Poor feeding, dyspnea, and poor weight gain or signs of acute circulatory shock may develop in the first 6 weeks of life. Figure 13–13 provides an explanation for hemodynamic deterioration in the newborn period. The newborn discharge examination may have been normal as a result of incomplete obliteration of the aortic end of the ductus, which would permit blood flow to the descending aorta. After ductal obliteration, the aortic lumen narrows with loss of the space provided by the aortic end of the ductus.

Physical Examination

1. Infants with COA are pale and experience varying degrees of respiratory distress. Oliguria or anuria, general circulatory shock, and severe acidemia are common. Differential cyanosis may be present; for example, only the lower half of the body is cyanotic because of a right-to-left ductal shunt (particularly after PGE$_1$ infusion).

2. Peripheral pulses may be weak and thready as a result of CHF. A blood pressure differential may become apparent only after improvement of cardiac function with administration of rapidly acting inotropic agents.

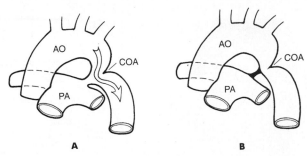

Figure 13–13. *Explanation for hemodynamic deterioration seen in some infants with coarctation of the aorta (COA) in the first days of life. **A,** Coarctation is at the juxtaductal position, so that space is added to the narrowed aorta (AO) by the ductus. **B,** After ductal obliteration, the added lumen is lost, and the aorta becomes severely obstructed, although the severity of the coarctation is unchanged. PA, pulmonary artery.*

3. The S2 is single and loud; a loud S3 gallop is usually present. No heart murmur is present in 50% of sick infants. A nonspecific ejection systolic murmur is audible over the precordium. The heart murmur may become louder after treatment.

Electrocardiography. A normal or rightward QRS axis and RVH or right bundle branch block (RBBB) are present in most infants with COA, rather than LVH; LVH is seen in older children (see Chapter 10) (Fig. 13–14).

X-ray Studies. Marked cardiomegaly and pulmonary edema or pulmonary venous congestion are usually present.

Echocardiography. Two-dimensional echo and color flow Doppler studies usually show the site and extent of the coarctation (Fig. 13–15).

1. In the suprasternal notch view, a thin wedge-shaped "posterior shelf" is imaged in the posterolateral aspect of the upper descending aorta, which is distal to the left subclavian artery.

2. Varying degrees of isthmic hypoplasia are present. The mean normal internal dimension of the aortic isthmus at 40 weeks of gestation is approximately 6.2 mm with a third percentile value of 5.4 mm (Hornberger et al, 1992). The ratio of isthmus to ascending aorta, which remained relatively constant, was 0.81 ± 0.09 (SD) according to the same study.

3. The transverse aortic arch may also be hypoplastic. A bicuspid aortic valve is frequently present. Other associated defects such as VSD can be imaged.

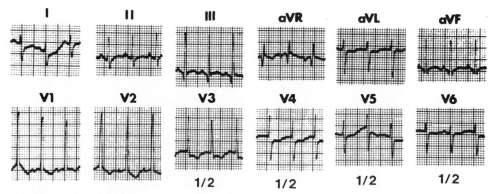

Figure 13–14. *Tracing from a 3-week-old infant with coarctation of the aorta. Note a marked right ventricular hypertrophy.*

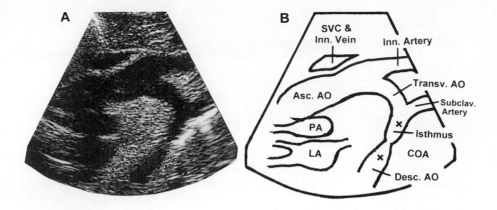

Figure 13–15. *Echocardiogram (**A**) and diagram (**B**) of a suprasternal long-axis view of coarctation of the aorta (COA). A narrowing is present in the upper descending aorta, distal to the left subclavian artery. The transverse aortic arch and aortic isthmus are mildly to moderately hypoplastic. Doppler estimation of pressure gradients should be obtained at two X marks, proximal and distal to the coarctation for accurate estimation of the pressure gradient. AO, aorta; Inn., innominate; LA, left atrium; PA, pulmonary artery; SVC, superior vena cava.*

4. Doppler studies above and below the coarctation site should be obtained, as shown in Figure 13–15, in assessing the severity of the coarctation (see "Echocardiography" in Chapter 6 for further discussion).

5. Reduced left ventricular function may be present.

Natural History

1. About 20% to 30% of all patients with COA develop CHF by 3 months of age.

2. If it is undetected or untreated, early death may result from CHF and renal shutdown in symptomatic infants with COA.

Management

Medical

1. In symptomatic neonates, PGE_1 infusion should be started to reopen the ductus arteriosus and establish flow to the descending aorta and the kidneys during the first weeks of life.

2. Intensive anticongestive measures with short-acting inotropic agents (e.g., dopamine, dobutamine), diuretics, and oxygen should be started.

3. Balloon angioplasty can be a useful procedure for sick infants in whom standard surgical management carries a high risk. This is controversial, however. Balloon angioplasty is associated with a higher rate of recoarctation than surgical repair, and the rate of complications (including femoral artery injury) is high during infancy.

Surgical

Indications and Timing

1. If CHF or circulatory shock develops early in life, surgery should be performed on an urgent basis. A short period of medical treatment, as described earlier, improves the patient's condition before surgery.

2. If there is a large associated VSD, which occurs in 17% to 33% of patients with COA, one of the following procedures may be performed:
   a. COA and VSD can be repaired in the same operative setting if the VSD is nonrestrictive. Both are performed through a median sternotomy.

b. Only coarctation repair is performed if the VSD appears restrictive. Approximately 40% of restrictive VSDs close spontaneously. If CHF cannot be managed medically, the VSD is surgically closed within days or weeks after the initial coarctation surgery.

c. Pulmonary artery banding is performed if the PA pressure remains high after completing COA surgery. This approach is necessary only for infants with multiple VSDs, large apical VSD, single ventricle, or other complex lesions. Later the VSD is closed, and the PA band is removed between 6 and 24 months of age.

Procedures. Surgical procedures vary greatly from institution to institution, but the following procedures are popular (Fig. 13–16).

1. Resection and end-to-end anastomosis consists of resecting the coarctation segment and anastomosing the proximal and distal aortas (see Fig. 13–16, top). Because most symptomatic neonatal COA is associated with hypoplasia of the isthmus and occasionally of the aortic arch, extended resection with end-to-end anastomosis has been performed with a lower recurrence rate (<10%).

2. Subclavian flap aortoplasty consists of dividing the distal subclavian artery and inserting a flap of the proximal portion of this vessel between the two sides of the longitudinally split aorta throughout the coarctation segment (see Fig. 13–16, middle). The recurrence rate is lower (10% to 40%) than with patch aortoplasty.

3. With patch aortoplasty, the aorta is opened longitudinally through the coarctation segment and extending to the left subclavian artery, and the fibrous shelf and any existing membrane are excised. An elliptic woven Dacron patch is inserted to

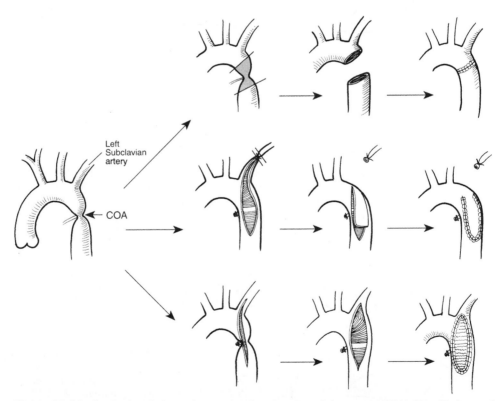

Figure 13–16. *Surgical techniques for repair of coarctation of the aorta (COA). Top, End-to-end anastomosis. A segment of coarctation is resected, and the proximal and distal aortas are anastomosed end to end. Middle, Subclavian flap procedure. The distal subclavian artery is divided, and the flap of the proximal portion of this vessel is used to widen the coarcted segment. Bottom, Patch aortoplasty. An elliptic woven Dacron patch is inserted to expand the diameter of the lumen. Regardless of the type of operative procedure, the ductus arteriosus is always ligated and divided.*

expand the diameter of the lumen (see Fig. 13–16, bottom). Patch aortoplasty has the highest recurrence rate (up to 50%).

4. A conduit insertion between the ascending and descending aorta may be performed for severe, long-segment COA (not shown).

Mortality. The mortality rate for COA patients is less than 5%. The mortality rate for repair of COA and VSD at the same time is less than 10%.

Complications

1. Postoperative renal failure is the most common cause of death.

2. Residual obstruction or recoarctation occurs in 6% to 33% of all patients, but the recurrence rate is lower after surgery than that after balloon angioplasty.

Postoperative Follow-up

1. An examination every 6 to 12 months to check for recurrence of COA is necessary, especially when surgery is performed in the first year of life.

2. SBE prophylaxis should be continued because of the frequently associated bicuspid aortic valve and residual coarctation.

3. Balloon angioplasty (with or without stent) may be performed if a significant recoarctation develops.

4. Physicians should watch for and treat systemic hypertension.

ASYMPTOMATIC INFANTS AND CHILDREN

Clinical Manifestations

History. Most children are asymptomatic. Occasionally, a child complains of weakness or pain in the legs, or both, after exercise.

Physical Examination (Fig. 13–17)

1. Patients grow and develop normally.

2. Arterial pulses in the leg are either absent or weak and delayed. There is hypertension in the arm, or the leg systolic pressure is equal to or lower than the arm systolic pressure. In normal children, the oscillometric systolic pressure in the thigh or calf is 5 to 10 mm Hg higher than that in the arm. With use of the auscultatory method, the leg systolic pressure may be as much as 20 mm Hg higher than in the arm in normal children (see Chapter 2).

3. A systolic thrill may be present in the suprasternal notch. The S2 splits normally, and the A2 is accentuated. An ejection click is frequently audible at the apex and/or at the base, which originates in the associated bicuspid aortic valve or from systemic hypertension. An ejection systolic murmur grade 2 to 4/6 is heard at the upper right sternal border and middle or lower left sternal border. A well-localized systolic murmur is also audible in the left interscapular area in the back. Occasionally, an early diastolic decrescendo murmur of AR from the bicuspid aortic valve may be audible in the third left intercostal space (see Fig. 13–17).

Electrocardiography. Leftward QRS axis and LVH are commonly found. The ECG appears normal in 20% of patients.

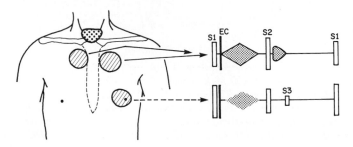

Figure 13–17. Cardiac findings of coarctation of the aorta. A systolic thrill may be present in the suprasternal notch (area shown by dots). EC, ejection click.

X-ray Studies

1. The heart size may be normal or slightly enlarged.
2. Dilatation of the ascending aorta may be seen.
3. An E-shaped indentation on the barium-filled esophagus or a "3 sign" on overpenetrated films suggests COA (see Fig. 4–10).
4. Rib notching between the fourth and eighth ribs may be seen in older children but rarely in children younger than 5 years (see Fig. 4–9).

Echocardiography

1. The suprasternal notch two-dimensional echo demonstrates a discrete shelf-like membrane in the posterolateral aspect of the descending aorta. Associated findings such as isthmus hypoplasia, poststenotic dilatation, and diminished pulsation in the descending aorta may be present. Bicuspid aortic valve is frequently present. Cardiac catheterization is unnecessary in children with clinically uncomplicated COA.
2. Doppler examination often demonstrates a pattern of diastolic runoff, especially in patients with robust collaterals or tight stenosis. The Doppler flow profile distal to the coarctation is composed of two superimposed signals representing low-velocity flow in the proximal descending aorta and high-velocity flow across the coarctation. As discussed earlier, a more accurate estimation of the gradient is obtained with the expanded Bernoulli equation, in which the peak velocities obtained from the segments proximal and distal to the coarctation site are used (see Fig. 13–15). In severe COA with extensive collaterals, the Doppler-estimated gradient may underestimate the severity of the coarctation because the blood flow through the coarctation site is decreased.

Natural History

1. A bicuspid aortic valve may cause stenosis and/or regurgitation with age.
2. SBE can occur on either the aortic valve or the coarctation.
3. LV failure, rupture of the aorta, intracranial hemorrhage (i.e., rupture of a berry aneurysm of the arterial circle of Willis), hypertensive encephalopathy, and hypertensive cardiovascular disease are rare complications seen in adulthood.

Management

Medical

1. Children with mild COA should be watched closely for hypertension in the arm or for increasing pressure differences between the arm and leg.
2. Balloon angioplasty for native unoperated coarctation is controversial, although most centers perform balloon dilatation for recurrent coarctation. Some centers continue to use the balloon procedure for the native COA, whereas other centers prefer a surgical approach. The most common acute complication of balloon angioplasty has been femoral artery injury and thrombosis, especially in small children. There is a possibility of aortic aneurysm formation with serious late complications.

   A single-center analysis of balloon angioplasty versus surgical repair of native coarctation in children 3 to 20 years of age suggests the superiority of surgical repair over a balloon procedure in terms of aortic aneurysm formation (0% versus 35%), with some aneurysms developing 5 years after the procedure (Cowley et al, 2005).

3. A balloon-expandable stainless-steel stent implanted concurrently with balloon angioplasty is in the early stage of experience. Stents may prove to reduce residual pressure gradients or recoarctation following the balloon procedure and diminish the incidence of late aneurysm formation. Currently, the aortic stent is used only in older children, at least 8 to 10 years old, to reduce complications of using a large arterial sheath and to minimize the need to redilate it and make it larger after the child has grown.

4. An absorbable metal stent is in the experimental stage. The Magnesium Biocorrodible Stent (Biotroniks, Bulach, Switzerland) is an innovative stent made of a magnesium alloy (which also contains zirconium, yttrium, and rare earths) that can be deliverable through a 5 French sheath (Peuster et al, 2001). This could be used in infants and small children, in whom repeated dilatation of the stent may be necessary. The degradable metal did not result in significant obstruction of the stented vessel caused by inflammation, neointimal proliferation, or thrombotic events. This stent has been successfully implanted in the left PA in a preterm infant.

5. Good dental hygiene and precautions against SBE are important.

Surgical

Indications and Timing

1. COA with hypertension in the upper extremities or with a large systolic pressure gradient equal to or greater than 20 mm Hg between the arms and the legs indicates that elective surgical correction is necessary between the ages of 2 and 4 years. Reduction of aortic diameter by 50% at the level of COA is also an indication for surgery. Older children are operated on soon after the diagnosis is made. A lower incidence of hypertension is found in patients who had COA repair before 1 year of age, usually at 2 to 3 months of age. However, some reports suggest that early surgery (i.e., before 1 year of age) increases the chance of recoarctation.

2. In asymptomatic children, surgery is performed by age 4 to 5; late surgery may increase the risk of developing early essential hypertension.

3. If severe hypertension, CHF, or cardiomegaly is present, surgery is performed at an earlier age.

4. Children with mild COA (<20 mm Hg gradient) may be considered for surgery if a prominent gradient develops with exercise.

Procedures

1. Resection of the coarctation segment and end-to-end anastomosis is the procedure of choice for discrete COA in children (see Fig. 13–16).

2. Occasionally, subclavian artery aortoplasty or circular or patch grafts may be performed.

Mortality. The mortality rate is less than 1% in older children.

Complications

1. Spinal cord ischemia producing paraplegia may develop after cross-clamping of the aorta during surgery, which is probably related to limited collateral circulation. This develops in 0.4% of cases.

2. Rebound hypertension may occur in the immediate postoperative period as a result of increased sympathetic activity (with elevated norepinephrine level).

Postoperative Follow-up

1. Annual examinations should pay attention to the following during childhood:
   a. Blood pressure differences in the arm and leg, which suggest recoarctation. If coarctation recurs after either surgery or balloon angioplasty, balloon dilatation of the COA is the procedure of choice.
   b. Persistence or resurgence of hypertension in the arms and legs of some patients. The cause of the hypertension is not completely understood. Its occurrence appears to be proportional to the age of the child at the time of the operative repair.
   c. Associated abnormalities such as bicuspid aortic valve or mitral valve disease. The physician should emphasize the need to continue SBE prophylaxis as indicated.
   d. Persistent myocardial dysfunction that was present before surgery.
   e. Subaortic stenosis evolving years after the initial surgery in some patients.

2. Lifelong follow-up is indicated because COA is not a localized disease of the aorta but is a diffuse aortopathy and because there is a frequent association of bicuspid aortic valve. Operation for COA should not be considered a correction.

    a. Systemic hypertension is common in adults and may predispose patients with cerebral aneurysm to rupture with resulting stroke. They should be treated with β-blockers.

    b. Aneurysm formation and likelihood of dissection and rupture. Magnetic resonance angiography or computed tomography imaging is better than echo studies and should be performed every 2 to 5 years.

    c. All patients with bicuspid aortic valve require SBE prophylaxis, and some of these patients may require aortic valve replacement.

Interrupted Aortic Arch

PREVALENCE

Interrupted aortic arch accounts for about 1% of all critically ill infants who have congenital heart defects.

PATHOLOGY

1. This is an extreme form of COA in which the aortic arch is atretic or a segment of the arch is absent.

2. Depending on the location of the interruption, the defect is divided into the following three types (Fig. 13–18):

    a. Type A: The interruption is distal to the left subclavian artery (occurs in 30% of cases).

    b. Type B: The interruption is between the left carotid and left subclavian arteries (occurs in 43% of cases). An aberrant right subclavian artery is common. DiGeorge syndrome is reported in about 50% of patients with type B.

    c. Type C: The interruption is between the innominate and left carotid arteries (occurs in 17% of cases).

3. Interrupted aortic arch is usually associated with PDA and VSD (occurring in >90% of cases). A bicuspid aortic valve occurs in 60% of all cases. Often there is mitral valve deformity (10% of cases), persistent truncus arteriosus (10% of cases), or subaortic stenosis (20% of cases).

4. DiGeorge syndrome occurs in at least 15% of these patients.

CLINICAL MANIFESTATIONS

1. Respiratory distress, variable degrees of cyanosis, poor peripheral pulses, and signs of CHF or circulatory shock develop during the first days of life. Differential cyanosis is uncommon because of the frequent association of VSD.

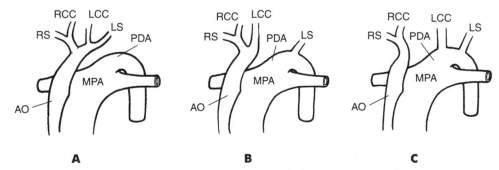

A   **B**   **C**

Figure 13–18. Three types of aortic arch interruption. A, Type A. B, Type B. C, Type C (see text). AO, aorta; LCC, left common carotid; LS, left subclavian; MPA, main pulmonary artery; PDA, patent ductus arteriosus; RCC, right common carotid; RS, right subclavian.

2. Chest x-ray films show cardiomegaly, increased pulmonary vascular markings, and pulmonary venous congestion or pulmonary edema. The upper mediastinum may be narrow because of the absence of the thymus, as is commonly found with DiGeorge syndrome. The ECG may show RVH in uncomplicated cases.

3. Echo is useful in the diagnosis of the interruption and associated defects. Angiocardiography is usually indicated for accurate diagnosis of the anatomy before surgery.

MANAGEMENT

1. Medical treatment consists of PGE_1 infusion (preferably before 4 days of age) with intubation and oxygen administration. Workup for DiGeorge syndrome (i.e., serum calcium) should be done. Hyperventilation that causes respiratory alkalosis and tetany should be avoided, and citrated blood (which causes hypocalcemia by chelation) should not be transfused in patients with DiGeorge syndrome. Blood should be irradiated before the transfusion.

2. Primary complete repair of the interruption and the VSD is recommended if the interruption is associated with a simple VSD. If it is associated with complex anomalies, the initial procedures should be banding the PA and repairing the interruption. Debanding and repair of the VSD and other cardiac anomalies should be done at a later date. A primary anastomosis, Dacron vascular graft, or venous homograft may be used to repair the interruption. Surgical mortality can be as low as 10% for initial surgery.

Chapter 14

Cyanotic Congenital Heart Defects

This chapter discusses well-known congenital heart defects that produce cyanosis. Defects discussed in this chapter include complete transposition of the great arteries (D-TGA), tetralogy of Fallot (TOF), total anomalous pulmonary venous return (TAPVR), tricuspid atresia, pulmonary atresia with intact ventricular septum, hypoplastic left heart syndrome (HLHS), Ebstein's anomaly, persistent truncus arteriosus, single ventricle, double-outlet right ventricle (DORV), and heterotaxia (or splenic syndromes). Although uncomplicated cases of congenitally corrected transposition of the great arteries (L-TGA) do not produce cyanosis, they are included in this chapter because the majority of cases are associated with other cardiac defects, some of which produce cyanosis. Although persistent pulmonary hypertension of the newborn is a resolvable condition, it is included in this chapter because it manifests with cyanosis requiring differentiation from other cyanotic congenital heart diseases (CHDs). Occasional patients may present with a combination of more than one form of cyanotic and noncyanotic cardiac defects, especially in the setting of heterotaxy (splenic syndrome or atrial isomerism).

Most cyanotic CHDs manifest during the neonatal period, requiring a correct diagnosis for appropriate management. Therefore, before discussing each cyanotic lesion, we begin with general approaches to cyanotic neonates.

Approach to a Cyanotic Neonate

Central cyanosis with arterial desaturation requires a thorough, immediate investigation to rule out cyanotic congenital heart defects. Three common causes of central cyanosis are cardiac disease, pulmonary disease, and central nervous system (CNS) depression. Clinical findings often direct physicians to the correct system that causes cyanosis. Table 14–1 lists some of the differentiating clinical findings of central cyanosis associated with the three common causes of cyanosis. Crying may improve the cyanosis caused by lung diseases or CNS depression; however, crying usually worsens cyanosis in patients with cyanotic heart defects.

The following are some of the tools commonly used in the investigation of cyanotic newborns. Box 14–1 lists suggested steps in the management of cyanotic newborns.

1. *ECG and chest x-ray films.* Although the routine tools of cardiac evaluation (physical examination, ECG, and chest x-ray films) are not very helpful in diagnosing a specific cyanotic heart defect, these tools are often useful in reducing the diagnostic possibilities. Tables 14–2 and 14–3 summarize the differential diagnosis of cyanotic heart defects, based on pulmonary vascular markings and ECG findings. Other clinical information can further reduce the diagnostic possibilities.

Table 14–1. **Causes and Clinical Findings of Central Cyanosis**

Systems	Causes	Clinical Findings
CNS depression	Perinatal asphyxia Heavy maternal sedation Intrauterine fetal distress	Shallow irregular respiration Poor muscle tone Cyanosis that disappears when the patient is stimulated or oxygen is given
Pulmonary disease	Parenchymal lung disease (e.g., hyaline membrane disease) Pneumothorax or pleural effusion Diaphragmatic hernia PPHN	Tachypnea and respiratory distress with retraction and expiratory grunting Crackles and/or decreased breath sounds on auscultation Chest x-ray films may reveal causes (such as those listed under causes in this table) Oxygen administration may improve or abolish cyanosis
Cardiac disease	Cyanotic CHD with right-to-left shunt	Tachypnea usually without retraction Lack of crackles or abnormal breath sounds unless CHF supervenes Heart murmurs may be absent in serious forms of cyanotic CHD A continuous murmur (of PDA) is audible in a cyanotic neonate Chest x-ray films may show cardiomegaly, abnormal cardiac silhouette, increased or decreased pulmonary vascular markings Little or no increase in Po_2 with oxygen administration.

CHD, congenital heart defect; CHF, congestive heart failure; CNS, central nervous system; PDA, patent ductus arteriosus; PPHN, persistent pulmonary hypertension of newborn.

2. *Hyperoxitest.* This test helps differentiate cyanosis caused by cardiac disease from that caused by pulmonary disease. When central cyanosis has been confirmed by arterial partial pressure of oxygen (Po_2), one tests the response of arterial Po_2 to 100% oxygen inhalation (hyperoxitest). Oxygen should be administered through a plastic hood (such as an oxyhood) for at least 10 minutes in order to fill the alveolar space completely with oxygen. With pulmonary disease, arterial Po_2 usually rises to more than 100 mm Hg. When there is a significant intracardiac right-to-left shunt, the arterial Po_2 does not exceed 100 mm Hg, and the rise is usually

---

BOX 14–1	SUGGESTED STEPS IN THE MANAGEMENT OF CYANOTIC NEWBORNS

1. Chest x-ray films.
   Chest x-ray films may reveal pulmonary causes of cyanosis and the urgency of the problem. They can also hint at the presence or absence of cardiac defects and the type of defect.

2. ECG if cardiac origin of cyanosis is suspected.

3. Arterial blood gases in room air.
   Arterial blood gases in room air confirm or reject central cyanosis.
   An elevated Pco_2 suggests pulmonary or CNS problems.
   A low pH may be seen in sepsis, circulatory shock, or severe hypoxemia.

4. Hyperoxitest.
   Repeating arterial blood gases while the patient breathes 100% oxygen helps separate cardiac causes of cyanosis from pulmonary or central nervous system causes.

5. Umbilical artery line.
   A Po_2 value in a preductal artery (such as the right radial artery) that is 10 to 15 mm Hg higher than that in a postductal artery (an umbilical artery line) suggests a right-to-left ductal shunt.

6. Prostaglandin E_1.
   If a cyanotic defect is suspected that depends on the patency of the ductus for survival, prostaglandin E_1 (Prostin VR Pediatric) should be started or made available.

Table 14–2. **Differential Diagnosis of Cyanotic Newborns with Increased Pulmonary Vascularity**

Conditions	Other Important Clinical Findings
RVH on ECG	
D-TGA	Severe cyanosis in a large newborn*
	Male preponderance* (3:1)
	Single S2
	Signs of CHF (±)
	Usually no heart murmur*
	"Egg-shaped" heart with narrow waist (on x-ray film)*
	ECG: Normal or RVH
TAPVR with obstruction	Male preponderance* (4:1)
	Quadruple or quintuple rhythm*
	Usually no heart murmur
	Pulmonary crackles (±)
	Pulmonary venous congestion or pulmonary edema on x-ray film*
	ECG: RVH, Q waves in V1*
DORV with subpulmonary VSD (Taussig-Bing anomaly)	Resembles TGA (severe cyanosis, signs of CHF [±])*
	Systolic murmur at ULSB, grade 2-3/6*
	ECG: RVH, RAH (±)
PPHN	Meconium stain or birth asphyxia
	Marked tachypnea and cyanosis*
	Usually no heart murmur
	Differential Po$_2$ between preductal and postductal arterial sites*
	Cardiomegaly, "ground-glass" appearance, normal vascularity, or lung pathology on x-ray films*
	Normal ECG
LVH or BVH on ECG	
Persistent truncus arteriosus (type I)	Mild cyanosis
	Bounding peripheral pulses*
	Systolic ejection click at apex*
	Harsh systolic murmur of VSD
	Early diastolic murmur of truncal valve regurgitation* (±)
	Signs of CHF (±)
	Right aortic arch on x-ray film* (30%)
Single ventricle (without PS)	Mild cyanosis
	Signs of CHF and cardiomegaly on x-ray film (±)
	Loud systolic murmur along LSB
	ECG: (1) no Q waves in precordial leads or Q waves in V4R or V1 and (2) stereotype QRS (RS, rS, or QR) across most precordial leads
TGA and VSD	Mild cyanosis
	Signs of CHF* (±)
	Harsh systolic murmur of VSD
Polysplenia syndrome	Mild cyanosis
	Midline liver* (on palpation, x-ray films)
	Superior QRS axis and superior P axis* (ECG)
	ECG: RVH, LVH, or no hypertrophy

*Findings that are particularly important in the diagnosis of the condition.

BVH, biventricular hypertrophy; CHF, congestive heart failure; D-TGA, complete TGA; DORV, double-outlet right ventricle; ECG, electrocardiogram; LSB, left sternal border; LVH, left ventricular hypertrophy; PPHN, persistent pulmonary hypertension of the newborn; PS, pulmonary stenosis; RAH, right atrial hypertrophy; RVH, right ventricular hypertrophy; TAPVR, total anomalous pulmonary venous return; TGA, transposition of the great arteries; ULSB, upper left sternal border; VSD, ventricular septal defect.

not more than 10 to 30 mm Hg (see Chapter 11 for details). However, some infants with cyanotic defects with a large pulmonary blood flow, such as TAPVR, may have a rise in arterial Po$_2$ to 100 mm Hg or higher. Conversely, infants with a massive intrapulmonary shunt from lung disease (but with a normal heart) may not have a rise in arterial Po$_2$ to 100 mm Hg. Therefore, the response of Po$_2$ to 100% oxygen inhalation should be interpreted in light of clinical pictures, especially the degree of pulmonary pathology seen on chest x-ray films.

Table 14–3. **Differential Diagnosis of Cyanotic Newborns with Decreased Pulmonary Vascularity**

Conditions	Other Important Clinical Findings
RVH on ECG	
TOF	Long systolic murmur, grade 2–3/6, at ULSB*
	Soft continuous murmur in neonates with TOF with pulmonary atresia*
	Concave main PA segment (or "boot-shaped" heart) (on x-ray film)*
	Right aortic arch on x-ray film* (25%)
DORV with PS	Resemblance to TOF*
	Systolic murmur along LSB, grade 3–4/6
	ECG: RVH, first-degree AV block
Asplenia syndrome	Midline liver* (on palpation, x-ray films)
	Superior QRS axis* (ECG)
	ECG: RVH or LVH
	Howell-Jolly body or Heinz body on blood smear
RBBB on ECG	
Ebstein's anomaly	Triple or quadruple rhythm*
	Soft TR murmur
	Extreme cardiomegaly with oligemic lung fields (±)* (on x-ray film)
	ECG: RAH, WPW syndrome, first-degree AV block
LVH on ECG	
Pulmonary atresia	Severe cyanosis
	Usually no heart murmur, but possible soft PDA murmur*
	ECG: normal QRS axis, LVH, RAH
	X-ray examination: right atrial enlargement and oligemic lungs
Tricuspid atresia	Severe cyanosis*
	Murmur of VSD or PDA
	Superior QRS axis* (ECG)
	Boot-shaped heart* (on x-ray film)
BVH on ECG	
TGA and PS	Moderate cyanosis
	No signs of CHF
	Systolic murmur (of PS) at ULSB
Persistent truncus arteriosus (type II or III)	Severe cyanosis
	Systolic ejection click*
	Soft systolic murmur
Single ventricle and PS	Physical findings resembling TOF*
	Systolic murmur along LSB

*Findings that are particularly important in the diagnosis of the condition.
AV, atrioventricular; BVH, biventricular hypertrophy; CHF, congestive heart failure; DORV, double-outlet right ventricle; ECG, electrocardiogram; LSB, left sternal border; LVH, left ventricular hypertrophy; PA, pulmonary artery; PDA, patent ductus arteriosus; PS, pulmonary stenosis; RAH, right atrial hypertrophy; RBBB, right bundle branch block; RVH, right ventricular hypertrophy; TAPVR, total anomalous pulmonary venous return; TGA, transposition of the great arteries; TOF, tetralogy of Fallot; TR, tricuspid regurgitation; ULSB, upper left sternal border; VSD, ventricular septal defect; WPW, Wolff-Parkinson-White.

3. *Arterial Po_2 in preductal and postductal arteries.* It is important that one obtains arterial blood samples from the right upper body (right radial, brachial, or temporal artery), rather than from the descending aorta, to avoid false low values caused by a right-to-left ductal shunt. If a low arterial Po_2 is obtained from an umbilical artery line (or from a lower extremity site), another sample from the right upper body should be obtained and the Po_2 values from the two sites should be compared to see if there is a right-to-left ductal shunt. Arterial Po_2 from the right radial artery that is 10 to 15 mm Hg higher than that from an umbilical artery catheter is significant. In severe cases of right-to-left ductal shunt, differential cyanosis may be noticeable, with a pink upper and a cyanotic lower body. Such a right-to-left ductal shunt is caused not only by persistent pulmonary hypertension of the newborn (PPHN) but also by other serious cardiovascular conditions, including severe obstructive lesions of the LV (e.g., severe AS) or aortic obstructive lesions (such as interrupted aortic arch, coarctation of the aorta [COA]).

4. *Prostaglandin E_1 (PGE$_1$) infusion.* If a cyanotic congenital heart defect or a ductus-dependent cardiac defect (e.g., pulmonary atresia with or without VSD, tricuspid atresia, HLHS, interrupted aortic arch, severe COA) is suspected or confirmed, a PGE$_1$ (Prostin VR Pediatric) intravenous infusion should be started. The starting dose is 0.05 to 0.1 μg/kg per minute, administered in a continuous intravenous drip. When the desired effects (increased Po$_2$, increased systemic blood pressure, improved pH) are achieved, the dose should be reduced step by step to 0.01 μg/kg per minute. When the initial starting dose has no effect, it may be increased up to 0.4 μg/kg per minute. Three common side effects of intravenous infusion of PGE$_1$ are apnea (12%), fever (14%), and flushing (10%). Less common side effects include tachycardia or bradycardia, hypotension, and cardiac arrest.

Complete Transposition of the Great Arteries

PREVALENCE

D-TGA occurs in about 5% to 7% of all congenital heart defects. It is more common in males than in females (male/female ratio of 3:1).

PATHOLOGY

1. In D-TGA the aorta arises anteriorly from the right ventricle (RV) carrying desaturated blood to the body, and the pulmonary artery (PA) arises posteriorly from the left ventricle (LV) carrying oxygenated blood back to the lungs. Unlike the situation in a normal heart, there is a fibrous continuity between the pulmonary and mitral valves and subaortic conus is present. (In normal hearts there are aortic-mitral fibrous continuity and subpulmonary conus and the aorta arises from the LV and lies posterior to and right of the pulmonary valve.) The result of D-TGA is complete separation of the pulmonary and systemic circulations. This results in hypoxemic blood circulating throughout the body and hyperoxemic blood circulating in the pulmonary circuit, which is not compatible with survival (see Fig. 11–4). Defects that permit mixing of the two circulations (e.g., atrial septal defect [ASD], ventricular septal defect [VSD], and patent ductus arteriosus [PDA]) are necessary for survival.

2. About half of these infants do not have associated defects other than a patent foramen ovale (PFO) or a small PDA (i.e., simple TGA).

3. In about 5% of the patients, left ventricular outflow tract (LVOT) obstruction (or subpulmonary stenosis) occurs. The obstruction may be dynamic or fixed. Dynamic obstruction of the LVOT, which occurs in about 20% of such patients, results from bowing of the interventricular septum to the left because of a high RV pressure. Anatomic (or fixed) subpulmonary stenosis or abnormal mitral chordal attachment rarely causes obstruction of the LVOT

4. VSD is present in 30% to 40% of patients with D-TGA and may be located anywhere in the ventricular septum. A combination of VSD and significant LVOT obstruction (or pulmonary stenosis) occurs in about 10% of all patients with D-TGA. Infants with TGA and VSD more commonly have associated defects than those without associated VSD. Such associated defects include COA, interrupted aortic arch, pulmonary atresia, and an overriding or straddling of the atrioventricular (AV) valve.*

Overriding is an abnormal relationship between the AV valve annulus and the ventricular septum. The AV valve annulus commits to both ventricular chambers, and it is the result of malalignment of the atrial and ventricular septa. *Straddling* is present when the chordae tendineae insert into the contralateral ventricle through a septal defect. Type A straddling is a mild form in which the chordae insert near the crest of the ventricular septum. In type B, the insertion is along the ventricular septum. In type C straddling, the chordae insert into the free wall of the contralateral ventricle. Overriding and straddling may occur independently or coexist in the same valve.

5. The classic complete TGA is called *D-transposition*, in which the aorta is located anteriorly and to the right (dextro) of the PA. This is why the prefix *D* is used. When the transposed aorta is located to the left of the PA, it is called *L-transposition* (see Fig. 16–4).

CLINICAL MANIFESTATIONS

History
1. History of cyanosis from birth is always present.
2. Signs of congestive heart failure (CHF) with dyspnea and feeding difficulties develop during the newborn period.

Physical Examination (Fig. 14–1)
1. Moderate to severe cyanosis is present, especially in large, male newborns. Such an infant is tachypneic but without retraction unless CHF supervenes.
2. The S2 is single and loud. No heart murmur is heard in infants with an intact ventricular septum. An early or holosystolic murmur of VSD may be audible in less cyanotic infants with associated VSD. A soft midsystolic murmur of pulmonary stenosis (PS or LVOT obstruction) may be audible.
3. If CHF supervenes, hepatomegaly and dyspnea develop.

Laboratory Studies
1. Severe arterial hypoxemia usually with acidosis is present. Hypoxemia does not respond to oxygen inhalation. (See Hyperoxitest earlier in this chapter.)
2. Hypoglycemia and hypocalcemia are occasionally present.

Electrocardiography (Fig. 14–2)
1. There is a rightward QRS axis (i.e., +90 to +200 degrees).
2. Right ventricular hypertrophy (RVH) is usually present after the first few days of life. The QRS voltages and the QRS axis may be normal in some newborns with the defect. After 3 days of life, an upright T wave in V1 may be the only abnormality suggestive of RVH.
3. Biventricular hypertrophy (BVH) may be present in infants with large VSD, PDA, or pulmonary vascular obstructive disease because all these conditions produce an additional left ventricular hypertrophy (LVH).
4. Occasionally right atrial hypertrophy (RAH) is present.

X-ray Studies
1. Cardiomegaly with increased pulmonary vascularity is typically present.
2. An egg-shaped cardiac silhouette with a narrow, superior mediastinum is characteristic (Fig. 14–3).

Echocardiography. Two-dimensional echo and color flow Doppler studies usually provide all the anatomic and functional information needed for the management of infants with D-TGA.

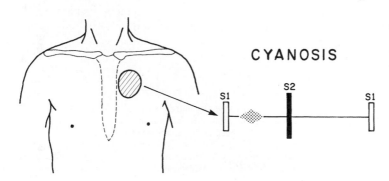

Figure 14–1. Cardiac findings of transposition of the great arteries. Heart murmur is usually absent, and the S2 is single in the majority of patients.

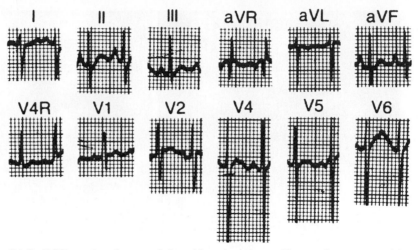

Figure 14–2. *ECG tracing from a 6-day-old male infant with complete transposition of the great arteries. The QRS axis is +140 degrees. Note the deep S waves in V5 and V6 and an upright T wave in V1.*

1. In the parasternal long-axis view, the great artery arising from the posterior ventricle (LV) has a sharp posterior angulation toward the lungs, which suggests that this artery is the PA (Fig. 14–4A). In contrast to the normal intertwining of the great arteries, the proximal portions of the great arteries run parallel.

2. In the parasternal short-axis view, the "circle and sausage" appearance of the normal great arteries is not visible. Instead, the great arteries appear as "double circles" (see Fig. 14–4B). The PA is in the center of the heart, and the coronary arteries do not arise from this great artery. The aorta is usually anterior and slightly to the right of the PA, and the coronary arteries arise from the aorta.

3. In the apical and subcostal five-chamber views, the PA (i.e., the artery that bifurcates) arises from the LV, and the aorta arises from the RV.

4. The status of atrial communication, both before and after balloon septostomy, is best evaluated in the subcostal view. Doppler examination and color flow mapping should aid in the functional evaluation of the atrial shunt.

5. Frequently, associated defects such as VSD, LVOT obstruction (dynamic or fixed), or pulmonary valve stenosis are found. Subaortic stenosis or COA rarely occurs.

6. The coronary arteries can be imaged in most patients by using parasternal and apical views (Fig. 14–5).

Figure 14–3. *Posteroanterior view of the chest roentgenogram from a 2-month-old infant with complete transposition of the great arteries. Note cardiomegaly (cardiothoracic ratio of 0.7), "egg-shaped" heart with narrow waist, and increased pulmonary vascular markings, which are characteristic of this condition.*

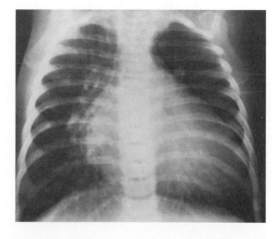

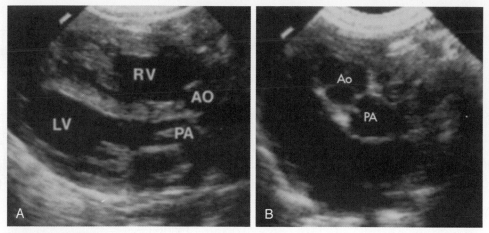

Figure 14–4. Parasternal echo views in complete transposition of the great arteries. **A,** In this parasternal long-axis view, the great arteries are seen in parallel alignment. The posterior artery is directed posteriorly, bifurcates into two branches, and is therefore a pulmonary artery (PA). **B,** In the parasternal short-axis view, the aorta (AO) and the PA are seen in cross section as double circles. LV, left ventricle; RV, right ventricle. (From Snider AR, Serwer GA: Echocardiography in Pediatric Heart Disease. St. Louis, Mosby, 1990.)

NATURAL HISTORY

1. Progressive hypoxia, acidosis, and heart failure result in death in the newborn period. Without surgical intervention, death occurs in 90% of patients before they reach 6 months of age.

2. Infants with an intact ventricular septum are the sickest group but demonstrate the most dramatic improvement after the Rashkind balloon atrial septostomy.

3. Infants with VSD are the least cyanotic group but the most likely to develop CHF and pulmonary vascular obstructive disease. Many infants with TGA and a large VSD develop moderate pulmonary vascular obstructive disease by 3 to 4 months of age. Thus, surgical procedures are recommended before that age.

4. Infants with a significant PDA are similar to those with a large VSD, in terms of their development of CHF and pulmonary vascular obstructive disease.

5. The combination of VSD and PS allows considerably longer survival without surgery because the pulmonary vascular bed is protected from developing pulmonary hypertension, but this combination carries a high surgical risk for correction.

MANAGEMENT

Medical

1. The following measures should be carried out to stabilize the patient before an emergency cardiac catheterization (if performed) or a surgical procedure is carried out:
   a. Arterial blood gases and pH should be obtained and metabolic acidosis should be corrected. Hypoglycemia and hypocalcemia, if present, should be treated.
   b. PGE_1 infusion should be started to improve arterial oxygen saturation by reopening the ductus (see earlier section, "Approach to a Cyanotic Neonate," or Appendix E for the dosage). This should be continued throughout the cardiac catheterization and until the time of surgery.
   c. Oxygen should be administered for severe hypoxia. Oxygen may help lower pulmonary vascular resistance (PVR) and increase pulmonary blood flow (PBF), which in turn increases systemic arterial oxygen saturation.

2. Before surgery, cardiac catheterization and a balloon atrial septostomy (i.e., the Rashkind procedure) are often carried out to have some flexibility in planning surgery. If adequate interatrial communication exists and the anatomic diagnosis of TGA

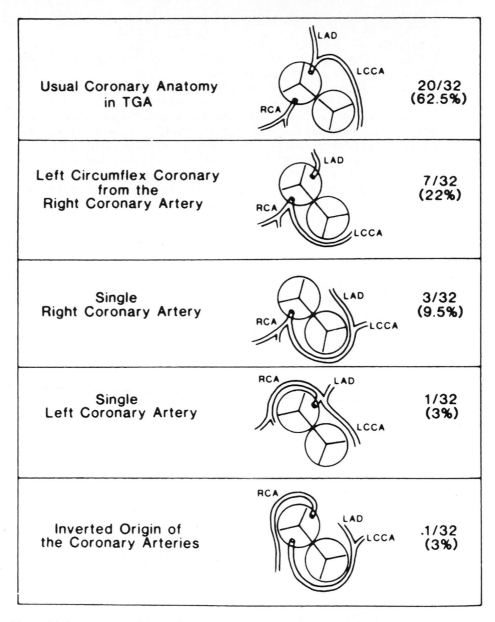

Figure 14–5. *Diagram of the coronary artery anatomy in 32 patients with transposition of the great arteries (TGA). The orientation of the figures is that of a parasternal short-axis echo view. LAD, left anterior descending artery; LCCA, left circumflex coronary artery; RCA, right coronary artery. (From Pasquini L, Sanders SP, Parness IA, et al: Diagnosis of coronary artery anatomy by two-dimensional echocardiography in patients with transposition of the great arteries. Circulation 75:557–564, 1987.)*

is clear by echo examination, the patient may go to surgery without cardiac catheterization or the balloon atrial septostomy. In the balloon atrial septostomy, a balloon-tipped catheter is advanced into the left atrium (LA) through the PFO. The balloon is inflated with diluted radiopaque dye and abruptly and forcefully withdrawn to the right atrium (RA) under fluoroscopic or echo monitoring. This procedure creates a large defect in the atrial septum through which improved intracardiac mixing occurs. An increase in the oxygen saturation of 10% or more and a minimal interatrial pressure gradient are considered satisfactory results of the procedure.

3. CHF may be treated with digoxin and diuretics.

Surgical

Palliative Procedure. No palliative procedure is performed unless an arterial switch operation cannot be performed early in life.

Definitive Repair. Historically, definitive surgeries performed for TGA were procedures that switched right- and left-sided blood at three levels: the atrial level (intra-atrial repair surgeries such as the Senning or Mustard operation), the ventricular level (Rastelli operation), and the great artery level (arterial switch operation). At this time, the arterial switch operation is clearly the procedure of choice and intra-atrial repair surgeries are rarely performed, only in unusual situations. The Damus-Kaye-Stansel operation in conjunction with the Rastelli operation can be performed in patients with VSD and subaortic stenosis. Because of a relatively poor long-term result of the Rastelli operation, other options such as the Nikaidoh operation or réparation à l'étage ventriculaire (REV) procedure have become more popular.

Procedures

1. Atrial baffle operations (Mustard and Senning operations). These procedures reroute pulmonary and systemic venous returns at the atrial level with resulting physiologic correction. The pulmonary venous blood eventually goes to the aorta and the systemic venous blood goes to the PA (see Fig. 14–6 for the hemodynamic results of the atrial baffle operation). The Mustard operation uses a pericardial or a prosthetic baffle, and the Senning operation uses the patient's own atrial septal flap and the RA free wall to redirect the venous returns.

   A number of long-term problems have been reported, including superior vena cava (SVC) obstruction (<5% of all cases), baffle leak (<20%), absence of sinus rhythm (>50%), frequent atrial and ventricular arrhythmias with occasional sudden death, tricuspid valve insufficiency (rare), and RV (i.e., systemic ventricular) dysfunction or failure. The arterial switch operation has largely replaced the atrial baffle operation. There are, however, rare indications for atrial baffle operations, including a situation in which relative contraindications to the arterial switch operation exist (such as coronary arteries that are difficult to transfer).

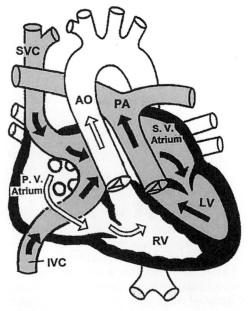

Figure 14–6. Atrial baffle operation. The hemodynamic results of the Mustard and Senning operations are shown. Systemic venous blood (shaded) is redirected to the anatomic LA and LV and eventually to the pulmonary circulation. Pulmonary venous blood is redirected to the anatomic RA and RV through the tricuspid valve and to the aorta. AO, aorta; IVC, inferior vena cava; LV, left ventricle; PA, pulmonary artery; P. V. atrium, pulmonary venous atrium; S. V. atrium, systemic venous atrium; SVC, superior vena cava.

2. Rastelli operation. In patients with VSD and severe PS, redirection of the pulmonary and systemic venous blood is carried out at the ventricular level. The LV is directed to the aorta by creating an intraventricular tunnel between the VSD and the aortic valve. A valved conduit or a homograft is placed between the RV and the PA (Fig. 14–7). Most surgeons prefer to delay this procedure until after the first year of life. The mortality rate is between 10% and 29%.

Complications after the Rastelli operation include conduit obstruction (especially in those containing porcine heterograft valves) and complete heart block (rarely occurs). The conduit needs to be replaced as the child grows. Occasionally, LVOT obstruction occurs at the level of the VSD or at the level of the intraventricular tunnels. More important, the long-term results are not optimal with the 20-year survival about 50%. Two alternative procedures are now available, the REV procedure and the Nikaidoh procedure (see later for discussion of these procedures).

3. Arterial switch operation. The arterial switch operation is now firmly established as the procedure of choice. There are almost no situations that would justify the performance of a Senning or Mustard procedure for D-TGA. The coronary arteries are transplanted to the PA, and the proximal great arteries are connected to the distal end of the other great artery, resulting in an anatomic correction (Fig. 14–8). This procedure has advantages over the atrial baffle operations because it is an anatomic (not physiologic) correction and long-term complications are infrequent. This procedure is indicated not only for simple TGA but also for TGA with other associated anomalies (such as VSD or PDA) and the Taussig-Bing type of DORV with subpulmonary VSD. The operative mortality for neonates with TGA and an intact ventricular septum is down to around 6%.

Complications after the arterial switch operation are infrequent. Normal sinus rhythm is usually present, arrhythmias are extremely rare, and LV function is usually normal. The following complications may occur after the arterial switch operation:
   a. Coronary artery obstruction, which may lead to myocardial ischemia, infarction, and even death, is a serious complication.
   b. Supravalvar PS at the anastomosis site (~12%) is the most common cause for reoperation, although the incidence has decreased.

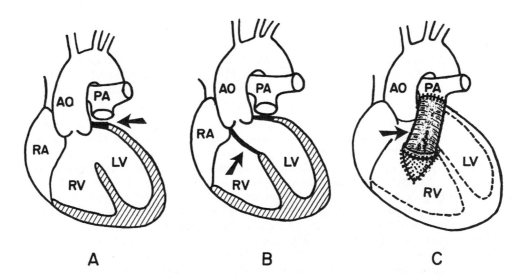

A   **B**   **C**

Figure 14–7. *The Rastelli operation.* ***A,*** *The pulmonary artery (PA) is divided from the left ventricle (LV), and the cardiac end is oversewn (arrow).* ***B,*** *An intracardiac tunnel (arrow) is placed between the large ventricular septal defect and the aorta (AO) so that the LV communicates with the aorta.* ***C,*** *The right ventricle (RV) is connected to the divided PA by a valved conduit or an aortic homograft.*

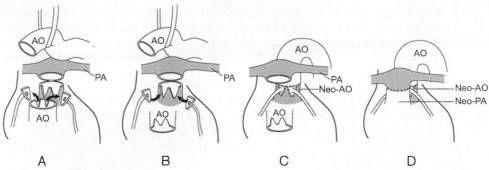

Figure 14–8. *Arterial switch operation.* **A,** *The aorta (AO; unshaded) is transected slightly above the coronary ostia, and the pulmonary artery (PA; shaded) is also transected at about the same level. The ascending aorta is lifted, and both coronary arteries are removed from the aorta with triangular buttons.* **B,** *Triangular buttons of similar size are made at the proper position in the PA trunk.* **C,** *The coronary arteries are transplanted to the PA trunk. The ascending aorta is brought behind the PA and is connected to the proximal PA, to form a neoaorta.* **D,** *The triangular defects in the proximal aorta are repaired, and the proximal aorta is connected to the distal portion of the divided PA. Note that the neo-PA is in front of the neoaorta.*

    c. Neoaortic valvar regurgitation and supravalvar neoaortic stenosis are rare complications.

    The following factors are important for a successful arterial switch operation.

    1). Left ventricular pressure. An LV that can support the systemic circulation after surgery must exist. The LV pressure should be near systemic levels at the time of surgery, therefore the arterial switch operation should be performed shortly after birth. The time limit is 3 weeks of age (although some suggest an upper limit of 8 weeks of age).

    2). Coronary artery anatomy. Almost all coronary artery patterns in TGA are amenable to the arterial switch operation. However, the risk is slightly higher when either one or both coronary arteries passed between the great arteries. The single coronary artery is transferable by various surgical techniques.

    Currently, other associated anomalies are repaired at the time of the arterial switch operation in the neonatal period.

    1). For patients with associated VSD, the VSD is repaired through an atrial approach or through the pulmonary valve. The mortality rate is around 6%.

    2). For patients with PDA and VSD, PDA is ligated and the VSD is closed.

    3). Mild pulmonary valve stenosis or dynamic subpulmonary stenosis does not preclude a successful arterial switch operation.

Two-Stage Switch Operation. In patients whose LV pressure is low (because of missing of early arterial switch operation), it can be raised by PA banding, either with or without a shunt procedure, for 7 to 10 days (in cases of a "rapid two-stage switch operation") or for several months before undertaking the switch operation. LV pressure greater than 85% of the RV pressure appears to be satisfactory for the switch operation. The rapid switch is preferable to a longer waiting period, which results in scarring and adhesions of the PA following PA banding. Scarring makes PA reconstruction and anastomosis of the great arteries difficult and adhesions obscure coronary artery anatomy.

Staged Conversion to Arterial Switch Operation. Some patients who received an atrial baffle operation develop RV failure with severe tricuspid valve regurgitation. For these patients, staged conversion to an arterial switch operation can be done. Initially, a PA band is placed to raise the LV pressure. This is followed by an arterial switch operation with a higher mortality rate (around 25% to 33%). Alternatively, following the PA band, a Damus-Kaye-Stansel operation can be performed, which does not require transfer of coronary arteries. Transfer of coronary arteries is much more difficult in these patients because of dense adhesions.

4. REV procedure (réparation à l'étage ventriculaire). This procedure, first reported by Lecompte, may be performed for patients with D-TGA associated with VSD and severe PS. The procedure comprises the following. (1) infundibular resection to enlarge the VSD, (2) intraventricular baffle to direct LV output to the aorta, (3) aortic transection in order to perform the Lecompte maneuver (by which the right pulmonary artery [RPA] is brought anterior to the ascending aorta), and (4) direct RV-to-PA reconstruction by using an anterior patch (Fig. 14–9). This may require fewer reoperations than the Rastelli procedure. Lecompte reported 50 cases (4 months to 15 years) with an 18% operative mortality.

5. Nikaidoh procedure: This procedure is another surgical option for patients with D-TGA, VSD, and severe PS. In this procedure, the aortic root is mobilized and translocated to the pulmonary position. The repair consists of the following: (1) harvesting the aortic root from the RV (with attached coronary arteries in the original procedure), (2) relieving the LVOT obstruction (by dividing the outlet

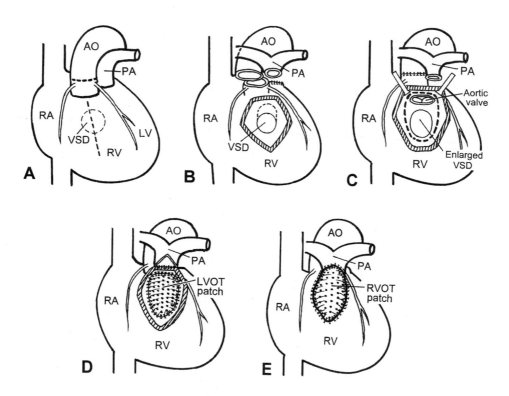

Figure 14–9. *Réparation à l'étage ventriculaire (REV) procedure for patients with complete transposition of the great arteries (D-TGA), ventricular septal defect (VSD), and severe pulmonary stenosis (PS). **A**, A schematic drawing of D-TGA with VSD and severe PS (with relatively small PA). The broken lines indicate the planned aortic and RV incision sites. The broken circle indicates a VSD. **B**, The aorta and PA have been transected and the RPA is brought anterior to the aorta (Lecompte maneuver). The proximal PA has been oversewn. The VSD is exposed through the right ventriculotomy (note that the figures have expanded ventriculotomy to allow visualization of intracardiac structures). Dotted lines indicate the portion of the infundibular septum to be excised to enlarge the VSD. **C**, The aortic valve is well shown by retractors. The broken line indicates the planned site of a patch placement for the LV-AO connection. The transected aorta has been reconnected behind the RPA. **D**, The completed LV-to-AO tunnel is shown. The superior portion of the right ventriculotomy is sutured directly to the posterior portion of the main PA. **E**, A pericardial or synthetic patch is used to complete the RV-to-PA reconstruction. AO, aorta; LPA, left pulmonary artery; LV, left ventricle; LVOT, left ventricular outflow tract; PA, pulmonary artery; RA, right atrium; RPA, right pulmonary artery; RV, right ventricle; RVOT, right ventricular outflow tract.*

septum and excising the pulmonary valve), (3) reconstructing the LVOT (with posteriorly translocated aortic root and the VSD patch), and (4) reconstructing the RVOT (with a pericardial patch or a homograft). In the modified Nikaidoh procedure, one or both coronary arteries are moved to a more favorable position as necessary (not shown) and the Lecompte maneuver is also performed (Fig. 14–10). The hospital mortality is less than 10%.

6. Damus-Kaye-Stansel operation. Infants with a large VSD and significant subaortic stenosis may receive the Damus-Kaye-Stansel operation at 1 to 2 years of age. In this procedure, the coronary arteries are not transferred to a neoaorta. Instead, the subaortic stenosis is bypassed by connecting the proximal PA trunk to the ascending aorta. The VSD is closed, and a conduit is placed between the RV and the distal PA (Fig. 14–11). The mortality rate is considerable, ranging from 15% to 30%.

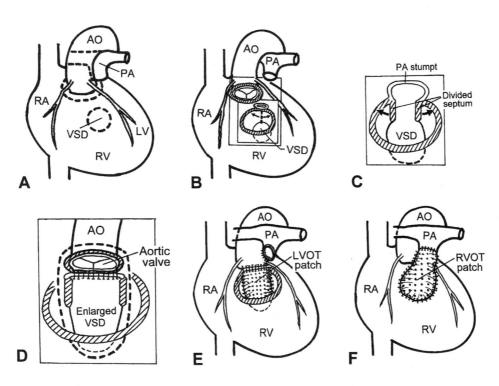

Figure 14–10. Nikaidoh procedure for patients with complete transposition of the great arteries (D-TGA), ventricular septal defect (VSD), and severe pulmonary stenosis (PS). *A,* Schematic drawing of D-TGA with VSD and severe PS (with relatively small PA) is shown. The circular broken line around the aorta is the planned incision site for aortic root mobilization. The smaller broken circle indicates a VSD. *B,* The aortic root has been mobilized by a circular incision around the aortic root, which leaves an opening in the RV free wall. The main PA is also transected. Through the opening, part of the VSD, ventricular septum, and the hypoplastic PA stump are seen. The dotted vertical line in the ventricular septum (in the smaller inset in *B*) is the planned incision through the infundibular septum. *C,* In the inset, the incision in the infundibular septum has created a large opening, which includes the PA annulus and stump and the VSD. *D,* In the large inset, the posterior portion of the aorta is directly sutured to the PA stump, which results in a large VSD. This completes translocation of the aorta to the original PA position. The thick oval-shaped broken line that goes through the front of the transected aortic root is the planned site for placement of the LV outflow tract patch, which will direct the LV flow to the aorta. *E,* The completed tunnel is shown (LVOT patch that directs the LV flow to the aorta). The distal segment of the main PA is fixed to the aorta. Some surgeons use Lecompte maneuver to bring the RPA in front of the ascending aorta (as shown here). *F,* A pericardial patch is oversewn to complete the RV-to-PA connection (RVOT patch). Abbreviations are the same as those in Figure 14–9.

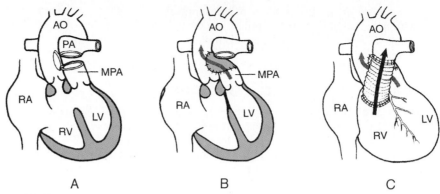

A   B   C

Figure 14–11. *Damus-Kaye-Stansel operation for complete transposition of the great arteries (D-TGA) plus ventricular septal defect (VSD) plus subaortic stenosis.* ***A,*** *D-TGA with VSD and subaortic stenosis is illustrated. The main pulmonary artery (MPA) is transected near its bifurcation. An appropriately positioned and sized incision is made in the ascending aorta (AO).* ***B,*** *The proximal MPA is anastomosed end to side to the ascending aorta using either a Dacron tube or Gore-Tex. This channel will direct left ventricular blood to the aorta. The aortic valve is either closed or left unclosed. The VSD is closed (through a right ventriculotomy).* ***C,*** *A valved conduit is placed between the right ventricle (RV) and the distal pulmonary artery (PA). This channel will carry RV blood to the PA. AO, aorta; LV, left ventricle; MPA, main pulmonary artery; PA, pulmonary artery; RA, right atrium; RV, right ventricle.*

The Damus-Kaye-Stansel operation is also applicable in patients with single ventricle and TGA with an obstructive bulboventricular foramen or DORV with subaortic stenosis (see Fig. 14–62).

Surgical management for TGA is summarized in Figure 14–12.

Postoperative Follow-up

Arterial Switch. Although the complication rate is much lower for arterial switch than for atrial baffle repair, regular follow-up is needed to detect possible complications, such

Transposition of the Great Arteries

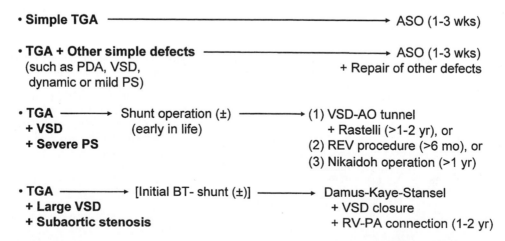

Figure 14–12. *Surgical approaches to transposition of the great arteries. ASO, arterial switch operation; BT, Blalock-Taussig; PDA, patent ductus arteriosus; PS, pulmonary stenosis; REV, réparation à l'étage ventriculaire; TGA, transposition of the great arteries; VSD, ventricular septal defect.*

as stenosis of the PA or aorta in the supravalvular regions, coronary artery obstruction with myocardial ischemia or infarction, ventricular dysfunction, arrhythmias, and/or semi-lunar valve regurgitation. These complications are, for the most part, hemodynamically insignificant or infrequent.

Congenitally Corrected Transposition of the Great Arteries

PREVALENCE

L-TGA (or ventricular inversion) occurs in less than 1% of all patients with congenital heart defects.

PATHOLOGY

1. In this condition, the visceroatrial relationship is normal but there is ventricular inversion. The RA is to the right of the LA and receives systemic venous blood. The RA empties into the anatomic LV through the mitral valve, and the LA empties into the RV through the tricuspid valve. For this to occur, the RV is located to the left of the LV (or the LV is located to the right of the RV), which is called *ventricular inversion* (Fig. 14–13). The great arteries are transposed, with the aorta rising from the RV and the PA rising from the LV. The aorta is located anterior to and left of the PA; thus, the prefix of L is used (see Fig. 16–4D). The result is functional correction in that oxygenated blood coming into the LA goes to the anatomic RV and then flows out to the aorta. This is why the term *corrected* is used to describe this condition.

2. Theoretically, no functional abnormalities exist, but, unfortunately, most cases are complicated by associated intracardiac defects, AV conduction disturbances, and arrhythmias.
   a. VSD occurs in 80% of all cases.
   b. PS, both valvular and subvalvular, occurs in 50% of patients and is usually associated with VSD.
   c. Systemic AV valve (tricuspid valve) regurgitation occurs in 30% of patients.
   d. Occasionally, complex associated defects are present with hypoplastic ventricle, AV valve abnormalities, or multiple VSDs.
   e. Both varying and progressive degrees of AV block and paroxysmal supraventricular tachycardia (SVT) frequently occur.

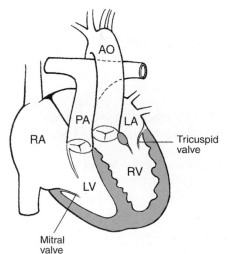

Figure 14–13. *Diagram of congenitally corrected TGA (L-TGA). There is an inversion of ventricular chambers with their corresponding atrioventricular valves. The great arteries are transposed, but functional correction results, with oxygenated blood going to the aorta. Unfortunately, a high percentage of the patients with L-TGA have associated defects, some of which may cause cyanosis. AO, aorta; LA, left atrium; LV, left ventricle; PA, pulmonary artery; RA, right atrium; RV, right ventricle.*

3. The cardiac apex is in the right chest (dextrocardia) in about 50% of cases.

4. The coronary arteries show a mirror-image distribution. The right coronary artery supplies the anterior descending branch and gives rise to a circumflex; the left coronary artery resembles a right coronary artery.

CLINICAL MANIFESTATIONS

History

1. Patients are asymptomatic when L-TGA is not associated with other defects.

2. During the first months of life, most patients with associated defects become symptomatic with cyanosis resulting from VSD and PS or CHF resulting from a large VSD.

3. Exertional dyspnea and easy fatigability may develop with regurgitation of the systemic AV valve (i.e., anatomic tricuspid valve).

Physical Examination

1. The patient is cyanotic if PS and VSD are present.

2. Hyperactive precordium occurs in the presence of a large VSD. Systolic thrill occurs in the presence of PS, with or without VSD.

3. The S2 is loud and single at the upper left or right sternal border. A grade 2 to 4/6 harsh, holosystolic murmur along the lower left sternal border indicates the presence of VSD or systemic AV valve regurgitation. A grade 2 to 3/6 ejection systolic murmur is present at the upper left or right sternal border if PS is present. An apical diastolic rumble may be audible if a large VSD or significant TR is present.

4. Bradycardia, tachycardia, or irregular rhythm requires an investigation for AV conduction disturbances or arrhythmias.

Electrocardiography

1. The absence of Q waves in V5 and V6 or the presence of Q waves in V4R or V1 is characteristic of the condition (Fig. 14–14). This is because the direction of ventricular septal depolarization is from the embryonic LV to RV.

2. Varying degrees of AV block are common. First-degree AV block is present in about 50% of patients. Second-degree AV block may progress to complete heart block.

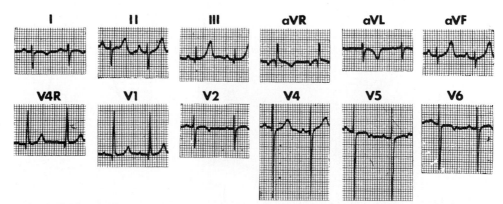

Figure 14–14. *Tracing from an 8-year-old girl with congenitally corrected transposition of the great arteries, ventricular septal defect, and pulmonary stenosis. Note that no Q waves are seen in leads V5 and V6. Instead, the Q waves are seen in V4R and V1. This suggests ventricular inversion. The electrocardiogram also suggests hypertrophy of the right-sided ventricle (anatomic left ventricle).*

3. Atrial arrhythmias and Wolff-Parkinson-White (WPW) preexcitation are occasionally present.

4. Atrial or ventricular hypertrophy, or both, may be present in complicated cases (see Fig. 14–14).

X-ray Studies

1. A straight, left upper cardiac border, formed by the ascending aorta, is a characteristic finding (Fig. 14–15).

2. Cardiomegaly and increased pulmonary vascular markings are present when the condition is associated with VSD.

3. Pulmonary venous congestion and left atrial enlargement may be seen with severe left-sided AV valve regurgitation.

4. Positional abnormalities (e.g., dextrocardia, mesocardia) may be present.

Echocardiography. With use of the segmental approach (see Chapter 16), the diagnosis of L-TGA can be made easily, and associated anomalies can be detected and quantitated.

1. The parasternal long-axis view is obtained from a more vertical and leftward scan than with a normal heart. The aorta, which arises from the posterior ventricle, is not in fibrous continuity with the AV valve.

2. In the parasternal short-axis scan, a double circle is imaged instead of the normal "circle and sausage" pattern. The posterior circle is the PA without demonstrable coronary arteries. The aorta is usually anterior to and left of the PA. The LV, which has two well-defined papillary muscles, is seen anteriorly and on the right and is connected to the characteristic "fish mouth" appearance of the mitral valve.

3. In the apical and subcostal four-chamber views, the LA is connected to the tricuspid valve (which has a more apical attachment to the ventricular septum than the other) and the RA is connected to the mitral valve. The anterior artery (aorta) arises from the left-sided morphologic RV, and the posterior artery with bifurcation (PA) arises from the right-sided morphologic LV.

4. The situs solitus of the atria is confirmed by the drainage of systemic veins (i.e., inferior and superior venae cavae) to the right-sided atrium and the drainage of pulmonary veins to the left-sided atrium.

5. The following associated abnormalities should be looked for, and their functional significance should be assessed by Doppler and color flow studies: type and severity of PS, size and location of VSD, straddling of the AV valve, and so forth.

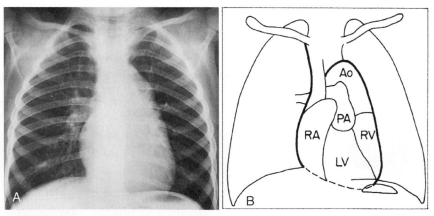

Figure 14–15. *Posteroanterior view of an actual chest roentgenogram (**A**) and a diagrammatic representation (**B**) from a 10-year-old child with congenitally corrected transposition of the great arteries. Note the straight left cardiac border formed by the ascending aorta. AO, aorta; LV, left ventricle; PA, pulmonary artery; RA, right atrium; RV, right ventricle.*

NATURAL HISTORY

The clinical course is determined by the presence or absence of associated defects and complications.

1. Some palliative surgeries are usually needed in infancy when L-TGA is associated with other defects—for example, PA banding for a large VSD or a systemic-to-PA shunt for PS. Without these procedures, 20% to 30% of patients die in the first year. CHF is the most common cause of death.

2. Regurgitation of the systemic AV valve (anatomic tricuspid valve) develops in about 30% of patients. This is often associated with dysplastic or Ebstein-like tricuspid valves.

3. Progressive AV conduction disturbances may occur, including complete heart block in up to 30% of cases. These disturbances occur more often in patients without VSD than in those with VSD. Sudden death rarely occurs.

4. Occasional adult patients without major associated defects are asymptomatic.

MANAGEMENT

Medical

1. Treatment with anticongestive agents is necessary if CHF develops.

2. Antiarrhythmic agents are used for arrhythmias.

3. Prophylaxis against subacute bacterial endocarditis (SBE) should be observed when indications arise.

Surgical

Palliative Procedures

1. A modified Blalock-Taussig shunt is necessary for patients with severe PS (usually associated with VSD).

2. PA banding may be needed for uncontrollable CHF in early infancy.

Definitive Procedures. There are two major approaches to surgical management of L-TGA: classic repair and anatomic repair. The surgical approach for L-TGA is summarized in Figure 14–16.

1. Classic repair leaves the anatomic RV as the systemic ventricle. Competent tricuspid valve (or left AV valve) and good RV function are required. Even after repair, progressive TR and RV failure may develop.

   a. In patients with VSD, the VSD is closed through an atrial approach. Complete heart block is a complication of the surgery, occurring 15% to 30% of the time. The mortality rate is 5% to 10%, which is higher than that for a simple VSD.

   b. In patients with VSD and PS (or LVOT obstruction), the VSD is closed and an LV-to-PA conduit is placed. The surgical mortality rate is higher (10% to 15%).

2. Anatomic repair makes the anatomic LV the systemic ventricle, which may reduce the likelihood of TR and RV failure. This repair is technically more difficult than the classic repair and carries a higher risk, but this procedure is a better choice for patients with TR or RV dysfunction, or both.

   a. A combination of the Senning procedure (which is an atrial switch operation; see Fig. 14–6) and an arterial switch operation (see Fig. 14–8), called a "double switch" operation, is performed in patients with VSD. A PA banding is initially placed to delay the procedure until after 1 year of age. Closure of a VSD, if present, is performed through the RA. Hospital mortality for the double switch operation is approximately 10% with complete heart block occurring in 0% to 23%.

   b. In patients with VSD and PS (or LVOT obstruction), a combination of the Senning operation and Rastelli operation is performed. VSD is closed through a right ventriculotomy in such a way as to connect the VSD to the aorta. Enlargement of the VSD is often necessary. RV-to-PA continuity is established with an extracardiac

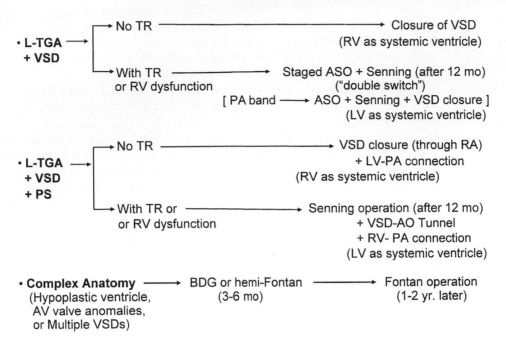

L-Transposition of the Great Arteries

Figure 14–16. *Surgical summary of congenitally corrected transposition of the great arteries (L-TGA). AO, aorta; ASO, arterial switch operation; OP, operation; PA, pulmonary artery; RV, right ventricle; PS, pulmonary stenosis (= LV outflow tract obstruction). TGA, transposition of the great arteries; TR, tricuspid regurgitation (= left-sided atrioventricular valve regurgitation); VSD, ventricular septal defect.*

valved conduit. The hospital mortality is around 10%. TR improved following the procedure.

3. *Fontan-type operation.* In patients with complex intracardiac anatomies, including hypoplasia of one ventricle, straddling AV valves, or multiple VSDs, a bidirectional Glenn operation (BDG) or full Fontan procedure is indicated.

4. *Other Procedures.*
   a. *Valve replacement.* For patients with significant TR, valve replacement is required in about 15% of patients, including those without other associated defects.
   b. *Pacemaker implantation* is required for either spontaneous or postoperative complete heart block.
   c. *Cardiac transplantation.* Some patients with complex L-TGA eventually become candidates for cardiac transplantation.

Postoperative Follow-up

1. Follow-up every 6 to 12 months is required for a possible progression of AV conduction disturbances, arrhythmias, or worsening of anatomic tricuspid valve regurgitation.

2. Antibiotic prophylaxis against SBE is indicated.

3. Routine pacemaker care, if a pacemaker is implanted, should be conducted.

4. Activity restriction is indicated if significant hemodynamic abnormalities persist.

Tetralogy of Fallot

PREVALENCE

TOF occurs in 5% to 10% of all congenital heart defects. This is probably the most common cyanotic heart defect.

PATHOLOGY

1. The original description of TOF included the following four abnormalities: a large VSD, right ventricular outflow tract (RVOT) obstruction, RVH, and overriding of the aorta. In actuality, only two abnormalities are required—a VSD large enough to equalize pressures in both ventricles and an RVOT obstruction. The RVH is secondary to the RVOT obstruction and the VSD. The overriding of the aorta varies (Fig. 14–17).
2. The VSD in TOF is a perimembranous defect with extension into the subpulmonary region.
3. The RVOT obstruction is most frequently in the form of infundibular stenosis (45%). The obstruction is rarely at the pulmonary valve level (10%). A combination of the two may also occur (30%). The pulmonary valve is atretic in the most severe form of the anomaly (15%).
4. The pulmonary annulus and main PA are variably hypoplastic in most patients. The PA branches are usually small, although marked hypoplasia is uncommon.

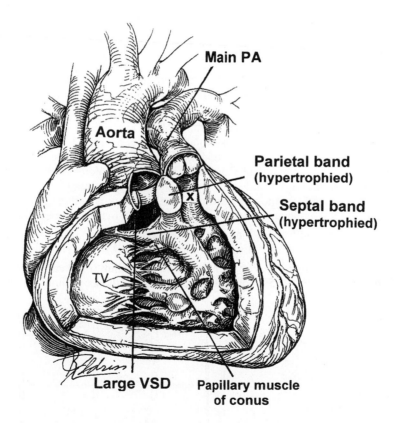

Figure 14–17. *Pathologic anatomy of tetralogy of Fallot viewed with the right ventricular (RV) free wall removed. A large ventricular septal defect (VSD) is present underneath the aortic valve. Hypertrophied parietal and septal bands produce infundibular stenosis (marked x). A stenotic and hypoplastic main pulmonary artery is shown. The RV muscle is hypertrophied. PA, pulmonary artery; TV, tricuspid valve. (From Hirsch JC, Bove EL: Tetralogy of fallot. In Mavroudis C, Backer CL (eds): Pediatric Cardiac Surgery, 3rd ed. Philadelphia, Mosby, 2003, pp 383–397. Reproduced with permission.)*

Stenosis at the origin of the branch PAs, especially the left PA, is common. Occasionally, systemic collateral arteries feed into the lungs, especially in severe cases of TOF.

5. Right aortic arch is present in 25% of cases.

6. In about 5% of TOF patients, abnormal coronary arteries are present. The most common abnormality is the anterior descending branch arising from the right coronary artery and passing over the right ventricular outflow tract, which prohibits a surgical incision in the region.

7. Complete AV septal defect occurs in approximately 2% of patients with TOF, more commonly among patients with Down syndrome. The VSD has a large outlet component in addition to the inlet portion associated with the AV canal.

CLINICAL MANIFESTATIONS

History

1. A heart murmur is audible at birth.

2. Most patients are symptomatic with cyanosis at birth or shortly thereafter. Dyspnea on exertion, squatting, or hypoxic spells develop later, even in mildly cyanotic infants (see Chapter 11).

3. Occasional infants with *acyanotic* TOF may be asymptomatic or may show signs of CHF from a large left-to-right ventricular shunt.

4. Immediately after birth, severe cyanosis is seen in patients with TOF and pulmonary atresia.

Physical Examination (Fig. 14–18)

1. Varying degrees of cyanosis, tachypnea, and clubbing (in older infants and children) are present.

2. An RV tap along the left sternal border and a systolic thrill at the upper and mid-left sternal borders are commonly present (50%).

3. An ejection click that originates in the aorta may be audible. The S2 is usually single because the pulmonary component is too soft to be heard. A long, loud (grade 3 to 5/6) ejection-type systolic murmur is heard at the middle and upper left sternal borders. This murmur originates from the PS but may be easily confused with the holosystolic regurgitant murmur of a VSD. The more severe the obstruction of the RVOT, the shorter and softer the systolic murmur. In a deeply cyanotic neonate with TOF with pulmonary atresia, heart murmur is either absent or very soft, although a continuous murmur representing PDA may be occasionally audible.

4. In the acyanotic form, a long systolic murmur, resulting from VSD and infundibular stenosis, is audible along the entire left sternal border, and cyanosis is absent. Thus, auscultatory findings resemble those of a small-shunt VSD (but, unlike VSD, the ECG shows RVH or BVH).

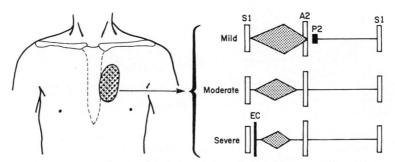

Figure 14–18. *Cardiac findings in cyanotic tetralogy of Fallot (TOF). A long ejection systolic murmur at the upper and mid-left sternal border and a loud, single S2 are characteristic auscultatory findings of TOF. EC, ejection click.*

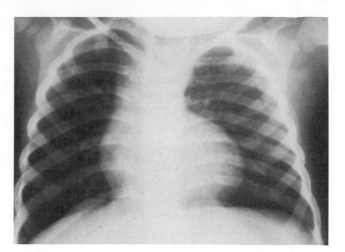

Figure 14–19. Posteroanterior view of chest roentgenogram in tetralogy of Fallot. The heart size is normal, and pulmonary vascular markings are decreased. A hypoplastic main pulmonary artery segment contributes to the formation of the "boot-shaped" heart.

Electrocardiography

1. Right axis deviation (RAD) (+120 to +150 degrees) is present in cyanotic TOF. In the acyanotic form, the QRS axis is normal.
2. RVH is usually present, but the strain pattern is unusual (because RV pressure is not suprasystemic). BVH may be seen in the acyanotic form. RAH is occasionally present.

X-ray Studies

Cyanotic Tetralogy of Fallot

1. The heart size is normal or smaller than normal, and pulmonary vascular markings are decreased. "Black" lung fields are seen in TOF with pulmonary atresia.
2. A concave main PA segment with an upturned apex (i.e., "boot-shaped" heart or coeur en sabot) is characteristic (Fig. 14–19).
3. Right atrial enlargement (25%) and right aortic arch (25%) may be present.

Acyanotic Tetralogy of Fallot. X-ray findings of acyanotic TOF are indistinguishable from those of a small to moderate VSD (but patients with TOF have RVH rather than LVH on the ECG).

Echocardiography. Two-dimensional echo and Doppler studies can make the diagnosis and quantitate the severity of TOF.

1. A large, perimembranous infundibular VSD and overriding of the aorta are readily imaged in the parasternal long-axis view (Fig. 14–20).

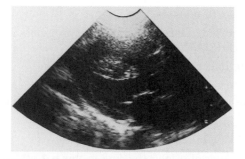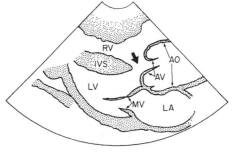

Figure 14–20. Parasternal long-axis view in a patient with tetralogy of Fallot. Note a large subaortic ventricular septal defect (arrow) and a relatively large aorta (AO) overriding the interventricular septum (IVS). AV, aortic valve; LA, left atrium; LV, left ventricle; MV, mitral valve; RV, right ventricle.

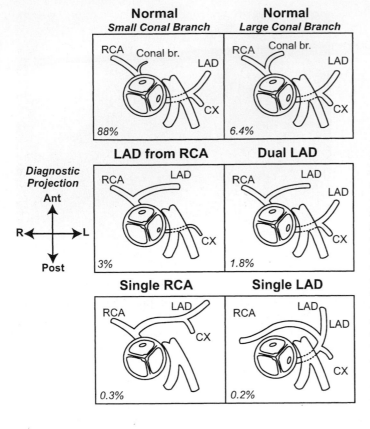

Figure 14–21. Patterns of coronary artery anatomy in tetralogy of Fallot (TOF) as imaged from the parasternal short-axis view. The percentage of each pattern seen in 598 patients with TOF is indicated in the lower left corner of each box. Ant, anterior; CX, left circumflex branch; L, left; LAD, left anterior descending coronary artery; R, right; RCA, right coronary artery; Post, posterior. (From Need LR, Powell AJ, del Nide P, Geva T: Coronary echocardiography in tetralogy of Fallot: Diagnostic accuracy, resource utilization and surgical implications over 13 years. J Am Coll Cardiol 36:1371–1377, 2000.)

2. Anatomy of the right ventricular outflow tract, the pulmonary valve, the pulmonary annulus, and the main PA and its branches are imaged in the parasternal short-axis view.

3. Doppler studies estimate the pressure gradient across the obstruction.

4. Anomalous coronary artery distribution can be imaged accurately by echo studies (Fig. 14–21). Thus, preoperative cardiac catheterization solely for the diagnosis of coronary artery anatomy is not necessary.

5. Associated anomalies such as ASD and persistence of the left superior vena cava can be imaged.

NATURAL HISTORY

1. Infants with acyanotic TOF gradually become cyanotic. Patients who are already cyanotic become more cyanotic as a result of the worsening condition of the infundibular stenosis and polycythemia.

2. Polycythemia develops secondary to cyanosis.*

3. Physicians need to watch for the development of relative iron-deficiency state (i.e., hypochromia) (see Chapter 11).*

4. Hypoxic spells may develop in infants (see Chapter 11).

5. Growth retardation may be present if cyanosis is severe.*

6. Brain abscess and cerebrovascular accident rarely occur (see Chapter 11).*

7. SBE is occasionally a complication.*

8. Some patients, particularly those with severe TOF, develop AR.

9. Coagulopathy is a late complication of a long-standing cyanosis.*

---

* This occurs in all types of cyanotic congenital heart defects.

HYPOXIC SPELL

Hypoxic spell (also called cyanotic spell, hypercyanotic spell, "tet" spell) of TOF requires immediate recognition and appropriate treatment because it can lead to serious complications of the CNS.

Hypoxic spells are characterized by a paroxysm of hyperpnea (i.e., *rapid* and *deep* respiration), irritability and prolonged crying, increasing cyanosis, and decreasing intensity of the heart murmur. Hypoxic spells occur in infants, with a peak incidence between 2 and 4 months of age. These spells usually occur in the morning after crying, feeding, or defecation. A severe spell may lead to limpness, convulsion, cerebrovascular accident, or even death. There appears to be no relationship between the degree of cyanosis at rest and the likelihood of having hypoxic spells (see Chapter 11).

Treatment of the hypoxic spell strives to break the vicious circle of the spell (see Fig. 11–11). Physicians may use one or more of the following to treat the spell.

1. The infant should be picked up and held in a knee-chest position.

2. Morphine sulfate, 0.2 mg/kg administered subcutaneously or intramuscularly, suppresses the respiratory center and abolishes hyperpnea (and thus breaks the vicious circle).

3. Oxygen is usually administered, but it has little demonstrable effect on arterial oxygen saturation.

4. Acidosis should be treated with sodium bicarbonate ($NaHCO_3$), 1 mEq/kg administered intravenously. The same dose can be repeated in 10 to 15 minutes. $NaHCO_3$ reduces the respiratory center–stimulating effect of acidosis.

With the preceding treatment, the infant usually becomes less cyanotic, and the heart murmur becomes louder, which indicates an increased amount of blood flowing through the stenotic RVOT. If the hypoxic spells do not fully respond to these measures, the following medications can be tried:

1. Vasoconstrictors such as phenylephrine (Neo-Synephrine), 0.02 mg/kg administered intravenously, may be effective (by raising systemic arterial pressure).

2. Ketamine, 1 to 3 mg/kg (average of 2 mg/kg) administered intravenously over 60 seconds, works well. It increases the systemic vascular resistance and sedates the infant.

3. Propranolol, 0.01 to 0.25 mg/kg (average 0.05 mg/kg) administered by slow intravenous push, reduces the heart rate and may reverse the spell.

MANAGEMENT

Medical

1. Physicians should recognize and treat hypoxic spells (see the preceding section and Chapter 11). It is important to educate parents to recognize the spell and know what to do.

2. Oral propranolol therapy, 0.5 to 1.5 mg/kg every 6 hours, is occasionally used to prevent hypoxic spells while waiting for an optimal time for corrective surgery in countries where open-heart surgical procedures are not well established for small infants.

3. Balloon dilatation of the right ventricular outflow tract and pulmonary valve, although not widely practiced, has been attempted to delay repair for several months.

4. Maintenance of good dental hygiene and practice of antibiotic prophylaxis against SBE are important (see Chapter 19).

5. A relative iron deficiency state should be detected and treated. Iron-deficient children are more susceptible to cerebrovascular complications. Normal hemoglobin or hematocrit values or decreased red blood cell indices indicate an iron deficiency state in cyanotic patients.

Surgical

Palliative Shunt Procedures

Indications. Shunt procedures are performed to increase PBF (Fig. 14–22). Indications for shunt procedures vary from institution to institution. Many institutions, however, prefer primary repair without a shunt operation regardless of the patient's age. However, when the following situations are present, a shunt operation may usually be chosen rather than primary repair.

1. Neonates with TOF and pulmonary atresia
2. Infants with hypoplastic pulmonary annulus, which requires a transannular patch for complete repair
3. Children with hypoplastic PAs
4. Unfavorable coronary artery anatomy
5. Infants younger than 3 to 4 months old who have medically unmanageable hypoxic spells
6. Infants weighing less than 2.5 kg

Procedures, Complications, and Mortality. Although several other procedures were performed in the past (see Fig. 14–22), a modified Blalock-Taussig (Gore-Tex interposition) shunt is the only popular procedure performed at this time. Occasionally, a classic Blalock-Taussig shunt is performed.

1. Classic Blalock-Taussig shunt, anastomosed between the subclavian artery and the ipsilateral PA, is usually performed for infants older than 3 months (see Fig. 14–22) because the shunt is often thrombosed in younger infants with smaller arteries. A right-sided shunt is performed in patients with left aortic arch; a left-sided shunt is performed for right aortic arch.

2. Modified Blalock-Taussig (BT) shunt. A Gore-Tex interposition shunt is placed between the subclavian artery and the ipsilateral PA. This is the most popular procedure for any age, especially for small infants younger than 3 months of age (see Fig. 14–22). A left-sided shunt is preferred for patients with a left aortic arch, whereas a right-sided shunt is preferred for patients with a right aortic arch. The surgical mortality rate is 1% or less.

3. The Waterston shunt, anastomosed between the ascending aorta and the right PA, is no longer performed because of a high incidence of surgical complications (see Fig. 14–22). Complications resulting from this procedure included too large a shunt leading to CHF or pulmonary hypertension, of both, and narrowing and kinking of the right PA at the site of the anastomosis. This created difficult problems in closing the shunt and reconstructing the right PA at the time of corrective surgery.

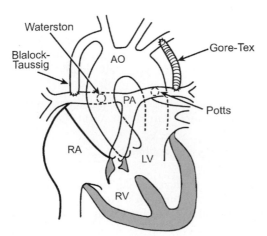

Figure 14–22. Palliative procedures that can be performed in patients with cyanotic cardiac defect with decreased pulmonary blood flow. The Gore-Tex interposition shunt (or modified Blalock-Taussig shunt) is the most popular systemic–to–pulmonary artery shunt procedure. AO, aorta; LV, left ventricle; PA, pulmonary artery; RA, right atrium; RV, right ventricle.

4. The Potts operation, anastomosed between the descending aorta and the left PA, is no longer performed either (see Fig. 14–22). It may result in heart failure or pulmonary hypertension, as in the Waterston operation. A separate incision (i.e., left thoracotomy) is required to close the shunt during corrective surgery, which is performed through a midsternal incision.

Complete Repair Surgery. Timing of this operation varies greatly from institution to institution, but early surgery is generally preferred.

Indications and Timing

1. Oxygen saturation less than 75% to 80% is an indication for surgery by most centers. The occurrence of a hypoxic spell is generally considered an indication for operation.

2. Symptomatic infants who have favorable anatomy of the RVOT and PAs may have primary repair at any time after 3 to 4 months of age, with some centers performing it even before 3 months of age. Most centers prefer primary elective repair by 1 to 2 years of age, even if the patients are asymptomatic, acyanotic (i.e., "pink tet"), or minimally cyanotic.

   Advantages cited for early primary repair include diminution of hypertrophy and fibrosis of the RV, normal growth of the PAs and alveolar units, and reduced incidence of postoperative premature ventricular contractions and sudden death. Early repair obviates the need for additional surgical procedures and thereby reduces hospital stay and the cost of operation.

3. Mildly cyanotic infants who have had previous shunt surgery may have total repair 1 to 2 years after the shunt operation.

4. Asymptomatic children with coronary artery anomalies may have the repair after 1 year of age because a conduit placement may be required between the RV and the PA.

Procedure. Total repair of the defect is carried out under cardiopulmonary bypass, circulatory arrest, and hypothermia. The procedure includes patch closure of the VSD, preferably through a transatrial and transpulmonary artery approach (rather than right ventriculotomy, which is shown in Fig. 14–23); widening of the RVOT by division and/or resection of the infundibular tissue; and pulmonary valvotomy, avoiding placement of a fabric patch whenever possible (see Fig. 14–23). Widening of the RVOT without placement of patch is more likely to be accomplished if the repair is done in early infancy. However, if the pulmonary annulus and main PA are hypoplastic, transannular patch placement is unavoidable. Some centers advocate placement of a monocusp valve at the time of initial repair, and others advocate pulmonary valve replacement at a later time if indicated.

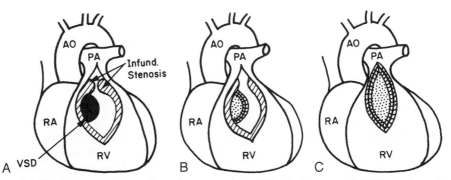

Figure 14–23. *Total correction of tetralogy of Fallot (TOF). **A,** Anatomy of TOF showing a large ventricular septal defect (VSD) and infundibular stenosis seen through a right ventriculotomy. Note that the size of the ventriculotomy has been expanded to show the VSD. **B,** Patch closure of the VSD and resection of the infundibular stenosis. **C,** Placement of a fabric patch on the outflow tract of the right ventricle (RV). AO, aorta; PA, pulmonary artery; RA, right atrium.*

The surgical approach for TOF is summarized in Figure 14–24.

Mortality. For patients with uncomplicated TOF, the mortality rate is 2% to 3% during the first 2 years. Patients at risk are those younger than 3 months and older than 4 years as well as those with severe hypoplasia of the pulmonary annulus and trunk. Other risk factors may include multiple VSDs, large aortopulmonary collateral arteries, and Down syndrome.

Complications

1. Bleeding problems may occur during the postoperative period, especially in older polycythemic patients.

2. Pulmonary valve regurgitation may occur, but mild regurgitation is well tolerated.

3. CHF, although usually transient, may require anticongestive measures.

4. Right bundle branch block (RBBB) on the ECG caused by right ventriculotomy, which occurs in over 90% of patients, is well tolerated.

5. Complete heart block (i.e., <1%) and ventricular arrhythmia are both rare.

Anomalous Coronary Artery. Anomalous anterior descending coronary artery arising from the right coronary artery is considered a contraindication to a primary repair because it may require placement of a conduit between the RV and PA, which is usually performed after 1 year of age. However, it is often possible to enlarge the outflow tract through a transatrial approach and by placing a short outflow patch either above or below the anomalous coronary artery. Alternatively, when a small conduit is necessary between the RV and the PA, the native outflow tract should be made as large as possible through an atrial approach, so that a "double outlet" (the native outlet and the conduit) results from the RV.

Postoperative Follow-up

1. Long-term follow-up with office examinations every 6 to 12 months is recommended, especially for patients with residual VSD shunt, residual obstruction of the RVOT, residual PA obstruction, arrhythmias, or conduction disturbances.

2. Significant pulmonary valve regurgitation may require surgical insertion of a homograft pulmonary valve at a later time. It may be due to stenosis of the MPA or branch PA stenosis (natural or secondary to shunt operations). In such cases, relief of PA stenosis by balloon or stent procedure, or both, may improve pulmonary

Tetralogy of Fallot

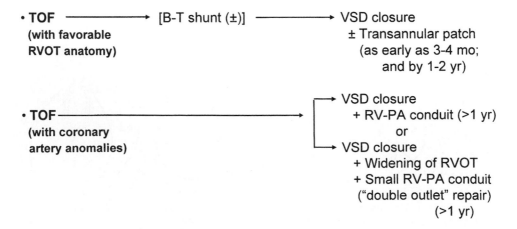

Figure 14–24. Surgical approaches for tetralogy of Fallot. B-T, Blalock-Taussig; RVOT, right ventricular outflow tract; RV-PA, right ventricle–to–pulmonary artery; TOF, tetralogy of Fallot; VSD, ventricular septal defect.

regurgitation (PR). Surgery is indicated for PR when the child is symptomatic or when it is associated with significant TR, poor RV function, or progressive RV dilatation. Even asymptomatic children with significant PR may have a decreased exercise test.

3. Some patients, particularly those who had a Rastelli operation using a valved conduit, develop valvular stenosis or regurgitation. Valvular stenosis may improve after balloon dilatation but PR may worsen. A nonsurgical percutaneous pulmonary valve implantation technique has been developed by Bonhoeffer and colleagues, and the technique has been used successfully in Europe (see further discussion under TOF with pulmonary atresia in this chapter).

4. Some children develop late arrhythmias, particularly ventricular tachycardia, which may result in sudden death. Arrhythmias are primarily related to persistent RVH as a result of unsatisfactory repair. Complaints of dizziness, syncope, or palpitation may suggest arrhythmias. A 24-hour Holter monitor, event recorder, or exercise test may be needed.

5. Pacemaker therapy is indicated for surgically induced complete heart block or sinus node dysfunction. Pacemaker follow-up care is required for these patients.

6. Varying levels of activity limitation may be necessary.

7. For patients who have had TOF repair, SBE prophylaxis should be observed throughout life.

Tetralogy of Fallot with Pulmonary Atresia (Pulmonary Atresia and Ventricular Septal Defect)

PREVALENCE

Pulmonary atresia occurs in about 15% to 20% of patients with TOF.

PATHOLOGY

1. The intracardiac pathology resembles that of TOF in all respects except for the presence of pulmonary atresia, the extreme form of right ventricular outflow tract obstruction. The atresia may be at the infundibular or valvular level.

2. The PBF is most commonly mediated through a PDA (70%) and less commonly through multiple systemic collaterals (30%), which are referred to as multiple aortopulmonary collateral arteries (MAPCAs). Both PDA and collateral arteries may coexist as the source of PBF. The subgroup, in which MAPCAs supply PBF and the central pulmonary arteries are nonconfluent, is designated as pulmonary atresia and ventricular septal defect (PA-VSD).

3. PA anomalies are common in the form of hypoplasia, nonconfluence, and abnormal distribution.
   a. The central and branch PAs are hypoplastic in most patients, but this occurs more frequently in patients with MAPCAs than in those with PDA (see later for further discussion of hypoplasia of the pulmonary arteries*).

---

* The McGoon ratio and the Nakata index are used to quantitate the degree of PA hypoplasia. Small values of these measurements may adversely affect the outcome of surgeries in patients with small pulmonary arteries.
1. The McGoon ratio is the ratio of the sum of the diameter of the immediately prebranching portion of the RPA plus LPA divided by the diameter of the descending aorta just above the diaphragm. Normal values of the McGoon ratio are 2.0 to 2.5. Most survivors of TOF with pulmonary atresia have a McGoon ratio >1. Good Fontan candidates should have a ratio of >1.8.
2. The Nakata index is the cross-sectional area of the RPA and LPA (in mm^2) divided by the body surface area (BSA). The average diameters of both RPA and LPA are measured at the points immediately proximal to the origin of the first lobar branches at maximal and minimal during one cardiac cycle in the anteroposterior view of the pulmonary arteriogram. The cross-sectional area is calculated by using the formula $\pi \times 2/1$ diameter $\times$ magnification coefficient and expressed per body surface area. Normal Nakata index is 330 ± 30 mm^2/BSA. Patients with TOF with PS should have an index >100 for survival. A good Fontan candidate should have an index >250 and a good Rastelli candidate should have an index >200. (Those with index <200 should have a shunt operation rather than the Rastelli.)

   b. The central PAs are confluent in 85% of patients; they are nonconfluent in 15%. The central PAs are usually confluent in patients with PDA (70%). In patients with MAPCAs, the central PA is frequently nonconfluent, with the right upper lobe frequently supplied by a collateral from the subclavian artery and the left lower lobe by a collateral from the descending aorta.

   c. Incomplete arborization (distribution) of one or both PAs is found in 50% of patients with confluent PAs and in 80% of patients with nonconfluent PAs.

4. Collateral arteries arise most commonly from the descending aorta (occurring in two thirds of patients), less commonly from the subclavian arteries, and rarely from the abdominal aorta or its branches.

5. The ductus is small and long and arises from the transverse aortic arch and courses downward ("vertical" ductus) (Fig. 14–25).

CLINICAL MANIFESTATIONS

1. These patients are cyanotic at birth. The degree of cyanosis depends on whether the ductus is patent and how extensive the systemic collateral arteries are.

2. Usually a heart murmur cannot be heard. However, a faint, continuous murmur may be audible from the PDA or collaterals. The S2 is loud and single. A systolic click is occasionally present.

3. The ECG shows RAD and RVH.

4. Chest x-ray films show a normal heart size. The heart often appears as a boot-shaped silhouette (see Fig. 14–19), and the pulmonary vascularity is usually markedly decreased (i.e., black lung field). Rarely, children with MAPCAs and excessive PBF develop CHF.

5. Echo studies show all the anatomic findings of TOF plus absence of a direct connection between the RV and the PA. The small branch PAs and vertical ductus (see Fig. 14–25) are well imaged from a high parasternal or suprasternal transducer position. Sometimes differentiation between severe stenosis and atresia of the pulmonary valve is difficult on echo studies. Some of the multiple collateral arteries are also imaged (but angiograms are needed for a complete delineation of the collaterals).

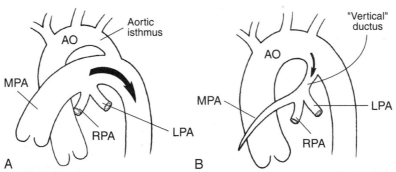

Figure 14–25. Anatomy of the ductus arteriosus in pulmonary atresia. The size and direction of the ductus arteriosus are different between a normal fetus and a fetus with pulmonary atresia. **A,** In a normal fetus, the ductus is large and joins the aorta (AO) at an obtuse angle. The aortic isthmus (the portion of the aorta between the left subclavian artery and the ductus) is narrower than the descending aorta. **B,** In pulmonary atresia, the ductus is small because flow to the descending aorta does not go through the ductus. Furthermore, because flow is from the aorta to the pulmonary artery, the connection of the ductus with the aorta has an acute inferior angle (sometimes called vertical ductus). The aortic isthmus has the same diameter as the descending aorta. This type of ductus arteriosus is also found in some patients with tricuspid atresia. LPA, left pulmonary artery; MPA, main pulmonary artery; RPA, right pulmonary artery.

NATURAL HISTORY

1. Without immediate attention to the establishment of PBF during the newborn period, most neonates who have this condition die during the first 2 years of life; however, infants with extensive collaterals may survive for a long time, perhaps for more than 15 years.

2. Occasionally, patients with excessive collateral circulation develop hemoptysis during late childhood.

MANAGEMENT

Medical

1. PGE$_1$ infusion should be started as soon as the diagnosis is made or suspected to keep the ductus open for cardiac catheterization and to prepare for surgery. The starting dose of alprostadil (Prostin VR Pediatric) solution is 0.05 to 0.1 µg/kg per minute. When the desired effect is obtained, the dosage should be gradually reduced to 0.01 µg/kg per minute.

2. Emergency cardiac catheterization is usually performed to delineate the anatomy of the PAs and systemic arterial collaterals.

Surgical. A connection must be established between the RV and true PA as early in life as possible. This may make tiny central PAs enlarge rapidly during the first year of life with improved arborization (distribution) of the pulmonary arteries with concurrent development of alveolar units. To achieve this goal, some centers initially use a central shunt procedure and others proceed with an RV-PA connection.

1. Central shunt operation. Some centers use a central shunt directly connecting the ascending aorta and the hypoplastic main PA to achieve growth of the peripheral PAs (Mee procedure) (Fig. 14–26). A classic or modified Blalock-Taussig shunt is avoided because it is difficult to perform on tiny PAs and may cause stenosis or distortion. This is followed by unifocalization (see later for explanation), RV-PA connection, and closure of VSD. Other centers skip the shunt procedure and proceed with the connection of the RV and the main PA (see later).

2. RV-to-PA Connection
   a. *Single-stage repair.* Complete, primary surgical repair in patients with TOF and pulmonary atresia is possible only when the true PAs provide most or all PBF

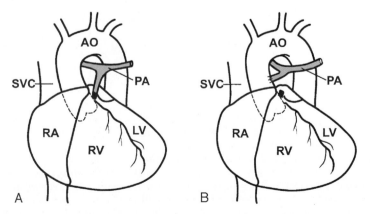

Figure 14–26. *Central end-to-side shunt (Mee procedure). A, Diagram of tetralogy of Fallot with pulmonary atresia. B, The hypoplastic pulmonary artery (PA) is anastomosed to the ascending aorta (AO) as posteriorly as possible. LV, left ventricle; RA, right atrium; RV, right ventricle; SVC, superior vena cava. (From Watterson KG, Wilkinson JL, Karly TR, Mee RBB: Very small pulmonary arteries: Central end-to-side shunt. Ann Thorac Surg 52:1131–1137, 1991.)*

(with O_2 saturation of >75%) and the central PA connects without obstruction to sufficient regions of the lungs (i.e., at least equal to one whole lung). If additional major collaterals are identified, one tests the level of arterial O_2 saturation after occlusion of the collateral in the catheterization laboratory. If the O_2 saturation remains greater than 70% to 75%, coil occlusion of the collaterals is carried out.

Primary repair of this condition consists of closing the VSD, establishing continuity between the RV and the unifocalized PA (see later for unifocalization procedure) using either an aortic or pulmonary homograft (9 to 10 mm internal diameter), and interrupting collateral circulation. The mortality rate varies between 5% and 20%. Good candidates for the repair are those with the Nakata index greater than 200. If the index is less than 200, a shunt procedure is preferable.

b. *Multiple-stage repair.* When the requirements for single-stage repair are not met, three sequential steps are used to repair this condition. These steps are summarized in Figures 14–27 and 14–28.

1). *Stage 1.* RV–to–hypoplastic PA conduit, using a relatively small homograft conduit (6 to 8 mm internal diameter) (see Fig. 14–27).

Interventional catheterization is carried out 3 to 6 months later to identify and coil occlude remaining aortic collaterals, to define the PA distribution, and to identify whether certain bronchopulmonary segments are receiving a duplicate blood supply.

2). *Stage 2.* A unifocalization procedure is carried out. Unifocalization is a surgical procedure in which aortopulmonary collaterals are divided from their

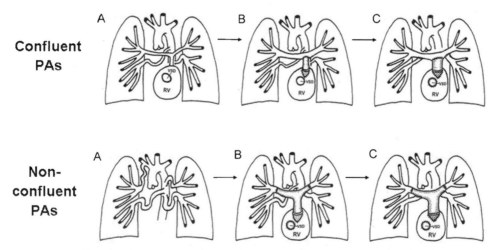

Figure 14–27. Diagram of multiple-stage repair. Upper row: *A, Confluent pulmonary arteries as seen in patients with tetralogy of Fallot (TOF) with pulmonary atresia with a hypoplastic but confluent central pulmonary artery (PA) and multiple collaterals are diagrammatically shown. B, A small right ventricle (RV)-to-PA connection is made with pulmonary homograft (shown in shade), with collaterals left alone. C, The PA has grown to a larger size. Collateral arteries are now anastomosed to the originally hypoplastic PA branches. Ventricular septal defect (VSD) may be closed at a later time, usually 1 to 3 years of age. The pulmonary homograft is usually replaced with a larger graft at this time.* Bottom row: *A, Nonconfluent pulmonary arteries as seen in patients with pulmonary atresia and VSD with absent central PA and multiple collateral arteries (MAPCAs) are shown. B, A small pulmonary homograft (6 to 8 mm internal diameter, shown in shade) is used to establish RV-to-PA connection (performed at 3 to 6 months). Some collaterals are not unifocalized at this time. C, The homograft conduit has been replaced with a larger one. Remaining collateral arteries are anastomosed to the pulmonary homograft to complete unifocalization procedure. VSD is closed with or without fenestration, usually at 1 to 3 years of age.*

Tetralogy of Fallot with Pulmonary Atresia
(or Pulmonary Atresia and VSD)

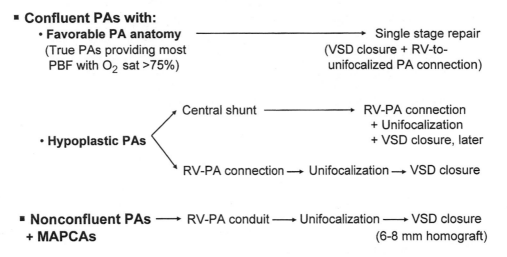

■ **Confluent PAs with:**

• **Favorable PA anatomy** ──────────────→ Single stage repair
(True PAs providing most   (VSD closure + RV-to-
PBF with O$_2$ sat >75%)   unifocalized PA connection)

Central shunt ──────→ RV-PA connection
                       + Unifocalization
• **Hypoplastic PAs**   + VSD closure, later

RV-PA connection ──→ Unifocalization ──→ VSD closure

■ **Nonconfluent PAs** ──→ RV-PA conduit ──→ Unifocalization ──→ VSD closure
+ MAPCAs   (6-8 mm homograft)

Figure 14–28. Surgical approaches for tetralogy of Fallot with pulmonary atresia (or pulmonary atresia and VSD). MAPCAs, multiple aortopulmonary collateral arteries; PA, pulmonary artery; PBF, pulmonary blood flow; RV-PA, right ventricle–to–pulmonary artery; VSD, ventricular septal defect.

aortic origin and are anastomosed to the true pulmonary arteries or main PA conduit (see Fig. 14–27).

Postunifocalization catheterization is carried out 3 to 6 months later to identify multiple peripheral stenosis in both the true and unifocalized collaterals and do balloon dilatation with or without stenting and to assess the need for further unifocalization procedures.

3). *Stage 3.* Closure of VSD with or without fenestration, usually at 1 to 3 years of age (see Fig. 14–27). The homograft conduit may need to be replaced at the same time. If the RV pressure is 10% to 20% greater than the systemic pressure, a central fenestration of 3 to 4 mm is created. Multiple ballooning and stenting procedures are often necessary to reduce RV pressure to less than 50% systemic if possible.

Surgical steps used in patients with TOF with pulmonary atresia are summarized in Figure 14–28.

Postoperative Follow-up

1. Frequent follow-up is needed to assess the palliative surgery and decide on appropriate times for further surgeries.

2. Valved conduits or homografts may develop valve degeneration requiring conduit replacement at a later time. Valvular stenosis can be dilated with a balloon to reduce the pressure gradient but this often results in a significant valve regurgitation, eventually leading to RV dysfunction. Many of these patients require surgical replacement of the conduit.

3. Bonhoeffer and his colleagues (2000) have successfully replaced the dysfunctional valve by percutaneous replacement of a pulmonary valve, and more than 50 cases of children and adults have had this procedure done successfully in Europe (Khambadkone et al, 2005). A bovine jugular venous valve was mounted into the platinum stent and loaded in the delivery system. The assembly was delivered (implanted) in the RV outflow tract according to standard stent-placing technique

using an 18 French long sheath through a right femoral approach. The patients were mostly adults but included some children as young as 9 years with weight as low as 25 kg. Although most of the patients had TOF variant, other patients had TGA plus VSD plus PS, Ross operation, or truncus arteriosus surgeries.

4. Antibiotic prophylaxis for SBE should be observed for an indefinite period.

5. A certain level of activity restriction is needed because many of these children have exercise intolerance. Most survivors after complete repair are in New York Heart Association class I or II symptomatically.

Tetralogy of Fallot with Absent Pulmonary Valve

PREVALENCE

TOF with absent pulmonary valve occurs in approximately 2% of patients with TOF.

PATHOLOGY AND PATHOPHYSIOLOGY

1. The pulmonary valve leaflets are completely absent or have an uneven rim of rudimentary valve tissue present. The annulus of the valve is stenotic and displaced distally. A massive aneurysmal dilatation of the PAs is present. This anomaly is usually associated with a large VSD, similar to that seen in TOF. It rarely occurs with an intact ventricular septum.

2. The massive PA aneurysm (Fig. 14–29) results from severe PR and an associated increase in RV stroke volume. The aneurysmal PAs compress anteriorly the lower end of the developing trachea and bronchi throughout fetal life, producing hypoplasia of the compressed airways. This produces signs of airway obstruction and respiratory distress during infancy. Pulmonary complications (e.g., atelectasis, pneumonia) are the usual causes of death, rather than the intracardiac defect.

3. The ductus arteriosus is frequently (but not invariably) absent in patients with more severe aneurysmal dilatation of the PAs.

4. Because the stenosis at the pulmonary valve ring is only moderate, an initial bidirectional shunt becomes predominantly a left-to-right shunt after the newborn period.

5. In some infants, tufts of PAs entwine and compress the intrapulmonary bronchi, resulting in reduced numbers of alveolar units. This may preclude successful surgical correction.

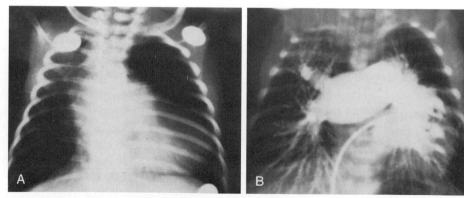

Figure 14–29. A, *Posteroanterior view of plain chest film showing hyperinflated areas in the left upper lobe and right lower portion of the chest in a 1-month-old infant who had tetralogy of Fallot with absence of the pulmonary valve.* **B,** *Anteroposterior view of pulmonary arteriogram showing massive aneurysmal dilatation of both the right and left pulmonary arteries.*

CLINICAL MANIFESTATIONS

1. Mild cyanosis may be present as a result of a bidirectional shunt during the newborn period when the PVR is relatively high. Cyanosis disappears, and signs of CHF may develop, after the newborn period. Respiratory symptoms vary greatly, ranging from neonates with severe respiratory compromise to those with wheezing or frequent respiratory infection and to those with no respiratory symptoms at all.

2. A to-and-fro murmur (with a "sawing-wood" sound) at the upper and mid-left sternal borders is a characteristic auscultatory finding of the condition. This murmur occurs because of mild PS and free PR. The S2 is loud and single. The RV hyperactivity is palpable.

3. The ECG shows RAD and RVH.

4. Chest x-ray images reveal a noticeably dilated main PA and hilar PAs. The heart size is either normal or mildly enlarged, and pulmonary vascular markings may be slightly increased. The lung fields may show hyperinflated areas, representing partial airway obstruction (see Fig. 14–29A).

5. Echo reveals a large, subaortic VSD with overriding of the aorta, distally displaced pulmonary annulus (with thick ridges instead of fully developed pulmonary valve leaflets), and gigantic aneurysm of the PA and its branches. The RV is markedly dilated, often with paradoxical motion of the ventricular septum. Doppler studies reveal evidence of stenosis at the annulus and PR. Cardiac catheterization and angiocardiography (see Fig. 14–29B) are usually unnecessary for accurate anatomic assessment of the PAs.

6. A computed tomography or magnetic resonance imaging (MRI) scan can define the relationship between sites of airway obstruction and dilatation of the central PA. Bronchoscopy provides the degree of airway compression.

NATURAL HISTORY

1. More than 75% of infants with severe pulmonary complications (e.g., atelectasis, pneumonia) die during infancy if treated only medically. The surgical mortality of infants with pulmonary complications is 20% to 40%.

2. Infants who survive infancy without serious pulmonary problems do well for 5 to 20 years and have fewer respiratory symptoms during childhood. They become symptomatic later and die from intractable right-sided heart failure.

MANAGEMENT

Medical. In the past, medical management was preferred because of poor surgical results in newborns; however, the mortality rate of medical management is much higher than that of surgical management. Once the pulmonary symptoms appear, neither surgical nor medical management has good results.

Surgical. Symptomatic neonates should have corrective surgery on an urgent basis. Even an asymptomatic child should have elective surgery in the first 3 to 6 months of life.

Primary Repair. Complete primary repair is the procedure of choice. VSD is closed through right ventriculotomy (across the pulmonary annulus). In symptomatic neonates, a pulmonary homograft to replace the dysplastic pulmonary valve and the dilated main and branch PAs is indicated. Alternatively, a valved conduit may be used to restore competence of the pulmonary valve and the aneurysmal PAs are plicated. Some surgeons advocate aortic transection to achieve good exposure of the PAs for an extensive pulmonary arterioplasty into the hila of both lungs. An early surgical mortality is as high as over 20% with a 1-year survival rate of 75%.

Total Anomalous Pulmonary Venous Return

PREVALENCE

TAPVR accounts for 1% of all congenital heart defects. There is a marked male preponderance for the infracardiac type (male/female ratio of 4:1).

PATHOLOGY AND PATHOPHYSIOLOGY

1. No direct communication exists between the pulmonary veins and the LA. Instead, they drain anomalously into the systemic venous tributaries or into the RA. Depending on the drainage site of the pulmonary veins, the defect may be divided into the following four types (Fig. 14–30):

    a. Supracaordiac: This type accounts for 50% of TAPVR patients. The common pulmonary venous sinus drains into the right SVC through the left vertical vein and the left innominate vein (see Fig. 14–30A).

    b. Cardiac: This type accounts for 20% of TAPVR patients. The common pulmonary venous sinus drains into the coronary sinus (see Fig. 14–30C), or the pulmonary veins enter the RA separately through four openings (only two openings are illustrated in Fig. 14–30B).

    c. Infracardiac: This type accounts for 20% of TAPVR patients. The common pulmonary venous sinus drains to the portal vein, ductus venosus, hepatic vein, or inferior vena cava (IVC). The common pulmonary vein penetrates the diaphragm through the esophageal hiatus (see Fig. 14–30D).

    d. Mixed type: This type, which is a combination of the other types, accounts for 10% of TAPVR patients.

2. Many patients with supracardiac and cardiac types of TAPVR and most patients with the infracardiac type have pulmonary hypertension secondary to obstruction of the pulmonary venous return. Either the length of the venous channels or the resistance caused by the hepatic sinusoids is the cause of obstruction.

3. In patients with pulmonary venous obstruction, pulmonary arterial hypertension develops. These patients develop progressive pulmonary venous congestion, hypoxemia, and systemic hypoperfusion.

4. An interatrial communication, either an ASD or PFO, is necessary for survival. Most patients do not have restricted flow across the atrial septum.

5. The left side of the heart is relatively small.

CLINICAL MANIFESTATIONS

Clinical manifestations differ, depending on whether there is obstruction to the pulmonary venous return.

Without Pulmonary Venous Obstruction

History

1. CHF with growth retardation and frequent pulmonary infection are common in infancy.

2. A history of mild cyanosis from birth is present.

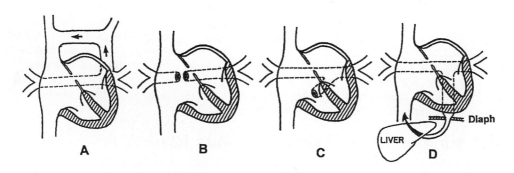

Figure 14–30. Anatomic classification of total anomalous pulmonary venous return. **A,** Supracardiac. **B** and **C,** Cardiac. **D,** Infracardiac. Diaph, diaphragm.

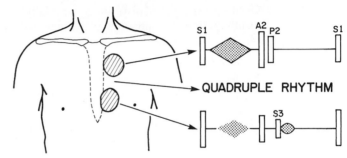

Figure 14–31. Cardiac findings of total anomalous pulmonary venous return without obstruction to pulmonary venous return.

Physical Examination

1. The infant is undernourished and mildly cyanotic. Signs of CHF (e.g., tachypnea, dyspnea, tachycardia, hepatomegaly) are present.
2. Precordial bulge with hyperactive RV impulse is present. Cardiac impulse is maximal at the xyphoid process and the lower left sternal border.
3. Characteristic quadruple or quintuple rhythm is present. The S2 is widely split and fixed, and the P2 may be accentuated. A grade 2 to 3/6 ejection systolic murmur is usually audible at the upper left sternal border. A mid-diastolic rumble is always present at the lower left sternal border (because of increased flow through the tricuspid valve) (Fig. 14–31).

Electrocardiography. RVH of the so-called volume overload type (i.e., rsR′ in V1) and occasional RAH are present.

X-ray Studies

1. Moderate to marked cardiomegaly involving the RA and RV is present with increased pulmonary vascular markings.
2. "Snowman" sign or figure-of-8 configuration may be seen in the supracardiac type, but rarely before 4 months of age (Fig. 14–32).

With Pulmonary Venous Obstruction

History

1. Marked cyanosis and respiratory distress develop in the neonatal period with failure to thrive.

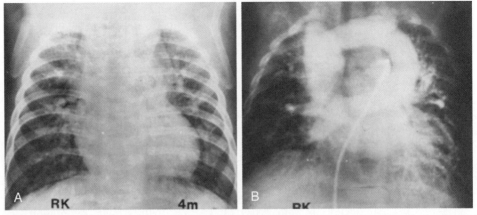

Figure 14–32. Posteroanterior view of plain chest film demonstrating the "snowman" sign (**A**) and angiocardiogram demonstrating anatomic structures that participate in the formation of the snowman sign (**B**). The vertical vein (left superior vena cava), the dilated left innominate vein, and the right superior vena cava are opacified.

2. Cyanosis worsens with feeding, especially in infants with the infracardiac type, resulting from compression of the common pulmonary vein by the food-filled esophagus.

Physical Examination

1. Moderate to marked cyanosis and tachypnea with retraction are present in newborns or undernourished infants.

2. Cardiac findings may be minimal. A loud, single S2 and gallop rhythm are present. Heart murmur is usually absent. If present, however, it is usually a faint ejection-type systolic murmur at the upper left sternal border.

3. Pulmonary crackles and hepatomegaly are usually present.

Electrocardiography. Invariably, RVH in the form of tall R waves in the right precordial leads is present. RAH is occasionally present.

X-ray Studies. The heart size is normal or slightly enlarged. The lung fields reveal findings of pulmonary edema (i.e., diffuse reticular pattern and Kerley's B lines). These findings may be confused with those of pneumonia or hyaline membrane disease.

Echocardiography

Common Features

1. A large RV with a compressed LV (i.e., relative hypoplasia of the LV) is the most striking initial finding. A large RA and a small LA, with deviation of the atrial septum to the left and dilated PAs, are also present.

2. An interatrial communication is usually present with a right-to-left shunt. PFO occurs in 70% of patients, and secundum ASD occurs in 30%.

3. A large, common chamber (i.e., common pulmonary venous sinus) may be imaged posterior to the LA in the parasternal long-axis view.

4. An M-mode echo may show signs of RV volume overload, which includes abnormal (paradoxical or flat) motion of the interventricular septum.

5. Doppler studies reveal an increased flow velocity in the PA, an increased flow velocity or continuous flow at the site of the pulmonary venous drainage, and findings suggestive of pulmonary hypertension.

Features of the Supracardiac Type. The most common site of connection is the left SVC (i.e., left vertical vein), with subsequent drainage to the dilated left innominate vein and right SVC. These abnormal pathways can be imaged in the suprasternal notch short-axis view. Color flow mapping and Doppler ultrasound are helpful in defining the direction of the flow in the left SVC.

Features of the Cardiac Type. The most common site of entry is to the coronary sinus, occurring in 15% of cases. A dilated coronary sinus, best imaged in the parasternal long-axis view and the apical four-chamber view, may be the first clue to this condition.

Features of the Infracardiac Type. A dilated vein descending to the abdominal cavity through the diaphragm is imaged using the subcostal sagittal and transverse scans. All four pulmonary veins that connect to the confluence must be imaged. They are best imaged on the subcostal coronal scan or the suprasternal notch short-axis view.

Possibility of the Mixed Type. Unless it is demonstrated that all four pulmonary veins connect to the confluence, the possibility of the mixed type of TAPVR cannot be eliminated. In the most common mixed type, the left lung, usually the upper lobe, drains to the left SVC, and the remaining pulmonary veins in both lungs drain to the coronary sinus.

NATURAL HISTORY

1. CHF occurs in both types of TAPVR with growth retardation and repeated pneumonias.

2. Without surgical repair, two thirds of the infants without obstruction die before reaching 1 year of age. They usually die from superimposed pneumonia.

3. Patients with the infracardiac type rarely survive for longer than a few weeks without surgery. Most die before 2 months of age.

MANAGEMENT

Medical

1. Intensive anticongestive measures with digitalis and diuretics should be provided for infants without pulmonary venous obstruction.
2. Metabolic acidosis should be corrected, if present.
3. Infants with severe pulmonary edema (resulting from the infracardiac type and from other types with obstruction) should be intubated and receive ventilator support with oxygen and positive end-expiratory pressure, if necessary, before cardiac catheterization and surgery.
4. In some patients with pulmonary hypertension, PGE_1 can increase systemic flow by keeping the ductus open. In the infracardiac type, PGE_1 may be helpful in maintaining the ductus venosus open.
5. If the size of the interatrial communication appears small and immediate surgery is not indicated, balloon atrial septostomy or blade atrial septostomy may be performed to enlarge the communication.

Surgical

Indications and Timing. Corrective surgery is necessary for all patients with this condition. No palliative procedure exists.

1. All infants with pulmonary venous obstruction should be operated on soon after diagnosis, in the newborn period.
2. Infants who do not have pulmonary venous obstruction but do have heart failure that is difficult to control are usually operated on between 4 and 6 months of age.

Procedures. Although procedures vary with the site of the anomalous drainage, all procedures are intended to redirect the pulmonary venous return to the LA (Fig. 14–33). Surgical techniques used vary from surgeon to surgeon; some use the right atrial approach to reach the LA and others reach the posterior wall of the LA directly. Some favor use of deep hypothermic (18°C to 20°C) circulatory arrest.

Supracardiac Type. A large, side-to-side anastomosis is made between the common pulmonary venous sinus and the LA. The vertical vein is ligated. The ASD is closed with a cloth patch (see Fig. 14–33A).

TAPVR to the Right Atrium. The atrial septum is excised and a patch is sewn in such a way that the pulmonary venous return is diverted to the LA (see Fig. 14–33B). The ASD may have to be enlarged.

TAPVR to the Coronary Sinus. An incision is made in the anterior wall of the coronary sinus ("unroofing") to make a communication between the coronary sinus and the LA. A single patch closes the original ASD and the ostium of the coronary sinus.

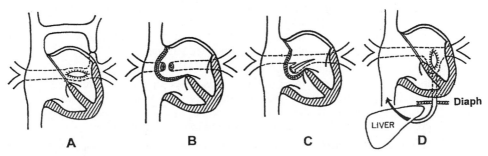

Figure 14–33. *Surgical approaches to various types of total anomalous pulmonary venous return (see text). Diaph, diaphragm.*

This results in the drainage of coronary sinus blood with low oxygen saturation into the LA (see Fig. 14–33C).

Infracardiac Type. A large vertical anastomosis is made between the common pulmonary venous sinus and the LA. The common pulmonary vein, which descends vertically to the abdominal cavity, is ligated above the diaphragm (see Fig. 14–33D).

Mortality. The surgical mortality rate is between 5% and 10% for infants with the unobstructed type. This rate can be as high as 20% for infants with the infracardiac type. Two common causes of death are postoperative paroxysms of pulmonary hypertension and the development of pulmonary vein stenosis.

Complications

1. Paroxysms of pulmonary hypertension, which relate to a small and poorly compliant left heart, with resulting cardiac failure and pulmonary edema, may require prolonged respiratory support postoperatively.
2. Postoperative arrhythmias are usually atrial.
3. Obstruction at the site of anastomosis or pulmonary vein stenosis rarely occurs.

Postoperative Follow-up

1. An office evaluation every 6 to 12 months is recommended for such late complications as pulmonary vein obstruction and atrial arrhythmias.
2. Pulmonary vein obstruction at the anastomosis site or delayed development of pulmonary vein stenosis may occur in about 10% of patients and requires reoperation. These complications are usually evident within 6 to 12 months after the repair. The possibility of pulmonary vein stenosis requires cardiac catheterization and angiocardiography. If present, it is nearly impossible to correct.
3. Some patients develop atrial arrhythmias, including sick sinus syndrome, that require medical treatment or pacemaker therapy.
4. Activity restriction is usually unnecessary unless pulmonary venous obstruction occurs.
5. SBE prophylaxis is usually not needed unless an obstruction is present.

Tricuspid Atresia

PREVALENCE

Tricuspid atresia accounts for 1% to 3% of congenital heart defects.

PATHOLOGY

1. The tricuspid valve is absent, and the RV is hypoplastic, with absence of the inflow portion of the RV. The associated defects such as ASD, VSD, or PDA are necessary for survival.
2. Tricuspid atresia is usually classified according to the presence or absence of PS and TGA (Fig. 14–34). The great arteries are normally related in about 70% of cases and are transposed in 30% of cases. In 3% of cases, the L form of transposition occurs
3. In patients with normally related great arteries, the VSD is usually small, and PS is present with resulting hypoplasia of the pulmonary arteries (and reduced PBF). This is the most common type, occurring in about 50% of all patients with tricuspid atresia. Occasionally, the VSD is large with normal-sized PAs, or the ventricular septum is intact with pulmonary atresia.
4. When TGA is present, the pulmonary valve is normal with increased PBF in two thirds of cases. In one third of cases, it is either stenotic or atretic with decreased PBF. Patients with TGA need a fairly large VSD to maintain normal systemic cardiac output. Less than adequate size or spontaneous reduction of the VSD creates problems with a decreased systemic cardiac output.
5. COA or interrupted aortic arch is a frequently associated anomaly that is more commonly seen in patients with TGA. Occasionally, subaortic stenosis occurs in patients with TGA.

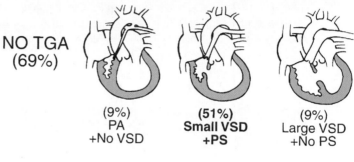

NO TGA
(69%)

(9%)
PA
+No VSD

**(51%)
Small VSD
+PS**

(9%)
Large VSD
+No PS

Figure 14–34. Anatomic classification of tricuspid atresia. In about 70% of cases the great arteries are normally related, and there is a small ventricular septal defect (VSD) with associated hypoplasia of the pulmonary artery (PA). When the great arteries are transposed, the VSD is usually large, and the PAs are large with increased pulmonary blood flow. AS, aortic stenosis; D-TGA, complete TGA; L-TGA, congenitally corrected TGA; PA, pulmonary atresia; PS, pulmonary stenosis; Sub AS, subaortic stenosis; Sub PS, subpulmonary stenosis; TGA, transposition of the great arteries; VSD, ventricular septal defect. (Data from Keith JD, Rowe RD, Vlad P: Heart Disease in Infancy and Childhood, 3rd ed. New York, Macmillan, 1978.)

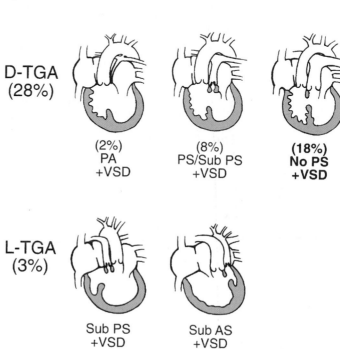

D-TGA
(28%)

(2%)
PA
+VSD

(8%)
PS/Sub PS
+VSD

**(18%)
No PS
+VSD**

L-TGA
(3%)

Sub PS
+VSD

Sub AS
+VSD

CLINICAL MANIFESTATIONS

History

1. Cyanosis is usually severe from birth. Tachypnea and poor feeding usually manifest.

2. History of hypoxic spells may be present in infants with this condition.

Physical Examination (Fig. 14–35)

1. Cyanosis, either with or without clubbing, is always present.

2. A systolic thrill is rarely palpable when associated with PS.

Figure 14–35. Cardiac findings of tricuspid atresia associated with patent ductus arteriosus and ventricular septal defect. "Superior" QRS axis on the ECG and cyanosis are characteristic of the defect.

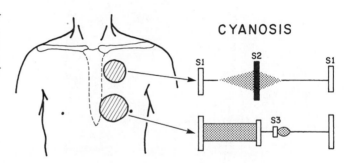

CYANOSIS

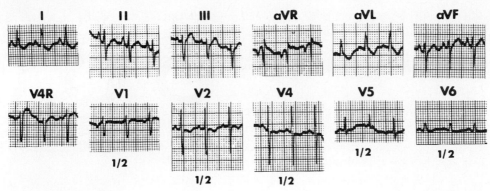

Figure 14–36. *Tracing from a 6-month-old girl with tricuspid atresia showing left anterior hemiblock (−30 degrees), right atrial hypertrophy, and left ventricular hypertrophy.*

3. The S2 is single. A grade 2 to 3/6 holosystolic (or early systolic) murmur of VSD is usually present at the lower left sternal border. A continuous murmur of PDA is occasionally present. An apical diastolic rumble is rarely audible in patients with large PBF.

4. Hepatomegaly may indicate an inadequate interatrial communication or CHF.

Electrocardiography

1. "Superior" QRS axis (between 0 and −90 degrees) is characteristic. It appears in most patients without TGA (Fig. 14–36). The superior QRS axis is present in only 50% of patients with TGA.

2. LVH is usually present; RAH or biatrial hypertrophy (BAH) is common.

X-ray Studies. The heart size is normal or slightly increased, with enlargement of the RA and LV. Pulmonary vascularity decreases in most patients (Fig. 14–37), although it may increase in infants with TGA. Occasionally, the concave PA segment may produce a boot-shaped heart, like the x-ray findings of TOF.

Echocardiography. Two-dimensional echo readily establishes the diagnosis of tricuspid atresia.

1. Absence of the tricuspid orifice, marked hypoplasia of the RV, and a large LV can be imaged in the apical four-chamber view.

2. The bulging of the atrial septum toward the left and the size of the interatrial communication are easily imaged in the subcostal four-chamber view.

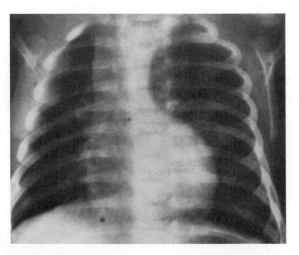

Figure 14–37. *Posteroanterior view of chest roentgenogram in an infant with tricuspid atresia with normally related great arteries. The heart is minimally enlarged. The pulmonary vascular markings are decreased, and the main pulmonary artery segment is somewhat concave.*

3. The size of the VSD, the presence and severity of PS, and the presence of TGA should all be investigated.

4. Patients with TGA should be examined for possible subaortic stenosis and aortic arch anomalies.

NATURAL HISTORY

1. Few infants with tricuspid atresia and normally related great arteries survive beyond 6 months of age without surgical palliation.

2. Occasionally, patients with increased PBF develop CHF and eventually pulmonary vascular obstructive disease.

3. For patients who survive into their second decade of life without a Fontan-type operation, the chronic volume overload of the LV usually produces secondary cardiomyopathy and reduced contractility of that ventricle. (A Fontan procedure should be performed before LV dysfunction develops.)

MANAGEMENT

Initial Medical Management

1. PGE$_1$ should be started in neonates with severe cyanosis to maintain the patency of the ductus before planned cardiac catheterization or cardiac surgery.

2. The Rashkind procedure (balloon atrial septostomy) may be performed as part of the initial catheterization to improve the RA-to-LA shunt, especially when the interatrial communication is considered inadequate by echo studies.

3. Treatment of CHF is rarely needed in infants with TGA and without PS.

4. Infants with normally related great arteries and adequate PBF through a VSD do not need any other procedures; rather, they need to be closely watched for decreasing oxygen saturation resulting from spontaneous reduction of the VSD.

Surgical. Most infants with tricuspid atresia require one or more palliative procedures before a Fontan-type operation, the definitive surgery, can be performed. Staged palliative surgical procedures are aimed at producing ideal candidates for a future Fontan procedure. Ideal candidates for a Fontan-type operation are those who have normal LV function and low pulmonary resistance.

1. Normal LV function results from prevention of excessive volume or pressure loading of the LV by:
   a. Preventing excessive volume load by using a relatively small systemic-to-pulmonary shunt (e.g., 3.5 mm for neonates).
   b. Avoiding ventricular hypertrophy (for example, by relieving outflow obstruction).

2. Low pulmonary resistance may result from:
   a. Providing adequate PBF that promotes the growth of PA branches (with resulting increase in the cross-sectional area of the vascular bed).
   b. Preventing distortion of the central pulmonary arteries. A shunt operation is preferably done on the right PA, which can be incorporated into the Fontan operation.
   c. Protecting the pulmonary vascular bed from overflow or pressure overload (by PA band when PBF is increased).

Palliative surgical procedures described subsequently and the Fontan procedure are not just for tricuspid atresia; they are also performed for other CHDs with functionally single ventricle, such as single ventricle (double-inlet ventricle), some cases of pulmonary atresia with intact ventricular septum, unbalanced AV canal, complicated DORV, HLHS, and heterotaxia (splenic syndromes). Because the Fontan operation is applicable to so many other defects, a staged approach to the Fontan operation is summarized in Box 14–2 for quick reference.

Stage I. The most frequently done first-stage operation is the Blalock-Taussig shunt. Under special circumstances, another procedure (such as the Damus-Kaye-Stansel operation)

BOX 14–2	FONTAN PATHWAY

Stage I. One of the following procedures is done in preparation for a future Fontan operation:

1. Blalock-Taussig shunt, when PBF is small

2. PA banding, when PBF is excessive

3. Damus-Kaye-Stansel plus shunt operation (for TA + TGA + restrictive VSD)

Medical follow-up after stage I. Watch for:

a. Cyanosis (O_2 saturation <75%)—cardiac catheterization or MRI to find out its cause.

b. Poor weight gain (CHF from too much PBF)—tightening of PA band may be necessary.

Stage II (at 3 months or by 6 months).

1. BDG operation or

2. The hemi-Fontan operation

Medical follow-up after stage II. Watch for the following:

a. A gradual decrease in O_2 saturation (<75%) may be caused by:

   1) Opening of venous collaterals

   2) Pulmonary AV fistula (due to the absence of hepatic inhibitory factor)

   Perform cardiac catheterization (to find and occlude collaterals) or
   Proceed with Fontan operation.

b. Transient hypertension—1 to 2 weeks postoperatively—may use ACE inhibitors

c. Cardiac catheterization by 12 months after stage II

The following are risk factors. Presence of two or more is a high-risk situation.

a. Mean PA pressure >18 mm Hg (or PVR >2 U/m^2)

b. LV end-diastolic pressure >12 mm Hg (or EF <60%)

c. AV valve regurgitation

d. Distorted PAs secondary to previous shunt operation

Stage III (Fontan operation)—within 1 to 2 years after stage II operation.

1. "Lateral tunnel" Fontan (with 4 mm fenestration)

2. An extracardiac conduit (with or without fenestration)

may have to be combined with the Blalock-Taussig shunt. On rare occasions, PA banding is indicated for infants with too much PBF.

1. *Blalock-Taussig shunt.* Most patients who have tricuspid atresia with decreased PBF need the Blalock-Taussig shunt soon after birth when the PVR is still high (see Fig. 14–22). This procedure results in the volume load on the LV because the LV supplies blood to both the systemic and pulmonary circulations. Thus, the shunt should be relatively small (e.g., 3.5 mm) and should not be left alone too long (before proceeding to stage II operation).

2. *Damus-Kaye-Stansel and shunt operation.* For infants with tricuspid atresia with TGA and restrictive VSD, the Damus-Kaye-Stansel procedure may be performed, in addition to a systemic-to-PA shunt. In the Damus-Kaye-Stansel operation, the main PA is transected, and the distal PA is sewn over. The proximal PA is connected end to side to the ascending aorta (see Fig. 14–11). A systemic-to-PA shunt is created to supply blood to the lungs. A Fontan-type operation is performed at a later time. This procedure also results in volume overload to the LV, and a stage II operation should be performed as early as possible.

3. *Pulmonary artery banding.* PA banding is rarely necessary for infants with CHF resulting from increased PBF. PA banding protects the pulmonary vasculature from

developing pulmonary hypertension, and it may be performed at any age with a mortality rate of less than 5%.

Follow-up Medical Management. After the stage I operation, the infant should be watched carefully until the time of the stage II palliation with emphasis on the following.

1. Cyanosis (with O_2 saturation <75%) should be investigated by cardiac catheterization or MRI.

2. Poor growth may indicate too large a PBF, and tightening of PA band should be considered.

Stage II. As a stage II operation, either a bidirectional Glenn shunt or the hemi-Fontan operation is performed in preparation for the final Fontan operation.

1. *Bidirectional Glenn operation (BDG).* An end-to-side SVC-to-RPA shunt (also called bidirectional superior cavopulmonary shunt) can be performed by 2.5 to 3 months of age (Fig. 14–38A). By this time, the PVR is sufficiently low to allow venous pressure to be the driving force for the pulmonary circulation. There appears to be no advantage in further delaying the second-stage operation beyond 6 months. For this procedure to be successful, the PVR has to be relatively low because the SVC blood flows passively into the pulmonary arteries. Any previous systemic-to-PA shunt is taken down at the time of the procedure. The azygos vein and, when present, the hemiazygos are divided. The IVC blood still bypasses the lungs. This procedure satisfactorily increases oxygen saturation, which averages 85%, without adding volume work to the LV. The mortality rate for this procedure is between 5% and 10%.

2. *The hemi-Fontan operation.* An incision is made along the most superior part of the right atrial appendage and is extended into the SVC (Fig. 14–39). A connection is made between this opening and the lower margin of the central portion of the PA. An intra-atrial baffle is placed to direct blood to the pulmonary arteries. The Blalock-Taussig shunt is taken down and the native pulmonary valve is oversewn.

Advantages of hemi-Fontan are that (1) it allows supplementation of the central PA area so as to optimize flow to the left lung and (2) it simplifies the subsequent Fontan operation. A major disadvantage may be that it involves extensive surgery in the region of the sinus node and sinus node artery, which may result in late sinus node dysfunction.

Medical follow-up after the stage II operation should focus on the following.

1. A remarkable improvement in O_2 saturation (approximately 85%) results after the procedure. However, a gradual deterioration in O_2 saturation may occur in the months postoperatively, which may be caused by:
   a. Opening of venous collaterals that decompress the upper body
   b. The development of pulmonary arteriovenous (AV) fistula, which may be related to absence of hepatic inhibitory factor (which may be vasoconstrictive prostaglandins)

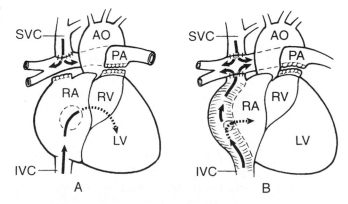

Figure 14–38. A popular modified Fontan operation. **A,** *Bidirectional Glenn operation or superior vena cava (SVC)–to–right pulmonary artery anastomosis.* **B,** *Cavocaval baffle–to–pulmonary artery (PA) connection, with or without fenestration. See text for description of these procedures. AO, aorta; IVC, inferior vena cava; LV, left ventricle; RA, right atrium; RV, right ventricle.*

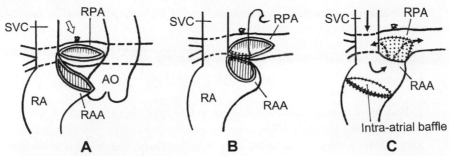

Figure 14–39. *Hemi-Fontan operation.* **A,** *A Blalock-Taussig shunt is taken down (arrow). An incision is made in the superior aspect of the right atrial appendage (RAA) extending it into the superior vena cava (SVC), and a horizontal incision is made in the right pulmonary artery (RPA).* **B,** *The lower margin of the RPA incision and the adjacent margin of the incision in the RAA and SVC are connected.* **C,** *The connection is completed using pulmonary allograft. An intra-atrial patch is placed to direct SVC blood to the pulmonary arteries. AO, aorta; RA, right atrium.*

Pulmonary AV fistulas develop commonly after the SVC-to-PA connection, in which hepatic venous blood does not reach the pulmonary circulation. It has been postulated that the liver may produce vasoconstrictor prostaglandins, which prevent pulmonary vasodilation and development of pulmonary arteriovenous fistula. Vasoconstrictor prostaglandins in blood from the liver bypassing the pulmonary circulation may lead to the pulmonary AV fistulas. Song and colleagues reported that long-term aspirin (a cyclooxygenase inhibitor) therapy has successfully prevented the development of cyanosis, possibly by preventing pulmonary AV fistula formation. A similar pulmonary AV fistula also occurs, with the clinical manifestation of cyanosis, in patients with liver dysfunction (hepatopulmonary syndrome). The diagnosis of pulmonary AV malformation requires pulmonary angiography or, even better, a bubble contrast echo with injection into branch pulmonary arteries (Chang et al, 1999).

2. If a child's O_2 saturation is 75% or less, it is preferable to proceed with a Fontan operation. Alternatively, cardiac catheterization may be performed to find a cause of desaturation (such as missed left SVC, which can be coil occluded).

3. A pre-Fontan cardiac catheterization is performed by 12 months after the second-stage operation.

Stage III. A modified Fontan operation is the definitive procedure for patients with tricuspid atresia. The whole premise of the Fontan operation is directing the entire systemic venous blood to the pulmonary arteries without an intervening pumping chamber. The Fontan operation is usually completed when the child is around 2 years of age. This procedure can even be performed on infants.

The following are risk factors for the Fontan operation: The presence of two or more of these risk factors constitutes a high-risk situation.

1. High PVR (>2 U/m^2) or high mean PA pressure (>18 mm Hg)

2. Distorted PAs secondary to previous shunt operations

3. Poor systolic or diastolic ventricular function, with LV end-diastolic pressure greater than 12 mm Hg or an ejection fraction less than 60%

4. AV valve regurgitation

Surgical technique of completing modified Fontan operation varies according to the type of the second-stage operation performed; bidirectional Glenn operation or hemi-Fontan operation.

1. *Following bidirectional Glenn procedure.* An intra-atrial tubular pathway is created from the orifice of the IVC to the orifice of the SVC (termed cavocaval baffle or a "lateral tunnel"). The cardiac end of the SVC is anastomosed to the undersurface of the RPA to complete the operation (see Fig. 14–38B).

Some centers routinely use fenestration (4 to 6 mm) in the baffle, and others use it only in high-risk patients. The fenestration needs to be closed later, usually with an ASD closure device in the catheterization laboratory. Cited advantages of fenestration include decompression of the systemic venous circulation and augmentation of cardiac output in the early postoperative period. Disadvantages include systemic arterial desaturation with possible systemic embolization from the systemic veins and the later need to close the fenestration. As an alternative to the previously described procedure, an extracardiac conduit may be used to complete the Fontan operation (see Fig. 14–41G). Fenestration is not necessary for the extracardiac conduit, but some surgeons create the fenestration with this approach.

Early survival rates have improved to over 90%. In a large series of 500 Fontan operations, the probability of survival was 85% at 1 month, about 80% at 1 and 5 years, and 70% at 10 years.

2. *Following the hemi-Fontan operation.* The intra-atrial patch that was used to direct SVC blood to the PAs is excised and a lateral atrial tunnel is constructed, directing flow from the IVC to the previously created amalgamation of the SVC with the RPA (Fig. 14–40).

Timing for surgery is the same as for the cavocaval baffle-to-PA anastomosis. The mortality rate of the Fontan procedure for children who have undergone a hemi-Fontan operation is reportedly lower than for those who had the BDG.

Complications of the Fontan-type Operation

Early complications: Early postoperative complications may include the following.

1. Low cardiac output, heart failure, or both are early postoperative complications.

2. Persistent pleural effusion. This is the result of a sudden rise in the systemic venous or RA pressure. It occurs more often on the right side. The presence of aortopulmonary collaterals increases the risk of prolonged pleural effusion. Coil occlusion of these vessels before surgery can ameliorate this problem. The following treatment can be used for this complication: prolonged chest tube drainage, a low-fat diet with a medium-chain triglyceride oil supplement or total parenteral nutrition, chemical or talc pleurodesis, a pleuroperitoneal shunt, and thoracic duct ligation, which is a major surgery.

3. Thrombus formation in the systemic venous pathways may result from sluggish blood flow, which can be diagnosed by transesophageal echo. Treatment consists of warfarin, streptokinase thrombolysis, or surgical removal.

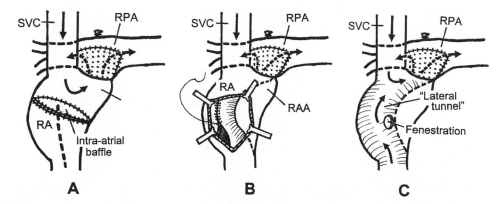

Figure 14–40. *From the hemi-Fontan to Fontan connection.* **A,** *A vertical incision (heavy broken line) is made in the anterior right atrial (RA) wall.* **B,** *The intra-atrial patch is removed and a lateral tunnel is constructed to direct the inferior vena cava (IVC) blood to the existing conglomerate of RA and right pulmonary artery (RPA).* **C,** *The direction of blood flow from the superior vena cava (SVC) and IVC is shown. RAA, right atrial appendage.*

4. Although rare, acute liver dysfunction with alanine transaminase greater than 1000 U/L can occur during the first week after surgery, possibly resulting from hepatic hypoperfusion (caused by low cardiac output).

Late complications: Regular follow-up is necessary to detect the following late complications:

1. Prolonged hepatomegaly and ascites require treatment with digitalis, diuretics, and afterload-reducing agents.

2. Supraventricular arrhythmia is one of the most troublesome complications. Early-onset arrhythmias occur in 15% of patients. The incidence of late-onset supraventricular arrhythmia continues to increase with longer follow-up after the Fontan procedure (6% at 1 year, 12% at 3 years, and 17% at 5 years).

3. A progressive decrease in arterial oxygen saturation may result from obstruction of the venous pathways, leakage in the intra-atrial baffle, or development of pulmonary AV fistula.

4. Protein-losing enteropathy can result from increased systemic venous pressure that subsequently causes lymphangiectasis. Increased PVR, decreased cardiac index, and increased ventricular end-diastolic pressure were coincident findings with the condition. The incidence of protein-losing enteropathy among survivors is 4%. The prognosis is poor; about half the patients die within 5 years, regardless of the type of treatment—medical or surgical. Heart transplantation should be considered for these patients.

Postoperative Medical Follow-up

1. Patients should maintain a low-salt diet.
2. Medications:
   a. Some patients need continued digoxin and diuretic therapy.
   b. An angiotensin-converting enzyme (ACE) inhibitor is generally recommended. Although not proved, it may augment LV output with consequent improvement in PBF.
   c. Aspirin (or even warfarin) is used to prevent thrombus formation in the RA.

3. Patients should not participate in competitive, strenuous sports.
4. Antibiotic prophylaxis against SBE should be observed when indications arise.
5. Among patients with tricuspid atresia, the 5-year survival rate is 80%, and the 10-year survival rate is 70%. During years 11 to 16 after surgery, the majority of patients have shown acceptable results, with 48% in New York Heart Association class I and 16% in class II (see Appendix A, Table A–4).

Evolution of the Fontan-Type Operation. The Fontan-type operation applies to many complex congenital heart defects, most of which are otherwise uncorrectable. Therefore, this procedure can be considered a major advancement in pediatric cardiac surgery during the last three decades. Castaneda (1992) has written an excellent review article on the historical aspect of the Fontan-type operations. Many modifications have been made since the original Fontan operation in 1971. The results of animal experiments conducted in the 1940s and 1950s suggested that the RV could be successfully bypassed (i.e., systemic venous pressure was an adequate force for PBF). The Glenn shunt (1958), which is an end-to-end anastomosis of the SVC to the distal end of the right PA, was the first such example, although it involved only one lung.

The original Fontan operation consisted of a Glenn shunt, connection of the RA and the right PA with insertion of an aortic homograft, insertion of another allograft valve in the IVC-RA junction, and closure of the ASD (Fig. 14–41A). At that time, RA contractions were thought to be important in pulsatile assistance to the pulmonary circulation. It became evident later that inlet and outlet valves were more problematic than beneficial.

Kreutzer and associates (1973) made a direct anastomosis between the right atrial appendage and the PA trunk using either a homograft or the patient's own pulmonary valve.

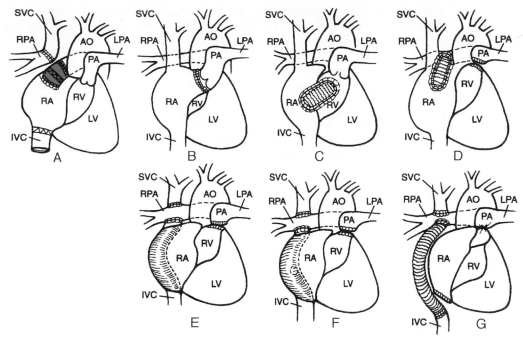

Figure 14–41. *Modifications of the Fontan operation.* **A,** *The original Fontan operation (Fontan and Baudet, 1971) consisted of an end-to-end anastomosis of the right pulmonary artery (RPA) to the superior vena cava (SVC), an end-to-end anastomosis of the right atrial appendage to the proximal end of the RPA by means of an aortic valve homograft, closure of the atrial septal defect (ASD), insertion of a pulmonary valve homograft into the inferior vena cava (IVC), and ligation of the main pulmonary artery (PA).* **B,** *Modification by Kreutzer et al (1973) consisted of an anastomosis of the right atrial appendage and the main PA with its intact pulmonary valve (which was excised from the right ventricle [RV]) after closure of the ASD and ventricular septal defect. A Glenn operation was not performed, and no IVC valve was used.* **C,** *A later modification by Bjork et al (1979) consisted of a direct anastomosis between the right atrial appendage and the right ventricular outflow tract in patients with a normal pulmonary valve, using a roof of pericardium to avoid a synthetic tube graft.* **D,** *Direct anastomosis of the right atrium (RA) to the RPA.* **E and F,** *Separate anastomosis of the two ends of the divided SVC to the RPA and insertion of IVC to SVC intra-atrial baffle (total cavopulmonary connection) with (**F**) and without (**E**) fenestration.* **G,** *Extracardiac conduit between the IVC and the RPA and a bidirectional Glenn operation. AO, aorta; LPA, left pulmonary artery; LV, left ventricle.*

The ASD was closed (see Fig. 14–41B). Subsequently, modifications of the connection were made between the RA and RV (see Fig. 14–41C), as well as between the RA and the main or right PA (see Fig. 14–41D), by direct anastomosis of the two structures or by the use of patches or conduits with or without an interposed valve. It became evident later that a direct connection between the right atrial appendage and the right PA without an interposed valve provided equally good hemodynamic results and that the incorporation of a portion of the RV was not beneficial.

Kawashima and associates (1984) reported a new operation in which the systemic venous return completely bypassed the RA and RV in patients with an interrupted IVC with azygos or hemiazygos continuation and other complex intracardiac anomalies. The right and left SVCs, which received blood from the entire systemic venous system, were connected end to side to the ipsilateral PAs. This procedure proved that the RA and RV can be completely bypassed in people.

In cavocaval baffle-to-PA connection, the latest modification of the Fontan operation, the RA and RV are both completely bypassed in patients with normal IVCs (see Fig. 14–41E). De Leval and associates have shown that the interposition of a compliant RA chamber between the systemic vein and the PA is a major cause of energy loss in the RA, and cavocaval baffle-to-PA anastomosis has significant hemodynamic advantages.

A two-stage Fontan operation was recommended for high-risk patients (see Fig. 14–41A). Initially, a bidirectional Glenn shunt was performed. This was later followed by the completion of the cavocaval baffle-to–right PA anastomosis. After the first procedure, there was often a noticeable improvement in oxygen saturation and symptoms, which raised questions about the necessity of the second procedure.

A fenestrated Fontan operation has been recommended for high-risk patients (see Fig. 14–41F). Reported advantages of fenestration include the following: lower early surgical mortality, reduced incidence or duration of postoperative pleural effusion, shorter hospital stay, and right-to-left shunt through the fenestration, which may help maintain cardiac output if blood flow through the lungs decreases. The following are possible disadvantages: paradoxical embolization and stroke, lower arterial oxygen saturation, and the need to close the fenestration.

Extracardiac right heart bypass with an IVC-to–right PA Dacron conduit and SVC-to-PA anastomosis has also been performed (see Fig. 14–41G). This procedure may reduce the incidence of late atrial arrhythmia, but the conduit does not have growth potential.

Surgical approaches in tricuspid atresia are shown in Figure 14–42.

Pulmonary Atresia with Intact Ventricular Septum

PREVALENCE

Pulmonary atresia with intact ventricular septum accounts for fewer than 1% of all congenital heart defects. It accounts for 2.5% of the critically ill infants with congenital heart defects.

PATHOLOGY

1. In 80% of these patients, the pulmonary valve is atretic with a diaphragm-like membrane. The infundibulum is atretic in 20% of these patients. The valve ring and the main PA are hypoplastic. The PA trunk is rarely atretic. The ventricular septum remains intact.

2. RV size varies and relates to survival. In 1982, Bull and associates divided this condition into three types, based on the presence or absence of the three portions

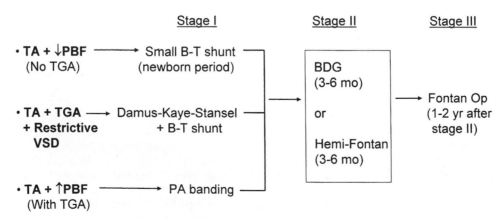

Figure 14–42. Surgical approaches in tricuspid atresia. BDG, bidirectional Glenn; B-T, Blalock-Taussig; Op, operation; PA, pulmonary artery; PBF, pulmonary blood flow; TA, tricuspid atresia; TGA, transposition of the great arteries; VSD, ventricular septal defect.

of the RV—inlet, trabecular, and infundibular portions (Fig. 14–43). All three of these portions are present and the RV is almost normal in size in the *tripartite type* of pulmonary atresia. In the *bipartite type*, the inlet and infundibular portions are present, but the trabecular portion is obliterated. The inlet is the only portion present, and the RV size is diminutive, in the *monopartite type*. The RV size is highly correlated with the size of the tricuspid valve.

3. This condition is frequently associated with important anomalies of the coronary arteries. The high pressure in the RV is decompressed through dilated coronary microcirculation (i.e., ventriculocoronary connection or coronary sinusoids) into the left or right coronary artery (see Fig. 14–45). Often the proximal coronary arteries are obstructed (approximately 10%). Rarely, proximal portions of the right or left coronary artery, or both, are absent. Sinusoid channels are demonstrable by a right ventriculogram in 30% to 50% of cases. If proximal coronary artery obstruction is present, coronary circulation is perfused entirely by desaturated RV blood (RV-dependent coronary circulation). Tricuspid valve z score less than −2.5 is a helpful predictor of coronary fistulas and RV-dependent coronary circulation. Such coronary sinusoids occur only in patients with hypertensive RV and not in patients with tricuspid regurgitation.

4. RV myocardium shows varying degrees of ischemia, infarction, fibrosis, and endocardial fibroelastosis, with poorly compliant RV, which may contribute to surgical mortality.

5. An interatrial communication (i.e., either ASD or PFO) and PDA (or collateral arteries) are necessary for the patient to survive.

6. PBF is provided usually through a PDA. Rarely, multiple aortopulmonary collaterals supply the PBF.

CLINICAL MANIFESTATIONS

History. A history of severe cyanosis since birth is present.

Physical Examination (Fig. 14–44)

1. Severe cyanosis and tachypnea are seen in distressed neonates.
2. The S2 is single. A heart murmur is usually absent, but a soft murmur of TR or a soft continuous murmur of PDA may be audible.
3. Inadequate interatrial communication causes hepatomegaly.

Electrocardiography

1. The QRS axis is normal (i.e., +60 to +140 degrees), in contrast to the superiorly oriented QRS axis seen in tricuspid atresia.
2. LVH is usually present. Occasionally, RVH is seen in infants with a relatively large RV cavity. RAH is common, occurring in 70% of cases.

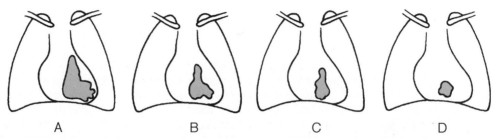

A   B   C   D

Figure 14–43. *Schematic diagrams of right ventriculograms that illustrate three types of pulmonary atresia with intact ventricular septum. **A**, Normal right ventricle (RV). **B**, Tripartite type that shows all three portions (inlet, trabecular, and infundibular) of the RV. **C**, Bipartite type in which only the inlet and infundibular portions are present. **D**, Monopartite type in which only the inlet portion of the RV is present.*

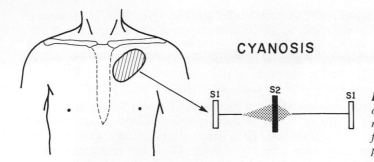

CYANOSIS

Figure 14–44. Cardiac findings of pulmonary atresia. These are nonspecific for the defect and may be found in tetralogy of Fallot with pulmonary atresia as well.

X-ray Studies. The heart size may be normal or large, resulting from right atrial enlargement. Pulmonary vascular markings are decreased with dark lung fields. The main PA segment is concave.

Echocardiography

1. Diagnostic features of the condition include (a) a thickened, immobile, atretic pulmonary valve with no Doppler evidence of blood flow through it; (b) hypertrophied RV wall with a small cavity; (c) patent, but small, tricuspid valve; (d) right-to-left atrial shunt through an ASD demonstrated by color flow and Doppler studies; and (e) ductus arteriosus running vertically from the aortic arch to the PA (i.e., vertical ductus) (see Fig. 14–25).

2. The size of the tricuspid valve should be carefully measured because this measurement correlates well with the size of the RV cavity (see Table D–6, Appendix D, for tricuspid and other valve annulus dimensions in neonates). The most severely stenotic tricuspid valve is associated with the most underdeveloped RV and with likelihood of RV-dependent coronary circulation.

3. The right and left PA branches are usually well developed.

4. Color Doppler flow mapping usually demonstrates coronary artery fistulas.

NATURAL HISTORY

Without appropriate management (which includes PGE_1 infusion and surgery), the prognosis is exceedingly poor. About 50% of these patients die by the end of the first month if not managed properly; about 80% die by 6 months of age. Death usually coincides with the spontaneous closure of the ductus arteriosus.

MANAGEMENT

Medical

1. PGE_1 (Prostin VR Pediatric solution) infusion should begin as soon as the diagnosis is suspected or confirmed so that the patency of the ductus arteriosus is maintained. Infusion is continued during cardiac catheterization and surgery. The starting dose of Prostin is 0.05 to 0.1 µg/kg per minute. When the desired effect is achieved, the dosage is gradually reduced to 0.01 µg/kg per minute.

2. For small premature infants, a prolonged course of PGE_1 infusion may be necessary before surgery is undertaken.

3. Cardiac catheterization and angiocardiography are required for proper management in most patients with pulmonary atresia. A right ventriculogram demonstrates the size of the RV cavity and the presence or absence of coronary sinusoids (Fig. 14–45). An ascending aortogram identifies stenosis or interruption of the coronary arteries. Both are important in surgical decision making. A balloon atrial septostomy may be performed as part of the cardiac catheterization to improve the right-to-left atrial shunt, but it is recommended only when a two-ventricular repair is considered not possible (e.g., the presence of RV sinusoids or too small an RV cavity).

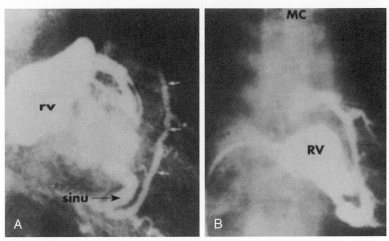

Figure 14–45. *Right ventriculograms in a patient with pulmonary atresia.* **A,** *Contrast medium filling the right ventricle (rv) passes into the ventricle-coronary fistula (sinu) and left anterior descending (LAD) coronary artery. Small white arrows point to multiple stenotic areas in the LAD.* **B,** *Massive filling of a dilated and irregular LAD coronary artery from the right ventricular injection (RV). (From Williams WG, Burrows P, Freedom RM, et al: Thromboexclusion of the right ventricle in children with pulmonary atresia and intact ventricular septum. J Thorac Cardiovasc Surg 101:222–229, 1991.)*

4. A laser-assisted pulmonary valvotomy with balloon pulmonary valvuloplasty may be a useful alternative surgical procedure that establishes an RV-PA continuity (Cheung et al, 2002).

5. For survivors, prophylaxis against SBE is required when indications arise.

Surgical. The size of the RV (or that of the tricuspid valve) and the presence or absence of coronary sinusoids or coronary artery anomalies dictate surgical procedures for infants with pulmonary atresia with intact ventricular septum. Surgical options are as follows.

1. Two-ventricular repair, which is the ultimate goal whenever feasible, is possible only when there is an adequate size of the RV cavity with adequate RV outflow tracts.

2. One and one-half ventricular repair—when the RV size is judged to be borderline for a two-ventricular repair but too good to be abandoned for Fontan-type repair.

3. One-ventricular repair (Fontan operation)—when an RV-dependent coronary circulation is present or when a monopartite RV (with a tricuspid valve z score <-4 to -5) is present.

4. Cardiac transplantation.

Procedures

1. *Staged two-ventricular repair.* The initial procedure, for the two-ventricular repair, consists of a connection between the RV and the PA (to promote growth of the RV) with a systemic-to-PA shunt performed at the same time. The RV-to-PA connection is established by one of the following procedures.

    a. Placement of a transannular RV outflow patch and a systemic-to-PA shunt seems most promising for a two-ventricular repair at a later date (Fig. 14–46). Balloon atrial septostomy is not recommended with this approach, so that a high RA pressure is maintained to maximize the forward RV output. The mortality rate is about 20%.

    b. For a patient with a well-formed pulmonary valve and adequate infundibulum, a closed transpulmonary valvotomy (without cardiopulmonary bypass) and a left-sided

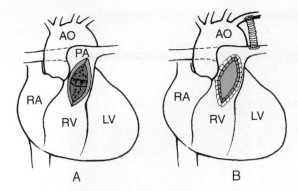

Figure 14–46. Initial surgery for tripartite or bipartite type of pulmonary atresia. **A,** A longitudinal incision is made across the pulmonary annulus. The pulmonary valve is incised, and the right ventricular outflow tract is carefully widened. **B,** A piece of pericardium is used for the transannular patch. A left-sided Gore-Tex shunt is made between the left subclavian artery and the left pulmonary artery (PA). AO, aorta; LV, left ventricle; RA, right atrium; RV, right ventricle.

modified Blalock-Taussig shunt procedure are performed. The mortality rate of these procedures is less than 5%.

c. An alternative to the closed surgical valvotomy is the use of laser wire and radiofrequency-assisted valvotomy and balloon dilatation during cardiac catheterization. The mortality rate of the procedure is about 5%.

Following one of these procedures, the growth of the RV is monitored in the following manner.

a. If the tricuspid valve size is within normal limit (z score >–2) and the child's O_2 saturation is stable or increasing, these are positive signs for two-ventricular repair.

b. Cardiac catheterization is performed within 6 to 18 months after the initial surgery to determine whether the surgical procedures have increased the RV size. An arterial oxygen saturation greater than 70%, a greater RV volume, and evidence of forward flow through the pulmonary valve are all positive signs. If the patient tolerates balloon occlusion of the shunt during cardiac catheterization, the patient is considered a candidate for a two-ventricular repair.

Right ventricular outflow tract reconstruction and closure of the ASD are carried out under cardiopulmonary bypass. The systemic-to-PA shunt is closed at the time of surgery. The mortality rate is about 15%.

2. *One and one-half ventricular repair.* The 1½ ventricular repair may be performed when the RV size is not quite large enough to have two-ventricular repair but the RV is too good to be abandoned for one-ventricular repair. In this repair, a bidirectional Glenn anastomosis is created to bring the SVC blood directly to the PA, bypassing the RV. The IVC blood goes to the lungs by the normal pathway through the RV, which is large enough to handle half of the systemic venous return. Following this procedure, the size of the tricuspid valve and the RV may actually increase with adequate RV function. Complications associated with the Fontan procedure (such as arrhythmias, protein-losing enteropathy) do not occur following this procedure. The surgical mortality rate is between 0% and 12% (similar to that of the Fontan procedure).

3. *One-ventricular repair* (Fontan operation). A two-ventricular repair is not possible for patients with monopartite RV (without adequate RV outflow tract) and those with coronary fistulas (see later).

a. For monopartite RV. A systemic-to-PA shunt without the RV outflow patch is recommended as the initial procedure. A staged Fontan operation is performed at a later time (see Fig. 14–38).

b. For patients who have rudimentary RV (with high RV pressure) and sinusoidal channels. Decompression of the RV by valvotomy or an outflow patch cannot be done because it results in a reversal of coronary flow into the RV, producing myocardial ischemia.

1). If coronary anomalies are identified by an aortogram, the sinusoids are left alone, and a systemic-to-PA shunt is performed for a future Fontan-type operation. After the Fontan operation, the sinusoids are perfused by highly oxygenated blood. (Enlargement of ASD may be done for easy drainage of pulmonary venous blood to the right side of the heart.)

2). Alternatively, the tricuspid valve is closed (converting it to tricuspid atresia, the Starnes procedure) and a systemic-to-PA shunt is created for a future Fontan operation.

3). When the proximal portion of the coronary arteries is not identified or severe anomalies of the coronary circulation are present, cardiac transplantation may be an option.

Postoperative Follow-up

1. Most patients require close follow-up because none of the surgical procedures available are curative.

2. Antibiotic prophylaxis against SBE is recommended.

The surgical approach to pulmonary atresia with intact ventricular septum is illustrated in Figure 14–47.

Hypoplastic Left Heart Syndrome

PREVALENCE

HLHS occurs in 1% of all congenital heart defects or 9% of such defects in critically ill newborns.

Pulmonary Atresia with Intact Ventricular Septum

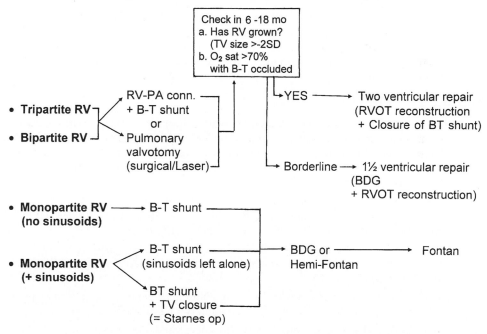

Figure 14–47. *Surgical approach to pulmonary atresia with intact ventricular septum. BDG, bidirectional Glenn; B-T, Blalock-Taussig; op, operation; Pulm., pulmonary; RV, right ventricle; RVOT, right ventricular outflow tract; RV-PA conn., right ventricle–to–pulmonary artery connection; TV, tricuspid valve.*

PATHOLOGY

1. HLHS includes a group of closely related anomalies characterized by hypoplasia of the LV and encompasses atresia or critical stenosis of the aortic or mitral valves, or both, and hypoplasia of the ascending aorta and aortic arch.

2. The LV is small and nonfunctional or totally atretic. The atrial septum may be intact with a normal foramen ovale, or the patient may have a true ASD (15%). A VSD appears in about 10% of patients. COA is frequently an associated finding (up to 75%).

3. A high prevalence of brain abnormalities has been reported. Up to 29% of the patients had a CNS abnormality. Overt CNS malformations (such as agenesis of the corpus callosum, holoprosencephaly) were seen in 10% of these infants. Micrencephaly was found in 27% of the infants, and an immature cortical mantle was seen in 21% of the patients. The presence or absence of dysmorphic physical features did not predict CNS malformations (Glauser et al, 1990).

PATHOPHYSIOLOGY

1. During fetal life, the PVR is higher than the systemic vascular resistance, and the dominant RV maintains normal perfusing pressure in the descending aorta and the placenta through the ductal right-to-left shunt. The proximal aorta and the coronary and cerebral circulations are adequately perfused retrogradely. The fetus tolerates this serious cardiac anomaly well in utero.

2. Difficulties arise after birth for two reasons: reduction of PVR (with the onset of respiration) and closure of the ductus arteriosus. The result is a marked reduction in the aortic perfusing pressure and systemic cardiac output, producing circulatory shock and metabolic acidosis.

3. Maintenance of adequate systemic blood flow (and, thus, survival of these infants) depends on an adequate size of the ductus arteriosus and maintenance of a high PVR to permit the RV to send adequate blood flow to the aorta. An adequate interatrial communication is also necessary to decompress the LA. In the presence of a large ASD that permits a left-to-right atrial shunt, pulmonary edema is not severe, and the arterial oxygen saturation may be in the 80s. With an inadequate atrial septal communication, pulmonary edema is severe, and the arterial oxygen saturation is low. Without treatment, the infant dies shortly after birth.

CLINICAL MANIFESTATIONS

1. A neonate with HLHS becomes critically ill within the first few hours to the first few days of life. Tachycardia, dyspnea, pulmonary crackles, weak peripheral pulses, and vasoconstricted extremities are characteristic. The patient may not have severe cyanosis but has a grayish blue color of the skin with poor perfusion.

2. The S2 is loud and single. Heart murmur is usually absent. Occasionally, a grade 1 to 2/6 nonspecific ejection systolic murmur may be heard over the precordium. Signs of CHF develop, with hepatomegaly and gallop rhythm.

3. The ECG almost always shows RVH. Rarely, the ECG suggests LVH. Large R waves may be recorded in V5 and V6 because these leads record over the dilated RV, not over the hypoplastic LV.

4. Chest x-ray films characteristically show pulmonary venous congestion or pulmonary edema (Fig. 14–48A). The heart is moderately or markedly enlarged.

5. Arterial blood gas levels reveal a slightly decreased Po_2 and a normal Pco_2. Severe metabolic acidosis out of proportion to the Pco_2 (caused by markedly decreased cardiac output) is characteristic of the condition.

6. Echo findings are diagnostic and usually obviate the need for cardiac catheterization and angiocardiography.

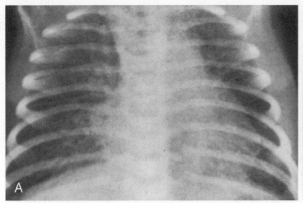
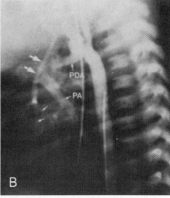

Figure 14–48. *Anteroposterior view of chest film (**A**) and lateral view of an aortogram (**B**) of a 1-day-old newborn with hypoplastic left heart syndrome. The heart is enlarged, and the pulmonary vascularity is increased, with marked pulmonary venous congestion and pulmonary edema (**A**). The aortogram, obtained with injection of a radiopaque dye through an umbilical artery catheter, shows a hypoplastic ascending aorta (thick arrows) with small coronary arteries (thin arrows) filling retrogradely, a large patent ductus arteriosus (PDA), and pulmonary artery (PA) branches.*

    a. The LV cavity is diminutive, but the RV cavity is markedly dilated, and the tricuspid valve is large.

    b. Imaging usually reveals severe hypoplasia of the aorta and aortic annulus and an absent or distorted mitral valve. COA is frequently an associated anomaly.

    c. The patient may have an ASD or a PFO with a left-to-right shunt. The patient occasionally has a VSD with a relatively large LV, aortic annulus, and ascending aorta.

    d. Color flow mapping and Doppler studies reveal retrograde blood flow in the aortic arch and ascending aorta.

NATURAL HISTORY

Pulmonary edema and CHF develop in the first week of life. Circulatory shock and progressive hypoxemia and acidosis result in death, usually in the first month of life.

MANAGEMENT

Medical

1. The patient should be intubated and ventilated appropriately with oxygen, and metabolic acidosis corrected.

2. Intravenous infusion of PGE_1 (Prostin VR Pediatric) may temporarily improve HLHS by reopening the ductus arteriosus (for the dosage, see Appendix E).

3. Balloon atrial septostomy may help decompress the LA and improve oxygenation but produces only a temporary benefit.

4. Infants with HLHS should have careful genetic, ophthalmologic, and neurologic evaluations, including imaging of their intracranial anatomy and long-term follow-up because of a high prevalence of neurodevelopmental abnormalities seen with the condition.

Surgical. Three options are available in the management of these infants: the Norwood operation (followed by a Fontan-type operation), cardiac transplantation, and support therapy only (which has been challenged). The surgical procedure of choice remains controversial, but the Norwood operation is more popular than cardiac transplantation.

1. Staged Norwood operation. The first-stage Norwood operation is performed initially and followed later by the Fontan-type operation.

    a. The first-stage Norwood operation is performed in the neonatal period. The reported mortality rate is around 25%. Noncardiac anomalies and severe pulmonary venous obstruction are risk factors for death. The operation consists of the following procedures (Fig. 14–49):

1). The main PA is divided, the distal stump is closed with a patch, and the ductus arteriosus is ligated.

2). A right-side Gore-Tex shunt is created (with a 4- to 5-mm tube) to provide PBF while preventing CHF and pulmonary hypertension. Some centers prefer a central shunt to promote symmetrical growth of the pulmonary arteries. An RV-to-PA shunt, using polytetrafluoroethylene graft, rather than the Gore-Tex shunt, was used recently by Sano and colleagues (4 mm for patients weighing <2 kg and 5 mm for those weighing >2 kg) (Sano modification). The cited advantage of the RV-to-PA shunt over the Gore-Tex shunt includes a higher aortic diastolic pressure (thus a higher coronary artery perfusing pressure) and a lower PA mean pressure.

3). The atrial septum is excised to allow adequate interatrial mixing.

4). Using an aortic or PA allograft, one connects the proximal PA and the hypoplastic ascending aorta and aortic arch.

b. Second-stage procedure. There are two choices of second-stage operation: the bidirectional Glenn procedure and the hemi-Fontan procedure.

1). Cavopulmonary shunt (also called the bidirectional Glenn operation) is an end-to-side anastomosis of the SVC to the right PA (see Fig. 14–38A) performed at 3 to 6 months of age in an effort to reduce the volume overload to the systemic RV. The mortality rate for this procedure is less than 5%.

2). The hemi-Fontan operation. This procedure includes augmentation of the central PA without dividing the SVC, while excluding IVC blood from the pulmonary arteries by means of a temporary intra-atrial patch (see Fig. 14–39).

c. A modified Fontan operation is performed at 12 to 18 months of age (see Fig. 14–38B). Five important hemodynamic and anatomic features considered essential to successful Fontan operation are (1) unrestrictive interatrial communication, (2) competence of the tricuspid valve, (3) unobstructed PA–to–descending aorta anastomosis (with pressure gradient less than 25 mm Hg), (4) undistorted PAs and low PVR, and (5) preservation of RV function.

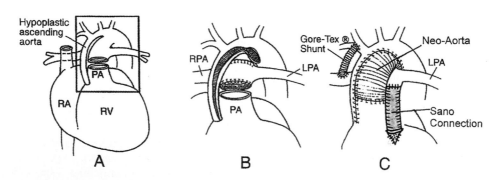

Figure 14–49. Schematic diagram of the Norwood procedure. A, The heart with aortic atresia and a hypoplastic ascending aorta and aortic arch are shown. The main pulmonary artery (PA) is transected. B, The distal PA is closed with a patch. An incision that extends around the aortic arch to the level of the ductus is made in the ascending aorta. The ductus is ligated. C, A modified right Blalock-Taussig shunt is created between the right subclavian artery and the right PA (RPA) as the sole source of pulmonary blood flow. Instead of the Blalock-Taussig shunt, a homograft conduit may be placed between the RV and PA bifurcation as shown (Sano modification). By the use of an aortic or pulmonary artery allograft (striped area), the main PA is anastomosed to the ascending aorta and the aortic arch to create a large new arterial trunk. The procedure to widen the atrial communication is not shown. LPA, left pulmonary artery; RA, right atrium; RV, right ventricle.

Significant TR appears to be an important predictor of poor outcome of the Fontan operation. The operative mortality of the Fontan procedure is about 15% to 20%. The overall survival rate after the Fontan operation is about 60% at 1 year and 55% at 4 years.

2. Infants with aortic atresia and normal-sized LV because of a large VSD can have a biventricular repair rather than a Fontan approach. The VSD is tunneled to the PA. The MPA is divided and the proximal MPA is connected to the ascending aorta. The RV is connected to the distal MPA using a valved conduit or a homograft.

3. Some centers consider cardiac transplantation the procedure of choice (see Chapter 35). If the diameter of the ascending aorta is less than 2.5 mm, cardiac transplantation, rather than the Norwood operation, is believed to provide a better result. The surgical technique of cardiac transplantation is presented in Chapter 35. Donor hearts must be harvested with all the ascending, transverse, and upper descending thoracic aortas intact.

For patients placed on a transplantation algorithm, it is necessary to keep the ductus open and to increase the size of the interatrial communication. An endovascular stent has been placed in a closing ductus to keep the ductus open. Blade atrial septostomy followed by balloon dilatation has been performed for the latter requirement.

Surgery for hypoplastic left heart syndrome is illustrated in Figure 14–50.

Ebstein's Anomaly

PREVALENCE

Ebstein's anomaly of the tricuspid valve occurs in less than 1% of all congenital heart defects.

PATHOLOGY

1. There is downward displacement of the septal and posterior leaflets of the tricuspid valve into the RV cavity so that a portion of the RV is incorporated into the RA (i.e., *atrialized* RV) and functional hypoplasia of the RV results (Fig. 14–51). Tricuspid regurgitation is usually present and redundant tricuspid valve tissues can rarely obstruct the RVOT, which results in dilatation and hypertrophy of the RA.

2. An interatrial communication (e.g., PFO, true ASD) with a right-to-left shunt is present in all patients.

3. The RV free wall is often dilated and thin. Fibrosis is present in both RV and LV free walls; this may be responsible for severe symptoms early in life and LV dysfunction in later life.

Hypoplastic Left Heart Syndrome

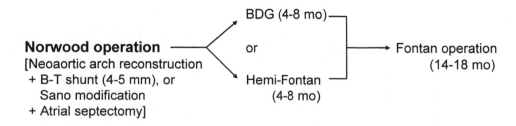

Figure 14–50. *Surgery for hypoplastic left heart syndrome. BDG, bidirectional Glenn; B-T, Blalock-Taussig.*

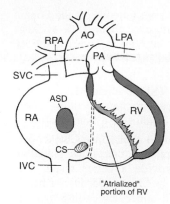

Figure 14–51. Diagram of Ebstein's anomaly of the tricuspid valve. There is a downward displacement of the tricuspid valve, usually the septal and posterior leaflets, into the right ventricle (RV). Part of the RV is incorporated into the right atrium (RA) ("atrialized" portion of the RV). Regurgitation of the tricuspid valve results in RA enlargement. An atrial septal defect (ASD) is usually present. AO, aorta; CS, coronary sinus; IVC, inferior vena cava; LPA, left pulmonary artery; RPA, right pulmonary artery; SVC, superior vena cava.

4. WPW preexcitation is frequently associated with the anomaly and predisposes the patient to SVT.

5. PS, pulmonary atresia, TOF, VSD, and other defects are occasionally associated with the anomaly.

CLINICAL MANIFESTATIONS

History

1. In severe cases, cyanosis and CHF develop during the first few days of life. Some subsequent improvement coincides with reduction of the PVR.

2. Children with milder cases may complain of dyspnea, fatigue, cyanosis, or palpitation on exertion.

3. A history of SVT is occasionally present.

Physical Examination

1. Mild to severe cyanosis is present, as well as clubbing of the fingers and toes in older infants and children.

2. Characteristic triple or quadruple rhythm is audible. This rhythm has a widely split S2, in addition to split S1, S3, and S4. A soft holosystolic (or early systolic) murmur of TR is usually audible at the lower left sternal border (Fig. 14–52). A soft, scratchy, mid-diastolic murmur is present at the same location.

3. Hepatomegaly is usually present.

Electrocardiography

1. Characteristic ECG findings of RBBB and RAH are present in most patients with this condition (Fig. 14–53).

2. First-degree AV block is frequent, occurring in 40% of patients. A WPW pattern of preexcitation syndrome is present in 15% to 20% of patients with occasional episodes of SVT.

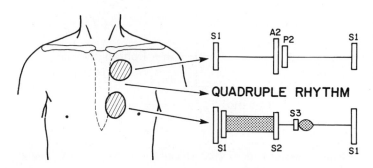

Figure 14–52. Cardiac findings of Ebstein's anomaly. Quadruple rhythm and a soft, regurgitant systolic murmur are characteristic of the defect.

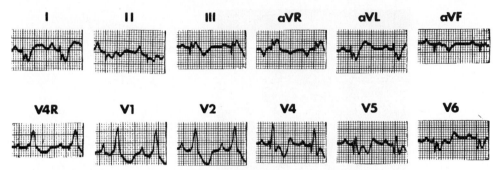

Figure 14–53. *Tracing from a 5-year-old child with Ebstein's anomaly. The tracing shows right atrial hypertrophy, right bundle branch block, and first-degree atrioventricular block.*

X-ray Studies. In mild cases, the heart is almost normal in size and has normal pulmonary vascular markings. In severe cases, an extreme cardiomegaly (principally involving the RA) with a balloon-shaped heart and decreased pulmonary vascular markings are present. Some of the largest heart sizes are found in newborns with this condition (Fig. 14–54).

Echocardiography. Two-dimensional echo with color flow Doppler study is the procedure of choice for morphologic and functional assessment of Ebstein's anomaly. An echo can replace cardiac catheterization and angiography.

1. The single most diagnostic feature is apical displacement of the hinge point of the septal leaflet of the tricuspid valve (Fig. 14–55). Normally, the septal leaflet of the tricuspid valve inserts on the ventricular septum slightly below the insertion of the mitral valve. In patients with Ebstein's anomaly, this normal displacement is exaggerated. A diagnosis of Ebstein's anomaly is made when the tricuspid valve is displaced toward the apex by more than 8 mm/m^2 of body surface area from the mitral valve insertion. This displacement is best seen in the apical four-chamber view.

2. The tricuspid valve leaflets are elongated, redundant, and dysplastic with abnormal chordal attachment.

3. A large RA, including the atrialized RV, and a small functional RV represent anatomic severity. Evidence of tricuspid valve regurgitation and tricuspid stenosis is present.

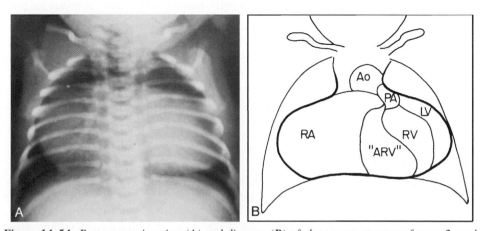

Figure 14–54. *Posteroanterior view (**A**) and diagram (**B**) of chest roentgenogram from a 2-week-old infant with severe Ebstein's anomaly. Note extreme cardiomegaly involving primarily the right atrium (RA) and diminished pulmonary vascularity. AO, aorta; ARV, atrialized right ventricle; LV, left ventricle; PA, pulmonary artery; RV, right ventricle.*

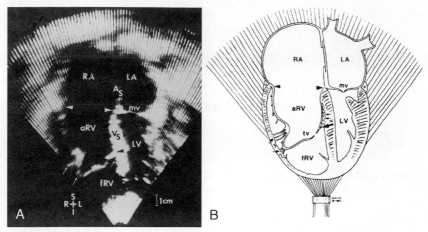

Figure 14–55. *Echocardiogram (**A**) and diagram (**B**) of an apical four-chamber view of a patient with Ebstein's anomaly. The septal leaflet is displaced into the right ventricle (RV; large dark arrow) and thus forms an atrialized RV (aRV). The anterior tricuspid leaflet is elongated. Both leaflets are tethered to underlying myocardium (small arrows). The tricuspid annulus and the right atrium (RA) are dilated. AS, atrial septum; fRV, functional right ventricle; LA, left atrium; LV, left ventricle; mv, mitral valve; tv, tricuspid valve; VS, ventricular septum. (From Shiina A, Serwer JB, Edwards WD, et al: Two-dimensional echocardiographic spectrum of Ebstein's anomaly: Detailed anatomic assessment. J Am Coll Cardiol 3:356–370, 1984.)*

4. RVOT obstruction may be present owing to the redundant anterior leaflet of the tricuspid valve.

5. A nonrestrictive ASD is commonly imaged.

6. Other anomalies may include mitral valve prolapse and left ventricular dysfunction.

NATURAL HISTORY

1. Some 18% of symptomatic newborns die in the neonatal period; 30% of patients die before the age of 10 years, usually from CHF. The median age at death is about 20 years.

2. Cyanosis tends to improve as the PVR falls during the newborn period. Cyanosis may reappear later.

3. Patients with a less severe anomaly may be either asymptomatic or mildly symptomatic.

4. Hemodynamic deterioration with increasing cyanosis, CHF, and LV dysfunction develops later in life. These developments foretell early death.

5. Attacks of SVT with associated WPW preexcitation occur in 15% to 20% of all patients. Sudden, unexpected death can occur, probably as a result of arrhythmias.

6. Other possible complications include infective endocarditis, brain abscess, and cerebrovascular accident.

MANAGEMENT

Medical

1. In severely cyanotic newborns, intensive treatment with mechanical ventilation, PGE_1 infusion, inotropic agents, and correction of metabolic acidosis may be necessary before proceeding with emergency surgery.

2. In infants who appear to have a mild form of Ebstein's anomaly and appear to be improving with the preceding management, treatment with PGE_1 and inotropic support is gradually withdrawn to observe the effect of ductal closure.

3. Asymptomatic children with mild Ebstein's anomaly require only regular observation. If CHF develops, anticongestive measures including digoxin and diuretics are indicated.

4. Acute episodes of SVT may be treated most effectively with adenosine (see Chapter 24). β-Blockers are the most appropriate first-line preventive therapy for SVT. For patients with recurrent SVT related to an AV reentrant mechanism, radiofrequency catheter ablation techniques have been successful. The success rate is 95% in those with isolated right-sided accessory pathways and 76% in those with multiple pathways (Cappato et al, 1996).

5. Maintenance of good dental hygiene and antibiotic prophylaxis for SBE are important.

6. Varying degrees of activity restriction may be necessary for children with this condition.

Surgical

Indications. Although surgical indications for Ebstein's anomaly are not completely defined, they may include the following:

1. Critically ill neonates who show symptoms within the first week of life (after a period of intensive medical treatment)

2. Occurrence of moderately severe or progressive cyanosis (arterial saturation of ≤80%), polycythemia (hemoglobin level ≥16 g/dL), or CHF

3. Right ventricular outflow tract obstruction by redundant tricuspid valve

4. Severe activity limitation (i.e., functional class Ill or IV) (see Appendix A, Table A–4)

5. History of paradoxical embolus

6. Repeated, life-threatening arrhythmias in patients with associated WPW syndrome

Procedures. Controversy exists concerning the type and timing of surgical procedures.

1. Palliative procedures. For critically ill neonates, if medical management does not result in signs of improvement, surgical intervention is indicated to avoid certain death.

   a. Blalock-Taussig shunt (with enlargement of ASD). This procedure can be lifesaving when there are obstructive lesions between the RV and the PA or stenotic or atretic tricuspid valve. Good LV function (with adequate LV size) is required to survive the procedure. A Fontan-type operation is performed later (see Fig. 14–38).

   b. If the LV is "pancaked" by a large RV or RA, a procedure to reduce the RV or RA may be considered, such as the Starnes operation (which includes pericardial closure of the tricuspid valve or plication of a large RA [atrialized RV], enlargement of ASD, and a Blalock-Taussig shunt using a 4-mm tube). A Fontan-type operation (see Fig. 14–38) is performed later.

   c. Classic Glenn anastomosis or its modification may be considered in severely cyanotic infants.

2. Definitive procedures. Children with good RV size and function are candidates for biventricular repair (with tricuspid valve repair or replacement). Inadequate RV size or function requires a Fontan operation. Surgical approaches for this anomaly are summarized in Figure 14–57 for quick reference.

   a. *Two-ventricular repair*: Reconstruction of the tricuspid valve (such as the Danielson and Carpentier procedures) is preferable to valve replacement. ASD is closed at the time of surgery.

      1). Danielson technique: For repair of the tricuspid valve, this technique is the most desirable and best tested, although it is frequently limited by anatomy. This technique can be applied in about 60% of patients (Fig. 14–56). It plicates the atrialized portion of the RV, narrows the tricuspid orifice in a selective manner, and results in a monoleaflet valve (by the anterior leaflet of

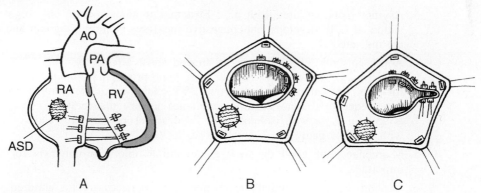

Figure 14–56. *Danielson technique for tricuspid valve repair.* **A,** *A series of interrupted mattress sutures are placed to obliterate the atrialized portion of the right ventricle (RV). The atrial septal defect (ASD) is closed with a patch.* **B,** *As the sutures are tied, the atrialized portion of the RV is obliterated (seen through a right atriotomy).* **C,** *Sutures are placed to further narrow the tricuspid orifice. The valve is now a monocusp valve (anterior leaflet of the tricuspid valve) that is mobile and opens widely during diastole. AO, aorta; PA, pulmonary artery; RA, right atrium.*

the tricuspid valve). Two other leaflets are often severely hypoplastic and cannot be made to function as a leaflet. The mortality rate is about 5%, which is lower than that for valve replacement.

2). Carpentier technique: As an alternative, Carpentier reconstructive surgery may be used. This repair also plicates the atrialized portion of the RV and the tricuspid annulus but in a direction that is at right angles to that used by Danielson. This repair can be applied in most patients with Ebstein's anomaly. The surgical mortality rate is 15%.

3). Tricuspid valve replacement and closure of the ASD is a less desirable surgical approach but may be necessary for 20% to 30% of patients with Ebstein's anomaly who are not candidates for reconstructive surgery. The replacement valve of choice is a stented, antibiotically treated semilunar valve allograft or a heterograft valve. A pulmonary allograft valve mounted in a short Dacron sleeve can be used in younger children. The surgical mortality rate ranges from 5% to 20%.

   b. *One-ventricular repair:* For patients with inadequate size of the RV, a Fontan-type operation is usually performed in stages following the initial palliative procedures such as bidirectional Glenn operation (see Fig. 14–38) or hemi-Fontan operation (see Fig. 14–39).

3. Other procedures. For patients with WPW syndrome and recurrent SVT, surgical interruption of the accessory pathway is recommended at the time of surgery.

Complications

1. Complete heart block is a rare complication.

2. Supraventricular arrhythmias persist in 10% to 20% of patients after surgery.

Postoperative Follow-up

1. Frequent follow-up is necessary because of the persistence of arrhythmias after surgery, which occurs in 10% to 20% of patients, and because of possible problems associated with tricuspid valve surgery that require reoperation.

2. Antibiotic prophylaxis against SBE should be observed.

3. The patient should not participate in competitive or strenuous sports.

Surgical approaches for Ebstein's anomaly are shown in Figure 14–57.

Ebstein's Anomaly

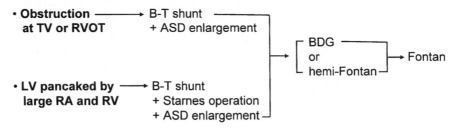

■ **Deeply Cyanotic Newborns:**

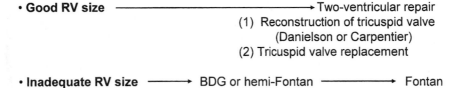

■ **Asymptomatic Children:**

Figure 14–57. Surgical approaches for Ebstein's anomaly of the tricuspid valve. ASD, atrial septal defect; BDG, bidirectional Glenn; B-T, Blalock-Taussig; LV, left ventricle; RA, right atrium; RV, right ventricle; RVOT, right ventricular outflow tract; TV, tricuspid valve.

Persistent Truncus Arteriosus

PREVALENCE

Persistent truncus arteriosus occurs in less than 1% of all congenital heart defects.

PATHOLOGY

1. Only a single arterial trunk with a truncal valve leaves the heart and gives rise to the pulmonary, systemic, and coronary circulations. A large perimembranous, infundibular VSD is present directly below the truncus (Fig. 14–58). The truncal valve may be bicuspid, tricuspid, or quadricuspid, and it is often incompetent.

2. This anomaly is divided into four types according to Collett and Edwards' classification (see Fig. 14–58). The PBF is increased in type I, nearly normal in types II and III, and decreased in type IV. Types I and II constitute 85% of cases. Type IV is not a true persistent truncus arteriosus; rather, it is a severe form of TOF with pulmonary atresia (i.e., pseudotruncus arteriosus), with aortic collaterals supplying the lungs.

3. Coronary artery abnormalities are quite common and may contribute to the high surgical mortality. The anomalies include stenotic coronary ostia, high and low takeoff of coronary arteries, and abnormal branching and course of coronary arteries.

4. Interrupted aortic arch is seen in 13% of cases (this is type A4 of the van Praagh classification). In this case, the interruption occurs distal to the takeoff of the left carotid artery and lower extremity flow is accomplished through the PDA.

5. A right aortic arch is present in 30% of patients.

6. Evidence of DiGeorge syndrome with hypocalcemia is present in 33% of patients.

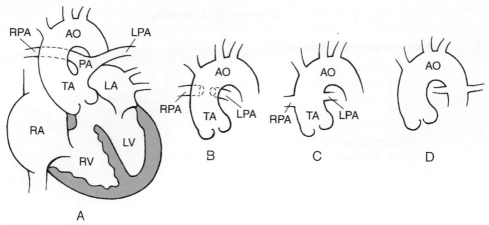

Figure 14–58. *The anatomic type of persistent truncus arteriosus (TA) is determined by the branching patterns of the pulmonary arteries.* **A,** *In type I, the main pulmonary artery (PA) arises from the truncus and then divides into the right (RPA) and left pulmonary artery (LPA) branches.* **B,** *In type II, the pulmonary arteries arise from the posterior aspect of the truncus.* **C,** *In type III, the pulmonary arteries arise from the lateral aspects of the truncus.* **D,** *In type IV, or pseudotruncus arteriosus, arteries arising from the descending aorta (AO) supply the lungs. LA, left atrium; LV, left ventricle; RA, right atrium; RV, right ventricle.*

CLINICAL MANIFESTATIONS

History

1. Cyanosis may be seen immediately after birth.
2. Signs of CHF develop within several days to weeks after birth.
3. History of dyspnea with feeding, failure to thrive, and frequent respiratory infections is usually present in infants.

Physical Examination

1. Varying degrees of cyanosis and signs of CHF with tachypnea and dyspnea are usually present.
2. The peripheral pulses are bounding, with a wide pulse pressure. The precordium is hyperactive and the apical impulse is displaced laterally.
3. A systolic click is frequently audible at the apex and upper left sternal border. The S2 is single. A harsh (grade 2 to 4/6), regurgitant systolic murmur, which suggests VSD, is usually audible along the left sternal border. An apical diastolic rumble with or without gallop rhythm may be present when the PBF is large. A high-pitched, early diastolic, decrescendo murmur of truncal valve regurgitation may be audible. Rarely is a continuous murmur heard over either side of the chest.

Electrocardiography. The QRS axis is normal (+50 to +120 degrees). BVH is present in 70% of cases; RVH or LVH is less common. Left atrial hypertrophy (LAH) is occasionally present.

X-ray Studies. Cardiomegaly is usually present, with increased pulmonary vascularity. A right aortic arch is seen in 30% of cases.

Echocardiography. Two-dimensional and Doppler echo show the following. The first three findings are diagnostic.

1. A large VSD is imaged directly under the truncal valve, similar to that seen in TOF.
2. A large, single great artery arises from the heart (i.e., truncus arteriosus). The type of persistent truncus arteriosus can be identified, and the size of the PAs can be determined. An artery, branching posteriorly from the truncus, is the PA.
3. The pulmonary valve cannot be imaged; only one semilunar valve (i.e., truncal valve) is imaged.

4. Cross-sectional imaging may determine the number of sinuses (usually three, although it may be two or four) of the truncal valve and the presence or absence of stenosis or regurgitation of the valve.

5. Right aortic arch is frequently present. Interruption of the aortic arch is occasionally present, which is difficult to image.

NATURAL HISTORY

1. Most infants present with CHF during the first 2 weeks; 85% of untreated children die by 1 year of age.

2. Clinical improvement occurs if the infant develops pulmonary vascular obstructive disease, which may begin to occur by 3 to 4 months of age. Death occurs around the third decade of life.

3. Truncal valve insufficiency worsens with time.

MANAGEMENT

Medical

1. Vigorous anticongestive measures with digitalis and diuretics should be pursued before an operation is undertaken.

2. Because of the frequent association of DiGeorge syndrome:
   a. Serum calcium and magnesium levels should be checked; their supplementation may be indicated.
   b. Only irradiated blood product should be used for an urgent surgery (because of insufficient time for evaluation of immune status accurately).
   c. Because of the thymus-based immune deficiency, treatment and prophylaxis against pneumococcal and streptococcal infections are important.
   d. Immunization with live vaccine should be avoided.

3. Prophylaxis against SBE should be observed when indications arise.

Surgical

Palliative Procedures. Although PA banding was performed in the past in small infants with large PBF and CHF, primary repair of the defect is currently recommended by many centers. The banding produces distortion of the PAs and does not necessarily prevent pulmonary vascular obstructive disease. The procedure is associated with a high mortality rate, as high as 30%.

Definitive Procedure

1. Various modifications of the Rastelli procedure are performed. Ideally, surgery should be undertaken within the first week of life. When the diagnosis is delayed, surgery should be performed on an urgent basis following 2 to 3 days of medical stabilization.

2. For all types, the VSD is closed in such a way that the LV ejects into the truncus. The surgical mortality rate is 10% to 30%. Careful investigation of coronary artery anomalies and avoidance of surgical interruption of the coronary arteries are important.
   a. For type I, an aortic homograft (with internal diameter of 9 to 11 mm) is placed between the RV and the PA (Fig. 14–59).
   b. For types II and III, a circumferential band of the truncus, which contains both PA orifices, is removed. This cuff is tailored and then connected to the RV by the use of a homograft. Aortic continuity is restored with a tubular Dacron graft (Fig. 14–60).
   c. When associated with an interrupted aortic arch, aortic reconstruction is done by anastomosis of the proximal and distal aortas. The RPA is brought anterior to the ascending aorta (Lecompte maneuver) to prevent compression on the RPA. Using a homograft, the RV and the PA are connected.

3. The regurgitant truncal valve is almost always amenable to various repair techniques. A prolapsing vestigial leaflet can be supported by suturing to the adjacent leaflet

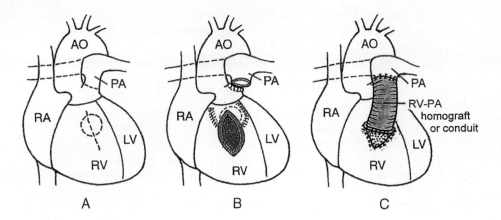

Figure 14–59. *Operative technique for type I truncus arteriosus.* **A,** *Truncus arteriosus type I is shown with a large ventricular septal defect (VSD; broken circle) directly under the truncal valve. The vertical broken line on the right ventricle (RV) is the site of the right ventriculotomy.* **B,** *The pulmonary artery (PA) trunk has been cut away from the truncal artery, and the opening in the truncal artery is sutured to the truncal artery. Patch closure of the VSD (which is visible through the ventriculotomy) is completed in such a way that only left ventricular blood goes out to the truncal artery (creating the left ventricle [LV]–to–truncal artery pathway).* **C,** *A valved conduit or homograft is anastomosed to the pulmonary trunk. The posterior half of the proximal conduit is anastomosed to the upper end of the ventriculotomy. A small pericardial patch is trimmed and sutured into place to fill the defect between the allograft and the lower end of the right ventriculotomy. AO, aorta; RA, right atrium.*

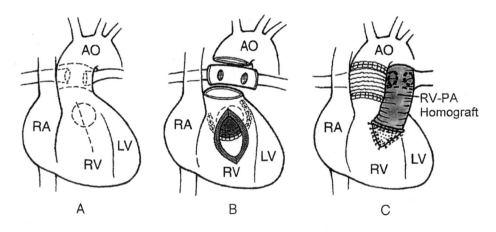

Figure 14–60. *Operative technique for types II and III truncus arteriosus.* **A,** *Two broken lines on the truncal artery indicate the sites of excision of the pulmonary arteries (PAs). The vertical broken line is the site of the right ventriculotomy. A ventricular septal defect (VSD) is under the truncal valve (broken circle).* **B,** *The VSD is closed with a patch through a right ventriculotomy (which is visible through the ventriculotomy) in such a way that the truncal artery receives blood only from the left ventricle (LV) (LV-to-truncus pathway). The cuff of truncal tissue, including the PA orifices, has been excised and trimmed.* **C,** *Continuity of the truncal artery, which is now the aorta (AO), has been restored with a Dacron graft. The lower end of a homograft has been anastomosed to the right ventriculotomy, and the upper end of the homograft has been anastomosed to the cuff containing the PAs. RA, right atrium; RV, right ventricle.*

(closure of a commissure). Truncal valve replacement is indicated if there is significant truncal valve insufficiency. It has an extremely high mortality rate of 50% or greater.

Postoperative Follow-up

1. Follow-up every 4 to 12 months is required to detect late complications, either natural or postoperative.
    a. Progressive truncal valve insufficiency may develop, and truncal valve repair or replacement may be needed.
    b. A small conduit needs to be changed to a larger size, usually by 2 to 3 years of age.
    c. Calcification of the valve in the conduit may occur within 1 to 5 years, which requires reoperation.
    d. Ventricular arrhythmias may develop because of right ventriculotomy.
2. Balloon dilatation and stent implantation in the RV-to-PA conduit can prolong conduit longevity and delay the need to replace the conduit surgically.
3. For older children who received a larger sized conduit and develop valvular regurgitation following balloon dilatation of the conduit valve, a nonsurgical percutaneous pulmonary valve implantation technique has been developed by Bonhoeffer and colleagues (2000), and this technique has been used successfully in Europe (see further discussion under TOF with pulmonary atresia in this chapter).
4. SBE prophylaxis should be observed throughout life.
5. The patient should not participate in competitive, strenuous sports.

Single Ventricle

PREVALENCE

Single ventricle (double-inlet ventricle) occurs in less than 1% of all congenital heart defects.

PATHOLOGY

1. Both AV valves are connected to a main, single ventricular chamber (i.e., double-inlet ventricle), and the main chamber is in turn connected to a rudimentary chamber through the bulboventricular foramen. One great artery arises from the main chamber, and the other arises from the rudimentary chamber (Fig. 14–61). In about 80% of cases, the main ventricular chamber has anatomic characteristics of the LV (i.e., double-inlet LV). Occasionally, the main chamber has anatomic characteristics of the RV (i.e., double-inlet RV). Rarely does the ventricle have an

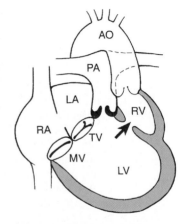

Figure 14–61. *Diagram of the most common form of single ventricle. The single ventricle is an anatomic left ventricle (LV). The great arteries are transposed, with the aorta (AO) anterior to and left of the pulmonary artery (PA) and arising from the rudimentary right ventricle (RV). Both atrioventricular valves open into the single ventricle (double inlet). The opening between the main and rudimentary ventricles is the bulboventricular foramen (thick arrow). Stenosis of the pulmonary valve is present in about 50% of cases (shown as thick valves). This type accounts for 70% to 75% of cases of single ventricle. LA, left atrium; MV, mitral valve; RA, right atrium; TV, tricuspid valve.*

intermediate trabecular pattern without a rudimentary chamber (i.e., common ventricle). Also, both atria rarely empty through a common AV valve into the main ventricular chamber with either LV or RV morphology (i.e., common-inlet ventricle).

2. Either D-TGA or L-TGA is present in 85% of cases. The most common form of single ventricle is double-inlet LV with L-TGA with the aorta arising from the rudimentary chamber. This type occurs in 70% to 75% of single ventricle (see Fig. 14–61). The mitral valve is right sided; the tricuspid valve is left sided. Pulmonary stenosis or pulmonary atresia is present in about 50% of cases. COA and interrupted aortic arch are also common. Less commonly, D-TGA is present with the aorta arising from the right and anterior rudimentary chamber.

3. The bulboventricular foramen is frequently obstructive.

4. Anomalies of the AV valves are common, which include stenosis, overriding, or straddling.

5. In double-inlet RV, either right or left atrial isomerism and straddling and/or overriding of the AV valves are common. The most frequently encountered ventriculoarterial connection is a double outlet from the main chamber. Pulmonary stenosis is frequently found.

PATHOPHYSIOLOGY

1. Because there is complete mixing in the single ventricle, the systemic arterial saturation is determined primarily by the amount of PBF.
   a. With PS, PBF is decreased and cyanosis is present (with arterial oxygen saturation <85%). With pulmonary atresia, cyanosis is intense at birth.
   b. When the pulmonary valve is not stenotic, the PBF is large and signs of CHF develop within days or weeks without cyanosis; arterial oxygen saturation is nearly 90%.

2. An obstructed bulboventricular foramen may either occur naturally with growth or, for unknown reasons, develop after PA banding. This condition occurs in 70% to 85% of banded patients. The occurrence of an obstructed foramen has a profound hemodynamic effect as well as major surgical implications in patients with the aorta arising from the anterior rudimentary chamber. The obstruction increases PBF and decreases systemic perfusion. The banding also causes excessive hypertrophy of the LV, resulting in decreased compliance of the ventricle, which places the patient at risk for a future Fontan operation.

3. When the dominant ventricle is anatomic LV, ventricular dysfunction is rare. However, when the dominant ventricle is anatomic RV, dilated cardiomyopathy may develop, especially when the condition is associated with progressive AV valve regurgitation.

CLINICAL MANIFESTATIONS

History

1. Cyanosis of varying degrees may be present from birth.

2. History of failure to thrive or pneumonia may be present in infants with increased PBF (signs of CHF).

Physical Examination. Physical findings depend on the magnitude of PBF.

1. With *increased* PBF, physical findings resemble those of TGA and VSD or even those of large VSD:
   a. Mild cyanosis and CHF with growth retardation are present in early infancy.
   b. The S2 is single or narrowly split with a loud P2. A grade 3 to 4/6 long systolic murmur is audible along the left sternal border. A loud S3 or an apical diastolic rumble may also be audible.
   c. A diastolic murmur of PR may be present along the upper left sternal border as a result of pulmonary hypertension.

2. With *decreased* PBF, physical findings resemble those of TOF:
   a. Moderate to severe cyanosis is present. CHF is not present. Clubbing may be seen in older infants and children.
   b. The S2 is loud and single. A grade 2 to 4/6 ejection systolic murmur may be heard at the upper right or left sternal border.

Electrocardiography

1. An unusual ventricular hypertrophy pattern with similar QRS complexes across most or all precordial leads is common (e.g., RS, rS, QR pattern).
2. Abnormal Q waves (representing abnormalities in septal depolarization) are also common and take one of the following forms: Q waves in the right precordial leads, no Q waves in any precordial leads, or Q waves in both the right and left precordial leads.
3. Either first- or second-degree AV block may be present.
4. Arrhythmias occur (e.g., SVT, wandering pacemaker).

X-ray Studies

1. With increased PBF the heart size enlarges and the pulmonary vascularity increases.
2. When PBF is normal or decreased, the heart size is normal and the pulmonary vascularity is normal or decreased.
3. A narrow upper mediastinum suggests that TGA may be present.

Echocardiography

1. The most important diagnostic sign is the presence of a single ventricular chamber into which two AV valves open.
2. The following anatomic and functional information is important from a surgical point of view and should be systematically obtained in each patient with a single ventricle:
   a. Morphology of the single ventricle (e.g., double-inlet LV? double-inlet RV?).
   b. Location of the rudimentary outflow chamber, which is usually left and anterior.
   c. Size of the bulboventricular foramen and whether there is an obstruction at the foramen. Obstruction of the foramen is considered present if the Doppler gradient is more than 1.5 m/sec or if the area of the foramen is less than 2 cm^2/m^2. A foramen that is nearly as large as the aortic annulus is considered ideal.
   d. Presence or absence of D-TGA or L-TGA, stenosis of the pulmonary or aortic valve, and size of the PAs.
   e. Anatomy of the AV valves. The position of the mitral and tricuspid valves, in addition to the presence of stenosis, regurgitation, hypoplasia, or straddling of these valves, should be checked.
   f. The size of the ASD.
   g. Associated defects such as COA, interrupted aortic arch, or PDA.

NATURAL HISTORY

1. In patients without PS, CHF and growth failure develop in early infancy, in association with pulmonary hypertension. Without surgery, about 50% of these patients die before reaching 1 year of age.
2. Patients with increased PBF develop pulmonary vascular obstructive disease after the first year of life with clinical improvement of CHF.
3. Cyanosis increases if PS worsens.
4. If the aorta arises from the rudimentary chamber, the bulboventricular foramen is often small or becomes obstructed. This results in increased PBF and decreased systemic perfusion.
5. Progressive AV valve regurgitation is poorly tolerated.
6. Complete heart block develops in about 12% of patients.

7. SBE or cerebral complications may develop as in TOF.

8. The cause of death can be CHF, arrhythmias, or sudden death.

MANAGEMENT

Initial Medical Management

1. Newborns with severe PS or pulmonary atresia and those with interrupted aortic arch or coarctation require PGE_1 infusion and other supportive measures before surgery.

2. Anticongestive measures with digoxin and diuretics should be taken if CHF develops.

Surgical

1. Initial surgical palliative procedures
   a. Blalock-Taussig shunt is necessary for cyanotic patients with PS or pulmonary atresia (see Fig. 14–22). A sternotomy approach is preferable to a thoracotomy approach as the former results in a lower rate of distortion of the PA. Shunt to the right PA is preferable because any distortion of the RPA can be incorporated later in the Fontan anastomosis. The mortality rate remains low (5% to 10%). In PGE_1-dependent neonates, PDA is ligated after placement of the shunt.
   b. PA banding is considered for infants with CHF and pulmonary edema resulting from increased PBF, although banding carries a high mortality rate—around 25% or even higher. The major risk factor is the presence or development of an obstructed bulboventricular foramen. Most infants with obstructed foramen do not tolerate the banding well. Therefore, PA banding is performed only when the bulboventricular foramen is *normal* or *unobstructed*. However, these patients should be watched for the development of obstruction after the banding.
   c. If the bulboventricular foramen is too *small*, one of the following two procedures may be performed, rather than the PA banding. A high mortality rate remains:
      1). The Damus-Kaye-Stansel operation is the preferred procedure in the absence of pulmonary or subpulmonary stenosis. It involves a PA-to-aorta anastomosis, which is accomplished by transection of the main PA and anastomosis of the proximal PA to the ascending aorta. This operation is combined with Blalock-Taussig shunt (Fig. 14–62), single ventricle to PA (Sano) shunt

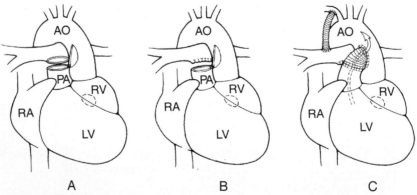

    A   B   C

Figure 14–62. Damus-Kaye-Stansel anastomosis for single ventricle and subaortic stenosis. A, The pulmonary artery (PA) is transected proximal to the bifurcation. An appropriately positioned and sized incision is made in the ascending aorta (AO). B, The distal end of the PA is oversewn and the proximal end of the PA is anastomosed to the opening in the aorta. C, An appropriately shaped hood (Dacron tube, pericardium, allograft, or Gore-Tex) is added to the anastomosis. A Blalock-Taussig shunt has been completed. A Sano shunt can be placed instead (not shown here). LV, left ventricle; RA, right atrium; RV, right ventricle.

(which has become more popular), or bidirectional Glenn shunt (see Fig. 14–38A). A Fontan-type operation can be performed later (see Fig. 14–38B).

2). Another option involves enlargement of the bulboventricular foramen by a transaortic approach and without cardiopulmonary bypass. This procedure is performed especially when PS is present. The surgical mortality rate is about 15%.

   d. Surgery for interrupted aortic arch or coarctation should be performed, if present.
   e. The infant should be watched carefully until the time of the second-stage pallia-tion for cyanosis (with O_2 saturation <75%) or signs of CHF (too large a PBF for which tightening of the PA band should be considered).

2. Second-stage surgical palliative procedures
   a. A bidirectional Glenn operation (or bidirectional cavopulmonary connection) (see Fig. 14–38) is carried out between the ages of 3 and 6 months, before proceed-ing with the Fontan operation. There appears to be no advantage in further delay-ing the second-stage operation beyond 6 months. Alternatively, a hemi-Fontan procedure can be performed (see Fig. 14–39) (see "Tricuspid Atresia" for further discussion of the procedures).
   b. After the second-stage surgical procedure, the child needs to be followed up with attention to the O_2 saturation. Initially there is a remarkable improvement in O_2 saturation (approximately 85%), but a gradual deterioration in O_2 saturation may occur in the months postoperatively (related to opening of venous collaterals that decompress the upper body and/or the development of pulmonary AV fistula). If the child's O_2 saturation is 75% or less, one may proceed with the Fontan procedure. Cardiac catheterization is performed by 12 months after the second-stage operation. Ideal candidates should have low mean PA pressure (<16 to 18 mm Hg), low PVR (<2 units), and low end diastolic pressure less than 12 mm Hg. (see Box 14–2).

3. Definitive procedures. The Fontan-type operation is performed at 18 to 24 months of age. Many centers consider a lateral tunnel Fontan procedure (also called cavopul-monary connection) the procedure of choice (see Figs. 14–38B and 14–40). Some cen-ters make a 4- to 6-mm fenestration in the baffle and others do not. Some centers prefer the extracardiac conduit modification of the Fontan procedure. If an AV valve is incompetent, it may need to be closed during surgery. The surgical mortality rate of the Fontan-type operation has been reduced to 5% to 10%, similar to that for tri-cuspid atresia.

   Some centers recommend device closure of the fenestration a year or so after the Fontan procedure. However, about 20% to 40% of fenestrations close spontaneously over the first year or two postoperatively.

Postoperative Follow-up

1. Close follow-up is necessary for early and late complications, which have been discussed in detail under "Tricuspid Atresia."

2. Some survivors of surgery, if performed late, remain symptomatic with cyanosis, dyspnea as a result of ventricular dysfunction, and arrhythmias. These symptoms require regular follow-up. Early surgery as outlined previously tends to reduce unfavorable results.

3. Antibiotic prophylaxis against SBE should be observed whenever necessary.

The surgical approach for single ventricle is shown in Figure 14–63.

Double-Outlet Right Ventricle

PREVALENCE

DORV occurs in less than 1% of all congenital heart defects. DORV occurs frequently in patients with heterotaxy in association with other complex cardiac defects.

Single Ventricle

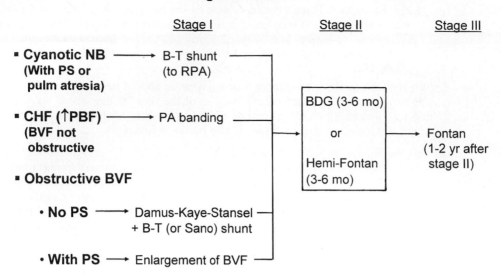

Figure 14–63. Surgical approach for single ventricle. BDG, bidirectional Glenn; B-T, Blalock-Taussig; BVF, bulboventricular foramen; CHF, congestive heart failure; NB, newborn; PBF, pulmonary blood flow, PS, pulmonary stenosis; RPA, right pulmonary artery.

PATHOLOGY

1. Both the aorta and the PA arise from the RV. The only outlet from the LV is a large VSD.

2. The great arteries usually lie side by side. The aorta is usually to the right of the PA, although one of the great arteries may be more anterior than the other. The aortic and pulmonary valves are at the same level. Conus septum is present between the aorta and the PA. The subaortic and subpulmonary coni separate the aortic and pulmonary valves from the tricuspid and mitral valves, respectively. This means that there is no fibrous continuity between the semilunar valves and the AV valves. In a normal heart, the aortic valve is lower than the pulmonary valve, and the aortic valve is in fibrous continuity with the mitral valve.

3. The position of the VSD and the presence or absence of PS (or RVOT obstruction) influence hemodynamic alterations and form the basis for dividing the defect into the following types of DORV (Fig. 14–64):
   a. Subaortic VSD. The VSD is closer to the aortic valve than to the pulmonary valve and lies to the right of the conus septum (see Fig. 14–64A). This is the most common type, occurring in 55% to 70% of cases. RVOT obstruction is common, occurring in about 50% of patients with this type of DORV (Fallot type). RVOT obstruction is most commonly due to infundibular stenosis, but rarely pure valvular pulmonary stenosis can occur with small annulus (see Fig. 14–64B).
   b. Subpulmonary VSD (i.e., Taussig-Bing syndrome) (see Fig. 14–64C). The VSD is closer to the pulmonary valve than to the aortic valve, and it usually lies above the crista supraventricularis and to the left of the conus septum. This type accounts for approximately 10% to 30% of cases.
   c. Doubly committed VSD. The VSD is closely related to both semilunar valves and is usually above the crista supraventricularis (<5% of cases).
   d. Noncommitted (or remote) VSD. The VSD is clearly away from the semilunar valves (about 10% of cases). It most commonly represents the AV canal–type VSD

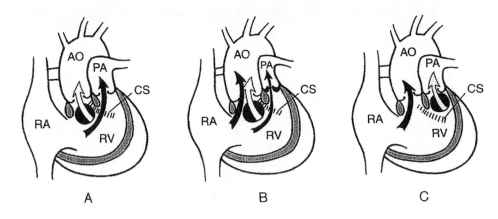

Figure 14–64. Diagram of three representative types of double-outlet right ventricle (RV), viewed with the free wall of the RV removed. **A,** Subaortic ventricular septal defect (VSD). **B,** Subaortic VSD with pulmonary stenosis. **C,** Subpulmonary VSD (Taussig-Bing syndrome). Doubly committed and remote VSDs are not shown. AO, aorta; CS, crista supraventricularis; PA, pulmonary artery; RA, right atrium.

and occasionally an isolated muscular VSD. Atrial isomerism is commonly seen with this type.

4. Sometimes, surgeons' and pathologists' definitions of DORV are different and are a source of confusion. Some cases of TOF with marked overriding of the aorta may be called DORV by surgeons because the mitral-aortic fibrous continuity is not always clear in the operating room. Surgeons use the so-called 50% rule: when the aortic annulus overlies the RV at least 50%, it is called DORV.

PATHOPHYSIOLOGY AND CLINICAL MANIFESTATIONS

The pathophysiology and clinical manifestations of DORV are determined primarily by the position of the VSD and the presence or absence of PS. Each type is presented separately.

1. Subaortic VSD without pulmonary stenosis. In subaortic VSD, oxygenated blood from the LV is directed to the aorta, and desaturated systemic venous blood is directed to the PA, producing mild or no cyanosis (see Fig. 14–64A). The PBF increases in the absence of PS, and CHF may result. Therefore, clinical pictures of this type resemble those of a large VSD with pulmonary hypertension and CHF.
   a. Growth retardation, tachypnea, and other signs of CHF are usually present. A hyperactive precordium, a loud S2, and a VSD-type (holosystolic or early systolic) murmur are present. An apical diastolic rumble may be audible.
   b. The ECG often resembles that of complete endocardial cushion defect. Superior QRS axis (i.e., −30 to −170 degrees) may be found in this type. RVH or BVH, as well as LAH, is common. Occasionally, first-degree AV block is present.
   c. Chest x-ray images show cardiomegaly with increased pulmonary vascular markings and a prominent PA segment.

2. Subaortic VSD with pulmonary stenosis (Fallot type). Even though the VSD is subaortic, in the presence of PS (or RVOT obstruction), some desaturated blood goes to the aorta. This causes cyanosis and a decrease in PBF. Clinical pictures resemble those of TOF (see Fig. 14–64B).
   a. Growth retardation and cyanosis are common. The S2 is loud and single. A grade 2 to 4/6 midsystolic (ejection) murmur along the left sternal border is present, either with or without a systolic thrill.
   b. The ECG shows RAD, RAH, RVH, or RBBB. First-degree AV block is frequent.

c. Chest x-ray images show normal heart size with an upturned apex. Pulmonary vascularity is decreased.

3. Subpulmonary VSD (Taussig-Bing syndrome). In subpulmonary VSD, or Taussig-Bing syndrome, oxygenated blood from the LV is directed to the PA, and desaturated blood from the systemic vein is directed to the aorta. This results in severe cyanosis (see Fig. 14–64C). The PBF increases with the fall of the PVR. Clinical pictures resemble those of TGA.

   a. Growth retardation and severe cyanosis with or without clubbing are common findings. The S2 is loud, and a grade 2 to 3/6 systolic murmur is audible at the upper left sternal border. An ejection click and an occasional PR murmur (as a result of pulmonary hypertension) may be audible.

   b. The ECG shows RAD, RAH, and RVH. LVH may be seen during infancy.

   c. Chest x-ray images show cardiomegaly with increased pulmonary vascular markings and a prominent PA segment.

4. Doubly committed or noncommitted ventricular septal defect. With the VSD close to both semilunar valves (called *doubly committed VSD*), or remotely located from these valves (*noncommitted VSD*), cyanosis of a mild degree is present and the PBF increases.

Echocardiography. Three diagnostic signs of DORV are the origin of both great arteries from the anterior RV, the absence of LV outflow other than the VSD, and the discontinuity of the mitral and semilunar valves.

1. In the parasternal long-axis view, all three diagnostic features of DORV are imaged. Typical subaortic or subpulmonary VSD can be demonstrated in this view for most patients (Fig. 14–65). No great artery is seen to arise from the posterior ventricle. The great arteries arising from the anterior ventricle are seen in parallel orientation. In addition, a mass of echo-positive tissue, usually more than 5 mm in length, is present between the mitral valve annulus and the semilunar valve (i.e., mitral-semilunar discontinuity).

2. In the parasternal short-axis view, a "double circle" rather than the normal "circle and sausage" appearance of the great arteries may be seen. Either the great arteries are side by side with the aorta to the right or the aorta is anterior and slightly to the right of the PA.

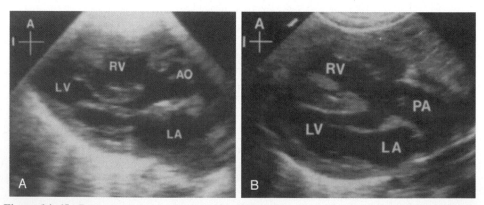

*Figure 14–65. Parasternal long-axis view of double-outlet right ventricle. **A**, Subaortic ventricular septal defect (VSD). The VSD is closely related to the aorta (AO). The marked separation between the anterior mitral valve leaflet and the aortic valve can be seen. The aorta overrides the ventricular septum by more than 50%. **B**, Subpulmonary VSD. The great artery that is closely related to the VSD has an immediate posterior sweep, suggesting that it is a pulmonary artery (PA). Note the separation between the anterior mitral valve leaflet and the pulmonary valve. The PA overrides the ventricular septum by more than 50%. LA, left atrium; LV, left ventricle; RV, right ventricle. (**A** from Snider AR, Serwer GA: Echocardiography in Pediatric Heart Disease. St. Louis, Mosby, 1990; **B** from Snider AR: Two-dimensional and Doppler echocardiographic evaluation of heart disease in the neonate and fetus. Clin Perinatol 15:523–565, 1988.)*

3. The size and position of the VSD should be determined in relation to the great arteries.
   a. Typical subpulmonary or subaortic VSD can be demonstrated by parasternal long-axis scanning in most patients (see Fig. 14–65).
   b. In the subcostal four-chamber view, the subaortic VSD is located to the right of the conus septum just beneath the aortic valve. The subpulmonary VSD is located to the left of the conus septum just beneath the pulmonary valve.
   c. Doubly committed VSD is recognized in the parasternal or the apical long-axis view.
   d. Noncommitted (remote) VSDs, either endocardial cushion type or apical muscular VSD, are best recognized in the apical four-chamber view.

4. Associated anomalies such as valvular and/or subvalvular PS and other left-to-right shunt lesions (e.g., ASD, PDA) should be looked for.

5. Occasionally, differentiation of DORV from TOF with a marked overriding of the aorta or from TGA is necessary. There is mitral-semilunar continuity in TOF and TGA (i.e., mitral-aortic continuity in TOF, and mitral-pulmonary continuity in TGA), but no mitral-semilunar continuity is present in DORV.

NATURAL HISTORY

1. Infants without PS may develop severe CHF and later pulmonary vascular obstructive disease if left untreated. Spontaneous closure of VSD, which is fatal, is rare.

2. When PS is present, complications common to cyanotic congenital heart defects (e.g., polycythemia, cerebrovascular accident) may develop.

3. In patients with the Taussig-Bing malformation, severe pulmonary vascular obstructive disease develops early in life, as seen in patients with D-TGA.

4. Associated anomalies (e.g., COA, LV hypoplasia) also contribute to the poor prognosis.

MANAGEMENT

Medical

1. Treatment of CHF with digoxin and diuretics is indicated.

2. Antibiotic prophylaxis against SBE should be observed.

Surgical

Palliative Procedures

1. PA banding for symptomatic infants with increased PBF and CHF is occasionally performed in infants with multiple muscular VSD or a remote VSD. However, this procedure is not recommended for infants with subaortic VSD or doubly committed VSD. Primary repair is a better choice.

2. For infants with the Taussig-Bing type, enlarging the interatrial communication is important for better mixing and for decompressing the LA, which causes pulmonary venous congestion. Balloon or blade atrial septostomy should be considered.

3. In infants with PS and decreased PBF with cyanosis, a systemic-to-PA shunt procedure is occasionally indicated.

Definitive Surgeries

Subaortic or Doubly Committed VSD. An intraventricular tunnel between the VSD and the subaortic outflow tract is created by means of a Dacron patch. This procedure is performed early in life, preferably during the neonatal period or at least in early infancy, without preliminary PA banding. Sometimes, the RVOT may have to be augmented with an outflow patch if the VSD-AO tunnel obstructs the RV outflow tract. The mortality rate is less than 5% for simple subaortic VSD; it is slightly higher for doubly committed VSD.

Fallot Type. There are three surgical options. Surgical repair is generally advised by 6 months of age, preferably during the neonatal period. However, if the patient's condition is poor or if there are major associated noncardiac anomalies, an initial shunt operation is an option.

1. Tunnel VSD closure plus Rastelli operation. An intraventricular tunnel between the VSD and the aorta is established and a Rastelli operation is performed to relieve PS using either a pulmonary or aortic homograft conduit.

2. REV procedure. The réparation à l'étage ventriculaire (REV), which is similar to an arterial switch operation, may be performed. In the REV procedure, the proximal ascending aorta and main PA are transected and the proximal stump of the PA is oversewn (see Fig. 14–9, which is performed for D-TGA plus VSD plus PS, a situation very similar to this one). The pulmonary arteries are translocated anterior to the aorta (Lecompte maneuver) and the ascending aorta is reconnected. The distal PA is anastomosed directly to the upper margin of the infundibular incision. Autologous pericardium forms the anterior portion of the pathway. The hospital mortality is 18%.

3. Nikaidoh procedure. This combines the principle of the Ross procedure and the Konno operation. The aortic root including the aortic valve is detached in the same manner as done to the pulmonary root in the Ross procedure. The PA is divided and the pulmonary valve is excised. The pulmonary root is divided and the conal septum above the VSD is excised, which creates a large opening to the LV cavity. The aortic root is translocated posteriorly and sutured to the open orifice of the pulmonary annulus. A pericardial patch is used to connect the lower margin of the VSD and the anterior circumference of the harvested aortic root, completing the LV to AO connection. A pericardial gusset completes the connection of the RV and the distal end of the MPA (see Fig. 14–10, which has been described for D-TGA plus VSD plus PS).

Taussig-Bing Anomaly (Subpulmonary Ventricular Septal Defect). There are four possible surgical approaches. These operations should be carried out by 3 to 4 months of age or sooner because of the rapid development of pulmonary vascular obstructive disease in this subtype.

1. The procedure of choice is the creation of an intraventricular tunnel between the VSD and the PA (resulting in TGA), which is then corrected by the arterial switch operation. The mortality rate is between 5% and 15%.

2. Creation of an intraventricular tunnel between the VSD and the PA is followed by the Senning operation. This is a less desirable approach because of a high mortality rate (>40%) and a higher late complication rate associated with the Senning procedure.

3. An intraventricular tunnel between the VSD and the aorta is desirable but often technically impossible. The surgical mortality rate is about 15%.

4. Creation of VSD-to-PA tunnel, followed by Damus-Kaye-Stansel operation and RV-to-PA conduit, is another possibility.

Noncommitted VSD. When possible, an intraventricular tunnel procedure between the AV canal–type VSD and the aorta is performed, but the mortality rate is high (30% to 40%). PA banding is usually needed in infancy to control CHF, and the surgery may be delayed until 2 to 3 years of age.

Postoperative Follow-up. Long-term, regular follow-up at 6- to 12-month intervals is necessary to detect and manage late complications of surgery.

1. In general, patients who had subaortic VSD without PS have an excellent long-term outlook.

2. Ventricular arrhythmia should be treated because it may cause sudden death.

3. About 20% of patients require reoperation of the intraventricular tunnel.

4. Continued SBE prophylaxis is necessary for most patients who have had repair of DORV.

The surgical approach for DORV is illustrated in Figure 14–66.

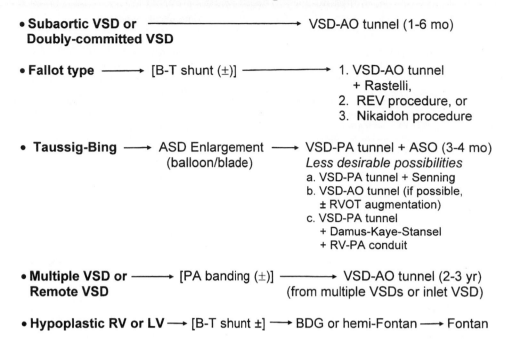

Figure 14–66. Surgical approach for double-outlet right ventricle. AO, aorta; ASD, atrial septal defect; ASO, arterial switch operation; B-T, Blalock-Taussig; PA, pulmonary artery; REV, réparation à l'étage ventriculaire; RV, right ventricle; RVOT, right ventricular outflow tract; RV-PA, RV–to–pulmonary artery; VSD, ventricular septal defect; VSD-AO, VSD-to-aorta; VSD-PA, VSD-to-PA.

Heterotaxia (Atrial Isomerism, Splenic Syndromes)

There is a failure of differentiation into right-sided and left-sided organs in heterotaxia (splenic syndrome or atrial isomerism), with resulting congenital malformations of multiple organ systems including complex malformation of the cardiovascular system. Asplenia syndrome (Ivemark's syndrome, right atrial isomerism) is associated with absence of the spleen, which is a left-sided organ, and a tendency for bilateral right-sidedness. In polysplenia syndrome (left atrial isomerism), multiple splenic tissues are present, with a tendency for bilateral left-sidedness.

There is a striking tendency for symmetrical development of normally asymmetrical organs or pairs of organs. Members of paired organs, such as the lungs, commonly show pronounced isomerism; unpaired organs, such as the stomach, seem to be located in a random fashion. Table 14–4 compares cardiovascular abnormalities in asplenia and polysplenia syndromes. Although the type and severity of cardiovascular malformations differ as a group between the two syndromes, the same types of defects are present in both. The abnormalities that help differentiate the two are shown with asterisks, but probably the most significant differential power is the IVC, which is almost always normal with asplenia syndrome but is interrupted (with azygos continuation) with polysplenia. In general, cardiovascular abnormalities are much more severe in patients with asplenia than in those with polysplenia.

There are some noncardiac findings that suggest heterotaxia. Because of the symmetry of paired organs, normally different right- and left-sided organs show the same morphology. Some clinical findings available to general physicians that may lead to the recognition of heterotaxia include the following.

Table 14–4. **Cardiovascular Malformations in Asplenia and Polysplenia Syndromes**

Structure	Asplenia Syndrome	Polysplenia Syndrome
Systemic veins	Bilateral SVC (65%); single SVC usually right (35%)	Bilateral SVC (33%); single SVC right or left (66%)
	Normal IVC in all, but may be left-sided (35%); (interrupted IVC extremely rare)	*Interrupted IVC (absent hepatic segment of IVC) with azygos continuation right or left (85%)
	†IVC and aorta on the same side, either right or left	Juxtaposition of IVC and aorta occasionally
	Normal hepatic veins to IVC (75%)	Bilateral, common hepatic vein to RA or LA
Pulmonary veins	*TAPVR with *extracardiac* connection—supracardiac or infracardiac—(>80%), often with PV obstruction	†Normal PV return (50%); Right PVs to right-sided atrium and left PVs to left-sided atrium (50%) (but not extracardiac)
Coronary sinus	Absent coronary sinus (most)	Absent coronary sinus (most)
Atrium and atrial septum	Bilateral right atria (with bilateral sinus node)	Bilateral left atria
	†Absent atrial septum (common atrium) common; primum ASD (100%), secundum ASD (66%)	Single (or common) atrium, primum ASD (60%), or secundum ASD (25%)
AV valve	*Common (single) AV valve (90%)	Normal AV valve (50%); single AV valve rare
	Complete AV canal, usually	Partial ECD common (with large primum defect)
Ventricles and cardiac apex	VSD always present	VSD frequent but not always.
	†Single ventricle (50%) usually morphologic RV or undetermined; two ventricles (50%) DORV (>80%)	*Two ventricles usually present; VSD (65%); DORV (20%)
	Left apex (60%); right apex (40%)	Left apex (60%); right apex (40%)
Semilunar valves	†Stenosis (40%) or atresia (40%) of pulmonary valve	Normal pulmonary valve (60%); PS or pulmonary atresia (40%)
Great arteries	*Transposition (70%), either D- or L-	†Normal great arteries (85%); transposition (15%)
ECG	Normal P axis or in the +90 to +180 degree quadrant	†Superior P axis (70%)

*Extremely important differentiating points.
†Important differentiating points.
ASD, atrial septal defect; AV, atrioventricular; DORV, double-outlet right ventricle; IVC, inferior vena cava; PS, pulmonary stenosis; PV, pulmonary venous or vein; RA, right atrium; RV, right ventricle; SVC, superior vena cava; TAPVR, total anomalous pulmonary venous return; VSD, ventricular septal defect.

1. Symmetrical "midline" liver (on palpation or x-ray films)
2. Discordant cardiac apex and stomach bubble (on chest x-ray films)
3. Biliary atresia in a neonate with congenital heart defects
4. Symmetrical main stem bronchi on chest x-rays,
5. Superior P axis (or coronary sinus rhythm) on the ECG

It is important to know which type of isomerism is present from the point of view of prophylaxis against bacterial infection for patients with asplenia syndrome. Patients with asplenia syndrome should be given prophylaxis against infection by encapsulated bacteria with penicillin or amoxicillin as a daily requirement. Immunization against pneumococcus is indicated at age 2 years.

ASPLENIA SYNDROME

Prevalence

Asplenia syndrome occurs in 1% of newborns with symptomatic congenital heart defects. This syndrome occurs more often in males than in females.

Pathology

1. The spleen is absent in asplenia syndrome. A striking tendency for bilateral right-sidedness characterizes malformations of the major organ systems. Bilateral, three-lobed lungs with bilateral, eparterial bronchi (Fig. 14–67); various gastrointestinal

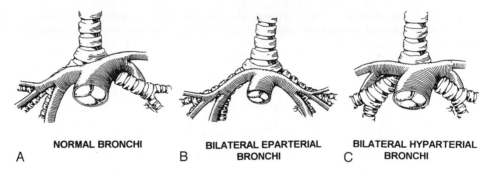

| A | NORMAL BRONCHI | B | BILATERAL EPARTERIAL BRONCHI | C | BILATERAL HYPARTERIAL BRONCHI |

Figure 14–67. Diagrams of normal bronchi (**A**); bilateral eparterial bronchi, usually seen in asplenia syndrome (**B**); and bilateral hyparterial bronchi, usually seen in polysplenia syndrome (**C**). (From Fyler DC, ed: Nadas' Pediatric Cardiology. St. Louis, Mosby, 1992.)

malformations (occurring in 20% of cases); a symmetrical, midline liver; and malrotation of the intestines are all present. The stomach may be located on either the right or the left.

2. Complex cardiac malformations are always present. Cardiovascular malformations involve all parts of the heart, systemic and pulmonary veins, and the great arteries. Two sinoatrial nodes are present. Table 14–4 summarizes and compares these malformations with those of polysplenia syndrome. Cardiovascular anomalies that help distinguish asplenia syndrome from polysplenia syndrome include the following:

  a. A normal IVC is present in asplenia syndrome, whereas the hepatic portion of the IVC is commonly absent (with azygos continuation draining into the SVC) in polysplenia syndrome.

  b. TGA with PS or pulmonary atresia occurs in about 80% of asplenia syndrome cases, producing severe cyanosis during the newborn period. TGA is present in only 15% of patients with polysplenia syndrome.

  c. Single ventricle and common AV valve occur with greater frequency in asplenia syndrome. In polysplenia syndrome, two ventricles are usually present.

  d. TAPVR to *extracardiac* structures occurs in more than 75% of cases of asplenia syndrome, although it is difficult to diagnose. Pulmonary venous return is normal in 50% of patients with polysplenia syndrome.

Pathophysiology

1. Complete mixing of systemic and pulmonary venous blood usually occurs because of the multiple cardiovascular abnormalities associated with this syndrome.

2. PBF is reduced because of stenosis or atresia of the pulmonary valve. This results in severe cyanosis shortly after birth.

3. Although rare, the absence of PS may result in CHF early in life.

Clinical Manifestations

Physical Examination

1. Cyanosis is usually the presenting sign and is often severe.

2. Auscultation of the heart is nonspecific. Heart murmurs of PS and VSD are frequently audible.

3. A symmetrical liver (midline liver) is palpable.

Electrocardiography

1. A superior QRS axis is present as a result of the presence of endocardial cushion defect.

2. The P axis is either normal (0 to +90 degrees) or alternating between the lower left and lower right quadrants. This occurs because two sinus nodes alternate the pacemaker function.

3. RVH, LVH, or BVH is present.

X-ray Studies

1. The heart size is usually normal or slightly increased, with decreased pulmonary vascular markings.

2. The heart is in the right chest, left chest, or midline (mesocardia).

3. A symmetrical liver is a striking feature (see Fig. 4–8).

4. Tracheobronchial symmetry with bilateral, eparterial bronchi is usually identified.

Echocardiography. When the systematic approach is used, two-dimensional echo and color flow Doppler studies can detect all or most of the anomalies described in the section on pathology. The anatomy of the IVC and great arteries and the presence or absence of PS or pulmonary atresia are important in differentiating the two splenic syndromes.

Laboratory Studies

1. Howell-Jolly and Heinz bodies seen on the peripheral smear suggest asplenia syndrome. However, these bodies may be found in some normal newborns and in septic infants, too.

2. A splenic scan may be useful in older infants but is of limited value in extremely ill neonates.

Natural History

Without palliative surgical procedures, more than 95% of patients with asplenia syndrome die within the first year of life. Fulminating sepsis is one cause of death.

Management

Medical

1. In severely cyanotic newborns, PGE_1 infusion is given to reopen the ductus. (If obstructive anomalous pulmonary venous return is suspected, a pulmonary angiogram should be obtained while the ductus is opened by PGE_1 infusion.)

2. The risk of fulminating infection, especially by *Streptococcus pneumoniae*, is high (Red Book, 2006). Continuous oral antibiotic therapy is recommended regardless of immunization status. Oral penicillin V (125 mg, twice a day for children younger than 5 years, and 250 mg, twice a day for children 5 years or older) is recommended. Some experts recommend amoxicillin (20 mg/kg per day, divided into two doses). Erythromycin is an alternative choice in patients who are allergic to penicillin. Prophylactic penicillin can be discontinued at 5 years of age, but other experts continue prophylactic penicillin throughout childhood and into adulthood.

3. Immunizations against *S. pneumoniae*, *Haemophilus influenzae* type b (Hib), and *Neisseria meningitidis* are recommended (Red Book, 2006).
   a. Heptavalent pneumococcal vaccine is indicated for all asplenic children. For children 5 years and younger at diagnosis, the conjugate vaccine (PCV7) is recommended beginning at 2 months of age, times 3 every 2 months, including reimmunization at 12 to 15 months. For children older than 5 years, a single dose of PCV7 or 23PS is recommended.
   b. Immunization against Hib infections should be initiated at 2 months of age, as recommended for otherwise healthy children and for previously unimmunized children with asplenia.
   c. Tetravalent meningococcal polysaccharide vaccine should also be administered to children 2 through 10 years of age. Meningococcal conjugate vaccine should be given to adolescents.

Surgical

1. A systemic-to-PA shunt is usually necessary during the newborn period or infancy. Surgical mortality for the shunt is higher in asplenia patients than in those with other defects, and it is probably related to regurgitation of the common AV valve and undiagnosed obstructive TAPVR.
   a. Patients with common AV valve, especially those with regurgitation of the valve, do not tolerate the volume overload that results from the shunt.
   b. Patients with the obstructive type of TAPVR may show evidence of the anomalous return, with signs of pulmonary edema, only after the systemic-to-PA shunt. Surgical mortality for both the shunt and repair of the TAPVR is unacceptably high in that death occurs in more than 90% of cases.
   c. Identification of infants with obstructive TAPVR by pulmonary angiography with PGE$_1$ infusion before surgery is important. In infants with the infracardiac type of TAPVR, a successful connection can be made between the pulmonary venous confluence and the RA with the use of a partial exclusion clamp and without cardiopulmonary bypass.

2. Although complete anatomic correction of the defect is impossible, a Fontan-type operation can be performed. The overall mortality rate for Fontan-type surgery is as high as 65%. Regurgitation of the AV valve is a high-risk factor, requiring repair or replacement of the valve.

POLYSPLENIA SYNDROME

Prevalence

Polysplenia syndrome (left atrial isomerism) occurs in less than 1% of all congenital heart defects. It occurs more often in females than males.

Pathology

1. Multiple splenic tissues are present. A tendency for bilateral left-sidedness characterizes this syndrome. Noncardiovascular malformations include bilateral, bilobed lungs (i.e., two left lungs); bilateral, hyparterial bronchi (see Fig. 14–67); symmetrical liver (25%); occasional absence of the gallbladder; and some degree of intestinal malrotation (80%).

2. Cardiovascular malformations are similar to those seen in asplenia syndrome but have a lower frequency of pulmonary valve stenosis or atresia. Occasionally, a normal heart or minimal malformation of the heart is present in patients with polysplenia syndrome (approximately 13%). Cardiovascular malformations are summarized and compared with those of asplenia syndrome in Table 14–4. Important features of polysplenia syndrome that distinguish it from asplenia syndrome include the following:
   a. Absence of the hepatic segment of the IVC with azygos (right side) or hemiazygos (left side) continuation is seen in 85% of patients. This abnormality is rarely present in asplenia syndrome.
   b. Two ventricles are usually present. On the contrary, single ventricle with a common AV valve is common in asplenia syndrome.
   c. TGA, PS or pulmonary atresia, and TAPVR occur less often than they do in asplenia syndrome.
   d. The ECG shows a superiorly oriented P axis (i.e., ectopic atrial rhythm), resulting from absence of the sinus node (Fig. 14–68).
   e. Polysplenia syndrome occurs more often in females (70%).

Pathophysiology

Because PS or pulmonary atresia occurs less frequently, cyanosis is not intense, if it is present at all. Rather, CHF often develops because of increased PBF.

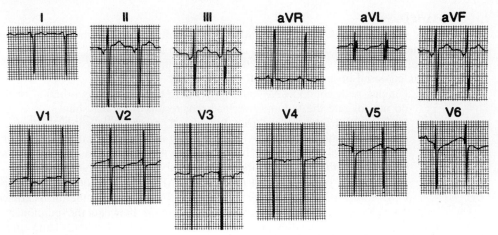

Figure 14–68. Tracing from a 1-week-old neonate with polysplenia syndrome. Both the P and the QRS axes are superiorly oriented (–45 and –150 degrees, respectively). The QRS voltages indicate right ventricular hypertrophy and possible additional left ventricular hypertrophy.

Clinical Manifestations

Physical Examination

1. Cyanosis is either absent or mild. Signs of CHF may develop during the neonatal period.
2. Heart murmur of VSD may be audible. A symmetrical liver is usually palpable.

Electrocardiography (see Fig. 14–68)

1. Ectopic atrial rhythm with a superiorly oriented P axis (–30 to –90 degrees) is seen in more than 70% of patients because there is no sinus node when two left atria are present.
2. A superior QRS axis is present as a result of the presence of endocardial cushion defect.
3. RVH or LVH is common.
4. Complete heart block occurs in about 10% of patients.

X-ray Studies. Mild to moderate cardiomegaly with increased pulmonary vascular markings, midline liver (see Fig. 4–8), and bilateral, hyparterial bronchi may be present.

Laboratory Studies

1. Some patients with splenic hypoplasia and hypofunction may have Howell-Jolly bodies but not in an excessive number.
2. The radioactive splenic scan may show multiple splenic tissues.

Echocardiography. Two-dimensional and Doppler echo studies reveal all or most of the cardiovascular malformations listed in Table 14–4 and help differentiate this syndrome from asplenia syndrome.

Natural History

1. The first-year mortality rate is 60%, in comparison with more than 95% in asplenia syndrome.
2. Most infants with severe cardiac malformations die within the first year without surgical palliation or repair.
3. The heart rate is lower than in normal children. Excessive junctional bradycardia may develop, resulting in CHF.

Management

Medical

1. If present, CHF should be treated.
2. PA banding should be performed if intractable CHF develops with large PBF.

Surgical

1. Occasionally, pacemaker therapy is required for children with excessive AV nodal bradycardia and CHF.
2. Total correction of the defect is possible in some children. If total correction is not possible, at least a Fontan-type operation can be performed. The surgical mortality rate of the Fontan-type operation in this group of children is about 25%, which is lower than that for asplenia but higher than that for tricuspid atresia.

Postoperative Follow-up. Periodic, regular follow-up is necessary because of continuing medical and surgical problems.

1. Although most patients are in New York Heart Association class I or II (see Appendix A, Table A–4), persistent ascites or edema occurs frequently and requires medications such as digoxin, diuretics, and others for several years after the Fontan-type operation.
2. Cardiac arrhythmias, usually supraventricular, are present in 25% of patients. Some require antiarrhythmic medications.

Persistent Pulmonary Hypertension of the Newborn

PREVALENCE

PPHN (or persistence of the fetal circulation) occurs in approximately 1 in 1500 live births.

PATHOLOGY AND PATHOPHYSIOLOGY

1. This neonatal condition is characterized by persistence of pulmonary hypertension, which in turn causes a varying degree of cyanosis from a right-to-left shunt through the PDA or PFO. No other underlying congenital heart defect is present.
2. Various causes have been identified, but they can be divided into three groups by the anatomy of the pulmonary vascular bed (Box 14–3).

BOX 14–3	CAUSES OF PERSISTENT PULMONARY HYPERTENSION OF THE NEWBORN

Pulmonary vasoconstriction in the presence of a normally developed pulmonary vascular bed may be caused by or seen in:
    Alveolar hypoxia (meconium aspiration syndrome, hyaline membrane disease, hypoventilation caused by central nervous system anomalies)
    Birth asphyxia
    Left ventricular dysfunction or circulatory shock
    Infections (such as group B hemolytic streptococcal infection)
    Hyperviscosity syndrome (polycythemia)
    Hypoglycemia and hypocalcemia
Increased pulmonary vascular smooth muscle development (hypertrophy) may be caused by:
    Chronic intrauterine asphyxia
    Maternal use of prostaglandin synthesis inhibitors (aspirin, indomethacin) resulting in early ductal closure
Decreased cross-sectional area of pulmonary vascular bed may be seen in association with:
    Congenital diaphragmatic hernia
    Primary pulmonary hypoplasia

   a. Intense pulmonary vasoconstriction in the presence of a normally developed pulmonary vascular bed. Clinical conditions such as perinatal asphyxia, meconium aspiration, ventricular dysfunction, group B streptococcal pneumonia, hyperviscosity syndrome, and hypoglycemia are frequent causes of pulmonary vasoconstriction. Alveolar hypoxia and acidosis are also important causes of pulmonary vasoconstriction. Thromboxane, vasoconstrictor prostaglandins, leukotrienes, and endothelin may also be important causes of pulmonary vasoconstriction.

   b. Hypertrophy (of the medial layer) of the pulmonary arterioles. Chronic intrauterine hypoxia and maternal ingestion of nonsteroidal anti-inflammatory agents may be important causes of pulmonary arteriolar hypertrophy.

   c. Developmentally abnormal pulmonary arterioles with decreased cross-sectional area of the pulmonary vascular bed. Congenital diaphragmatic hernia and primary pulmonary hypoplasia are examples.

   In general, pulmonary hypertension caused by the first group is relatively easy to reverse, and that caused by the second group is more difficult to reverse than that caused by the first group. Pulmonary hypertension caused by the third group is most difficult or impossible to reverse.

3. Varying degrees of myocardial dysfunction often occur in association with PPHN, manifested by a decrease in contractility or TR, which are caused by global or subendocardial ischemia and are worsened by hypoglycemia and hypocalcemia.

CLINICAL MANIFESTATIONS

1. Symptoms begin 6 to 12 hours after birth, with cyanosis and respiratory difficulties (with retraction and grunting). The idiopathic form usually affects full-term or post-term neonates. The patient usually has a history of meconium staining or birth asphyxia. A history of maternal ingestion of nonsteroidal anti-inflammatory drugs (in the third trimester) may be elicited.

2. A prominent RV impulse and a single and loud S2 are usually found. Occasional gallop rhythm (from myocardial dysfunction) and a soft regurgitant systolic murmur of TR may be audible. Severe cases of myocardial dysfunction may manifest with systemic hypotension.

3. Arterial desaturation is found in blood samples obtained from an umbilical artery catheter. Arterial Po_2 may be lower in the descending aorta (the umbilical artery line) than in the preductal arteries (the right radial, brachial, or temporal artery) by 5 to 10 mm Hg because of a right-to-left ductal shunt. In severe cases, differential cyanosis may appear (with a pink upper body and a cyanotic lower body). If there is a prominent right-to-left intracardiac shunt, usually through the PFO, the preductal and postductal arteries may not show a Po_2 difference.

4. The ECG is usually normal for age but occasional RVH is present. T-wave abnormalities suggestive of myocardial dysfunction may be seen.

5. Chest x-ray films reveal a varying degree of cardiomegaly. The lung fields may be free of abnormal findings or may show hyperinflation or atelectasis. The pulmonary vascular markings may appear normal, increased, or decreased.

6. Echo and Doppler studies are indicated to rule out congenital heart defects and to identify patients with myocardial dysfunction. Patients with PPHN have no evidence of cyanotic heart defect. The only structural abnormality is the presence of a large PDA with a right-to-left or bidirectional shunt. The RV is enlarged with a flattened interventricular septum. There is evidence of increased RA pressures (with the atrial septum bulging toward the left) with or without an ASD or PFO. The aortic arch is normal, with no evidence of COA or an interrupted aortic arch. Imaging shows normal drainage of pulmonary veins. (TAPVR can mimic PPHN.) The LV dimension may be increased, and its systolic function (fractional shortening or ejection fraction) may be decreased.

7. Cardiac catheterization is usually not indicated. If the diagnosis is unclear or the patient does not respond to therapy, cardiac catheterization and pulmonary arteriography are rarely considered.

MANAGEMENT

The goals of therapy are (1) to lower the PVR and PA pressure through the administration of oxygen, the induction of respiratory alkalosis, and the use of pulmonary vasodilators; (2) to correct myocardial dysfunction; and (3) to stabilize the patient and treat associated conditions.

1. General supportive therapy includes monitoring oxygen saturation; detecting and treating hypoglycemia, hypocalcemia, hypomagnesemia, and polycythemia; and maintaining body temperature between 98°F and 99°F (36.6°C and 37.2°C).

2. To increase arterial Po_2 levels, 100% oxygen is administered, initially without intubation. If this is not successful, intubation plus continuous positive airway pressure at 2 to 10 cm of water may be effective.

3. If the previous measures are not successful, mechanical ventilation with 100% oxygen is used to produce respiratory alkalosis. Ventilator settings are initially set to achieve Po_2 of 50 to 70 mm Hg and Pco_2 of 50 to 55 mm Hg. Extreme respiratory alkalosis with hypocarbia (with constriction of cerebral vasculature) has been associated with later neurologic deficit and sensorineuronal hearing loss. The patient is usually paralyzed with pancuronium (Pavulon) at 0.1 mg/kg intravenously. However, use of paralytic agents is controversial because it may promote atelectasis of dependent lung regions with resulting ventilation-perfusion mismatch. Paralysis may also be associated with sensorineuronal hearing loss. When relative normoxemia has been achieved for 12 to 24 hours, careful weaning can be begun, one ventilator setting at a time.

4. Maintaining a normal or alkaline pH level can also be achieved with the use of sodium bicarbonate, or tromethamine (Tham) infusion may promote pulmonary vasodilatation and improve oxygenation.

5. Tolazoline (Priscoline), a nonselective α-adrenergic antagonist, is sometimes used. A loading dose of 0.5 to 1.0 mg/kg by slow intravenous administration is followed by intravenous infusion of 2 to 4 mg/kg per hour. Tolazoline, being a nonselective vasodilator, also lowers systemic vascular resistance, resulting in systemic hypotension. One must carefully monitor blood pressure and maintain adequate circulating blood volume. Systemic hypotension is treated with volume expanders and dopamine infusion. Other side effects of tolazoline include increased gastric secretion, gastrointestinal bleeding, decreased platelet counts, and decreased urine output. Cimetidine (a histamine H_2 receptor antagonist) is not recommended because it may block the action of histamine, which is a known pulmonary vasodilator.

6. For myocardial dysfunction, the following therapy is provided:
   a. Dopamine is used with tolazoline to improve cardiac output. The usual dose of dopamine is 10 μg/kg per minute by intravenous infusion.
   b. Dobutamine (a β-adrenergic agent) may be used if signs of CHF are present. The usual starting dose is 5 to 8 μg/kg per minute by continuous intravenous infusion.
   c. Correction of acidosis, hypocalcemia, and hypoglycemia helps improve myocardial function.
   d. Diuretics may be included in the regimen. For chronic myocardial dysfunction, digoxin may be added at a later stage.

7. A high-frequency oscillatory ventilator is effective in patients with severe PPHN. Through the use of this device, about 40% of patients who would be candidates for extracorporeal membrane oxygenation can avoid this procedure.

8. Inhalation nitric oxide (iNO) is a potent and selective pulmonary vasodilator. The usual starting dose is 20 ppm. Prolonged low-dose NO therapy has caused sustained improvement in oxygenation without systemic hypotension. Most newborn infants require iNO for fewer than 5 days. In general, the dose can be weaned to 5 ppm

after 6 to 24 hours of therapy. The dose is then slowly discontinued when the fraction of inspired oxygen (FiO_2) is less than 0.6 and the iNO dose is 1 ppm. The use of iNO in PPHN has decreased the need for ECMO by approximately 40%. In some cases, the response to iNO has been augmented by the use of high-frequency oscillatory ventilation.

When administered by inhalation, NO diffuses to vascular smooth muscle, stimulating the production of cyclic guanosine monophosphate and causing vasodilatation. Its selectivity for the pulmonary circulation is due to the rapid and avid binding of NO by hemoglobin, decreasing its availability to the systemic circulation.

9. ECMO has been shown to be effective in the management of selected patients with severe PPHN. However, this treatment may require ligation of a carotid artery and the jugular vein, and cerebrovascular accidents have been reported.

PROGNOSIS

1. Prognosis generally is good for neonates with mild PPHN who respond quickly to therapy. Most of these neonates recover without permanent lung damage or neurologic impairment.

2. For those requiring a maximal ventilator setting for a prolonged time, the chance of survival is smaller, and many survivors develop bronchopulmonary dysplasia and other complications.

3. Patients with developmental decreases in cross-sectional areas of the pulmonary vascular bed usually do not respond to therapy, and their prognosis is poor.

4. Neurodevelopmental abnormalities may manifest. Patients have a high incidence of hearing loss (up to 50%). This is positively related to the degree of alkalosis, the duration of ventilator support, and possibly the use of furosemide and aminoglycosides. An abnormal electroencephalogram (up to 80%) and cerebral infarction (45%) have been reported.

Chapter 15

Vascular Ring

Prevalence

Vascular ring reportedly represents less than 1% of all congenital cardiovascular anomalies, but this may be an underestimate because some conditions are asymptomatic.

Pathology

1. *Vascular ring* refers to a group of anomalies of the aortic arch that cause respiratory symptoms or feeding problems. A rare anomaly of the left pulmonary artery (PA) that causes symptoms is also included in this group. The vascular ring may be divided into two groups: complete (or true) and incomplete.
   a. *Complete vascular ring* refers to conditions in which the abnormal vascular structures form a complete circle around the trachea and esophagus. These include double aortic arch and right aortic arch with left ligamentum arteriosum.
   b. *Incomplete vascular ring* refers to vascular anomalies that do not form a complete circle around the trachea and esophagus but do compress the trachea or esophagus. These include anomalous innominate artery, aberrant right subclavian artery, and anomalous left PA ("vascular sling").

2. Double aortic arch is the most common vascular ring (40%) (Fig. 15–1). This anomaly is due to a failure of regression of both the right and left fourth branchial arches, resulting in right and left aortic arches, respectively. These two arches completely encircle and compress the trachea and esophagus, producing respiratory distress and feeding problems in early infancy. The right arch gives off two arch vessels, the right common carotid and the right subclavian, whereas the left arch gives off the left common carotid and left subclavian arteries. The right aortic arch is usually larger than the left arch, but on rare occasions partial obstruction or complete atresia of the left arch may exist. Double aortic arch is commonly an isolated anomaly but is occasionally associated with a variety of congenital heart defects such as transposition of the great arteries, ventricular septal defect (VSD), persistent truncus arteriosus, tetralogy of Fallot (TOF), and coarctation of the aorta (COA).

3. Right aortic arch with left ligamentum arteriosum is the second most common vascular ring (30%) (see Fig. 15–1). This results from persistence of the right fourth branchial arch (forming the right aortic arch). There are two common variations: retroesophageal left subclavian artery originating from the descending aorta and coursing behind the esophagus (65%), with the ligamentum connecting the descending aorta and the left PA, and mirror-image branching as in double aortic arch (35%), with the ligamentum connecting the descending aorta and the left PA. In addition, some patients have a Kommerell diverticulum at the origin of the left subclavian

	Anatomy	Ba-Esophagogram	Other X-Ray Findings	Symptoms	Treatment
Double Aortic Arch	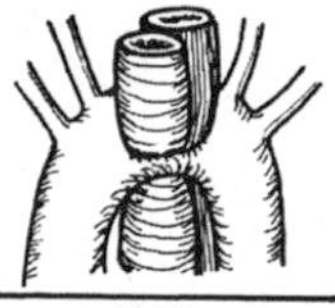	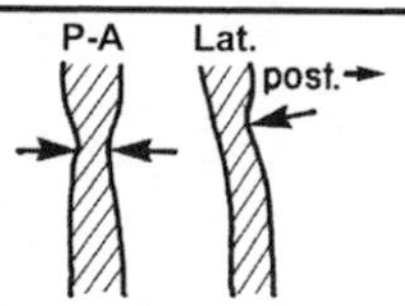	Anterior compression of trachea	Respiratory difficulty (onset < 3 mos.) Swallowing dysfunction	Surgical division of a smaller arch
Right Aortic Arch with Left Lig. Arteriosum	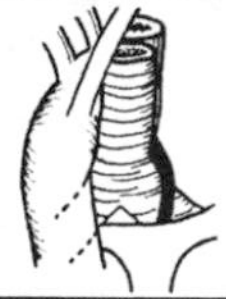	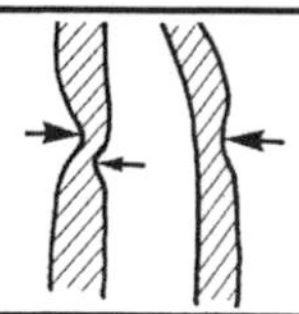		Mild respiratory difficulty (onset > 1 year) Swallowing dysfunction	Surgical division of the lig. arteriosum
Anomalous Innominate Artery	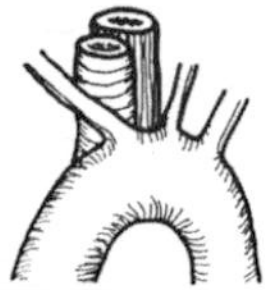	Normal	Anterior compression of trachea	Stridor and/or cough in infancy	Conservative management, or Surgical suturing of the artery to the sternum
Aberrant Right Subclavian Artery	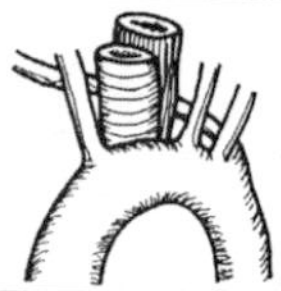	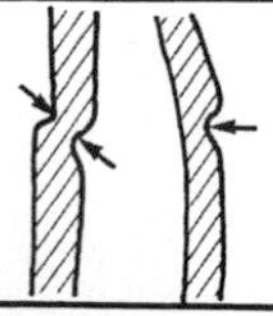		Occasional swallowing dysfunction	Usually no treatment is necessary
"Vascular Sling"	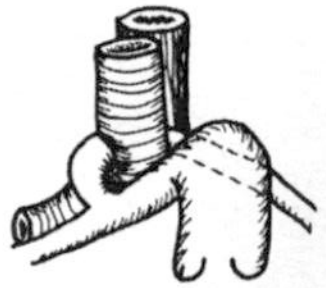	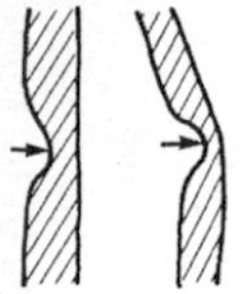	Right-sided emphysema or atelectasis. Posterior compression of trachea or Rt. main-stem bronchus	Wheezing and cyanotic episodes since birth	Surgical division of the anomalous LPA (from the RPA) and anastomosis to the MPA

Figure 15–1. Summary and clinical features of vascular ring. Lat, lateral view; Lig, ligamentum; LPA, left pulmonary artery; MPA, main pulmonary artery; P-A, posteroanterior view; post, posterior; RPA, right pulmonary artery.

artery from the descending aorta. This diverticulum may enlarge and independently compress the esophagus or trachea. This condition is highly associated with congenital heart defects (98% of cases), particularly TOF (48% of cases). Approximately 25% of patients with cyanotic congenital heart defects and right aortic arch have left ligamentum arteriosum.

4. Anomalous innominate artery occurs in about 10% of patients with vascular ring (see Fig. 15–1). If the innominate artery takes off too far to the left from the aortic arch or more posteriorly, it may compress the trachea, producing mild respiratory symptoms. This anomaly is commonly associated with other congenital heart defects such as VSD.

5. Aberrant right subclavian artery is the most common arch anomaly (accounting for 0.5% of general population, but its true incidence may be higher if asymptomatic patients are included). Its incidence is very high (38%) in Down syndrome with congenital heart defect. When the right subclavian artery arises independently from the descending aorta, it courses behind the esophagus, compressing the posterior aspect of the esophagus and producing mild feeding problems (Fig. 15–2; see Fig. 15–1). Often, a larger compression is found behind the esophagus by an aortic diverticulum at the takeoff of the right subclavian artery. This anomaly is usually an isolated anomaly but may be associated with TOF with left aortic arch, COA, or interrupted aortic arch. Most cases are asymptomatic.

6. Anomalous left PA (vascular sling) is a rare anomaly in which the left PA arises from the right PA (Fig. 15–3; see Fig. 15–1). To reach the left lung, the anomalous artery courses over the proximal portion of the right main-stem bronchus, behind the trachea, and in front of the esophagus to the hilum of the left lung. Therefore, both respiratory symptoms and feeding problems (such as coughing, wheezing, stridor,

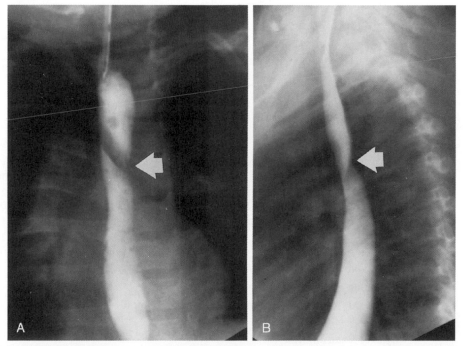

*Figure 15–2. Barium esophagogram of a child with aberrant right subclavian artery. **A,** Anteroposterior view shows an oblique indentation of the esophagus (arrow) at a level slightly higher than the carina produced by the subclavian artery. The indentation proceeds upward and to the right toward the right shoulder. **B,** Lateral projection shows a relatively shallow, long retroesophageal impression produced by the aberrant artery.*

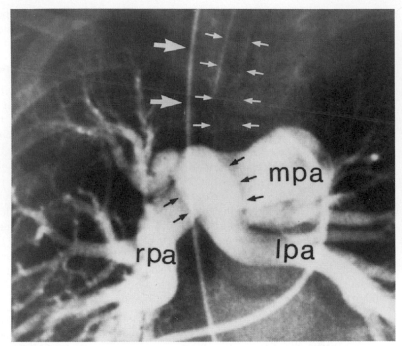

Figure 15–3. Pulmonary arteriogram in an infant with "vascular sling." The left pulmonary artery (lpa) arises from the posterosuperior aspect of the right pulmonary artery (rpa) (black arrows) rather than from the main pulmonary artery (mpa). The origin of the lpa is to the right of the trachea, which is easily identifiable by an endotracheal tube (small white arrows). The esophagus is directly behind the proximal portion of the aberrant lpa, which caused an anterior indentation on the barium esophagogram. The esophagus is identifiable by an orogastric tube that was inserted at the time of cardiac catheterization (large white arrows).

and episodes of choking, cyanosis, or apnea) may occur. This anomaly is associated with other cardiac defects, such as patent ductus arteriosus, VSD, atrial septal defect, atrioventricular canal, single ventricle, or aortic arch anomalies, in more than half of all cases.

Clinical Manifestations

History

1. Inspiratory stridor and feeding problems of varying severity are present, beginning at different ages. In double aortic arch, symptoms tend to appear in the newborn period or in early infancy (younger than 3 months), and they are more severe than in right aortic arch with left ligamentum arteriosum. Symptoms are often made worse by feeding. Affected infants frequently hyperextend their necks to reduce tracheal compression.

2. Respiratory symptoms or feeding problems are milder with incomplete forms of vascular ring than with the complete form.

3. A history of pneumonia is frequently elicited.

4. A history of atelectasis, emphysema, or pneumonia of the right lung is found with vascular sling.

Physical Examination

1. Physical examination is not revealing, except for a varying degree of rhonchi when the vascular ring is an isolated anomaly.

2. Cardiac examination is usually normal, except in about 25% of patients in whom associated cardiac anomalies are present.

Electrocardiography. The ECG is normal unless the vascular ring is associated with other congenital heart defects.

X-ray Studies

1. With the complete form of vascular ring, compression of the air-filled trachea may be visible on posteroanterior or lateral chest x-ray films, or both. Aspiration pneumonia or atelectasis may be present.

2. Barium esophagogram is usually diagnostic, except in anomalous innominate artery (see Fig. 15–1).
   a. In double aortic arch, two large indentations are present in both sides (with the right one usually larger) in the posteroanterior view, and a posterior indentation is seen on the lateral view.
   b. In right aortic arch with left ligamentum arteriosum, a large right-sided indentation and a much smaller left-sided indentation are present. A posterior indentation, either small or large, is also present on the lateral view.
   c. Barium esophagogram is normal in anomalous left innominate artery.
   d. In aberrant right subclavian artery, there is a small oblique indentation extending toward the right shoulder on the posteroanterior view. There is a small posterior indentation on the lateral view (see Figs. 15–1 and 15–2). Indentations may be large if the compression is made by an aortic diverticulum.
   e. In vascular sling, an anterior indentation of the esophagus seen in the lateral view at the level of the carina is characteristic. This is the only vascular ring that produces an anterior esophageal indentation. A right-sided indentation is usually seen on the posteroanterior view. The right lung is either hyperlucent or atelectatic with pneumonic infiltrations.

Echocardiography. Echo is helpful, both for excluding intracardiac defects and for diagnosing vascular ring. One should perform a careful segmental investigation of the aortic arch and arch vessels. The suprasternal notch views are especially useful in establishing the diagnosis.

Diagnosis

1. Vascular ring is suspected on the basis of clinical symptoms.
2. Barium esophagogram is probably the most useful noninvasive diagnostic tool (see Fig. 15–1).
3. Computed tomography (CT) and magnetic resonance imaging (MRI) are very accurate in the identification of vascular anomalies of the aortic arch and great vessels. However, these two tests cannot reveal ligamentum arteriosum. Digital subtraction angiography may provide almost the same information as angiography.
4. Echo studies can support the diagnosis of vascular ring and delineate associated intracardiac defects, but these studies usually do not provide detailed anatomic information about the vascular anomaly.
5. Occasionally, angiography is indicated to confirm the diagnosis. Combination of barium esophagogram, CT or MRI, and echo studies can substitute for angiography.
6. Tracheography and bronchoscopy usually add little information and may be hazardous in some patients. However, external compression of the trachea at different levels would help suggest either a double aortic arch or right aortic arch with left ligamentum arteriosum. These tests may be useful in delineating tracheobronchial malacia associated with vascular ring in some patients.

Management

Medical

1. Asymptomatic patients need no surgical treatment, even when the anomalies are found incidentally.

2. Medical management for infants with mild symptoms includes careful feeding with soft foods and aggressive treatment of pulmonary infections.

Surgical

Indications and Timing. Respiratory distress and a history of recurrent pulmonary infections and apneic spells are indications for surgical intervention. The timing of surgery depends on the severity of symptoms, and surgery may be performed during infancy.

Procedures and Mortality

Double Aortic Arch. Division of the smaller of the two arches (usually the left) is performed through a left thoracotomy. The surgical mortality rate is less than 5%.

Right Aortic Arch and Left Ligamentum Arteriosum. Ligation and division of the ligamentum are performed through a left thoracotomy. If a Kommerell diverticulum is found, the diverticulum is resected and the left subclavian artery is transferred to the left carotid artery. The mortality rate is less than 5%.

Anomalous Innominate Artery. Through right anterolateral thoracotomy, the innominate artery is suspended to the posterior sternum.

Aberrant Right Subclavian Artery. Surgical interruption of the artery is rarely performed in symptomatic patients with dysphagia.

Anomalous Left Pulmonary Artery. Surgical division and reimplantation of the left PA to the main PA are performed, usually through a median sternotomy and with the use of cardiopulmonary bypass. The surgical mortality rate is nearly zero.

Complications. In infants who have had surgery for severe symptoms, airway obstruction may persist for weeks or months. Careful respiratory management is required in the postoperative period. A period of months to 1 year may be required before disappearance of the noisy respiration, which is caused by preexisting tracheomalacia. This fact should be anticipated and clearly explained to the parents preoperatively. This complication is more likely in patients who have had double aortic arch, vascular sling, or right aortic arch with left ligamentum arteriosum.

Chapter 16

Chamber Localization and Cardiac Malposition

In this chapter, clinical methods of locating cardiac chambers using chest x-ray films, ECGs, echocardiography, and physical examination are discussed. This is followed by application of a principle that may aid in the anatomic diagnosis of the heart in the right chest (dextrocardia) or in the midline (mesocardia). Although these methods are valid, many false-positive and false-negative results are possible. Two-dimensional echo usually reveals the correct diagnosis, but occasionally cardiac catheterization and angiography may be needed.

Chamber Localization

The heart and great arteries can be viewed as three separate segments: the atria, the ventricles, and the great arteries. These three segments can vary from their normal positions either independently or together, resulting in many possible sets of abnormalities. The *segmental approach* of Van Praagh is useful in determining the relationship at each segment. This approach also simplifies the description of complex cardiac defects and abnormal positions of the heart (e.g., dextrocardia, levocardia, mesocardia).

LOCALIZATION OF THE ATRIA

The atria can be localized accurately by three noninvasive methods: chest x-ray films, ECG, and echocardiography. The x-ray method relies on the fact that the atrial situs is almost always the same as the type of visceral situs; the right atrium (RA) is on the same side as the liver or on the opposite side of the stomach bubble. The ECG method is based on the principle that the sinus node is always located in the RA and that the site of the sinus node can be determined by the P axis. Echo clarifies the relationship between systemic and pulmonary veins and the atria.

Chest X-ray Films. The clinician should locate the liver shadow and the stomach bubble.

1. Right-sided liver shadow and left-sided stomach bubble (situs solitus) indicate situs solitus of the atria (the RA on the right of the left atrium [LA], as in normal) (Fig. 16–1A). Left-sided liver shadow and right-sided stomach bubble (situs inversus) indicate situs inversus of the atria (the RA on the left of the LA) (see Fig. 16–1B).

2. A midline (symmetrical) liver shadow with a variable location of stomach bubble suggests heterotaxia (or splenic syndromes) in which either two RAs or two LAs (situs ambiguus) and other complex cardiac anomalies are present (see Fig. 16–1C; see also sections on heterotaxia in Chapter 14).

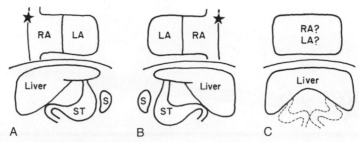

Figure 16–1. *The visceroatrial relationship. **A,** Situs solitus. **B,** Situs inversus. **C,** Situs ambiguus. The right atrium (RA) is either on the same side as the liver or on the opposite side of the stomach (ST). The sinoatrial node (star) is always in the RA. LA, left atrium; S, spleen.*

Electrocardiography. The sinus node is always located in the RA. Therefore, the P axis of the ECG can be used to locate the atria; the RA is located on the opposite side of the P axis.

1. When the P axis is in the lower left quadrant of the hexaxial reference system (0 to +90 degrees), the RA is on the right side (the RA to the right of the LA, or situs solitus of the atria) (Fig. 16–2).

2. When the P axis is in the lower right quadrant (+90 to +180 degrees), the RA is on the left side (the RA on the left of the LA, or situs inversus of the atria) (see Fig. 16–2).

3. With heterotaxia, the P axis may be superiorly directed (polysplenia syndrome) or may change between the lower left quadrant and lower right quadrant from time to time (asplenia syndrome).

Two-Dimensional Echocardiography and Other Methods. Two-dimensional echo identifies the inferior vena cava (IVC) or pulmonary veins, or both. The atrial chamber that is connected to the IVC is the RA, and the atrium that receives the pulmonary veins is the LA. Angiocardiogram, surgical inspection, or autopsy findings aid further in the diagnosis of atrial situs.

LOCALIZATION OF THE VENTRICLES

Ventricles can be localized noninvasively by the ECG and two-dimensional echo (or invasively by angiocardiograms).

Electrocardiography. The ECG method of localizing the ventricle is based on the fact that the depolarization of the ventricular septum moves from the embryonic left ventricle (LV) to the right ventricle (RV). This produces Q waves in the precordial leads that lie over the anatomic LV.

1. If Q waves are present in V5 and V6 but not in V1, D-loop of the ventricle, as in the normal person, is likely (Fig. 16–3A).

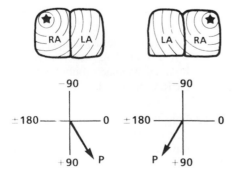

Figure 16–2. *Locating the atria by the use of the P axis. When the right atrium (RA) is on the right side, the P axis is in the left lower quadrant (0 to +90 degrees). When the RA is on the left side, the P axis is in the right lower quadrant (+90 to +180 degrees). LA, left atrium. (From Park MK, Guntheroth WG: How to Read Pediatric ECGs, 4th ed. Philadelphia, Mosby, 2006.)*

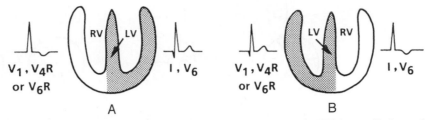

Figure 16–3. *Locating the ventricles from the ECG. The left ventricle (LV) is usually located on the same side as the precordial leads that show Q waves. If V6 shows a Q wave, the LV is on the left side (**A**). If V4R and V1 show a Q wave, the LV is to the right of the anatomic right ventricle (RV) (**B**). Note that Q waves are also present in V1 in severe right ventricular hypertrophy. (From Park MK, Guntheroth WG: How to Read Pediatric ECGs, 4th ed. Philadelphia, Mosby, 2006.)*

    2. If Q waves are present in V4R, V1, and V2 but not in V5 and V6, L-loop of the ventricles is likely (ventricular inversion) (see Fig. 16–3B).

    Two-Dimensional Echocardiography. The anatomic RV and LV are identified by the facts that the tricuspid valve leaflet usually inserts on the interventricular septum in a more apical position than the mitral septal leaflet and that the LV is invariably attached to the mitral valve and the RV to the tricuspid valve. A ventricular chamber that has two papillary muscles is the LV.

    Ventriculograms. The anatomic RV is coarsely trabeculated and triangular, and the anatomic LV is finely trabeculated and ellipsoid.

LOCALIZATION OF THE GREAT ARTERIES

    One can accurately determine the relationship between the two great arteries and the relationship of the great arteries to the ventricles noninvasively through echo (and invasively through angiocardiography). The ECG and chest x-ray films are not very helpful in determining the relationship between the great arteries and the ventricles. In many cases, however, one can deduce the relationship through the *loop rule* (of Van Praagh). The loop rule states that the D-loop of the ventricle (with the anatomic RV to the right of the LV) is usually associated with normally related great arteries or with complete transposition of the great arteries (D-TGA). The L-loop of the ventricle (with the anatomic RV to the left of the anatomic LV) is usually associated with the mirror image of normally related great arteries or with congenitally corrected transposition of the great arteries (L-TGA). There are four types of relationships between the two great arteries: (1) solitus, (2) inversus, (3) D-transposition, and (4) L-transposition (Fig. 16–4). One can deduce the relationship of the great artery. For example, when the situs solitus of the atria and the D-loop of the ventricle are confirmed, a situs solitus relationship is present if the patient is not cyanotic; if the patient is cyanotic, a D-TGA is present.

SEGMENTAL EXPRESSION

    The following symbols are used in describing the segmental relationship:

    1. Visceroatrial relationship: S (solitus), I (inversus), or A (ambiguus)

    2. Ventricular loop: D (D-loop), L (L-loop), or X (uncertain or indeterminate)

    3. Great arteries: S (solitus), I (inversus), D (D-transposition), or L (L-transposition)

    With these symbols, the segmental relationship of the heart can be expressed by three letters. The first letter signifies the visceroatrial relationship; the second letter, the ventricular loop; and the third letter, the relationship of the great arteries. The segmental approach to the diagnosis of cardiac malposition is independent of the location of the cardiac apex. Consequently, this approach applies to normally located hearts (levocardia in situs solitus) as well as to abnormally located hearts, such as dextrocardia

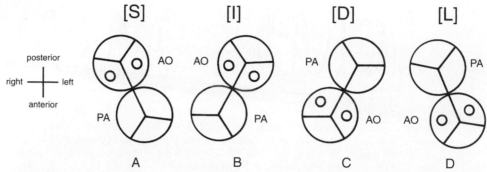

Figure 16–4. *Four types of relationships between the great arteries, viewed in the horizontal section.* **A,** *Solitus (S) relationship is present when the aortic valve is posterior and to the right of the pulmonary valve.* **B,** *In inversus (I) relationship, the aortic valve is posterior to and to the left of the pulmonary valve (mirror image of normal).* **C,** *Complete transposition (D) is present when the aortic valve is anterior and to the right of the pulmonary valve.* **D,** *Congenitally corrected transposition (L) is present when the aortic valve is anterior and to the left of the pulmonary valve. AO, aorta; PA, pulmonary artery.*

and mesocardia. A few examples of normal and well-known abnormal segmental relationships can be expressed as follows:

Normal heart with situs solitus: (S, D, S)
Normal heart with situs inversus (mirror image of normal): (I, L, I)
D-TGA: (S, D, D)
D-TGA with situs inversus: (I, L, L)
L-TGA with situs solitus: (S, L, L)
Normally formed heart that is displaced to the right side of the chest secondary to hypoplasia of the right lung ("dextroversion"): (S, D, S)

Dextrocardia and Mesocardia

Dextrocardia refers to a condition in which the heart is located on the right side of the chest. *Mesocardia* indicates that the heart is located approximately on the midline of the thorax; that is, the heart lies predominantly neither to the right nor to the left on the posteroanterior chest x-ray film. The terms *dextrocardia* and *mesocardia* express the position of the heart as a whole but do not specify the segmental relationship of the heart.

The four common types of dextrocardia are classic mirror-image dextrocardia (Fig. 16–5A), normal heart displaced to the right side of the chest (see Fig. 16–5B), L-TGA (see Fig. 16–5C), and single ventricle. Less commonly, asplenia and polysplenia syndromes with situs ambiguus and complicated cardiac defects cause dextrocardia (see Fig. 16–5D). All these abnormalities may result in mesocardia.

With chest x-ray studies and the ECG, one can deduce the location of the atria and the ventricles in dextrocardia (as well as in mesocardia). One can gain a more conclusive diagnosis of the segmental relationship through two-dimensional echo and angiocardiography.

1. Classic mirror-image dextrocardia (I, L, I) (see Fig. 16–5A) shows:
   a. The liver shadow on the left and the stomach bubble on the right on x-ray films and the P axis between +90 and +180 degrees on the ECG (situs inversus)
   b. Q waves in V5R and V6R (V5R and V6R are right-sided precordial leads, the mirror-image positions of V5 and V6, respectively)
2. Normal heart shifted toward the right side of the chest with the normal right-to-left relationship maintained (dextroversion) (S, D, S) (see Fig. 16–5B) shows:
   a. The liver shadow on the right and the stomach bubble on the left on x-ray films and the P axis between 0 and +90 degrees on the ECG (situs solitus)
   b. Q waves in V5 and V6

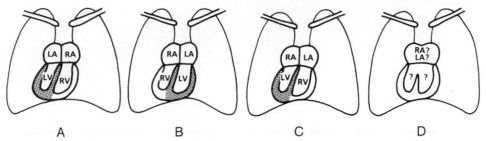

Figure 16–5. *Examples of common conditions in which the apex of the heart is in the right chest.* **A,** *Classic mirror-image dextrocardia.* **B,** *Normally formed heart shifted toward the right side of the chest.* **C,** *Congenitally corrected transposition of the great arteries with situs solitus.* **D,** *Situs ambiguus seen with splenic syndromes. LA, left atrium; LV, left ventricle; RA, right atrium; RV, right ventricle. (From Park MK, Guntheroth WG: How to Read Pediatric ECGs, 4th ed. Philadelphia, Mosby, 2006.)*

3. L-TGA with situs solitus (S, L, L) (see Fig. 16–5C) shows:

   a. Situs solitus of abdominal viscera on x-ray films and the P axis in the normal quadrant (0 to +90 degrees) on the ECG

   b. Q waves in V5R and V6R

4. Undifferentiated cardiac chambers (see Fig. 16–5D) are often associated with complicated cardiac defects and may show:

   a. Midline liver on x-ray films and shifting P axis or superiorly oriented P axis on the ECG

   b. Abnormal Q waves in the precordial leads (similar to those described for single ventricle; see Chapter 14)

Chapter 17

Miscellaneous Congenital Cardiac Conditions

In this chapter, congenital heart defects with a relatively low prevalence that have not been discussed previously are presented briefly.

Aneurysm of the Sinus of Valsalva

In aneurysm of the sinus of Valsalva (congenital aortic sinus aneurysm), there is a gradual downward protrusion of the aneurysm into a lower pressure cardiac chamber and eventually rupture. Most of the aneurysm arises from the right coronary sinus (80%) and less frequently from the noncoronary cusp (20%). When a sinus of Valsalva aneurysm ruptures, a sinus of Valsalva fistula is formed. The fistula communicates most frequently with the right ventricle (RV) (75%) and less frequently with the right atrium (RA) (25%). Associated anomalies are common and include ventricular septal defect (VSD) (50%), aortic regurgitation (AR) (20%), and coarctation of the aorta (COA). This rare anomaly has been reported primarily in the Asian population.

Unruptured aneurysm produces no symptoms or signs. Small sinus of Valsalva fistulas may develop without symptoms. The aneurysm ruptures during the third or fourth decade, usually into the RA or RV. The rupture is often characterized by sudden onset of chest pain, dyspnea, a continuous heart murmur over the right or left sternal border, and bounding peripheral pulses. Severe congestive heart failure (CHF) eventually develops. Chest x-ray films show cardiomegaly and increased pulmonary vascularity. The ECG may show biventricular hypertrophy (BVH), first- or second-degree atrioventricular (AV) block, or AV nodal rhythm.

Small to moderate-sized unruptured aneurysms probably do not need surgery. Unruptured aneurysms of the sinus of Valsalva that produce hemodynamic derangement should be repaired. When an aneurysm of the sinus of Valsalva has ruptured or is associated with a VSD with or without AR, prompt operation is advisable.

Anomalous Origin of the Left Coronary Artery from the Pulmonary Artery (Bland-White-Garland Syndrome, ALCAPA Syndrome)

In anomalous origin of the left coronary artery from the pulmonary artery (PA), the left coronary artery arises abnormally from the PA. Patients are usually asymptomatic in the newborn period until the PA pressure falls to a critical level after birth. The direction of blood flow is from the right coronary artery, through intercoronary collaterals, to the left coronary artery and into the PA. This results in left ventricular insufficiency or infarction.

Symptoms appear at 2 to 3 months of age and consist of recurring episodes of distress (anginal pain), marked cardiomegaly, and CHF. Significant heart murmur is usually absent, with a rare exception of a heart murmur of mitral regurgitation (MR) secondary to myocardial infarction. The ECG shows an anterolateral myocardial infarction pattern consisting of abnormally deep and wide Q waves, inverted T waves, and an ST-segment shift in leads I and aVL and the precordial leads (see Fig. 3–27). Cardiac enzyme changes probably occur, but the relatively slow development of myocardial infarction and the uncertainty of the exact time of infarction may make it difficult to interpret laboratory data. However, knowledge of cardiac enzyme changes seen in adult cases of myocardial infarction helps in the diagnosis of this condition (see Appendix A, Fig. A–2). Cardiac troponin I levels may also increase. The normal level of cardiac troponin I in children is 2 ng/mL or less and is frequently below the level of detection for the assay.

MANAGEMENT

Medical treatment alone carries an unacceptably high mortality (80% to 100%). Therefore, all patients with this diagnosis need operation. The optimal operation in infancy remains controversial, but most centers prefer definitive surgery unless the patient is critically ill.

Palliative Surgery

In critically ill infants, simple ligation of the anomalous left coronary artery close to its origin from the PA may be performed to prevent steal into the PA. This should be followed by a later elective bypass procedure (as described subsequently).

Definitive Surgery

Even for infants who are critically ill, many centers prefer to create a two-coronary system by performing one of the following procedures.

Intrapulmonary Tunnel Operation (Takeuchi Repair). Intrapulmonary tunnel operation is the most popular among two-coronary repair surgeries (Fig. 17–1). Two circular openings are made in the contiguous wall of the aorta and the pulmonary trunk, and a 5- to 6-mm aortopulmonary window is created by suturing together these

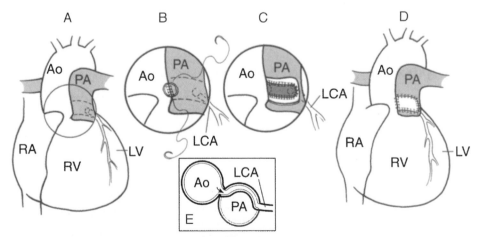

Figure 17–1. Intrapulmonary artery tunnel repair for anomalous origin of the left coronary artery (LCA) from the pulmonary artery (PA) (Takeuchi repair). **A,** Two dashed lines on the anterior wall of the PA are the proposed incision sites to create a flap of the PA. **B,** An aortopulmonary shunt is created, after making a punch hole (5 to 6 mm in size) in the contiguous wall of the aorta (Ao) and PA. **C,** The flap of the PA is sutured in place to form the convex roof of a tunnel through which aortic blood passes to the anomalous orifice of the left coronary artery. **D,** A piece of pericardium is used to close the opening in the anterior wall of the PA. **E,** Cross-sectional view of the tunnel operation when completed. LV, left ventricle; RA, right atrium; RV, right ventricle.

two openings. Two horizontal incisions are made in the anterior wall of the PA directly over the aortopulmonary window to create the flap of the PA wall. The flap is sutured in the posterior wall of the PA, and a tunnel is created that connects the opening of the aortopulmonary window and the orifice of the anomalous left coronary artery. The opening in the anterior wall of the PA is closed by a piece of pericardium. The mortality rate is near 0%, but mortality as high as over 20% has been reported.

Late complications of the procedure include supravalvar PA stenosis (75%), baffle leak (52%) causing coronary-PA fistula, and aortic insufficiency.

Left Coronary Artery Implantation. Left coronary artery implantation, with direct transfer of the anomalous left coronary artery into the aortic root, appears to be the most advisable procedure, but it is not always possible. The anomalous coronary artery is excised from the PA along with a button of PA wall, and the artery is reimplanted into the anterior aspect of the ascending aorta. If the direct implantation may result in excessive tension in the coronary artery, flaps can be developed from the anterior main PA wall and ascending aorta. These flaps are sutured to form a tube extension for the left coronary artery, which is then implanted to the aorta. The early surgical mortality rate is 15% to 20%.

Tashiro Repair. Tashiro and colleagues (1993) reported a repair technique that was performed in adult patients. In this procedure, a narrow cuff of the main PA, including the orifice of the left coronary artery, is transected; the upper and lower edges of the cuff are closed to form a new left main coronary artery; and the aorta and the newly creased left coronary artery are anastomosed side to end. The divided main PA is anastomosed end to end. This creates no obstruction to the PA. This technique has a potential application in the pediatric population, including small infants.

Subclavian–to–Left Coronary Artery Anastomosis. In subclavian–to–left coronary artery anastomosis, the end of the left subclavian artery is turned down and anastomosed end to side to the anomalous left coronary artery through a left thoracotomy approach. Aortic cross-clamping, which could be the source of ventricular impairment with postoperative low cardiac output and a high mortality rate, is avoided.

The need for simultaneous mitral valve reconstruction at the time of definitive surgery is controversial because spontaneous improvement of MR occurs following surgical revascularization. After successful two-coronary artery repair, LV systolic function and heart failure improve markedly and the severity of the MR also decreases. Even the infarct pattern on ECG may eventually disappear.

Aortopulmonary Septal Defect

In aortopulmonary septal defect (aortopulmonary window, aortopulmonary fenestration), a large defect is present between the ascending aorta and the main PA (Fig. 17–2). This condition results from failure of the spiral septum to divide completely the embryonic truncus arteriosus.

Hemodynamic abnormalities are similar to those of persistent truncus arteriosus and are more severe than those of patent ductus arteriosus (PDA). CHF and pulmonary hypertension appear in early infancy. Peripheral pulses are bounding, but the heart

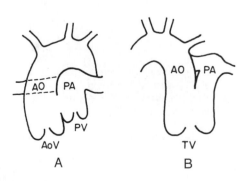

*Figure 17–2. Diagram of aortopulmonary window (**A**) and persistent truncus arteriosus (**B**). These two conditions are similar from a hemodynamic point of view. Anatomically, however, there are two separate semilunar valves (aortic valve [AoV] and pulmonary valve [PV]) without associated ventricular septal defect (VSD) in aortopulmonary window, whereas there is only one truncal valve (TV) with associated VSD in persistent truncus arteriosus. AO, aorta; PA, pulmonary artery.*

murmur is usually of the systolic ejection type (rather than continuous murmur) at the base.

The natural history of this defect is similar to that of a large untreated PDA, with development of pulmonary vascular disease in surviving patients. This defect has no known tendency to close spontaneously. Prompt surgical closure of the defect under cardiopulmonary bypass is indicated when the diagnosis is made. The surgical mortality rate is very low.

Arteriovenous Fistula, Coronary

Coronary artery fistulas are the most common congenital anomalies of the coronary artery, representing nearly one half of all coronary artery anomalies. They can be isolated or associated with other congenital heart diseases (CHDs), such as tetralogy of Fallot (TOF), atrial septal defect (ASD), PDA, and VSD. The right coronary artery is much more frequently involved than the left, and rarely both coronary arteries are involved.

These fistulas occur in one of two patterns. They may represent a branching tributary from a coronary artery coursing along a normal anatomic distribution ("true" coronary arteriovenous fistula), occurring in only 7% of cases (Fig. 17–3). In the majority of cases (over 90% of patients), the coronary fistula results from an abnormal coronary artery system with aberrant termination (coronary artery fistula or coronary-cameral fistula) rather than arteriovenous fistula. In more than 90% of reported cases, the fistula terminates in the right side of the heart (approximately 40% in the RV, 30% in the RA, and 20% in the PA). It rarely terminates in the left side of the heart, but when it does, the majority enter the left atrium (LA).

Patients are usually asymptomatic. However, CHF may develop if the shunt through the fistula is large. With a significant shunt, a continuous murmur, similar to the murmur of PDA, is audible over the precordium (rather than in the left infraclavicular area).

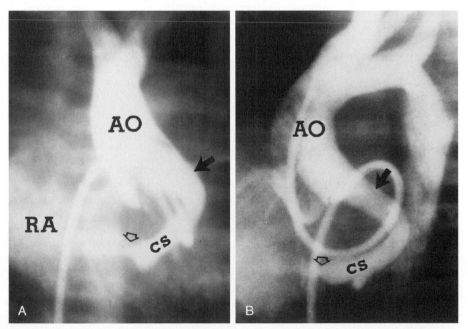

Figure 17–3. Aortogram showing coronary arteriovenous fistula in the distribution of the left circumflex artery (solid arrows). *A,* Anteroposterior projection. *B,* Lateral projection. The fistula empties through the coronary sinus (cs) and eventually into the right atrium (RA). The point of entry into the RA is marked by an open arrow. AO, aorta.

The ECG is usually normal but may show RVH or LVH if the fistula is large. Chest x-ray films show a normal heart size. Echo studies usually suggest the site and type of the fistulas. A tiny coronary artery fistula to the PA, which produces no symptoms, can be detected only incidentally by an echo study.

Except for the very small coronary-to-PA fistula, which has no hemodynamic significance, elective surgery is indicated for most fistulas as soon as the diagnosis is made to prevent complications such as subacute bacterial endocarditis (SBE), fistula rupture, myocardial infarction, and possible sudden death. Using cardiopulmonary bypass, the fistula is ligated as proximally as can be done without jeopardizing flow in the normal arteries and also ligated near its entrance to the cardiac chamber. The surgical mortality rate is zero to 5%. Successful nonsurgical closure of the fistula with the use of Gianturco coils or a double-umbrella device has been reported in selected patients.

Arteriovenous Fistula, Pulmonary

In this condition, the pulmonary arteries and veins communicate directly, bypassing the pulmonary capillary circulation. The fistulas may take the form of either multiple tiny angiomas (telangiectasis) or a large PA-to-pulmonary vein communication. About 60% of patients with pulmonary arteriovenous fistulas have Rendu-Osler-Weber syndrome (see Table 2–1). Rarely, chronic liver disease may be the cause of the fistula, but the mechanism of this remains an enigma. Desaturated systemic blood from the PAs reaches the pulmonary veins, bypassing the lung tissue and resulting in systemic arterial desaturation and cyanosis. The pulmonary blood flow and pressure remain unchanged, and there is no volume overload to the heart.

Physical examination may reveal cyanosis and clubbing. The peripheral pulses are not bounding. A faint systolic or continuous murmur may be audible over the affected area in about 50% of patients. Polycythemia is usually present, and arterial oxygen saturation runs between 50% and 85%. Chest x-ray films show a normal heart size. One or more rounded opacities of variable size may be present in the lung fields. The ECG is usually normal. Occasional complications include stroke, brain abscess, rupture of the fistula with hemoptysis or hemothorax, and infective endocarditis.

Although pulmonary angiography remains the definitive method for locating pulmonary arteriovenous fistulas, the diagnosis can be made through contrast two-dimensional echo by the appearance of microcavitations in the LA. The echo study can also be used to monitor the effectiveness of embolotherapy. Surgical resection of the lesions, with preservation of as much healthy lung tissue as possible, may be attempted in symptomatic children, but the progressive nature of the disorder calls for a conservative approach. Recently, selective embolotherapy has been proposed as an alternative to surgical resection.

Arteriovenous Fistula, Systemic

In this type of fistula, there is direct communication (either a vascular channel or angiomas) between the artery and a vein without the interposition of the capillary bed. The two most common sites of systemic arteriovenous fistulas are the brain and liver. In the liver, hemangioendotheliomas (densely vascular benign tumors) are more common than fistulous arteriovenous malformations. Because of decreased peripheral vascular resistance, an increase in stroke volume (with a wide pulse pressure) and tachycardia result, leading to increased cardiac output, volume overload to the heart, and even CHF.

Physical examination reveals a systolic or continuous murmur over the affected organ. An ejection systolic murmur may be present over the precordium because of increased blood flow through the semilunar valves. The peripheral pulses may be bounding during the high-output state but weak when CHF develops. A gallop rhythm may be present with CHF. Chest x-ray films show cardiomegaly and increased pulmonary vascular markings. The ECG may show hypertrophy of either or both ventricles.

Most patients with large cerebral arteriovenous fistulas and CHF die in the neonatal period, and surgical ligation of the affected artery to the brain is rarely possible without infarcting the brain. Surgical treatment of hepatic fistulas is often impossible because they are widespread throughout the liver. However, hemangioendotheliomas may undergo spontaneous involution after treatment with corticosteroids, interferon, or partial embolization.

Atrial Septal Aneurysm

An aneurysmal tissue is present in part or all of the atrial septum that shows phasic septal excursion (of 10 to 15 mm in the adult) protruding into either atrium. Atrial septal aneurysm (ASA) is present in 4% of the neonates using different criteria (of marked mobility of the atrial septum). The prevalence of ASA varies between 0.2% and 1.9% of normal adult patients and up to 8% to 15% of adult stroke patients by transesophageal echo studies. It is commonly associated with patent foramen ovale (PFO), and together they may play a role in cryptogenic stroke in adult patients. ASA may prove to be a cause of atrial arrhythmias in some patients. See "Patent Foramen Ovale" in this chapter for further discussion of PFO or ASA versus stroke.

Cervical Aortic Arch

In this rare anomaly, the aortic arch is elongated, usually into the neck just above the clavicle. The aortic arch is usually right sided and sometimes with the descending aorta on the left, producing an anatomic vascular ring. Sometimes it is associated with arch hypoplasia or abnormal branching of the arch (such as anomalous subclavian artery, separate origin of the internal and external carotid arteries, and common origin of both carotid arteries). Rarely, discrete aortic coarctation or stenosis or atresia of the left subclavian artery is seen.

Infants with this condition may present with stridor, dyspnea, or repeated lower respiratory infection, similar to the signs of vascular ring. In adults, dysphagia is a common presenting complaint. A pulsating mass with associated thrill is present in the right supraclavicular fossa. A presumptive diagnosis of cervical aortic arch is made by noting loss of femoral pulses during brief compression of the pulsating mass. Chest x-rays may show a wide upper mediastinum with absence of the aortic knob. Echocardiogram, computed tomography, and magnetic resonance imaging may be diagnostic. However, an aortogram is often necessary to make an accurate diagnosis of the condition with arch vessel abnormalities.

Treatment is necessary if the cervical arch is complicated by arch hypoplasia, symptomatic vascular ring, or, rarely, aneurysm of the cervical arch itself.

Common Atrium

In common atrium (single atrium, cor triloculare biventriculare), either the atrial septum is completely absent or only the vestigial element of a poorly developed atrial septum is present. This is a form of endocardial cushion defect with cleft mitral valve. Symptoms may include shortness of breath and easy fatigability. Occasional infants may be critically ill with heart failure. Cyanosis varies from constant and obvious to very mild and present only with exertion. The ECG shows left anterior hemiblock ("superior" QRS axis), as in endocardial cushion defect, and an rsR′ pattern in the right precordial leads, as in ASD. This condition is most commonly seen with Ellis–van Creveld syndrome (see Table 2–1). Successful creation of a polyvinyl septum is possible.

Cor Triatriatum

Cor triatriatum is a rare congenital cardiac anomaly in which the LA is divided into two compartments by an abnormal fibromuscular septum with an opening (Fig. 17–4A), producing varying degrees of obstruction of pulmonary venous return. Pulmonary venous and pulmonary arterial hypertension result. Embryologically, this condition results from failure of incorporation of the embryonic common pulmonary vein into the LA.

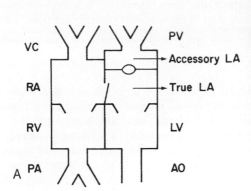

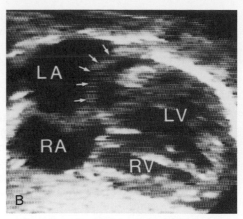

*Figure 17–4. Cor triatriatum. **A,** Diagrammatic drawing. **B,** Subcostal four-chamber view of an echocardiogram demonstrating a membrane (arrows) in the left atrium (LA). AO, aorta; LV, left ventricle; PA, pulmonary artery; PV, pulmonary vein; RA, right atrium; RV, right ventricle; VC, vena cava.*

Therefore, the upper compartment (accessory LA) is a dilated common pulmonary vein, and the lower compartment is the true LA. Hemodynamic abnormalities of this condition are similar to those of mitral stenosis in that both conditions produce pulmonary venous and pulmonary arterial hypertension (see Chapter 10).

Important physical findings include dyspnea, basal pulmonary crackles, a loud S2, and a nonspecific systolic murmur. The ECG shows right axis deviation and severe right ventricular hypertrophy (RVH) and occasional right atrial hypertrophy. Chest x-ray films show evidence of pulmonary venous congestion or pulmonary edema, a prominent PA segment, and right-sided heart enlargement. Echo demonstrates a linear structure within the LA cavity (see Fig. 17–4B). Surgical correction is always indicated. Pulmonary hypertension regresses rapidly in survivors if the correction is made early.

DiGeorge Syndrome

Although DiGeorge syndrome does not always involve a single cardiac defect, it is presented in this chapter because the great majority of patients with DiGeorge syndrome have serious congenital heart defects.

Common clinical features exist among DiGeorge syndrome, velocardiofacial syndrome (or Shprintzen's syndrome), and conotruncal anomaly face (CTAF) syndrome. These syndromes share a common genetic cause in most cases, a chromosome 22q11 deletion, and therefore currently the term 22q11 deletion syndrome is used. The same syndrome has been described by different researchers in different areas of expertise. Angelo DiGeorge, MD, an endocrinologist, reported DiGeorge syndrome in the 1960s, and Robert Shprintzen, PhD, a speech pathologist, reported velocardiofacial syndrome in the 1970s. A group of Japanese cardiologists called it CTAF syndrome in 1978. Clinical features in these syndromes include abnormal facies, congenital heart defects, and absence or hypoplasia of the thymus (with congenital immune deficiency and increased susceptibility to infection) and parathyroid gland (with hypocalcemia). Clinical features of the syndrome are collectively grouped under the acronym CATCH-22 (*c*ardiac, *a*bnormal facies, *t*hymic hypoplasia, *c*left palate, and *h*ypocalcemia resulting from 22q11 deletion).

Approximately 90% of patients have a deletion of the long arm of chromosome 22 (22q11) detectable with current cytogenetic and fluorescence in situ hybridization (FISH) techniques. In 90% of cases, the disorder occurs as the result of a new mutation, and in 10% the disorder is inherited from a parent in an autosomal dominant fashion. Rarely, the syndrome may be caused by other chromosomal abnormalities or maternal environmental factors (such as alcohol, retinoids).

CLINICAL MANIFESTATIONS

1. Facies. Abnormal facies are characterized by hypertelorism, micrognathia, short philtrum with fish-mouth appearance, antimongoloid slant, telecanthus with short palpebral fissures, and low-set ears, often with defective pinnae.

2. Cardiac. Many patients (85%) have cardiac defects. The most common cardiac anomalies include TOF (25%); interrupted aortic arch (15%); VSD, usually perimembranous, malaligned VSD (15%); persistent truncus arteriosus (9%); and isolated aortic arch anomalies (5%). Less common anomalies include pulmonary stenosis, ASD, AV canal defect, and transposition of the great arteries.

3. Anomalies in the palate are common (70% to 80%), with speech and feeding disorders. The palatal abnormalities may be overt or submucosal clefts. Occasionally, a bilateral cleft lip and palate may be present. Velopharyngeal insufficiency with delayed and hypernasal speech may be present.

4. Metabolic. Hypocalcemia (observed in 60%) is due to hypoparathyroidism.

5. Immunologic. Thymic hypoplasia or aplasia leads to mild to moderate decreases in T-cell number. Occasionally, humoral deficits, including immunoglobulin A deficiency, have been observed (~10%).

6. Recurrent infections are common and an important cause of later mortality.

7. General. Short stature, mental retardation, and hypotonia in infancy are frequent. Occasionally, psychiatric disorders (e.g., schizophrenia and bipolar disorder) develop.

8. Lateral view of chest x-ray films shows a defective thymic shadow.

9. Cytogenetic analysis detects only 20% of the deletion in the region. The deletion is identified by FISH.

MANAGEMENT

1. Correction of cardiac malformation as discussed in other sections. Cardiac defects are major causes of early death.

2. Irradiated, cytomegalovirus-negative blood products must be administered because of the risk of graft-versus-host disease with nonirradiated products.

3. Monitoring of serum calcium levels and supplementation of calcium and vitamin D are important.
   a. Calcium gluconate (Kalcinate), 500 to 750 mg/kg/day, by mouth four times a day, or calcium carbonate (Os-Cal, Titralac, Oystercal, Caltrate), 112.5 to 162.5 mg/kg/day, four times a day.
   b. Ergocalciferol, vitamin D, 25,000 to 200,000 U by mouth every day.

4. Live vaccines are contraindicated in patients with DiGeorge syndrome and in household members because of the risk of shedding live organisms.

5. The usual prophylactic regimen for T- and B-cell deficiency is carried out.

6. Early thymus transplantation may promote successful immune reconstitution.

   Prognosis. The prognosis depends on cardiac and immune system disorders. Prognosis is poor with complex cyanotic heart defects, with a 1-month mortality rate of 55% and 6-month mortality rate of 86%.

Double-Chambered Right Ventricle

Double-chambered RV (anomalous muscle bundle of the RV) is characterized by aberrant hypertrophied muscle bands that divide the RV cavity into a proximal high-pressure chamber and a distal low-pressure chamber. In the majority of patients, VSD or pulmonary valve stenosis is also present.

Clinical manifestations closely resemble those of pulmonary valvular or infundibular stenosis: a loud, grade 3 to 5/6 ejection systolic murmur along the upper and mid-left sternal border is present. Surgical resection of the bundle, as well as repair of other anomalies, is usually indicated as soon as the diagnosis is made.

Ectopia Cordis

In this extremely rare condition, the heart is partially or totally outside the thorax. Most reported cases of ectopia cordis are either thoracic (60%) or thoracoabdominal (40%); rarely, a case may be cervical or abdominal. The thoracic type is characterized by a sternal defect, absence of the parietal pericardium, cephalic orientation of the cardiac apex, epigastric omphalocele, and small thoracic cavity. The thoracoabdominal type has partial absence or cleft of the lower sternum, an anterior diaphragmatic defect through which a portion of the ventricle protrudes into the abdominal cavity, a defect of the parietal pericardium, and an omphalocele. Intracardiac abnormalities are common but not invariable; ASD, VSD, TOF, and tricuspid atresia are the most common intracardiac defects. One reported case of the abdominal type (1806) was a healthy French soldier, the father of three children, who died of pyelonephritis.

The treatment and prognosis of the defect are determined by the location of the defect, the extent of the cardiac displacement, and the presence or absence of intracardiac anomalies. Simple sternal cleft with minimal cardiac protrusion can be successfully treated in early infancy. However, in more severe cases, most surgical efforts to put the heart into the thorax have failed because of the smallness of the thorax and kinking of the blood vessels. Patients without omphalocele or intracardiac defects may remain largely asymptomatic and can undergo surgical repair later in childhood.

Hemitruncus Arteriosus

In hemitruncus arteriosus (origin of one PA from the ascending aorta), one of the PAs, usually the right PA, arises from the ascending aorta (Fig. 17–5). Associated defects such as PDA, VSD, and TOF are occasionally present. Hemodynamically, one lung receives blood directly from the aorta, as in PDA, with resulting volume or pressure overload or both, and the other lung receives the entire RV output, resulting in volume overload of that lung. Therefore, pulmonary hypertension of both lungs develops. CHF develops early in infancy, with respiratory distress and poor weight gain.

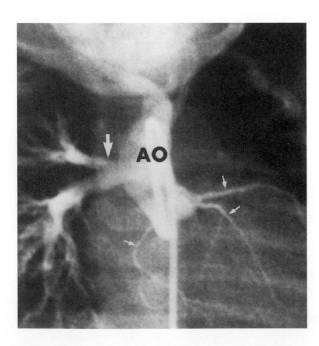

Figure 17–5. Hemitruncus. Aortogram showing the right pulmonary artery (large arrow) originating anomalously from the ascending aorta (AO). Coronary arteries are also opacified (small arrows).

A continuous murmur and bounding pulses may be present. The ECG shows combined ventricular hypertrophy, and chest x-ray films show cardiomegaly and increased pulmonary vascular markings. Early surgical correction (anastomosis of the anomalous PA to the main PA) is indicated.

Idiopathic Dilatation of the Pulmonary Artery

In idiopathic dilatation of the PA (congenital pulmonary insufficiency), pulmonary regurgitation is present in the absence of pulmonary hypertension in asymptomatic children or adolescents. Many regard this as a very mild pulmonary valve stenosis with resulting poststenotic dilatation but subsequent loss of pressure gradient and the murmur of pulmonary stenosis.

A characteristic auscultatory finding is a grade 1 to 3/6 low-frequency, decrescendo diastolic murmur at the upper and mid-left sternal borders. The S2 is normal. The ECG is usually normal, but occasional right bundle branch block is present. Chest x-ray films show a prominent main PA segment with normal peripheral pulmonary vascularity. Echo studies reveal a poststenotic dilatation of the main PA with little or no pressure gradient across the pulmonary valve but with a whirling of blood flow in the PA. The prognosis is generally good, but right-sided heart failure may occur in adult life.

Kartagener's Syndrome

Kartagener's syndrome consists of the triad of situs inversus (with dextrocardia), paranasal sinusitis, and bronchiectasis. This disorder is inherited as an autosomal recessive trait; males and females are affected with equal frequency. The dextrocardia is a mirror image of normal and is functionally normal. Bronchiectasis is believed to result from a functional defect of the mucociliary epithelium with immotility of the cilia. In addition, affected males are infertile as a result of immobile spermatozoa.

Parachute Mitral Valve

Parachute mitral valve is a severe form of congenital mitral valve stenosis. In this anomaly, all chordae tendineae are thickened and shortened and they attach to a single posteriorly located papillary muscle, producing severe mitral stenosis. The anterior papillary muscle is usually absent. The diagnosis can be suspected by two-dimensional echo on the parasternal views. In the parasternal short-axis view, only one papillary muscle is imaged. Commonly associated conditions include supramitral ring, subvalvular and/or valvular AS, and COA or the complete "Shone complex," which is the combination of all or some of these abnormalities.

Patent Foramen Ovale

PFO is a tunnel between the septum secundum and the superior margin of the septum primum. The septum secundum is a thick, concave, muscular structure that expands from the posterosuperior wall and partially partitions the atria. The septum primum, a thin flap, extends inferiorly and makes a tunnel. During fetal life, the tunnel (foramen ovale) is open and allows a direct flow of inferior vena cava (IVC) blood into the LA, sending blood with higher oxygen saturation to the brain and coronary circulation.

Postnatally, when the pressure in the LA exceeds that in the RA as the result of lung expansion and resulting increase in pulmonary venous return, the thin flap of the superior end of the septum primum is forced to shut against the septum secundum, resulting in functional closure of the foramen. In most individuals, the foramen ovale is sealed shortly after birth, but for some reason, functional closure does not always occur, with a small left-to-right atrial shunt detectable by color Doppler study. This condition is called incompetent foramen ovale and is quite common in the newborn, present in 75% of neonates. Probe patency of a competent foramen ovale is found in 25% of normal adults.

PFOs versus Strokes. There are controversies regarding the management of PFO, which has been proposed as a potential cause of cryptogenic stroke in adult patients. Some retrospective observational reports have shown a strong association (but not cause-effect relationship) between cryptogenic strokes and both PFO and ASA in adults. PFO prevalence was 4 times higher in stroke patients (40%) than in control subjects (10%) and it was much higher (33 times) in patients with both PFO and ASA. Thus, paradoxical embolism through a PFO has been postulated as a cause of stroke. The proponents of the hypothesis of paradoxical embolization have advocated closing PFO for secondary prevention of stroke in patients with PFO and also in high-risk adult patients without stroke.

However, there is evidence casting doubts about this hypothesis, and thus the rationale for closing PFO to prevent recurrence of stroke remains controversial.

1. In these observational studies, transient atrial fibrillation (with left atrial thrombus formation), emboli from aortic atherosclerotic plaques, and the hypercoagulable state were not ruled out (although the ability to rule out the hypercoagulable state is quite limited at this time).

2. Several studies (including a meta-analysis [Overell et al, 2000], a prospective case-control study [Mas et al, 2001], and a prospective population study [Meissner et al, 2006]), suggest that PFO alone does not appear to increase the odds ratio for stroke. ASA alone or in combination with PFO appears to increase substantially the odds ratio for stroke. In patients with isolated ASA (without PFO), paradoxical embolization cannot be the cause of stroke.

3. However, patients with ASA have been found to have higher vulnerability to atrial fibrillation than those without it (Berthet et al, 2000). Atrial fibrillation, even a transient one, is a known cause of cardiogenic embolism.

4. Unless the RA pressure is elevated and frequent venous thrombus formation is demonstrated, hemodynamics does not favor paradoxical embolization in normal individuals with normal RA pressure.

Given these findings, the cause of stroke is more likely systemic embolization rather than paradoxical embolization through PFO, and, thus, closing of an isolated PFO may not be an effective or justifiable procedure for prevention of stroke. In fact, there is no evidence that closure of a PFO (surgical or by device) is superior to medical management (aspirin or warfarin or both) in preventing recurrence of strokes.

A guideline from the American Heart Association and American Stoke Association (Goldstein et al, 2006), which has been endorsed by the American Academy of Neurology, does not support closure of PFO for prevention of recurrent stroke at this time. Rather, it recommends antithrombotic therapy with aspirin or warfarin. PFO closure may be considered for patients with recurrent cryptogenic stroke despite medical therapy.

With regard to pediatric patients, in the absence of convincing evidence for PFO as a cause of paradoxical embolization and in the absence of superiority of PFO closure to medical therapy in adult patients, the rationale for closing PFOs in pediatric patients is at best controversial and may not be justified. It appears prudent to wait until this controversy is cleared before adopting the practice of closing PFOs in pediatric patients.

Pericardial Defect, Congenital

This rare congenital anomaly of the pericardium may be partial or complete. The majority of these cases occur on the left side (85%), and they are more often complete (65%) than partial. Thirty percent to 50% of cases are associated with congenital anomalies of the heart (PDA, ASD, TOF, and mitral stenosis), lung, chest wall, or diaphragm. Pleural defect is almost always present.

Unless an associated cardiac anomaly is present, most patients are asymptomatic. Occasionally, a *partial* defect may produce chest pain, syncope, or systemic embolism secondary to herniation and strangulation of the left atrial appendage. A *complete* defect may produce vague positional discomfort in the supine or left lateral position.

Congenital pericardial defects are difficult to diagnose preoperatively. Occasionally, chest x-ray films may show a prominence of the left hilum or the PA caused by herniation of these structures through the partial defect. Complete absence of the left pericardium may be characterized by leftward displacement of the heart and aortic knob or a prominent PA. Echo findings of complete absence of the left pericardium include unusual cardiac hypermobility (cardioptosis), abnormal swing motion of the heart with each cardiac beat, and an abnormal systolic anterior motion of the ventricular septum (on M-mode). (These findings are similar to the echo findings of the transplanted heart, in which the donor heart is untethered and is placed in a large potential space.) Traditionally, the appearance of pneumopericardium after the introduction of air into the left pleural cavity was diagnostic. More recently, noninvasive procedures, such as two-dimensional echo, computed tomography, and magnetic resonance imaging, have been successfully applied for the diagnosis of this condition.

Surgical treatment is recommended only for symptomatic patients. Surgical procedures used in this condition include longitudinal pericardiotomy, partial pericardiectomy, primary closure, partial appendectomy (of the left atrial appendage), and pericardioplasty with pleural flaps, Teflon, or porcine pericardium.

Pseudocoarctation of the Aorta

Pseudocoarctation of the aorta is a condition in which the distal portion of the aortic arch and the proximal portion of the descending aorta are abnormally elongated and tortuous, giving the x-ray film the appearance of COA. There is a tendency for dilatation and aneurysm formation related to turbulent flow across the kink, and the condition may progress to show a substantial pressure difference between the arms and legs. Physical examination and the ECG are normal. Surgical intervention may be required if dilatation compresses surrounding structures (e.g., esophagus) or aneurysm formation is present.

Pulmonary Artery Stenosis

Stenosis of the PA occurs most frequently near the bifurcation, but occasionally it may involve more peripheral branches.

1. This may be an isolated anomaly but is more often seen with other CHDs such as valvular PS, ASD, VSD, PDA, or TOF (in which 20% of the patients have associated peripheral PA stenosis).

2. It may also be seen in association with other conditions such as rubella syndrome, Williams syndrome, and Alagille syndrome.

3. When associated with cyanotic CHDs (such as pulmonary atresia with intact ventricular septum or TOF with pulmonary atresia), the stenosis usually involves multiple branches and multiple sites.

4. Some PA stenosis is secondary to surgical procedures, such as previous systemic-to-PA shunts.

5. This condition should be distinguished from the normally small PA branches (with a relatively large main PA) seen in normal newborn infants, which produce the innocent pulmonary flow murmur of newborns.

Mild stenosis of the PAs causes no hemodynamic abnormalities. If the stenosis is severe, the RV may hypertrophy. An ejection systolic murmur grade 2 to 3/6 is audible at the upper left sternal border, with good transmission to the ipsilateral axilla and back. Occasionally, a continuous murmur is audible with severe stenosis. The S2 is either normal or more obviously split. The murmur is louder than the innocent pulmonary flow murmur of newborns and persists beyond 6 months of age. The ECG is normal with mild stenosis, but it shows RVH with severe stenosis. Chest x-ray films are usually normal. The echo may show stenosis in the main PA or near the bifurcation, but those in smaller branches cannot be imaged by echo. Stenosis of the peripheral PA branches may require pulmonary angiography for accurate diagnosis.

No treatment is necessary for isolated mild PA stenosis. The central (extraparenchymal) type is surgically correctable, but the multiple peripheral (intraparenchymal) type is not amenable to surgery. Balloon angioplasty alone has a limited success rate, approximately 50% with a 16% recurrence rate. In contrast, expandable metal stents can overcome an obstruction, with an acute angiographic success rate close to 100% and a recurrence rate of only 2% to 3%. However, the need for stent reexpansion as the child grows remains problematic.

Scimitar Syndrome

All or some of the pulmonary veins from the lower lobe and sometimes the middle lobe of the right lung drain anomalously into the IVC, making a peculiar scimitar-shaped, vertical radiographic shadow along the lower right cardiac border.

In symptomatic infants, associated anomalies (e.g., ASD, PDA, hypoplasia of the right lung and right PA, pulmonary venous obstruction, systemic arterial supply to the lung) are frequent. Left-sided obstructive lesions (e.g., hypoplastic LV, subaortic stenosis, aortic arch obstruction) are also frequently present. An anomalous systemic arterial supply originates in the descending aorta, usually supplies the right lung, and rarely supplies the left lung (pulmonary sequestration). Dextrocardia is also frequently found. For symptomatic infants, embolization or ligation of the systemic arterial supply to the right lung, if present, may result in improvement of pulmonary hypertension and signs of CHF. Most symptomatic infants require additional surgery for associated defects, with a high surgical mortality rate (near 50%).

Children and adults with the syndrome are either minimally symptomatic or asymptomatic, probably because they have a low incidence of associated anomalies. For older children, the anomalous pulmonary venous return can be redirected to the LA, but in patients with associated pulmonary sequestration, the involved lobes of the right lung may need to be resected.

Systemic Venous Anomalies

A wide variety of abnormalities appear in the systemic venous system; some of these have little physiologic importance, and others produce cyanosis. Developments in the diagnosis and treatment of cardiovascular disorders have brought these anomalies to the attention of cardiologists and thoracic surgeons. Some of these abnormalities produce difficulties in the manipulation of catheters during cardiac catheterization, and preoperative knowledge of systemic venous anomalies is important in cardiac surgery. Therefore, the search for common abnormalities of the systemic veins has become routine in the evaluation of pediatric cardiac patients during echo and cardiac catheterization.

Two well-known anomalies of systemic veins are persistent left superior vena cava (SVC) and infrahepatic interruption of the IVC with azygos continuation. Rarely, either persistent left SVC or interrupted IVC drains into the LA, producing cyanosis.

ANOMALIES OF SUPERIOR VENA CAVA

Persistent left SVC occurs in 3% to 5% of children with congenital heart defects. The persistent left SVC is connected to the RA in 92% of cases and to the LA (producing cyanosis) in the remainder.

Persistent Left Superior Vena Cava Draining into the Right Atrium. In the most common type, the left SVC is connected to the coronary sinus (Fig. 17–6A). As a rule, persistent left SVC is part of a bilateral SVC, but rarely the right SVC is absent (see Fig. 17–6B). A bridging innominate vein is present in 60% of cases.

Isolated persistent left SVC (see Fig. 17–6A and B) does not produce symptoms or signs. Cardiac examination is entirely normal. Chest x-ray films may show the shadow of the left SVC along the upper left border of the mediastinum. A high prevalence of leftward P axis (+15 degrees or less) has been reported on the ECG.

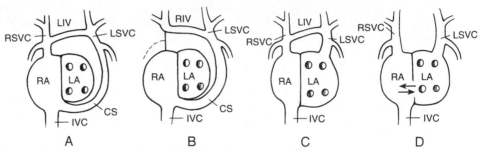

Figure 17–6. *Schematic diagram of persistent left superior vena cava (LSVC). **A,** Left SVC drains through the coronary sinus (CS) into the right atrium (RA). The left innominate vein (LIV) and the right SVC (RSVC) are adequate. **B,** Uncommonly, the RSVC may be atretic. The coronary sinus is large because it receives blood from both the right and left upper parts of the body. **C,** The coronary sinus is absent, and the LSVC drains directly into the left atrium (LA). The atrial septum is intact. **D,** The LSVC connects to the LA, and there is a posterior atrial septal defect, which allows a predominant left-to-right atrial shunt. IVC, inferior vena cava; RIV, right innominate vein.*

The enlarged coronary sinus may be imaged by an echo study. The diagnosis is suspected from two-dimensional echo studies, and angiocardiography confirms the diagnosis. Treatment for isolated persistent left SVC is not necessary.

Persistent Left Superior Vena Cava Draining into the Left Atrium. Rarely (in 8% of cases), persistent left SVC drains into the LA, resulting in systemic arterial desaturation (see Fig. 17–6C and D). This is due to failure of invagination between the left sinus horn and LA; therefore, the coronary sinus is absent. Associated cardiac anomalies almost invariably are present. Complex defects, such as cor biloculare, conotruncal abnormalities, and asplenia syndrome, are commonly found. Defects of the atrial septum (single atrium, secundum ASD, primum ASD) are also frequently found.

Clinical manifestations are dominated by the associated complex cardiac defects. In the absence of complex defects, cyanosis is more marked when there is no atrial communication (see Fig. 17–6C) than when there is an ASD. When there is an ASD (see Fig. 17–6D), clinical findings resemble those of ASD with left-to-right shunt, with only mild arterial desaturation. Surgical correction is necessary. When there is an adequate-sized bridging vein that connects two SVCs, simple ligation of the left SVC is performed. If the right SVC is absent or a bridging vein is inadequate, the left SVC is transposed to the RA.

ANOMALIES OF THE INFERIOR VENA CAVA

Many abnormalities in the formation of the IVC have been reported. Among the significant anomalies are infrahepatic interruption of the IVC with azygos continuation and anomalous drainage of the IVC into the LA, producing cyanosis (Fig. 17–7).

Interrupted IVC with azygos continuation (see Fig. 17–7A) has been reported in about 3% of children with congenital heart defects. The IVC below the level of the renal veins is normal, but the hepatic portion of the IVC is absent. Instead of receiving the hepatic veins and entering the RA, the IVC drains through an enlarged azygos system into the right SVC and eventually to the RA. The hepatic veins connect directly to the RA. Bilateral SVC is also common. Azygos continuation of the IVC is often associated with complex cyanotic heart defects, such as polysplenia syndrome, double-outlet RV, cor biloculare, and anomalies of pulmonary venous return. Less often, a simple cardiac defect is associated. No case has been reported in association with asplenia syndrome. This defect creates difficulties during cardiac catheterization and can complicate surgical correction of an underlying cardiac defect. This venous anomaly does not require surgical correction.

IVC connecting to the LA is an extremely rare condition in which the IVC receives the hepatic veins, curves toward the LA, and makes a direct connection with the

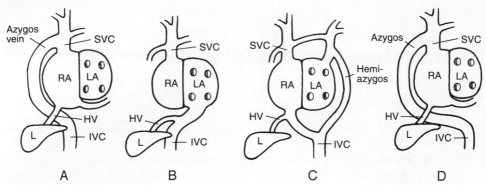

Figure 17–7. *Schematic diagram of selected abnormalities of the inferior vena cava (IVC).*
A, Interrupted IVC with azygos continuation, the most common abnormality of the IVC. The hepatic
veins (HVs) connect directly to the right atrium (RA). B, Right IVC draining into the left atrium (LA).
C, Absence of the lower right IVC. The IVC drains into the LA through the left superior vena cava
(SVC), and the RA drains through the hepatic portion of the IVC. D, Complete absence of the right
IVC with communicating vein draining to the azygos vein. L, liver.

chamber (see Fig. 17–7B). Pathologic persistence of the eustachian valve can result in
a clinically similar situation in which a membrane completely excludes the IVC from
the RA, with the IVC blood shunted to the LA through either an ASD or a PFO.

Two other extremely rare cases of IVC abnormalities are shown in Figure 17–7. In
one of them, the lower end of the right IVC is absent, and the dominant left IVC drains
into the LA (producing cyanosis) through the (left-sided) hemiazygos system and persistent left SVC (see Fig. 17–7C). In the other case, the lower end of the right IVC is
absent, and the left IVC drains through the (right-sided) azygos system (see Fig. 17–7D).

Part V

ACQUIRED HEART DISEASE

Among acquired heart diseases, emphasis is placed on the more common pediatric diseases, such as cardiomyopathies; cardiovascular infections, including myocarditis and infective endocarditis; acute rheumatic fever; and valvular heart disease. Although the cause of Kawasaki disease is not entirely clear, it is discussed in the chapter on cardiovascular infection. Mitral valve prolapse is discussed in the chapter on valvular heart disease. A chapter on cardiac involvement in some systemic diseases is also presented.

Chapter 18

Primary Myocardial Disease

Primary myocardial disease, or cardiomyopathy, is a disease of the heart muscle itself, not associated with congenital, valvular, or coronary heart disease or systemic disorders. It is distinct from the specific heart muscle diseases of known cause. Cardiomyopathy has been classified into three types based on anatomic and functional features: hypertrophic, dilated (or congestive), and restrictive (Fig. 18–1).

1. In hypertrophic cardiomyopathy (HCM), there is massive ventricular hypertrophy with a smaller than normal ventricular cavity. Contractile function of the ventricle is enhanced, but ventricular filling is impaired by relaxation abnormalities.

2. Dilated (or congestive) cardiomyopathy is characterized by decreased contractile function of the ventricle associated with ventricular dilatation. Endocardial fibroelastosis (seen in infancy) and doxorubicin cardiomyopathy (seen in children who

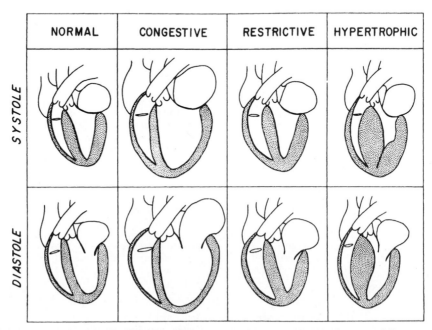

Figure 18–1. Diagram of the 50-degree left anterior oblique view of the heart in different types of cardiomyopathy at end systole and end diastole. "Congestive" corresponds to "dilated" cardiomyopathy as used in the text. (From Goldman MR, Boucher CA: Values of radionuclide imaging techniques in assessing cardiomyopathy. Am J Cardiol 46:1232–1236, 1980.)

have received chemotherapy for malignancies) have clinical features similar to those of dilated cardiomyopathy.

3. Restrictive cardiomyopathy denotes a restriction of diastolic filling of the ventricles (usually infiltrative disease). Contractile function of the ventricle may be normal, but there is marked dilatation of both atria.

The three types of cardiomyopathies are functionally different from one another, and the demands of therapy are also different. Table 18–1 summarizes clinical characteristics of the three types of cardiomyopathy.

Hypertrophic Cardiomyopathy

HCM is a heterogeneous, usually familial disorder of heart muscle. In about 50% of cases, HCM is inherited as a mendelian autosomal dominant trait and is caused by mutations in one of 10 genes encoding protein components of the cardiac sarcomere (such as β-myosin heavy chain, myosin binding protein C, and cardiac troponin-T). The remainder of the cases occurs sporadically. HCM is usually seen in adolescents and young adults, with equal gender distribution. It may be seen in children with LEOPARD syndrome (see Table 2–1). A usually transient form of HCM occurs in infants of diabetic mothers, which is presented under a separate heading in this chapter.

PATHOLOGY AND PATHOPHYSIOLOGY

1. The most characteristic abnormality is the hypertrophied left ventricle (LV), with the ventricular cavity usually small or normal in size. Although asymmetrical septal hypertrophy, a condition formerly known as idiopathic hypertrophic subaortic stenosis (Fig. 18–2), is most common, the hypertrophy may be concentric or

Table 18–1. **Summary of Clinical Characteristics of Cardiomyopathies**

Clinical Features	Hypertrophic	Dilated	Restrictive
Cause	Inherited (AD in about 50%) Sporadic (new mutation ±)	Pluricausal (e.g., toxic, metabolic, infectious, alcohol, doxorubicin)	Myocardial fibrosis, hypertrophy, or infiltration (amyloid, hemochromatosis)
Hemodynamic dysfunction	Diastolic dysfunction (with normal systolic function) (abnormally stiff LV with impaired ventricular filling)	Systolic contractile dysfunction ($\downarrow$ cardiac output, $\downarrow$ stroke volume, $\uparrow$ LVEDP)	Diastolic dysfunction (rigid ventricular walls impede ventricular filling)
Echo (morphology)	Thickened LV (and *occasionally* RV) wall	Biventricular dilatation ($\uparrow$ LVDD, $\uparrow$ LVSD)	Biatrial enlargement
	Small or normal LV chamber dimension	Atrial enlargement in proportion to ventricular enlargement	Normal LV and RV volume
	Supernormal LV contractility	Decreased LV contractility	Normal LV systolic function until advanced stage
	HOCM and/or ASH	Apical thrombus (±)	Atrial thrombus (±)
Doppler	Reduced relaxation pattern (see Fig. 18–6)	Reduced relaxation pattern (see Fig. 18–6)	"Restrictive" pattern (see Fig. 18–6)
Treatment	β-Adrenoreceptor blockers	Vasodilator therapy	Diuretics
	Calcium antagonists (Digitalis/catechols and nitrates contraindicated)	Digitalis plus diuretics β-Adrenoceptor blockers (±)	Anticoagulants (±) Corticosteroids (±)
		Anticoagulants	Permanent pacemaker for advanced heart block (±)
	(Diuretics may worsen symptoms)	Antiarrhythmics (±) Cardiac transplantation (±)	Cardiac transplantation (±)

AD, autosomal dominant; ASH, asymmetrical septal hypertrophy; HOCM, hypertrophic obstructive cardiomyopathy; LV, left ventricle; LVDD, left ventricular diastolic dimension; LVEDP, left ventricular end-diastolic pressure; LVSD, left ventricular systolic dimension; RV, right ventricle.

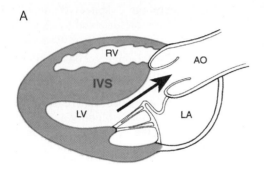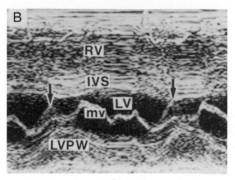

Figure 18–2. *Systolic anterior motion of the mitral valve.* **A,** *Diagram of systolic anterior motion in the presence of an asymmetrical septal hypertrophy. The Venturi effect may be important in the production of systolic anterior motion.* **B,** *M-mode echo of the mitral valve in a patient with hypertrophic cardiomyopathy. Systolic anterior motion of the anterior leaflet of the mitral valve is indicated by arrows. AO, aorta; IVS, interventricular septum; LA, left atrium, LV, left ventricle; LVPW, LV posterior wall; mv, mitral valve; RV, right ventricle.*

    localized to a small segment of the septum (Fig. 18–3). Microscopically, an extensive disarray of hypertrophied myocardial cells, myocardial scarring, and abnormalities of the small intramural coronary arteries are present.

2. In some patients, an intracavitary pressure gradient develops during systole, either at subaortic or less commonly (about 5%) at midcavity. Subaortic obstruction is caused by systolic anterior motion (SAM) of the mitral valve against the hypertrophied septum, which is called hypertrophic obstructive cardiomyopathy (HOCM) (see Fig. 18–2). The SAM is probably created by the high outflow velocities and Venturi forces with frequent association of mitral regurgitation. Midcavity obstruction is caused by anomalous direct insertion of anterolateral papillary muscle into the anterior mitral leaflet. In so-called apical HCM, hypertrophy is confined to the left ventricular apex, without intracavitary obstruction (and with giant negative T waves on the ECG). This subtype is present in about 25% of patients in Japan and less than 10% in other parts of the world.

3. The myocardium itself has an enhanced contractile state, but diastolic ventricular filling is impaired by abnormal stiffness of the LV, which may lead to left atrial enlargement and pulmonary venous congestion, producing congestive symptoms

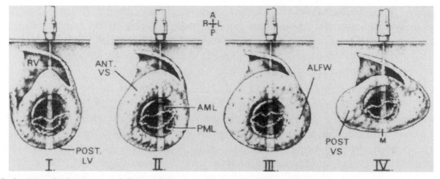

Figure 18–3. *Morphologic variability in hypertrophic cardiomyopathy seen on parasternal short-axis view of two-dimensional echo. In type I hypertrophy, relatively mild left ventricular hypertrophy confined to the anterior portion of the ventricular septum (VS) is present. In type II, hypertrophy of the anterior and posterior septum is present in the absence of free wall thickening. In type III, there is diffuse hypertrophy of substantial portions of both the ventricular septum and the anterolateral free wall (ALFW). In type IV, the M-mode echo beam (M) does not traverse the thickened portions of the left ventricle (LV) in the posterior septum and anterolateral free wall. A or ANT, anterior; AML, anterior mitral leaflet; L, left; LVFW, LV free wall; P or POST, posterior; PML, posterior mitral leaflet; R, right. (From Maron BJ: Asymmetry in hypertrophic cardiomyopathy: The septal to free wall thickness ratio revisited [editorial]. Am J Cardiol 55:835–838, 1985.)*

(exertional dyspnea, orthopnea, paroxysmal nocturnal dyspnea). Patients with left ventricular outflow tract (LVOT) obstruction are more disabled by elevated LV pressure and concomitant mitral regurgitation than by diastolic dysfunction.

4. A unique aspect of HOCM is the variability of the degree of obstruction from moment to moment, so that the intensity of the heart murmur varies from time to time. Because the obstruction of the LVOT results from SAM of the mitral valve against the hypertrophied ventricular septum, any influence that reduces the LV systolic volume (such as positive inotropic agents, reduced blood volume, or lowering of the systemic vascular resistance) increases the obstruction. On the other hand, any influence that increases the LV systolic volume (such as negative inotropic agents, leg raising, blood transfusion, or increasing systemic vascular resistance) lessens the obstruction.

5. A large portion of the stroke volume (about 80%) is ejected during the early part of systole when there is little or no obstruction, producing a sharp upstroke in the arterial pulse, a characteristic finding of HOCM. The obstruction occurs late in systole, producing a late systolic murmur.

6. Patients with severe hypertrophy and obstruction may experience anginal chest pain, lightheadedness, near syncope, or syncope. Patients are also likely to develop arrhythmias, which may lead to sudden death (presumably from ventricular tachycardia or fibrillation). Nearly 30% of children with HCM have myocardial bridging* (seen on coronary angiograms) with narrowing of the anterior descending coronary artery, which may have a key role in the development of ventricular arrhythmias. These patients may be more susceptible to sudden death.

CLINICAL MANIFESTATIONS

History

1. Easy fatigability, dyspnea, palpitation, dizziness, syncope, or anginal pain may be present.

2. Family history is positive for the disease in 30% to 60% of patients.

Physical Examination

1. A sharp upstroke of the arterial pulse is characteristic (in contrast to a slow upstroke seen with fixed aortic stenosis [AS]). A left ventricular lift and a systolic thrill at the apex or along the lower left sternal border may be present.

2. The S2 is normal, and an ejection click is generally absent. A grade 1 to 3/6 ejection systolic murmur of medium pitch is most audible at the middle and lower left sternal borders or at the apex. A soft holosystolic murmur of mitral regurgitation (MR) is often present. The intensity and even the presence of the murmur vary from examination to examination.

Electrocardiography. The ECG is abnormal in the majority of patients. Common ECG abnormalities include left ventricular hypertrophy (LVH), ST-T changes, and abnormally deep Q waves (owing to septal hypertrophy) with diminished or absent R waves in the left precordial leads (Fig. 18–4). Occasionally, "giant" negative T waves are seen in the left precordial leads, which may suggest apical HCM. Other ECG abnormalities may include cardiac arrhythmias and first-degree AV block.

X-ray Studies. Mild left ventricular enlargement with a globular-shaped heart may be present. The pulmonary vascularity is usually normal.

---

*Normally, the large epicardial coronary arteries run on the surface of the heart, with only their terminal branches penetrating the myocardium. When parts of the epicardial artery dip beneath the epicardial muscle so that there is a muscle bridge over the artery, it is called myocardial bridging.

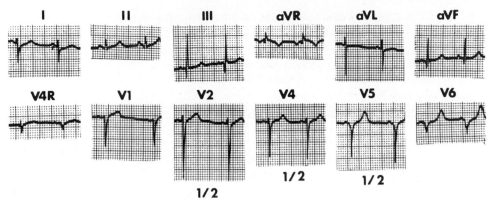

Figure 18–4. *Tracing from a 17-year-old girl with hypertrophic obstructive cardiomyopathy with marked septal hypertrophy. Note prominent Q waves with absent R waves in V5 and V6.*

Echocardiography

1. Echo is diagnostic. Two-dimensional echo demonstrates the wide morphologic spectrum of the disease, including concentric hypertrophy (Fig. 18–5), localized segmental hypertrophy, and asymmetrical septal hypertrophy (see Fig. 18–3). Apical HCM may be missed by two-dimensional echo. (If apical HCM is suspected, cardiac magnetic resonance imaging should be obtained.)

2. A diastolic LV wall thickness of 15 mm (or on occasion, 13 or 14 mm), usually with LV dimension less than 45 mm, is accepted for the clinical diagnosis of HCM in adults. For children, a z-score of 2 or more relative to body surface area is theoretically compatible with the diagnosis.

   The heart of some highly trained athletes may show hypertrophy of the LV wall, making the differentiation between the physiologic hypertrophy and HCM difficult. An LV wall thickness of 13 mm or greater is very uncommon in highly trained athletes and is always associated with an enlarged LV cavity (with LV diastolic dimension >54 mm, range 55 to 63 mm). Therefore, athletes with LV wall thickness greater than 16 mm and a nondilated LV cavity are likely to have HCM (Pelliccia et al, 1991).

3. M-mode echo may demonstrate an asymmetrical septal hypertrophy of the interventricular septum (with the septal thickness 1.4 times greater than the posterior

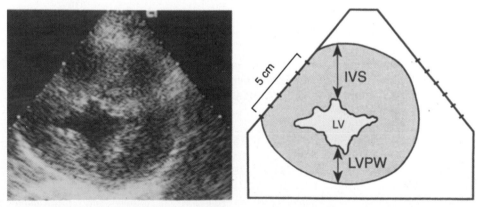

Figure 18–5. *Parasternal short-axis view of a 14-year-old boy with hypertrophic cardiomyopathy. Marked hypertrophy of the interventricular septum (IVS) as well as the posterior wall of the left ventricle (LVPW) is present. The left ventricle (LV) cavity is small. The interventricular septum is approximately 39 mm, and the LV posterior wall is 26 mm thick. The thickness of both structures does not exceed 10 mm in normal persons.*

LV wall) and occasionally SAM of the anterior mitral valve leaflet in the obstructive type (see Fig. 18–2).

4. Mitral inflow Doppler tracing demonstrates diastolic dysfunction with decreased E-wave velocity, increased deceleration time, and decreased E/A ratio of the mitral valve (usually less than 0.8) (Fig 18–6). LV systolic function is normal or supernormal.

5. Doppler peak gradient in the LVOT of 30 mm Hg indicates an obstructive type.

NATURAL HISTORY

1. The obstruction may be absent, stable, or slowly progressive. Genetically predisposed individuals often show striking increases in wall thickness during childhood.

2. Death is often sudden and unexpected and typically is associated with sports or vigorous exertion. Sudden death may occur most commonly in patients between 10 and 35 years of age. The incidence of sudden death may be as high as 4% to 6% a year in children and adolescents and 2% to 4% a year in adults. Ventricular fibrillation is the cause of death in the majority of sudden deaths. Even brief episodes of asymptomatic ventricular tachycardia on ambulatory ECG may be a risk factor for sudden death. Patients with myocardial bridging (occurring in about 30%) may be at risk for sudden death.

3. Atrial fibrillation may cause stroke or heart failure. Atrial fibrillation results from LA enlargement with loss of the atrial "kick" needed for filling the thick LV.

4. In a minority of patients, heart failure with cardiac dilatation ("burned out" phase of the disease) may develop later in life.

5. Subacute bacterial endocarditis (SBE) may affect the mitral valve, at the point of mitral-septal contact or aortic valve.

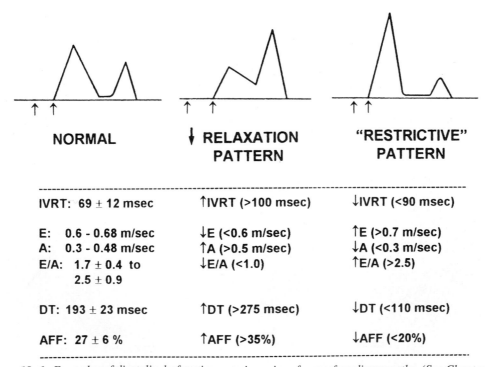

NORMAL	↓ RELAXATION PATTERN	"RESTRICTIVE" PATTERN
IVRT: 69 ± 12 msec	↑IVRT (>100 msec)	↓IVRT (<90 msec)
E: 0.6 - 0.68 m/sec	↓E (<0.6 m/sec)	↑E (>0.7 m/sec)
A: 0.3 - 0.48 m/sec	↑A (>0.5 m/sec)	↓A (<0.3 m/sec)
E/A: 1.7 ± 0.4 to 2.5 ± 0.9	↓E/A (<1.0)	↑E/A (>2.5)
DT: 193 ± 23 msec	↑DT (>275 msec)	↓DT (<110 msec)
AFF: 27 ± 6 %	↑AFF (>35%)	↓AFF (<20%)

Figure 18–6. *Examples of diastolic dysfunction seen in various forms of cardiomyopathy. (See Chapter 6 for further discussion.) A, A-wave velocity (the velocity of a second wave that coincides with atrial contraction); AFF, atrial filling fraction; DT, deceleration time; E, E-wave velocity (the velocity of an early peak); E/A, ratio of E-wave to A-wave velocity; IVRT, isovolumic relaxation time.*

6. Pregnancy is usually well tolerated, and most pregnant patients undergo normal vaginal delivery without the necessity for cesarean section.

MANAGEMENT

The goal of treatment is to reduce ventricular contractility, increase ventricular volume, increase ventricular compliance, and increase LV outflow tract dimensions. In the obstructive form of the condition, reduction of LV outflow tract pressure gradient is important. Unfortunately, most of the therapeutic modalities used do not appear to reduce mortality rate significantly. Surgical implantation of an automatic defibrillator may prove to be a very important modality to reduce sudden death.

1. General management:
   a. Moderate restriction of physical activity is recommended. Patients with the diagnosis of HCM should avoid strenuous exercise or competitive sports, regardless of age, gender, symptoms, LVOT obstruction, or treatment.
   b. Digitalis is contraindicated because it increases the degree of obstruction. Other cardiotonic drugs and vasodilators should be avoided because they tend to increase the pressure gradient. Diuretics are usually ineffective and can be harmful. However, judicious use can help improve congestive symptoms (e.g., exertional dyspnea, orthopnea) by reducing LV filling pressure.
   c. Prophylaxis against SBE is indicated.
   d. Clinical screening of first-degree relatives and other family members should be encouraged.
   e. Annual evaluation during adolescence (12 to 18 years of age) is recommended, with physical examination, ECG, and two-dimensional echo studies.

2. Patients with symptoms (dyspnea, chest discomfort, disability). Exertional dyspnea and disability are caused by diastolic dysfunction with impaired filling because of increased LV stiffness. Chest pain is probably due to myocardial ischemia of severely hypertrophied LV. β-Blockers and calcium channel blockers are effective therapies in children with HCM. These agents reduce hypercontractile systolic function and improve diastolic filling.
   a. A β-adrenergic blocker (such as propranolol, atenolol, or metoprolol) appears to be a preferred drug for symptomatic patients with outflow gradient, which develops only with exertion. This drug reduces the degree of outflow tract obstruction, decreases the incidence of anginal pain, and has antiarrhythmic effects.
   b. Calcium channel blockers (principally verapamil) may be equally effective in both the nonobstructive and obstructive forms. Adverse hemodynamic effects may occur, presumably as the result of vasodilating properties predominating over negative inotropic effects.
   c. Disopyramide (negative inotropic agent and type IA antiarrhythmic agent) has been shown to provide symptomatic benefit in patients with resting obstruction (by reducing the degree of SAM and mitral regurgitation volume as a result of the negative inotropic effect of the drug). Supplemental therapy with β-adrenergic blockers is advised because of accelerated AV conduction during atrial fibrillation.

3. Asymptomatic patients. Prophylactic therapy with either β-adrenergic blockers or the calcium channel blocker verapamil is controversial in asymptomatic patients without LV obstruction. Some favor prophylactic administration of these drugs to prevent sudden death or to delay progression of the disease process; others limit prophylactic drug therapy to young patients with a family history of premature sudden death and those with particularly marked LVH. The efficacy of empirical prophylactic drug treatment with these agents is unresolved.

4. Drug-refractory patients with obstruction. The Morrow procedure is the procedure of choice. Two other techniques, alcohol septal ablation and pacemaker implantation, can be considered alternatives to surgery for selected patients.

    a. Morrow's myotomy-myectomy. Transaortic LV septal myotomy-myectomy (the Morrow operation) is the procedure of choice for drug-refractory patients with LVOT obstruction. This operation is performed through an aortotomy without the benefit of complete direct visualization. Two vertical and parallel incisions are made (about 1 cm apart, 1 to 1.5 cm deep) into the hypertrophied ventricular septum. A third transverse incision connects the two incisions at their distal extent, and the bar of rectangular septal muscle is excised. An indication for the procedure is the presence of a resting pressure gradient greater than 50 mm Hg by continuous-wave Doppler study in patients who are symptomatic despite medical management.

    The mortality rate including children is 1% to 3%. Partial or complete left bundle branch block (LBBB) always results. Symptoms improve in most patients, but patients may later die of congestive symptoms and arrhythmias caused by the cardiomyopathy. Serious complications of the surgery such as complete heart block requiring permanent pacemaker and surgically induced ventricular septal defect have become uncommon (1% to 2%).

    b. Percutaneous alcohol septal ablation. The introduction of absolute alcohol into a target septal perforator branch of the left anterior descending coronary artery produces myocardial infarction within the proximal ventricular septum. This is analogous to surgical myomyectomy. A decrease in pressure gradient occurs after 6 to 12 months. A large proportion of patients demonstrate subjective improvement in symptoms and in quality of life. Increasing popularity of the procedure is probably unjustifiable. This procedure should not be considered a routine invasive procedure because selection of the appropriate perforator branch is crucially important.

    Procedure-related mortality is between 1% to 4%. Permanent pacemaker implantation occurs in 1% to 4%. This procedure commonly results in RBBB, rather than the LBBB seen with surgical myotomy.

    c. Pacemaker implantation. Dual-chamber pacing was shown in earlier studies to reduce symptoms and the pressure gradient across the LVOT, but more recent studies did not support earlier findings. There are currently no data to support the contention that pacing improves survival or quality of life. Therefore, pacing is not recommended as the primary treatment for most symptomatic patients with obstruction.

5. Implantable cardioverter-defibrillator (ICD). HCM has become one of the most frequent indications for ICD implantation in children, with proven efficacy to prevent sudden death from arrhythmias. ICD implantation is warranted when the risk for sudden death is judged to be unacceptably high. The following are risk factors for sudden death in HCM.
    a. Prior cardiac arrest (ventricular fibrillation)
    b. Spontaneous sustained ventricular tachycardia
    c. Family history of premature sudden death
    d. Unexplained syncope, particularly in young patients
    e. LV thickness of 30 mm and more, particularly in adolescents and young adults
    f. Abnormal exercise blood pressure (attenuated response or hypotension)
    g. Nonsustained ventricular tachycardia

    The ICD appears indicated in patients with HCM and spontaneously occurring VT, aborted sudden death, and malignant genotype or family history of sudden death. Special consideration may be given to adolescents for ICD implantation because it is the period of life consistently showing the greatest predilection for sudden death. For very young high-risk patients, the administration of amiodarone may be considered.

6. Cardiac arrhythmias.

    a. Ventricular arrhythmias may be treated with propranolol, amiodarone, and other standard antiarrhythmic agents guided by serial ambulatory ECG monitoring.
    b. Atrial fibrillation occurs more often in patients with LA enlargement. In certain patients, atrial fibrillation may trigger ventricular arrhythmias. For a new-onset

atrial fibrillation, electrical cardioversion followed by anticoagulation with warfarin (superior to aspirin) is recommended. Amiodarone is generally considered the most effective agent for preventing recurrence of atrial fibrillation.

7. Mitral valve replacement. Mitral valve replacement with a low-profile prosthetic valve may be indicated in selected patients in whom the basal anterior septum is relatively thin (<18 mm), the region of greatest septal thickness is inaccessible to a transaortic myotomy-myectomy, or there is severe MR. The operative mortality is about 6%. About 70% of patients show symptomatic improvement, but complications related to the prosthetic valve occur.

Infants of Diabetic Mothers

PREVALENCE

At least 1.3% of pregnancies are complicated by diabetes mellitus.

PATHOLOGY

1. The teratogenic action of diabetes mellitus is generalized, affecting multiple organ systems. The prevalence of major congenital malformations in infants of diabetic mothers is as high as 6% to 9% (i.e., three to four times that found in the general population). Congenital malformations of all types are increased in infants of diabetic mothers, but neural tube defects (anencephaly, myelomeningocele), congenital heart defects, and sacral dysgenesis or agenesis are common. Infants born to insulin-dependent diabetic mothers are at highest risk for developing congenital malformations; infants born to mothers with non–insulin-dependent, well-controlled diabetes do not appear to have an increased risk for congenital malformations.

2. Infants of diabetic mothers have a high prevalence of congenital heart defects, cardiomyopathy, and persistent pulmonary hypertension of the newborn (PPHN).

   a. The risk of a congenital heart defect is three to four times greater than that in the general population, with VSD, TGA, truncus arteriosus, tricuspid atresia, and coarctation of the aorta (COA) among the more common defects.

   b. HCM with or without obstruction is seen in 10% to 20% of these infants. The weight of the heart is increased by the increased myocardial fiber size and number (rather than by excess glycogen, as once thought); the hypertrophy is thought to be caused by hyperinsulinemia. Although free walls of both ventricles and the ventricular septum are hypertrophied, the ventricular septum characteristically is more hypertrophied than the LV posterior wall (asymmetrical septal hypertrophy) (Fig. 18–7).

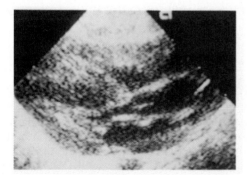 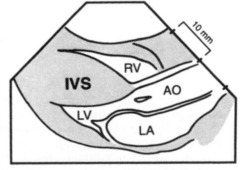

Figure 18–7. *Parasternal long-axis view of an infant of a diabetic mother. There is asymmetrical hypertrophy of the interventricular septum (IVS), which is at least two times as thick as the posterior wall of the left ventricle (LV). AO, aorta; LA, left atrium; RV, right ventricle.*

c. Infants of diabetic mothers also have an increased risk for PPHN. They are often affected by conditions that promote the persistence of pulmonary hypertension, such as hypoglycemia, perinatal asphyxia, respiratory distress, and polycythemia.

CLINICAL MANIFESTATIONS

The clinical manifestations only of cardiomyopathy are presented in this section. Congenital heart defects and PPHN are discussed under specific headings.

1. The history usually reveals gestational or insulin-dependent diabetes mellitus in the mother. The patient often has a history of progressive respiratory distress with tachypnea (80 to 100 breaths/minute) from birth.

2. These large-for-gestational-age babies are often plethoric and mildly cyanotic and may have tachypnea and tachycardia (>160 beats/minute). Signs of congestive heart failure (CHF) with gallop rhythm may be found in 5% to 10% of these babies. The patient may have a systolic murmur along the left sternal border, which may be caused by an outflow tract obstruction or an associated defect.

3. Chest x-ray films may reveal a varying degree of cardiomegaly. Pulmonary vascular markings are normal or mildly increased because of pulmonary venous congestion.

4. The ECG is usually nonspecific, but a long QT interval caused by a long ST segment secondary to hypocalcemia may be found. Occasionally, RVH, LVH, or biventricular hypertrophy (BVH) may be seen.

5. Echo may show the following:

   a. The ventricular septum is often disproportionately thicker than the LV free wall, but even free walls are thicker than normal (see Fig. 18–7). The degree of asymmetrical septal hypertrophy has no relationship to the severity of the maternal diabetes.

   b. Supernormal contractility of the LV and evidence of LVOT obstruction appear in about 50% of infants with cardiomyopathy.

   c. Rarely, the LV is dilated, and its contractility is decreased.

MANAGEMENT

1. General supportive measures are provided, such as intravenous fluids, correction of hypoglycemia and hypocalcemia, and ventilatory assistance, if indicated.

2. In most cases, the hypertrophy spontaneously resolves within the first 6 to 12 months of life. β-Adrenergic blockers, such as propranolol, may help the LVOT obstruction, but treatment is usually not necessary. Digitalis and other inotropic agents are contraindicated because they may worsen the obstruction.

3. If the LV is dilated with decreased LV contractility, the usual anticongestive measures (e.g., digoxin, diuretics) are indicated.

Transient Hypertrophic Cardiomyopathy in Neonates

Recently, transient HCM in neonates who had perinatal injury with acute fetal distress has been described. Initially, echo studies showed abnormal LV systolic and diastolic function but the LV wall thickness was normal. The hypertrophy of the LV occurred between days 2 and 7 and affected initially the interventricular septum and later the LV posterior wall, but it disappeared in all cases between 1 and 5 months of life. Acute fetal distress with myocardial ischemia is believed to have caused the hypertrophy. The prognosis of this type of HCM is good, in contrast to that of other primitive HCM occurring in neonates (Vaillant et al, 1997).

Dilated or Congestive Cardiomyopathy

CAUSE

Dilated cardiomyopathy is the most common form of cardiomyopathy. The most common cause of dilated cardiomyopathy is idiopathic (>60%), followed by familial cardiomyopathy, active myocarditis, and other causes. Many cases of unexplained dilated cardiomyopathy may, in fact, result from subclinical myocarditis. Among the familial type, an autosomal dominant inheritance pattern is most frequent, although X-linked, autosomal recessive, and mitochondrial inheritance patterns have been reported.

Other causes of dilated cardiomyopathy include infectious causes other than viral infection (bacterial, fungal, protozoal, rickettsial), as well as endocrine-metabolic disorders (hyper- and hypothyroidism, excessive catecholamines, diabetes, hypocalcemia, hypophosphatemia, glycogen storage disease, mucopolysaccharidoses) and nutritional disorders (kwashiorkor, beriberi, carnitine deficiency). Cardiotoxic agents such as doxorubicin and systemic diseases such as connective tissue disease can also cause dilated cardiomyopathy.

PATHOLOGY AND PATHOPHYSIOLOGY

1. In dilated cardiomyopathy, a weakening of systolic contraction is associated with dilatation of all four cardiac chambers. Dilatation of the atria is in proportion to ventricular dilatation. The ventricular walls are not thickened, although heart weight is increased. Intracavitary thrombus formation is common in the apical portion of the ventricular cavities and in atrial appendages and may give rise to pulmonary and systemic emboli.
2. Histologic examinations from endomyocardial biopsies show varying degrees of myocyte hypertrophy and fibrosis. Inflammatory cells are usually absent, but a varying incidence of inflammatory myocarditis has been reported.

CLINICAL MANIFESTATIONS

History

1. A history of fatigue, weakness, and symptoms of left-sided heart failure (dyspnea on exertion, orthopnea) may be elicited.
2. A history of prior viral illness is occasionally obtained.

Physical Examination

1. Signs of CHF (tachycardia, pulmonary crackles, weak peripheral pulses, distended neck veins, hepatomegaly) are present. The apical impulse is usually displaced to the left and inferiorly.
2. The S2 may be normal or narrowly split with accentuated P2 if pulmonary hypertension develops. A prominent S3 is present with or without gallop rhythm. A soft regurgitant systolic murmur (caused by mitral or tricuspid regurgitation) may be present.

Electrocardiography

1. Sinus tachycardia, LVH, and ST-T changes are the most common findings. Left or right atrial hypertrophy (LAH or RAH) may be present. Rarely, a healed anterior myocardial infarction pattern may be present.
2. Atrial or ventricular arrhythmias and atrioventricular (AV) conduction disturbances may be seen.

X-ray Studies. Generalized cardiomegaly is usually present, with or without signs of pulmonary venous hypertension or pulmonary edema.

Echocardiography. Echo is the most important tool in the diagnosis of the condition and is important in the longitudinal follow-up of patients.

1. Two-dimensional echocardiogram shows marked LV enlargement and poor contractility (Fig 18–8). The LA may also be enlarged. Occasionally, intracavitary

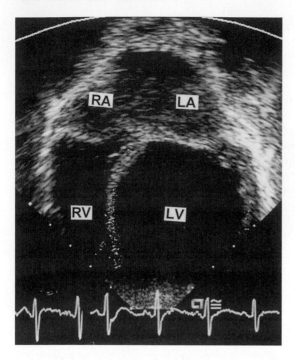

Figure 18–8. *Apical four-chamber view of two-dimensional echocardiogram showing a massively dilated left ventricular cavity in a 3-year-old child with dilated cardiomyopathy. LA, left atrium; LV, left ventricle; RA, right atrium; RV, right ventricle.*

thrombus may be found, especially in the left atrial appendage and cardiac apex. Pericardial effusion may be seen.

2. On the M-mode echo, the end-diastolic and end-systolic dimensions of the LV are increased, with a markedly reduced fractional shortening and ejection fraction of the LV (Fig. 18–9). The M-mode measurement provides a valuable technique for serial assessment of patients with dilated cardiomyopathy.

3. Mitral inflow Doppler tracing demonstrates a reduced E velocity and a decreased E/A ratio (ratio of E-wave to A-wave velocity) (see Fig. 18–6).

NATURAL HISTORY

1. Progressive deterioration is the rule rather than the exception. About two thirds of patients die from intractable heart failure within 4 years after the onset of symptoms of CHF.

2. Atrial and ventricular arrhythmias develop with time (in about 50% of patients studied by 24-hour Holter) but are not predictive of outcome.

3. Systemic and pulmonary embolism resulting from dislodgment of intracavitary thrombi occurs in the late stages of the illness.

4. Causes of death are CHF, sudden death resulting from arrhythmias, and massive embolization.

MANAGEMENT

1. Medical treatment is aimed at the underlying heart failure. Diuretics (furosemide, spironolactone), digoxin, and angiotensin-converting enzyme (ACE) inhibitors (captopril, enalapril) are an integral part of therapy, as is bed rest or restriction of activity.

2. Critically ill children may require intubation and mechanical ventilation. Rapidly acting intravenous inotropic support (dobutamine, dopamine) is often needed.

3. Use of β-adrenergic blocker therapy in children with chronic heart failure has been shown to improve LV ejection fraction. Carvedilol is a β-adrenergic blocker with additional vasodilating action. The beneficial effects of β-adrenergic blocking agents

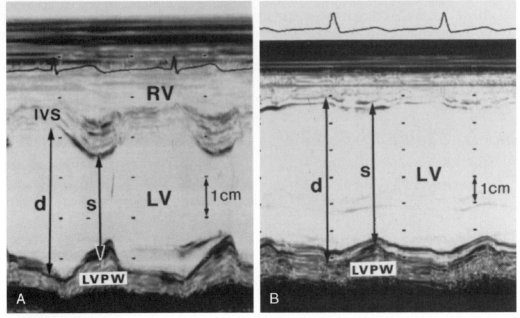

Figure 18–9. *M-mode echo in a child with dilated cardiomyopathy.* **A,** *M-mode echo from a 9-year-old normal child. The left ventricular (LV) diastolic dimension (d) is 36 mm, and the LV systolic dimension (s) is 24 mm, with resulting fractional shortening of 33%.* **B,** *M-mode echo from an 8-year-old child with dilated cardiomyopathy with a markedly decreased LV contractile function. The LV diastolic dimension (62 mm) and LV systolic dimension (52 mm) are markedly increased, with a marked decrease in the fractional shortening (16%). IVS, interventricular septum; LVPW, LV posterior wall; RV, right ventricle.*

(somewhat unorthodox, given poor contractility) have been reported in adult patients. Similar beneficial effects of β-blockers have been reported in children with dilated cardiomyopathy of various causes. Recent evidence suggests that activation of the sympathetic nervous system may have deleterious cardiac effects (rather than being an important compensatory mechanism, as traditionally thought). β-Adrenergic blockers may exert beneficial effects by a negative chronotropic effect, with reduced oxygen demand, reduction in catecholamine toxicity, inhibition of sympathetically mediated vasoconstriction, or reduction of potentially lethal ventricular arrhythmias.

4. Antiplatelet agents (aspirin) should be initiated. The propensity for thrombus formation in patients with dilated cardiac chambers and blood stasis may prompt use of anticoagulation with warfarin. If thrombi are detected, they should be treated aggressively with heparin initially and later switched to long-term warfarin therapy.

5. Patients with arrhythmias may be treated with amiodarone or other antiarrhythmic agents. Amiodarone is effective and relatively safe in children. For symptomatic bradycardia, a cardiac pacemaker may be necessary. An ICD may be considered, but there is limited experience with this device in children.

6. If carnitine deficiency is considered as the cause for the cardiomyopathy, carnitine supplementation should be started.

7. Following an interesting observation by Fazio and colleagues (1996), several small studies have shown beneficial effects of growth hormone in adult patients with dilated cardiomyopathy. Some of these studies reported that treatment with growth hormone for 3 to 6 months resulted in increased LV wall thickness, reduction of the chamber size, and improved cardiac output. However, some other studies did not find the same salutary effect of the hormone. A small study involving children (McElhinney et al, 2004) has reported that administration of recombinant

human growth hormone (0.025 to 0.04 mg/kg/day for 6 months) resulted in a trend toward improved LV ejection fraction, along with significant acceleration of somatic growth. Whether growth hormone treatment will finally find a place in the treatment of congestive cardiomyopathy remains to be established.

8. The utility of immunosuppressive agents, including steroids, cyclosporine, and azathioprine, remains unproved.

9. Many of these children may become candidates for cardiac transplantation.

Endocardial Fibroelastosis

PREVALENCE

The prevalence of the nonfamilial form of endocardial fibroelastosis is extremely rare. The prevalence has declined in the past three decades for unknown reasons; in the past, it accounted for 4% of cardiac autopsy cases in children.

PATHOLOGY

1. Primary endocardial fibroelastosis is a form of dilated cardiomyopathy seen in infants. The condition is characterized by diffuse changes in the endocardium with a white, opaque, glistening appearance. The heart chambers, primarily the left atrium (LA) and LV, are notably dilated and hypertrophied. Involvement of the right-sided heart chambers is rare. Deformities and shortening of the papillary muscles and chordae tendineae (resulting in MR) are often present late in the course. Similar pathology appears secondary to severe congenital obstructive lesions of the left heart, such as AS, COA, and hypoplastic left heart syndrome (HLHS) (called *secondary fibroelastosis*).

2. The cause of primary fibroelastosis is not known. It may be the result of a process of reaction to many different insults rather than a specific disease. Viral myocarditis and a sequel to interstitial myocarditis have received more attention than other proposed causes, including systemic carnitine deficiency and genetic factors. Several decades ago, mumps virus was once considered the possible causal agent for the disease. Recently, the mumps virus genome was found in the myocardium in a significant number of patients with the diagnosis, suggesting that endocardial fibroelastosis is a complication of myocarditis caused by the mumps virus (rather than enterovirus).

CLINICAL MANIFESTATIONS

History. Symptoms and signs of CHF (feeding difficulties, tachypnea, sweating, irritability, pallor, failure to thrive) develop in the first 10 months of life.

Physical Examination

1. Patients have tachycardia and tachypnea.

2. No heart murmur is audible in the majority of patients, although a gallop rhythm is usually present. Occasionally, a heart murmur of MR is audible.

3. Hepatomegaly is frequently present.

Electrocardiography. LVH with "strain" is typical of the condition. Occasionally, myocardial infarction patterns, arrhythmias, and varying degrees of AV block may be seen.

X-ray Studies. Marked generalized cardiomegaly with normal or congested pulmonary vascularity is usually present.

Echocardiography. A markedly dilated and poorly contracting LV in the absence of structural heart defects is characteristic. The LA is also markedly dilated. Bright endocardial echoes are typical of the condition.

MANAGEMENT

1. Early diagnosis and long-term (for years) treatment with digoxin, diuretics, and afterload-reducing agents are mandatory. Digoxin is continued for a minimum of

2 to 3 years and is then gradually discontinued if symptoms are absent, heart size is normal, and the ECG has reverted to normal.

2. An afterload-reducing agent (hydralazine up to 4 mg/kg per day, in four divided doses) has been reported to be beneficial.

3. SBE prophylaxis should be observed, especially when MR is present.

PROGNOSIS

When proper treatment is instituted, about one third of patients deteriorate and die of CHF. Another one third survive but experience persistent symptoms. The remaining one third exhibit complete recovery. Operative procedures are not available.

DIFFERENTIAL DIAGNOSIS

Infants with cardiomegaly on chest roentgenogram and no heart murmur often present a diagnostic challenge. The cardiomegaly may result from diseases that affect primarily the myocardium or coronary arteries, severe CHF from congenital heart defects, respiratory diseases, or other miscellaneous conditions. Box 18–1 contains partial lists of conditions that can arise with cardiomegaly without heart murmur in infants and young children. Most conditions listed under myocardial diseases and coronary artery diseases in Box 18–1 are discussed in other chapters, except for glycogen storage disease.

Glycogen Storage Disease. The classic glycogen storage disease that causes heart failure in infancy is Pompe's disease (Cori's type II), which is due to deficiency of α-1,4-glycosidase. This is an autosomal recessive disorder characterized by generalized muscle weakness, macroglossia, hepatomegaly, and signs of CHF or severe arrhythmias. The onset of CHF is around 2 to 3 months of age, with a fatal outcome usually during infancy.

BOX 18–1	DIFFERENTIAL DIAGNOSIS OF CARDIOMEGALY WITHOUT HEART MURMUR IN PEDIATRIC PATIENTS

MYOCARDIAL DISEASES
Endocardial fibroelastosis
Myocarditis (viral or idiopathic)
Glycogen storage disease

CORONARY ARTERY DISEASES RESULTING IN MYOCARDIAL INSUFFICIENCY
Anomalous origin of the left coronary artery from the pulmonary artery
Collagen disease (periarteritis nodosa)
Kawasaki disease

CONGENITAL HEART DEFECT WITH SEVERE HEART FAILURE
Critical aortic stenosis
Coarctation of the aorta in infants
Systemic arteriovenous fistula
Ebstein's anomaly (a soft tricuspid regurgitation murmur is frequently present)

MISCELLANEOUS CONDITIONS
Congestive heart failure (CHF) secondary to respiratory disease (upper airway obstruction, bronchopulmonary dysplasia)
Supraventricular tachycardia with CHF
Pericardial effusion
Tumors of the heart
Severe anemia
Endocrine disorders (thyrotoxicosis, pheochromocytoma)
Malnutrition (beriberi, kwashiorkor, carnitine deficiency)
Sensitivity/toxic reactions (sulfonamides, antibiotics, doxorubicin)
Muscular dystrophies
Familial dilated cardiomyopathies

The ECG may show a short PR interval, LVH in the majority of patients, occasional BVH, and ST-T changes in the left precordial leads. Excessive glycogen deposits in a skeletal muscle biopsy specimen are diagnostic. No treatment is available, but genetic counseling should be provided for the family.

Doxorubicin Cardiomyopathy

PREVALENCE

Doxorubicin cardiomyopathy is becoming the most common cause of chronic CHF in children. Its prevalence is nonlinearly dose related, occurring in 2% to 5% of patients who have received a cumulative dose of 400 to 500 mg/m^2 and up to 50% of patients who have received more than 1000 mg/m^2 of doxorubicin (Adriamycin).

CAUSE

1. Doxorubicin, which is commonly used in pediatric oncologic disorders, is the cause of the cardiomyopathy. C-13 anthracycline metabolites, which are inhibitors of adenosine triphosphatases of sarcoplasmic reticulum, mitochondria, and sarcolemma, have been implicated in the mechanism of cardiotoxicity.

2. Risk factors include age younger than 4 years and a cumulative dose exceeding 400 to 600 mg/m^2. A dosing regimen with larger and less frequent doses has been raised as a risk factor but not proved.

PATHOLOGY AND PATHOPHYSIOLOGY

1. Dilated LV, decreased contractility, elevated filling pressures of the LV, and reduced cardiac output characterize pathophysiologic features.

2. Microscopically, interstitial edema without evidence of inflammatory changes, loss of myofibrils within the myocyte, vacuolar degeneration, necrosis, and fibrosis are present.

CLINICAL MANIFESTATIONS

1. Patients are usually asymptomatic until signs of heart failure develop. Patients have a history of receiving doxorubicin, with the onset of symptoms 2 to 4 months, and rarely years, after completion of therapy. Tachypnea and dyspnea made worse by exertion are the usual presenting complaints. Occasionally, palpitation, cough, and substernal discomfort are complaints.

2. Signs of CHF are present, with hepatomegaly and distended neck veins. Gallop rhythm may be present, with occasional soft murmur of MR or tricuspid regurgitation (TR).

3. X-ray films show cardiomegaly with or without pulmonary congestion or pleural effusion.

4. The ECG shows sinus tachycardia with ST-T changes in a small number of patients (2% to 8%). A progressive increase in the basal (early morning) heart rate is reported.

5. Echo studies reveal the following:
   a. The size of the LV is slightly increased, and the thickness of the LV wall is decreased.
   b. LV contractility (either ejection fraction or fractional shortening) is decreased.
   c. Dobutamine stress echo is reported to be more sensitive than routine echo in examining the cardiac status of asymptomatic doxorubicin-treated patients.

MANAGEMENT

1. Attempts to reduce anthracycline cardiotoxicity have been directed toward (1) anthracycline dose limitation, (2) developing less cardiotoxic analogues, and (3) concurrently

administering cardioprotective agents to attenuate the cardiotoxic effects of anthracy-cline on the heart.

    a. Restriction of the total dose is controversial. Limiting the total cumulative dose to 400 to 500 mg/m^2 reduces the incidence of CHF to 5%, but this dose may not be effective in treating some malignancies. Continuous infusion therapy may reduce cardiac injury by avoiding peak levels, although such effects have not been observed.

    b. The analogues of doxorubicin, such as idarubicin and epirubicin, have cardiotoxicity similar to that of doxorubicin.

    c. Concurrent administration of cardioprotective agents, such as dexrazoxane (an iron chelator) (Lipshultz et al, 2004), carvedilol (a β-receptor antagonist with antioxidant property), and coenzyme Q10, has shown some protective effects without attenu-ating the antimalignancy effect of the drug.

2. In patients with clinical manifestations of doxorubicin cardiomyopathy, the following medications are used.

    a. Digoxin, diuretics, and afterload-reducing agents (ACE inhibitors) are useful.

    b. β-Blockers have been shown to be beneficial in some children with chemotherapy-induced cardiomyopathy, similar to what has been reported in adults. Metoprolol (starting at 0.1 mg/kg per dose twice a day and increasing to a maximal dose of 0.9 mg/kg per day) increases LV fractional shortening and ejection fraction and improves symptoms.

3. Cardiac transplantation may be an option for selected patients.

PROGNOSIS

Symptomatic cardiomyopathy carries a high mortality rate. The 2-year survival rate is about 20%, and all patients die by 9 years after the onset of the illness.

Carnitine Deficiency

Carnitine deficiency is a rare cause of cardiomegaly in infants and small children. Long-chain fatty acids are the primary and preferred substrate for the muscle. Carnitine is an essential cofactor for transport of long-chain fatty acids into mitochondria, where oxi-dation takes place. Carnitine deficiency leads to depressed mitochondrial oxidation of fatty acids, resulting in storage of fat in muscle and functional abnormalities of cardiac and skeletal muscle. Carnitine is synthesized predominantly in the liver.

Primary carnitine deficiency is an uncommon inherited disorder. The condition has been classified as either systemic or myopathic.

The systemic form of the disease manifests with low concentrations of carnitine in plasma, muscle, and liver. Symptoms are variable but include muscle weakness, cardiomyopathy, abnormal liver function, encephalopathy, impaired ketogenesis, and hypoglycemia during fasting. In systemic carnitine deficiency, patients may present with acute hepatic hypoglycemia and encephalopathy during the first year of life before the cardiomyopathy becomes symptomatic. Both hypertrophic and dilated cardiomyopathies have been reported with carnitine deficiency.

Myopathic disease is characterized primarily by muscle weakness. Fatty infiltration of muscle fiber is found at biopsy. The most common manifestation of myopathic carnitine deficiency is progressive cardiomyopathy, with or without skeletal muscle weakness that begins at 2 to 4 years of age.

The patients with cardiomyopathy may show bizarre T-wave spiking on the ECG. These children may die suddenly, presumably from arrhythmias.

Secondary forms of carnitine deficiency have been reported in renal tubular disorders (with excessive excretion of carnitine), chronic renal failure (excessive loss of carnitine from hemodialysis), inborn errors of metabolism with increased concentrations of organic acids, and occasional patients receiving total parenteral nutrition. Diagnosis of the condi-tion is established by extremely low levels of carnitine in plasma and skeletal muscle.

TREATMENT

1. Treatment with oral carnitine (L-carnitine: 50 to 100 mg/kg/day by mouth, divided twice or three times a day; maximum daily dose 3 g) may improve myocardial function, reduce cardiomegaly, and improve muscle weakness.

2. A recent multicenter study has shown that treatment of various forms of cardiomyopathy with L-carnitine, especially those with suggestive evidence of disorders of metabolism, provided clinical benefits.

3. Benefits of carnitine administration have been reported for other conditions with myocardial dysfunction, including prevention of diphtheric myocarditis in children and potential protective and therapeutic effects on doxorubicin-induced cardiomyopathy in rats.

Restrictive Cardiomyopathy

PREVALENCE AND CAUSE

Restrictive cardiomyopathy is an extremely rare form of cardiomyopathy, accounting for 5% of cardiomyopathy cases in children. It may be idiopathic, or it may be associated with a systemic disease such as scleroderma, amyloidosis, sarcoidosis, or an inborn error of metabolism (mucopolysaccharidosis). Malignancies or radiation therapy may result in restrictive cardiomyopathy.

PATHOLOGY AND PATHOPHYSIOLOGY

1. This condition is characterized by markedly dilated atria and generally normal ventricular dimensions. Ventricular diastolic filling is impaired, resulting from excessively stiff ventricular walls. Contractile function of the ventricle is normal. Therefore, this condition resembles constrictive pericarditis in clinical presentation and hemodynamic abnormalities.

2. There are areas of myocardial fibrosis and hypertrophy of myocytes, or the myocardium may be infiltrated by various materials. Infiltrative restrictive cardiomyopathy may be due to conditions such as amyloidosis, sarcoidosis, hemochromatosis, glycogen deposit, Fabry's disease (with deposition of glycosphingolipids), or neoplastic infiltration.

CLINICAL MANIFESTATIONS

1. The patients may have a history of exercise intolerance, weakness and dyspnea, or chest pain.

2. Jugular venous distention, gallop rhythm, and a systolic murmur of AV valve regurgitation may be present.

3. Chest x-ray films show cardiomegaly, pulmonary venous congestion, and occasional pleural effusion.

4. The ECG usually shows atrial hypertrophy. It may show atrial fibrillation and paroxysms of supraventricular tachycardia. AV block may be present in familial restrictive cardiomyopathy.

5. Echo studies reveal the following:
   a. Characteristic biatrial enlargement with normal dimension of the LV and RV is almost diagnostic.
   b. LV systolic function is normal (until the late stage of the disease).
   c. Atrial thrombus may be present.
   d. Findings of diastolic dysfunction are present (see Fig 18–6); the mitral inflow Doppler tracing shows an increased E velocity, shortened deceleration time, and increased E/A ratio.
   e. Differentiation from constrictive pericarditis can pose difficulties. In constrictive pericarditis, echo shows a thickened pericardium, and Doppler studies show a marked respiratory variation in the filling phase. Doppler studies also

show findings of diastolic dysfunction similar to those seen in restrictive pericarditis.

6. Cardiac catheterization reveals the following:
   a. PA pressure and RV and LV end-diastolic pressures are elevated.
   b. Endomyocardial biopsy may reveal a specific cause.

MANAGEMENT

Treatment is supportive because the prognosis is generally poor.

1. Diuretics are beneficial to relieve congestive symptoms, but they should be used judiciously because the resulting reduction in end-diastolic pressure may make symptoms worse. Digoxin is not indicated because systolic function is unimpaired. ACE inhibitors may reduce systemic blood pressure without increasing cardiac output and, therefore, should probably be avoided.

2. Calcium channel blockers may be used to increase diastolic compliance.

3. Anticoagulants (warfarin) and antiplatelet drugs (aspirin and dipyridamole) may help prevent thrombosis.

4. Corticosteroids and immunosuppressive agents have been suggested.

5. A permanent pacemaker is indicated for complete heart block.

6. Surgical options are limited to cardiac transplantation. Early transplantation is preferable before severe pulmonary hypertension develops. In patients with systemic disease (such as sarcoidosis), recurrence is a major concern after transplantation and it may not be a viable option.

Right Ventricular Dysplasia

PATHOLOGY

1. Right ventricular dysplasia, also called right ventricular cardiomyopathy, is a rare abnormality of unknown cause in which the myocardium of the RV is partially or totally replaced by fibrous or adipose tissue. The RV wall may assume a paper-thin appearance because of the total absence of myocardial tissue, but in others, RV wall thickness is normal or near normal. The LV is usually spared.

2. Most cases appear to be sporadic, although familial occurrences have been reported. Whether the disease is congenital or acquired is unknown, although evidence favors an acquired degenerative process. The disease appears to be prevalent in northern Italy.

CLINICAL MANIFESTATIONS

1. The onset is in infancy, childhood, or adulthood (but usually before the age of 20), with a history of palpitation, syncopal episodes, or both. Sudden death may be the first sign of the disease.

2. Presenting manifestations may be arrhythmias (ventricular tachycardia, supraventricular arrhythmias) or signs of CHF.

3. Chest x-ray films usually show cardiomegaly, and the ECG most often shows tall P waves in lead II (RAH), decreased RV potentials, T-wave inversion in the right precordial leads, and premature ventricular contractions or ventricular tachycardia of LBBB morphologies.

4. Echo shows selective RV enlargement and often areas of akinesia or dyskinesia.

5. A substantial portion of patients die before 5 years of age from CHF and intractable ventricular tachycardia.

MANAGEMENT

1. Various antiarrhythmic agents may be tried, but they are often unsuccessful in abolishing ventricular tachycardia.

2. Surgical intervention (ventricular incision or complete electrical disarticulation of the RV free wall) may be tried if antiarrhythmic therapy is unsuccessful.

3. An ICD may be indicated in selected cases.

Noncompaction Cardiomyopathy

Noncompaction cardiomyopathy, also known as left ventricular noncompaction, left ventricular hypertrabeculation, or spongy myocardium, results from an intrauterine arrest of normal compaction of the loose interwoven meshwork of the ventricular myocardium (which normally occurs during the first month of fetal life). This rare congenital cardiomyopathy was initially described in children, but it has been reported in adult population of all ages. The characteristic echo findings are segmental thickening of the LV wall consisting of two layers: a thin compacted epicardial layer and an extremely thickened noncompacted endocardial layer with prominent trabeculations and deep recesses. Apical and midventricular segments of both the inferior and lateral walls are most commonly affected.

The disease uniformly affects LV with or without concomitant RV involvement and results in systolic and diastolic ventricular dysfunction and clinical heart failure. There is usually no associated congenital anomaly of the heart, but facial dysmorphism may occur. Familial recurrence has been reported in up to 25% with a less severe form of abnormalities; evaluation of all members of the family has been recommended. The most common complication of the disease is heart failure. Less commonly, thromboembolic events, ventricular arrhythmias, and Wolff-Parkinson-White syndrome have been reported. The disease is usually progressive with worsening of heart failure despite optimal treatment. Treatment consists of anticongestive therapy (using digoxin, diuretic, ACE inhibitors). Oral anticoagulation, heart transplantation, and implantation of an ICD may be considered.

Mutations in the gene G4.5 on Xq28 may be responsible for noncompaction and may result in a wide spectrum of severe infantile cardiomyopathies, including isolated LV noncompaction as well as Barth syndrome. *Barth syndrome* consists of dilated cardiomyopathy (with endocardial fibroelastosis), skeletal myopathy, neutropenia (agranulocytopenia) with repeated infections, and abnormal mitochondria and has a sex-linked recessive inheritance pattern with females acting as carriers. Many patients with Barth syndrome die of cardiac failure during infancy.

Chapter 19

Cardiovascular Infections

Included in this chapter are infective endocarditis, myocarditis, pericarditis, Lyme carditis, and postperfusion syndrome. Other conditions in which the cause is not well established but the host's immune response to an infective agent is thought to play a role are also included, such as Kawasaki's disease and postpericardiotomy syndrome. Cardiac manifestations of human immunodeficiency virus (HIV) are also included.

Infective Endocarditis

PREVALENCE

Infective endocarditis (IE) accounts for 0.5 to 1 of every 1000 hospital admissions, excluding postoperative endocarditis. The frequency of IE among children seems to have increased in recent years. This is due in part to survivors of surgical repair of complex congenital heart disease and survivors of neonatal intensive care units, who are at an increased risk for IE.

PATHOGENESIS

1. Two factors are important in the pathogenesis of IE: a damaged area of endothelium and bacteremia, even transient. The presence of structural abnormalities of the heart or great arteries, with a significant pressure gradient or turbulence, produces endothelial damage. Such endothelial damage induces thrombus formation with deposition of sterile clumps of platelet and fibrin (nonbacterial thrombotic endocarditis), which provides a nidus for bacteria to adhere and eventually form an infected vegetation. Platelets and fibrin are deposited over the organisms, leading to enlargement of the vegetation.

2. Almost all patients who develop IE have a history of congenital or acquired heart disease. Drug addicts may develop endocarditis in the absence of known cardiac anomalies.

3. All congenital heart defects, with the exception of secundum-type atrial septal defect, predispose to endocarditis. More frequently encountered defects are tetralogy of Fallot, ventricular septal defect (VSD), aortic valve disease, transposition of the great arteries, and systemic–to–pulmonary artery (PA) shunt. Rheumatic valvular disease, particularly mitral insufficiency, is responsible in a small number of patients. Those with a prosthetic heart valve or prosthetic material in the heart are at particularly high risk for developing endocarditis. Patients with mitral valve prolapse (MVP) with mitral regurgitation (MR) and those with hypertrophic obstructive cardiomyopathy are also vulnerable to IE.

4. Any localized infection (e.g., abscess, osteomyelitis, pyelonephritis) can seed organisms into the circulation. Bacteremia frequently results after dental procedures,

especially in children who have carious teeth or disease of the gingiva. Bacteremia also occurs with activities such as chewing or brushing the teeth. Chewing with diseased teeth or gums may be the most frequent cause of bacteremia. (Therefore, good dental hygiene is more important in the prevention of IE than antibiotic coverage before dental procedures.)

PATHOLOGY

Vegetation of IE is usually found on the low-pressure side of the defect, either around the defect or on the opposite surface of the defect where endothelial damage is established by the jet effect of the defect. For example, vegetations are found in the PA in patent ductus arteriosus (PDA) or systemic-to-PA shunts, on the atrial surface of the mitral valve in MR, on the ventricular surface of the aortic valve and mitral chordae in aortic regurgitation (AR), and on the superior surface of the aortic valve or at the site of a jet lesion in the aorta in patients with aortic stenosis.

MICROBIOLOGY

1. In the past, *Streptococcus viridans*, enterococci, and *Staphylococcus aureus* were responsible for over 90% of the cases. This frequency has decreased to 50% to 60%, with a concomitant increase in cases caused by fungi and HACEK organisms (*Haemophilus*, *Actinobacillus*, *Cardiobacterium*, *Eikenella*, and *Kingella*). HACEK organisms are particularly common in neonates and immunocompromised children, accounting for 17% to 30% of cases.

2. α-Hemolytic streptococci (*S. viridans*) are the most common cause of endocarditis in patients who have had dental procedures or in those with carious teeth or periodontal disease.

3. Enterococci are the organisms most often found after genitourinary or gastrointestinal surgery or instrumentation.

4. The organisms most commonly found in postoperative endocarditis are staphylococci.

5. Intravenous drug abusers are at risk for IE caused by *S. aureus*.

6. Fungal endocarditis (which has a poor prognosis) may occur in sick neonates, in patients who are receiving long-term antibiotic or steroid therapy, or after open-heart surgery. Fungal endocarditis is often associated with very large friable vegetations; emboli from these vegetations frequently produce serious complications.

7. IE associated with indwelling vascular catheters, prosthetic material, and prosthetic valve is frequently caused by *S. aureus* or coagulase-negative staphylococci.

8. Among newborn infants, *S. aureus*, coagulase-negative staphylococci, and *Candida* species are the most common causes of IE.

9. Culture-negative endocarditis. A diagnosis of culture-negative endocarditis is made when a patient has clinical and/or echocardiographic evidence of endocarditis but persistently negative blood cultures. The most common cause of culture-negative endocarditis is current or recent antibiotic therapy or infection with a fastidious organism that grows poorly in vitro. Fungal endocarditis and IE caused by other rare organisms are rare causes of culture-negative endocarditis. At times, the diagnosis can be made only by removal of vegetation (during surgery). In the United States, about 5% to 7% of cases are culture-negative endocarditis.

CLINICAL MANIFESTATIONS

History

1. Most patients have a history of an underlying heart defect. However, some patients with bicuspid aortic valve may not have been diagnosed with the defect before the onset of the endocarditis.

2. A history of a recent dental procedure or tonsillectomy is occasionally present, but a history of toothache (from dental or gingival disease) is more frequent than a history of a procedure.

3. Endocarditis is rare in infancy; at this age, it usually follows open-heart surgery.

4. The onset is usually insidious with prolonged low-grade fever and somatic complaints, including fatigue, weakness, loss of appetite, pallor, arthralgia, myalgias, weight loss, and diaphoresis.

Physical Examination

1. Heart murmur is universal (100%). The appearance of a new heart murmur and an increase in the intensity of an existing murmur are important. However, many innocent heart murmurs are also of new onset.

2. Fever is common (80% to 90%). The temperature fluctuates between 101°F and 103°F (38.3°C and 39.4°C).

3. Splenomegaly is common (70%).

4. Skin manifestations (50%) (either secondary to microembolization or as an immunologic phenomenon) may be present in the following forms:
   a. Petechiae on the skin, mucous membranes, or conjunctivae are the most frequent skin lesions.
   b. Osler's nodes (tender, pea-sized red nodes at the ends of the fingers or toes) are rare in children.
   c. Janeway's lesions (small, painless, hemorrhagic areas on the palms or soles) are rare.
   d. Splinter hemorrhages (linear hemorrhagic streaks beneath the nails) are also rare.

5. Embolic or immunologic phenomena in other organs are present in 50% of cases:
   a. Pulmonary emboli may occur in patients with VSD, PDA, or a systemic-to-PA shunt.
   b. Seizures and hemiparesis are the result of embolization to the central nervous system (20%) and are more common with left-sided defects such as aortic and mitral valve disease or with cyanotic heart disease.
   c. Hematuria and renal failure may occur.
   d. Roth's spots (oval, retinal hemorrhages with pale centers located near the optic disc) occur in less than 5% of patients.

6. Carious teeth or periodontal or gingival disease is frequently present.

7. Clubbing of fingers in the absence of cyanosis develops rarely in more chronic cases.

8. Signs of heart failure may be present as a complication of the infection.

9. The clinical manifestations in a neonate with IE are nonspecific (respiratory distress, tachycardia) and may be indistinguishable from septicemia or congestive heart failure (CHF) from other causes. Embolic phenomena (such as osteomyelitis, meningitis, pneumonia) are common. There may be neurologic signs and symptoms (seizures, hemiparesis, apnea).

Laboratory Studies

1. Positive blood cultures are found in more than 90% of patients in the absence of previous antimicrobial therapy. Antimicrobial pretreatment reduces the yield of positive blood culture to 50% to 60%.

2. A complete blood cell count shows anemia, with hemoglobin levels lower than 12 g/100 mL (present in 80% of patients), and leukocytosis with a shift to the left. Patients with polycythemia preceding the onset of IE may have normal hemoglobin.

3. The sedimentation rate is increased unless there is polycythemia.

4. Microscopic hematuria is found in 30% of patients.

Echocardiography. Two-dimensional echo is the main modality for detecting endocardial infection (Fig. 19–1). It detects the site of infection, extent of valvular damage,

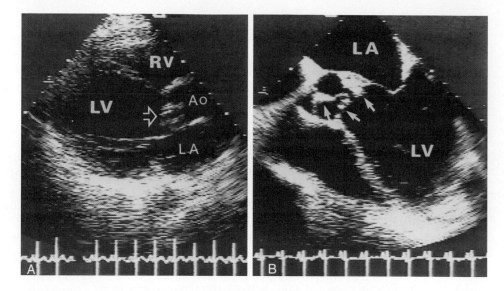

Figure 19–1. *Echoes of aortic valve vegetation.* ***A,*** *Parasternal long-axis view of a young adult patient with a bicuspid aortic valve demonstrating vegetation on the aortic valve (arrow). Severe aortic regurgitation was present, with a dilated left ventricle (LV).* ***B,*** *Five-chamber transverse plane of a transesophageal echo of the same patient that demonstrates vegetations and aortic valve anatomy more clearly than the ordinary two-dimensional echo. Ao, aorta; LA, left atrium; RV, right ventricle.*

and cardiac function. Baseline evaluation of ventricular function and cardiac chamber dimension is important for comparison later in the course of the infection. Color Doppler is a sensitive modality for detection of valvular regurgitation.

1. Certain echo findings are included as major criteria in the modified Duke criteria. They include:
   a. Oscillating intracardiac mass on valve or supporting structures, in the path of regurgitation jets, or on implanted material
   b. Abscesses
   c. New partial dehiscence of prosthetic valve
   d. New valvular regurgitation

2. Although standard transthoracic echo (TTE) is sufficient in most clinical circumstances, transesophageal echo (TEE) may be an important adjunct to TTE in obese or very muscular adolescents, in post–cardiac surgery patients, or in the presence of compromised respiratory function or pulmonary hyperinflation. TEE may be superior to TTE in identifying vegetations on prosthetic valves, detecting complications of left ventricular (LV) outflow tract endocarditis (either valvular or subvalvular), and in detecting aortic root abscess and involvement of the sinus of Valsalva.

3. The absence of vegetations on echo does not in itself rule out IE. Both TTE and TEE may produce false-negative results if vegetations are small or have already embolized, and they may miss initial perivalvular abscess. Repeated examinations are indicated if suspicion exists without diagnosis of IE or there is a worrisome clinical course during early treatment of IE.

4. Conversely, a false-positive diagnosis is possible. An echogenic mass may represent a sterile thrombus, sterile prosthetic material, or normal anatomic variation; an abnormal uninfected valve (previous scarring, severe myxomatous changes); or improper gain of the echo machine. Echo evidence of vegetation may persist for months or years after bacteriologic cure.

5. Certain echo features suggest a high-risk case or a need for surgery:
   a. Large vegetations (greatest risk when the vegetation is >10 mm)
   b. Severe valvular regurgitation
   c. Abscess cavities
   d. Pseudoaneurysm
   e. Valvular perforation or dehiscence
   f. Decompensated heart failure

DIAGNOSIS

The American Heart Association (Baddour et al, 2005) has recommended the modified Duke criteria in the diagnosis and management of IE. The usefulness of the criteria has been validated in clinical studies.

There are three categories of diagnostic possibilities using the modified Duke criteria: definite, possible, and rejected (Box 19–1).

1. A diagnosis of "definite" IE is made by pathologic evidence and fulfillment of certain clinical criteria.
   a. Pathologic evidence of IE includes demonstration of microorganism by culture, or histology in a vegetation or from an embolic site or an intracardiac abscess, or histologic evidence of active endocarditis demonstrated in vegetation or intracardiac abscess.

BOX 19–1	DEFINITION OF INFECTIVE ENDOCARDITIS ACCORDING TO THE MODIFIED DUKE CRITERIA

DEFINITE INFECTIVE ENDOCARDITIS

A. Pathologic criteria

   1. Microorganisms demonstrated by culture or histologic examination of a vegetation, a vegetation that has embolized, or an intracardiac abscess specimen; or

   2. Pathologic lesions; vegetation or intracardiac abscess confirmed by histologic examination showing active endocarditis

B. Clinical criteria

   1. Two major criteria (see Box 19–2); or

   2. One major criterion and three minor criteria; or

   3. Five minor criteria

POSSIBLE INFECTIVE ENDOCARDITIS

   1. One major criterion and one minor criterion; or

   2. Three minor criteria

REJECTED

   1. Firm alternative diagnosis explaining evidence of IE; or

   2. Resolution of IE syndrome with antibiotic therapy for <4 days; or

   3. No pathologic evidence of IE at surgery or autopsy, with antibiotic therapy for <4 days; or

   4. Does not meet criteria for possible IE as above

IE, infective endocarditis.
From Baddour LM, Wilson WR, Bayer AS, et al: Infective endocarditis: Diagnosis, antimicrobial therapy, and management of complications: A statement for healthcare professionals from the Committee on Rheumatic Fever, Endocarditis, and Kawasaki Disease, Council on Cardiovascular Disease in the Young, and the Councils on Clinical Cardiology, Stroke, and Cardiovascular Surgery and Anesthesia, American Heart Association: Endorsed by the Infectious Diseases Society of America. Circulation 111:e394–e433, 2005.

b. Fulfillment of clinical criteria is met by the presence of two major criteria, one major and three minor criteria, or five minor criteria as described in Box 19–2.

Major clinical criteria are positive blood cultures for microorganisms acceptable as a cause of endocarditis and evidence of endocardial involvement demonstrated by echo findings. A positive echo finding is considered a major criterion.

BOX 19–2	**DEFINITION OF TERMS USED IN THE MODIFIED DUKE CRITERIA FOR THE DIAGNOSIS OF INFECTIVE ENDOCARDITIS**

MAJOR CRITERIA

A. Blood culture positive for IE

1. Typical microorganisms consistent with IE from two separate blood cultures: viridans streptococci, *Streptococcus bovis*, HACEK group, *Staphylococcus aureus*, or community-acquired enterococci in the absence of a primary focus; or

2. Microorganisms consistent with IE from persistently positive blood cultures defined as follows: at least two positive cultures of blood samples drawn >12 hours apart; or all of three or a majority of four separate cultures of blood (with first and last samples drawn at least 1 hour apart)

3. Single positive blood culture for *Coxiella burnetii* or anti–phase 1 IgG antibody titer >1:800

B. Evidence of endocardial involvement

Echocardiogram positive for IE (TEE recommended for patients with prosthetic valves, rated at least "possible IE" by clinical criteria, or complicated IE [paravalvular abscess]; TTE as first test in other patients) defined as follows:

1. Oscillating intracardiac mass on valve or supporting structures, in the path of regurgitant jets, or on implanted material in the absence of an alternative anatomic explanation; or

2. Abscess; or

3. New partial dehiscence of prosthetic valve; or

4. New valvular regurgitation (worsening or changing or preexisting murmur not sufficient)

MINOR CRITERIA

1. Predisposition, predisposing heart condition, or injection drug users.

2. Fever, temperature >38°C

3. Vascular phenomena: major arterial emboli, septic pulmonary infarcts, mycotic aneurysm, intracranial hemorrhage, conjunctival hemorrhages, and Janeway's lesions

4. Immunologic phenomena: glomerulonephritis, Osler's nodes, Roth's spots, and rheumatoid factor

5. Microbiologic evidence: positive blood culture but does not meet a major criterion as noted above* or serologic evidence of active infection with organism consistent with IE

*Excludes single positive cultures for coagulase-negative staphylococci and organisms that do not cause endocarditis.

HACEK, *Haemophilus, Actinobacillus, Cardiobacterium, Eikenella*, and *Kingella*; IDUs, injection drug users; IE, infective endocarditis; TEE, transesophageal echocardiography; TTE, transthoracic echocardiography.

From Baddour LM, Wilson WR, Bayer AS, et al: Infective endocarditis: Diagnosis, antimicrobial therapy, and management of complications: A statement for healthcare professionals from the Committee on Rheumatic Fever, Endocarditis, and Kawasaki Disease, Council on Cardiovascular Disease in the Young, and the Councils on Clinical Cardiology, Stroke, and Cardiovascular Surgery and Anesthesia, American Heart Association: Endorsed by the Infectious Diseases Society of America. Circulation 111:e394–e433, 2005.

2. The category of "possible" IE exists when the following are present:
   a. One major criterion and one minor criterion, or
   b. Three minor criteria.

3. The other category of diagnosis is "rejected" IE, which is present:
   a. When an alternative diagnosis is established,
   b. When clinical manifestations of IE have resolved within 4 days of antibiotic therapy, or
   c. When no pathologic evidence is found on direct examination of the vegetation obtained from surgery or autopsy after antibiotic therapy for less than 4 days.
   d. When criteria for possible IE are not met.

MANAGEMENT

1. Blood cultures are indicated for all patients with fever of unexplained origin and a pathologic heart murmur, a history of heart disease, or previous endocarditis.
   a. Usually, three blood culture samples are drawn by separate venipunctures over 24 hours, unless the patient is very ill. In 90% of cases, the causative agent is recovered from the first two cultures.
   b. If there is no growth by the second day of incubation, two more may be obtained. There is no value in obtaining more than five blood cultures over 2 days unless the patient received prior antibiotic therapy.
   c. It is not necessary to obtain the cultures at any particular phase of the fever cycle.
   d. An adequate volume of blood must be obtained; 1 to 3 mL in infants and young children and 5 to 7 mL in older children are optimal.
   e. Aerobic incubation alone suffices because it is rare for IE to be due to anaerobic bacteria.

2. It is highly recommended that consultation with a local infectious disease specialist be obtained when IE is suspected or confirmed because antibiotics of choice are continually changing and there may be a special situation pertaining to the local area.

3. Initial empirical therapy is started with the following antibiotics while awaiting the results of blood cultures.
   a. The usual initial regimen is an antistaphylococcal semisynthetic penicillin (nafcillin, oxacillin, or methicillin) and an aminoglycoside (gentamicin). This combination covers against *S. viridans*, *S. aureus*, and gram-negative organisms. Some experts add penicillin to the initial regimen to cover against *S. viridans*, although a semisynthetic penicillin is usually adequate for initial therapy.
   b. If a methicillin-resistant *S. aureus* is suspected, vancomycin should be substituted for the semisynthetic penicillin.
   c. Vancomycin can be used in place of penicillin or a semisynthetic penicillin in penicillin-allergic patients.

4. The final selection of antibiotics depends on the organism isolated and the results of an antibiotic sensitivity test.
   a. Streptococcal IE
      1). In general, native cardiac valve IE caused by a highly sensitive *S. viridans* can be successfully treated with intravenous (IV) penicillin (or ceftriaxone given once daily) for 4 weeks. Alternatively, penicillin, ampicillin or ceftriaxone combined with gentamicin for 2 weeks may be used.
      2). For IE caused by penicillin-resistant streptococci, 4 weeks of penicillin, ampicillin, or ceftriaxone combined with gentamicin for the first 2 weeks are recommended.
   b. Staphylococcal endocarditis
      1). The drug of choice for native valve IE caused by methicillin-susceptible staphylococci is one of the semisynthetic β-lactamase–resistant penicillins (nafcillin, oxacillin, and methicillin) for a minimum of 6 weeks (with or without gentamicin for the first 3 to 5 days).

2). Patients with methicillin-resistant native valve IE are treated with vancomycin for 6 weeks (with or without gentamicin for the first 3 to 5 days).

c. Enterococcus-caused native valve endocarditis usually requires a combination of IV penicillin or ampicillin with gentamicin for 4 to 6 weeks. If patients are allergic to penicillin, vancomycin combined with gentamicin for 6 weeks is required.

d. HACEK organisms have begun to become resistant to ampicillin. Ceftriaxone or another third-generation cephalosporin alone or ampicillin plus gentamicin for 4 weeks is recommended. IE caused by other gram-negative bacteria (such as *Escherichia coli*, *Pseudomonas aeruginosa*, or *Serratia marcescens*) is treated with piperacillin or ceftazidime together with gentamicin for a minimum of 6 weeks.

e. Amphotericin B is the most effective agent for most fungal infections.

f. For culture-negative endocarditis, treatment is directed against staphylococci, streptococci, and the HACEK organisms using ceftriaxone and gentamicin. When staphylococcal IE is suspected, nafcillin should be added to the preceding therapy.

5. Patients with prosthetic valve endocarditis should be treated for 6 weeks based on the organism isolated and the results of the sensitivity test. Operative intervention may be necessary before the antibiotic therapy is completed if the clinical situation warrants (such as progressive CHF, significant malfunction of prosthetic valves, persistently positive blood cultures after 2 weeks of therapy). Bacteriologic relapse after an appropriate course of therapy also calls for operative intervention.

PROGNOSIS

The overall recovery rate is 80% to 85%; it is 90% or better for *S. viridans* and enterococci and about 50% for *Staphylococcus* organisms. Fungal endocarditis is associated with a very poor outcome.

PREVENTION

More important than the diagnosis and treatment of IE is its prevention. Maintenance of good oral hygiene is more important than antibiotic prophylaxis. The following is based on Prevention of bacterial endocarditis: Recommendations by the American Heart Association (Dajani et al, 1997).

Indications and Nonindications. Endocarditis prophylaxis is indicated for certain cardiac conditions and procedures, but it is not recommended for others. Box 19–3 lists cardiac conditions according to their level of risk for developing endocarditis. Box 19–4 shows which dental procedures need antibiotic prophylaxis and which procedures do not. Box 19–5 lists other surgical procedures or instrumentations that require antibiotic prophylaxis.

The incidence of endocarditis following most surgical and dental procedures in patients with underlying cardiac disease is low, and most cases of endocarditis are not attributable to a preceding procedure. In deciding whether to administer the prophylaxis, one should consider the risk level of underlying lesions and the risk of bacteremia following the procedure.

Some common dental procedures result in bacteremia in a large number of patients. For example, bacteremia results in about 60% to 80% of patients following tooth extraction and periodontal surgery. Tooth brushing or irrigation results in bacteremia in 40% of patients. The rate of bacteremia following tonsillectomy and rigid bronchoscopy is 35% and 15%, respectively. The rate of bacteremia following a normal vaginal delivery is about 3%.

Antibiotic Recommendations. The antibiotic prophylaxis is given orally 1 hour before a procedure. It should not be started several days before the procedure. Parenteral antibiotics are given within 30 minutes of starting a procedure.

1. Regimens for dental, oral, respiratory tract, or esophageal procedures: *S. viridans* (α-hemolytic streptococcus) is the most common cause of endocarditis following

BOX 19–3	INDICATIONS AND NONINDICATIONS OF ENDOCARDITIS PROPHYLAXIS BASED ON CARDIAC LESIONS

PROPHYLAXIS RECOMMENDED

High-Risk Category

Prosthetic cardiac valve, including bioprosthesis and homograft valves
Previous bacterial endocarditis
Complex cyanotic congenital heart defect (e.g., single ventricle, transposition of the great arteries, tetralogy of Fallot)
Surgically constructed systemic–to–pulmonary artery shunt or conduit

Moderate-Risk Category

Most other congenital heart defects (e.g., patent ductus arteriosus, ventricular septal defect, primum atrial septal defect, coarctation of the aorta, bicuspid aortic valve)
Acquired valvular dysfunction (e.g., rheumatic heart disease, collagen vascular disease)
Hypertrophic cardiomyopathy
Mitral valve prolapse with mitral regurgitation and/or thickened mitral valve leaflets

PROPHYLAXIS NOT RECOMMENDED

Negligible-Risk Category

Isolated secundum atrial septal defect
Surgical repair of atrial or ventricular septal defects or patent ductus arteriosus (without residua beyond 6 months)
Previous coronary artery bypass surgery
Mitral valve prolapse without mitral regurgitation
Innocent heart murmurs
Previous Kawasaki disease without valvular dysfunction
Previous rheumatic fever without valvular dysfunction
Cardiac pacemakers (intravascular and epicardial) and implanted defibrillators

---

dental, oral, respiratory tract, or esophageal procedures. Therefore, prophylaxis should be specifically directed against this organism (Table 19–1).

2. Regimens for genitourinary (GU) and nonesophageal gastrointestinal (GI) procedures: Bacterial endocarditis following surgery or instrumentation of the GU and GI tracts (excluding esophageal procedures) is most often caused by *Enterococcus faecalis*. Thus, antibiotic prophylaxis for these procedures is directed primarily against enterococci (Table 19–2).

    Parenteral antibiotics are recommended, particularly in high-risk patients. In medium-risk patients, a parenteral (ampicillin) or oral (amoxicillin) regimen is given. A smaller second dose of ampicillin or amoxicillin is recommended for high-risk patients. For procedures in which prophylaxis is not routinely recommended, physicians may choose to administer prophylaxis in high-risk patients.

3. Prophylaxis for special situations:

    a. Patients who are receiving rheumatic fever prophylaxis may have *S. viridans* in their oral cavities that is relatively resistant to penicillins. The penicillin dosage for the secondary prevention of rheumatic fever is inadequate for the prevention of bacterial endocarditis. In such cases, clindamycin or clarithromycin is recommended (see Table 19–1 for dosages).

    b. If patients are receiving antibiotics for other reasons, the procedure should be delayed, if possible, until at least 9 to 14 days after completion of the antibiotic. This allows the usual oral flora to be reestablished.

    c. For patients with MVP, antibiotic prophylaxis against subacute bacterial endocarditis is recommended only when evidence of MR is present by auscultation or Doppler studies.

BOX 19–4	DENTAL PROCEDURES AND ENDOCARDITIS PROPHYLAXIS

PROPHYLAXIS RECOMMENDED*

Dental extraction

Periodontal procedures including surgery, scaling and root planing, probing, and recall maintenance

Dental implant placement and reimplantation of avulsed teeth

Endodontic (root canal) instrumentation or surgery only beyond the apex

Subgingival placement of antibiotic fibers or strips

Initial placement of orthodontic bands but not brackets

Intraligamentary local anesthetic injections

Prophylactic cleaning of teeth or implants when bleeding is anticipated

PROPHYLAXIS NOT RECOMMENDED

Restorative dentistry[†] (operative and prosthodontic) with or without retraction cord[‡]

Local anesthetic injection (non-intraligamentary)

Intracanal endodontic treatment; post placement and buildup

Placement of rubber dams

Postoperative suture removal

Placement of removable prosthodontic or orthodontic appliances

Taking of oral impressions

Fluoride treatments

Taking of oral radiographs

Orthodontic appliance adjustment

Shedding of primary teeth

*Prophylaxis is recommended for patients with high- and moderate-risk cardiac conditions.

[†]This includes restoration of decayed teeth (filling cavities) and replacement of missing teeth.

[‡]Based on clinical judgment, antibiotic use may be indicated in selected circumstances in which there may be significant bleeding.

Myocarditis

PREVALENCE

Myocarditis severe enough to be recognized clinically is rare, but the prevalence of mild and subclinical cases is probably much higher.

PATHOLOGY

1. The principal mechanism of cardiac involvement in viral myocarditis is believed to be a cell-mediated immunologic reaction, not merely myocardial damage from viral replication. Isolation of virus from the myocardium is unusual at autopsy.

2. The inflamed myocardium is soft, flabby, and pale, with areas of scarring on gross examination. Microscopic examination reveals patchy infiltrations by plasma cells, mononuclear leukocytes, and some eosinophils during the acute phase and giant cell infiltration in the later stages.

CAUSE

1. In North America, viruses are probably the most common causes of myocarditis. Among viruses, adenovirus, coxsackievirus B, and echoviruses are the most common agents. Many other viruses (e.g., poliomyelitis, mumps, measles, rubella, cytomegalovirus, HIV, arboviruses, influenza) can cause myocarditis. In South America, Chagas' disease (caused by *Trypanosoma cruzi*, a protozoan) is a common cause of myocarditis. Rarely, bacteria, rickettsia, fungi, protozoa, and parasites are the causative agents.

2. Immune-mediated diseases, including acute rheumatic fever and Kawasaki disease, may be the cause.

BOX 19–5	OTHER SURGICAL PROCEDURES OR INSTRUMENTATIONS AND ENDOCARDIAL PROPHYLAXIS

PROPHYLAXIS RECOMMENDED

Respiratory tract
  Tonsillectomy and/or adenoidectomy
  Surgical operations that involve respiratory mucosa
  Bronchoscopy with a rigid bronchoscope
Gastrointestinal tract*
  Sclerotherapy for esophageal varices
  Esophageal stricture dilatation
  Endoscopic retrograde cholangiography with biliary obstruction
  Biliary tract surgery
  Surgical operations that involve intestinal mucosa
Genitourinary tract
  Prostatic surgery
  Cystoscopy
  Urethral dilatation

PROPHYLAXIS NOT RECOMMENDED

Respiratory tract
  Endotracheal intubation
  Bronchoscopy with a flexible bronchoscope, with or without biopsy[†]
  Tympanostomy tube insertion
Gastrointestinal tract
  Transesophageal echocardiography[†]
  Endoscopy with or without gastrointestinal biopsy[†]
Genitourinary tract
  Vaginal hysterectomy[†]
  Vaginal delivery[†]
  Cesarean section
  In uninfected tissue:
    Urethral catheterization
    Uterine dilatation and curettage
    Therapeutic abortion
    Sterilization procedure
    Insertion or removal of intrauterine devices
Other
  Cardiac catheterization, including balloon angioplasty
  Implanted cardiac pacemakers, implanted defibrillators, and coronary stents
  Incision or biopsy of surgically scrubbed skin
  Circumcision

*Prophylaxis is recommended for high-risk patients; it is optional for medium-risk patients.
[†]Prophylaxis is optional for high-risk patients.

3. Collagen vascular diseases can cause myocarditis.

4. Toxic myocarditis (from drug ingestion, diphtheria exotoxin, and anoxic agents) occurs.

CLINICAL MANIFESTATIONS

History

1. Older children may have a history of an upper respiratory infection.

2. The illness may have a sudden onset in newborns and small infants, with anorexia, vomiting, lethargy, and, occasionally, circulatory shock.

Physical Examination

1. The presentation depends on the patient's age and the acute or chronic nature of the infection. In neonates and infants, signs of CHF may be present; these include

Table 19–1. **Prophylactic Regimens for Dental, Oral, Respiratory Tract, or Esophageal Procedures**

Situation	Agent	Regimen*
Standard general prophylaxis	Amoxicillin	Children: 50 mg/kg orally 1 hr before procedure Adults: 2 g orally 1 hr before procedure
Unable to take oral medications	Ampicillin	Children: 50 mg/kg IM or IV within 30 min before procedure Adults: 2 g IM or IV within 30 min before procedure
Allergic to penicillin	Clindamycin, or cephalexin[†] or cefadroxil,[†] or azithromycin or clarithromycin	Clindamycin: children, 20 mg/kg; adults, 600 mg orally 1 hr before procedure Cephalexin or cefadroxil: children, 50 mg/kg orally; adults, 2 g orally 1 hr before procedure Azithromycin or clarithromycin: children, 15 mg/kg orally; adults, 500 mg orally; 1 hr before procedure
Allergic to penicillin and unable to take oral medications	Clindamycin or cefazolin	Clindamycin: children, 20 mg/kg IM or IV; adults, 600 mg IM or IV within 30 min before procedure Cefazolin: children, 25 mg/kg IM or IV; adults, 1 g IM or IV within 30 min before procedure

*The total children's dose should not exceed the adult dose.
[†]Cephalosporins should not be used in individuals with a history of immediate-type hypersensitivity reaction (urticaria, angioedema, or anaphylaxis) to penicillin.

poor heart tone, tachycardia, gallop rhythm, tachypnea, and, rarely, cyanosis. In older children, a gradual onset of CHF and arrhythmia is commonly seen.

2. A soft, systolic heart murmur and irregular rhythm caused by supraventricular or ventricular ectopic beats may be audible.

3. Hepatomegaly (evidence of viral hepatitis) may be present.

Electrocardiography. Any one or a combination of the following may be seen: low QRS voltages, ST-T changes, PR prolongation, prolongation of the QT interval, and arrhythmias, especially premature contractions.

Table 19–2. **Prophylactic Regimens for Genitourinary and Gastrointestinal (Excluding Esophageal) Procedures**

Situation	Agent	Regimen*
High-risk patients	Ampicillin plus gentamicin[†]	Children: ampicillin 50 mg/kg IM or IV (not to exceed 2 g) plus gentamicin 1.5 mg/kg within 30 min of starting the procedure; 6 hr later, ampicillin 25 mg/kg IM or IV or amoxicillin 25 mg/kg orally Adults: ampicillin 2 g IM or IV plus gentamicin 1.5 mg/kg (not to exceed 120 mg) within 30 min of starting the procedure; 6 hr later, ampicillin 1 g IM or IV or amoxicillin 1 g orally
High-risk patients allergic to ampicillin or amoxicillin	Vancomycin plus gentamicin[†]	Children: vancomycin 20 mg/kg IV over 1–2 hr plus gentamicin 1 mg/kg IM or IV; complete the injection or infusion within 30 min of starting procedure Adults: vancomycin 1g IV over 1–2 hr plus gentamicin 1.5 mg/kg IM or IV (not to exceed 120 mg); complete the injection or infusion within 30 min of starting procedure
Moderate-risk patients	Amoxicillin or ampicillin	Children: amoxicillin 50 mg/kg orally 1 hr before procedure, or ampicillin 50 mg/kg IM or IV within 30 min of starting procedure Adults: amoxicillin 2 g orally 1 hr before procedure, or ampicillin 2 g IM or IV within 30 min of starting procedure
Moderate-risk patients allergic to ampicillin or amoxicillin	Vancomycin[†]	Children: vancomycin 20 mg/kg IV over 1–2 hr; complete the infusion within 30 min of starting procedure Adult: vancomycin 1 g IV over 1–2 hr; complete the infusion within 30 min of starting procedure

*The total children's dose should not exceed the adult dose.
[†]No second dose of vancomycin or gentamicin is recommended.

X-ray Studies. Cardiomegaly of varying degrees is the most important clinical sign of myocarditis.

Echocardiography. Echo reveals cardiac chamber enlargement and impaired LV function, often regional in nature. Occasionally, increased wall thickness and LV thrombi are found.

Laboratory Studies

1. Cardiac troponin levels (troponin-I and -T) and myocardial enzymes (creatine kinase [CK], MB isoenzyme of CK [CK-MB]) may be elevated. In children, the normal value of cardiac troponin-I has been reported to be 2 ng/mL or less, and it is frequently below the level of detection for the assay. Troponin levels may be more sensitive than the cardiac enzymes.

2. Radionuclide scanning (after administration of gallium-67 or technetium-99m pyrophosphate) may identify inflammatory and necrotic changes characteristic of myocarditis.

3. Myocarditis can be confirmed by an endomyocardial biopsy.

NATURAL HISTORY

1. The mortality rate is as high as 75% in symptomatic neonates with acute viral myocarditis.

2. The majority of patients, especially those with mild inflammation, recover completely.

3. Some patients develop subacute or chronic myocarditis with persistent cardiomegaly (with or without signs of CHF) and ECG evidence of left ventricular hypertrophy (LVH) or biventricular hypertrophy (BVH). Clinically, these patients are indistinguishable from those with dilated cardiomyopathy. Myocarditis may be a precursor to idiopathic dilated cardiomyopathy in some cases.

MANAGEMENT

1. One should attempt virus identification by viral cultures from the blood, stool, or throat washing. Acute and convalescent sera should be compared for serologic titer rise.

2. Bed rest and limitation in activities are recommended during the acute phase (because exercise intensifies the damage from myocarditis in experimental animals).

3. Anticongestive measures include the following:
   a. Rapid-acting diuretics (furosemide or ethacrynic acid, 1 mg/kg, each one to three times a day).
   b. Rapid-acting inotropic agents, such as dobutamine or dopamine, are useful in critically ill children.
   c. Oxygen and bed rest are recommended. Use of a "cardiac chair" or "infant seat" relieves respiratory distress.
   d. Digoxin may be given cautiously, using half of the usual digitalizing dose (see Table 27–5), because some patients with myocarditis are exquisitely sensitive to the drug.

4. Beneficial effects of high-dose gamma globulin (2 g/kg, over 24 hours) have been reported. The gamma globulin was associated with better survival during the first year after presentation, echo evidence of smaller LV diastolic dimension, and higher fractional shortening compared with the control group. Myocardial damage in myocarditis is mediated in part by immunologic mechanisms, and a high dose of gamma globulin is an immunomodulatory agent, shown to be effective in myocarditis secondary to Kawasaki disease.

5. Angiotensin-converting enzyme inhibitors, such as captopril, may prove beneficial in the acute phase (as demonstrated in animal experiments).

6. Arrhythmias should be treated aggressively and may require the use of IV amiodarone.

7. The role of corticosteroids is unclear at this time, except in the treatment of severe rheumatic carditis (see Chapter 20).

8. Specific therapies include antitoxin in diphtheritic myocarditis.

Pericarditis

CAUSE

1. Viral infection is probably the most common cause of pericarditis, particularly in infancy. Many viruses similar to those listed in the section on myocarditis can cause pericarditis.

2. Acute rheumatic fever is a common cause of pericarditis, especially in certain parts of the world (see also Chapter 20).

3. Bacterial infection (purulent pericarditis) is a rare, serious form of pericarditis. Commonly encountered are *S. aureus*, *Streptococcus pneumoniae*, *Haemophilus influenzae*, *Neisseria meningitidis*, and streptococci.

4. Tuberculosis is an occasional cause of constrictive pericarditis, with an insidious onset.

5. Heart surgery is a possible cause (see "Postpericardiotomy Syndrome").

6. Collagen disease such as rheumatoid arthritis (see Chapter 23) can cause pericarditis.

7. Pericarditis can be a complication of oncologic disease or its therapy, including radiation.

8. Uremia (uremic pericarditis) is a rare cause.

PATHOLOGY

The parietal and visceral surfaces of the pericardium are inflamed. Pericardial effusion may be serofibrinous, hemorrhagic, or purulent. Effusion may be completely absorbed or may result in pericardial thickening or chronic constriction (constrictive pericarditis).

PATHOPHYSIOLOGY

The pathogenesis of symptoms and signs of pericardial effusion is determined by two factors: the speed of fluid accumulation and the competence of the myocardium. A rapid accumulation of a large amount of pericardial fluid produces more serious circulatory embarrassment. A slow accumulation of a relatively small amount of fluid may result in serious circulatory embarrassment (cardiac tamponade) if the extent of myocarditis is significant. Slow accumulation of a large amount of fluid may be accommodated by stretching of the pericardium, if the myocardium is intact.

With the development of pericardial tamponade, several compensatory mechanisms are triggered: systemic and pulmonary venous constriction to improve diastolic filling, an increase in systemic vascular resistance to raise falling blood pressure, and tachycardia to improve cardiac output.

CLINICAL MANIFESTATIONS

History

1. The patient may have a history of upper respiratory tract infection.

2. Precordial pain (dull, aching, or stabbing) with occasional radiation to the shoulder and neck may be a presenting complaint. The pain may be relieved by leaning forward and may be made worse by supine position or deep inspiration.

3. Fever of varying degrees may be present.

Physical Examination

1. Pericardial friction rub (a grating, to-and-fro sound in phase with the heart sounds) is the cardinal physical sign.

2. The heart is quiet and hypodynamic in the presence of a large amount of pericardial effusion.

3. Pulsus paradoxus is characteristic of pericardial effusion with tamponade (see Chapter 2 and Fig. 2–2).

4. Heart murmur is usually absent, although it may be present in acute rheumatic carditis (see Chapter 20).

5. In children with purulent pericarditis, septic fever (101°F to 105°F [38.3°C to 40.5°C]), tachycardia, chest pain, and dyspnea are almost always present.

6. Signs of cardiac tamponade may be present: distant heart sounds, tachycardia, pulsus paradoxus, hepatomegaly, venous distention, and occasional hypotension with peripheral vasoconstriction. Cardiac tamponade occurs more commonly in purulent pericarditis than in other forms of pericarditis.

Electrocardiography

1. The low-voltage QRS complex caused by pericardial effusion is characteristic but not a constant finding.

2. The following time-dependent changes secondary to myocardial involvement may occur (see Fig. 3–25):
   a. Initial ST-segment elevation.
   b. Return of the ST segment to the baseline with inversion of T waves (2 to 4 weeks after onset).

X-ray Studies

1. A varying degree of cardiomegaly is present.
2. A pear-shaped or water bottle–shaped heart is characteristic of a large effusion.
3. Pulmonary vascular markings may be increased if cardiac tamponade develops. Tamponade may occur without enlargement of the cardiac silhouette if it develops quickly.

Echocardiography. Echo is the most useful tool in establishing the diagnosis of pericardial effusion. It appears as an echo-free space between the epicardium (visceral pericardium) and the parietal pericardium.

1. Pericardial effusion first appears posteriorly in the dependent portion of the pericardial sac. The presence of a small amount of effusion posteriorly without anterior effusion suggests a small pericardial effusion. A small amount of fluid, which appears only in systole, is normal.

2. With larger effusion, the fluid also appears anteriorly. The larger the echo-free space, the larger is the pericardial effusion. With very large effusions, the swinging motion of the heart may be imaged.

3. In patients with chronic effusion, fibrinous strands and other organized materials can be seen in the pericardial fluid, which may lead to fluid loculations.

4. Echo is very helpful in detecting cardiac tamponade. Helpful two-dimensional echo findings of tamponade are as follows:
   a. Collapse of the right atrium in late diastole (Fig. 19–2) (because the pressure in the pericardial sac exceeds the pressure within the right atrium at end diastole when the atrium has emptied)
   b. Collapse or indentation of the right ventricular free wall, especially the outflow tract

MANAGEMENT

1. Pericardiocentesis or surgical drainage to identify the cause of the pericarditis is mandatory, especially when purulent or tuberculous pericarditis is suspected. A drainage catheter may be left in place with intermittent low-pressure drainage.

2. Pericardial fluid studies include cell counts and differential, glucose, and protein concentrations; histologic examination of cells; Gram and acid-fast stains; and viral, bacterial, and fungal cultures.

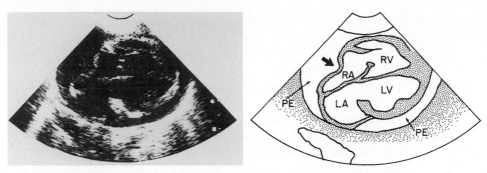

Figure 19–2. *Subcostal four-chamber view demonstrating pericardial effusion (PE) and collapse of the right atrial wall (large arrow), a sign of cardiac tamponade. LA, left atrium; LV, left ventricle; RA, right atrium; RV, right ventricle.*

3. For cardiac tamponade, urgent decompression by surgical drainage or pericardiocentesis is indicated. While getting ready for the procedure, fluid push with plasma protein fraction (Plasmanate) should be given to increase central venous pressure and thereby improve cardiac filling, which can provide temporary emergency stabilization.

4. Urgent surgical drainage of the pericardium is indicated when purulent pericarditis is suspected. This must be followed by IV antibiotic therapy for 4 to 6 weeks.

5. There is no specific treatment for viral pericarditis.

6. Treatment focuses on the basic disease itself (e.g., uremia, collagen disease).

7. Salicylates are given for precordial pain and nonbacterial or rheumatic pericarditis.

8. Corticosteroid therapy may be indicated in children with severe rheumatic carditis or postpericardiotomy syndrome.

9. Digitalis is contraindicated in cardiac tamponade because it blocks tachycardia, a compensatory response to impaired venous return.

Constrictive Pericarditis

Although rare in children, constrictive pericarditis may be associated with an earlier viral pericarditis, tuberculosis, incomplete drainage of purulent pericarditis, hemopericardium, mediastinal irradiation, neoplastic infiltration, or connective tissue disorders. In this condition, a fibrotic, thickened, and adherent pericardium restricts diastolic filling of the heart.

Diagnosis of constrictive pericarditis is suggested by the following clinical findings:

1. Signs of elevated jugular venous pressure occur.

2. Hepatomegaly with ascites and systemic edema may be present.

3. Diastolic pericardial knock, which resembles the opening snap, is often heard along the left sternal border in the absence of heart murmur.

4. Calcification of the pericardium, enlargement of the superior vena cava and left atrium, and pleural effusion are common on chest x-ray films.

5. The ECG may show low QRS voltages, T-wave inversion or flattening, and left atrial hypertrophy. Atrial fibrillation is occasionally seen.

6. M-mode echo may reveal two parallel lines representing the thickened visceral and parietal pericardia or multiple dense echoes. Two-dimensional echo shows (a) a thickened pericardium, (b) dilated inferior vena cava and hepatic vein, and (c) paradoxical septal motion and abrupt displacement of the interventricular septum during early diastolic filling ("septal bounce") (not specific for this condition). Doppler examination of the mitral inflow reveals findings of diastolic dysfunction (see Fig. 18–6) and a marked respiratory variation in diastolic inflow tracings.

7. Cardiac catheterization may document the presence of constrictive physiology.
   a. The right and left atrial pressures, ventricular end-diastolic pressures, and PA wedge pressure are all elevated and usually equalized.
   b. Ventricular pressure waveforms demonstrate the characteristic "square root sign" (in which there is an early rapid fall in diastolic pressure followed by a rapid rise to an elevated diastolic plateau).

The treatment for constrictive pericarditis is complete resection of the pericardium; symptomatic improvement occurs in 75% of patients.

Kawasaki Disease

CAUSE AND EPIDEMIOLOGY

1. The cause of Kawasaki disease (also called mucocutaneous lymph node syndrome) is not known. Most investigators believe that the disease is related to, if not caused by, an infectious disease. The disease is probably driven by abnormalities of the immune system initiated by the infectious insult.

2. Children of all racial and ethnic groups are affected, although it is more common in Asians and Pacific Islanders. The male/female ratio is 1.5:1. In the United States, Kawasaki disease is more common during the winter and early spring months.

3. It occurs primarily in young children, with a peak incidence between 1 and 2 years of age; 80% of patients are younger than 4 years of age, and 50% are younger than 2 years. Cases in children older than 8 years and younger than 3 months are uncommon.

PATHOLOGY

1. During the first 10 days after the onset of fever, generalized microvasculitis occurs throughout the body, with a predilection for the coronary arteries. Other arteries such as iliac, femoral, axillary, and renal arteries are less frequently involved.

2. Coronary artery aneurysm develops in 15% to 20% during the acute phase and persists for 1 to 3 weeks. It tends to develop most frequently in the proximal segment of the major coronary arteries and may assume fusiform, saccular, cylindrical, or beads-on-a-string appearance.

3. During the acute phase, there is pancarditis, with inflammation of the atrioventricular (AV) conduction system (which can produce AV block), myocardium (myocardial dysfunction, CHF), pericardium (pericardial effusion), and endocardium (with aortic and mitral valve involvement).

4. Late changes (after 40 days) consist of healing and fibrosis in the coronary arteries, with thrombus formation and stenosis in the postaneurysmal segment and myocardial fibrosis from old myocardial infarction.

5. The elevated platelet count seen in this condition contributes to coronary thrombosis.

CLINICAL MANIFESTATIONS

The clinical course of the disease can be divided into three phases: acute, subacute, and convalescent. Each phase of the disease is characterized by unique symptoms and signs. Only clinical features seen in the acute phase are important in making the diagnosis of the disease, and they are discussed in depth.

Acute Phase (First 10 Days)

1. Six signs that compose the principal clinical features of Kawasaki disease are present during the acute phase (Box 19–6).
   a. The onset of illness is abrupt, with a high fever, usually higher than 39°C (102°F) and in many cases above 40°C (104°F). Fever persists for a mean of 11 days without treatment. With appropriate therapy, the fever usually resolves

---

BOX 19–6	**PRINCIPAL CLINICAL FEATURES FOR DIAGNOSIS OF KAWASAKI DISEASE**

1. Fever persisting at least 5 days

2. Presence of at least four of the following principal features:

   a. Changes in extremities:

      Acute: Erythema of palms and soles; edema of hands and feet

      Subacute: Periungual peeling of fingers and toes in weeks 2 and 3

   b. Polymorphous exanthema

   c. Bilateral bulbar conjunctival injection without exudate

   d. Changes in the lips and oral cavity: erythema, lips cracking, strawberry tongue, diffuse injection of oral and pharyngeal mucosa

   e. Cervical lymphadenopathy (>1.5 cm in diameter), usually unilateral

3. Exclusion of other diseases with similar findings (see Box 19–7) is important.

Diagnosis of Kawasaki disease is made in the presence of ≥5 days of fever and at least four of the five principal clinical features listed above.

Patients with fever ≥5 days and less than four principal criteria can be diagnosed with Kawasaki disease when coronary artery abnormalities are detected by two-dimensional echo or angiography.

In the presence of four or more principal criteria plus fever, Kawasaki disease diagnosis can be made on day 4 of illness.

From Newburger JW, Takahashi M, Gerber MA, et al: Diagnosis, treatment, and long-term management of Kawasaki disease: A statement for health professionals from the Committee on Rheumatic Fever, Endocarditis, and Kawasaki Disease, Council on Cardiovascular Disease in the Young, American Heart Association. Pediatrics 114:1708–1733, 2004.

---

     within 2 days of treatment. Within 2 to 5 days after the onset of fever, other principal features develop.

  b. Conjunctivitis occurs shortly after the onset of fever. It is not associated with exudate, being different from that seen in other conditions such as measles, Stevens-Johnson syndrome, or viral conjunctivitis. Conjunctivitis resolves rapidly.

  c. Changes in the lips and oral cavity include (1) erythema, dryness, fissuring, peeling, cracking, and bleeding of the lips, (2) "strawberry tongue" that is indistinguishable from scarlet fever, and (3) diffuse erythema of the oropharyngeal mucosa. Oral ulceration and pharyngeal exudates are not seen.

  d. Changes in the hands and feet consist of erythema of the palms and soles, firm edema, and sometimes painful induration. Desquamation of hands and feet takes place within 2 to 3 weeks.

  e. The rash usually appears within 5 days of the onset of fever and may take many forms (except bullous and vesicular eruptions), even in the same patient. The most common is a nonspecific, diffuse maculopapular eruption. Its distribution is extensive, involving the trunk and extremities, with accentuation in the perineal region (where early desquamation may occur); desquamation usually occurs by days 5 to 7.

  f. Cervical lymph node enlargement is the least common of the principal clinical features, occurring in approximately 50% of patients. The firm swelling is usually unilateral, involves more than one node measuring more than 1.5 cm in diameter, and is confined to the anterior cervical triangle.

2. Cardiovascular abnormalities result from involvement of the pericardium, myocardium, endocardium, valves, and coronary arteries, with some or all of the following manifestations.

  a. Tachycardia, gallop rhythm, and/or other signs of heart failure

  b. Left ventricular dysfunction with cardiomegaly (myocarditis)

    c. Pericardial effusion

    d. Mitral valve regurgitation murmur

    e. Chest x-ray films may show cardiomegaly if myocarditis or significant coronary artery abnormality or valvular regurgitation is present.

    f. ECG changes may include arrhythmias, prolonged PR interval (occurring in up to 60%), and nonspecific ST-T changes. Abnormal Q waves (wide and deep) in the limb leads or precordial leads suggest myocardial infarction.

    g. Coronary artery abnormalities are seen initially at the end of the first week through the second week of illness (see later for further discussion).

3. Involvement of other organ systems is also frequent during the acute phase.

    a. Musculoskeletal system: arthritis or arthralgia of multiple joints (30%), involving small joints as well as large joints

    b. Genitourinary system: sterile pyuria (60%)

    c. Gastrointestinal system: abdominal pain with diarrhea (20%), liver dysfunction (40%), hydrops of the gallbladder (10%, demonstrable by abdominal ultrasonography) with jaundice

    d. Central nervous system: irritability, lethargy or semicoma, aseptic meningitis (25%), and sensory neuronal hearing loss

4. Laboratory studies. Even though laboratory results are nonspecific, they provide diagnostic support of the disease during the acute phase. For example, Kawasaki's disease is unlikely if acute phase reactants and platelet counts are normal after 7 days of the illness.

    a. Marked leukocytosis with a shift to the left and anemia are common.

    b. Acute phase reactant levels (C-reactive protein [CRP] levels, erythrocyte sedimentation rate [ESR]) are always elevated, which are uncommon with viral illnesses. An elevated sedimentation rate (but not CRP) can be caused by intravenous immunoglobulin (IVIG) infusion per se.

    c. Thrombocytosis (usually >450,000 /mm^3) occurs after day 7 of the illness, sometimes reaching 600,000 to more than 1 million/mm^3 during the subacute phase. Low platelet count suggests viral illnesses.

    d. Pyuria (related to urethritis) is common on microscopic examination.

    e. Liver enzymes are moderately elevated (more than two times the upper limit of normal) in 40% of patients; hypoalbuminemia and mild hyperbilirubinemia may be present in 10%.

    f. Elevated serum cardiac troponin-I may occur, which suggests myocardial damage.

    g. Lipid abnormalities are common. Decreased levels of high-density lipoprotein (HDL) are present during the illness and follow-up for more than 3 years, especially in patients with persistent coronary artery abnormalities. The total cholesterol level is normal, but the triglyceride level tends to be high. Repeated measurement is recommended a year later in patients with abnormal lipid profiles.

5. Echocardiography. The main purpose of an echo study during the acute phase is to detect coronary artery aneurysm and other cardiac dysfunction. For the initial examination, sedation with chloral hydrate (65 to 100 mg/kg, maximum 1000 mg) or other short-acting sedative or hypnotic agents is recommended.

    a. Coronary artery aneurysm rarely occurs before day 10 of illness. During this period, other echo findings may suggest cardiac involvement.

        1). Perivascular brightness, ectasia, and lack of normal tapering may represent coronary arteritis (before aneurysm formation).

        2). Decreased LV systolic function with increased LV dimensions.

        3). Mild mitral valve regurgitation (presumably from myocarditis, myocardial infarction, or coronary artery occlusion).

        4). Pericardial effusion.

    b. Multiple echo views should be obtained to visualize all major coronary artery segments [left main coronary artery (LMCA), left anterior descending (LAD), left circumflex coronary artery (LCXA), and right coronary artery (RCA)].

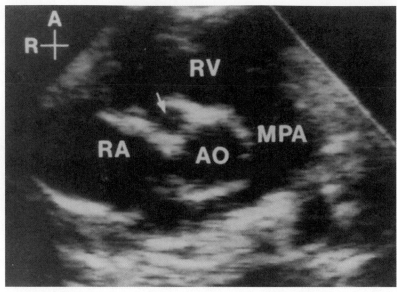

Figure 19–3. *Parasternal short-axis view from a patient with Kawasaki disease. There is a large circular aneurysm (arrow) of the right coronary artery. A, anterior; AO, aorta; MPA, main pulmonary artery; R, right; RA, right atrium; RV, right ventricle. (From Snider AR, Serwer GA: Echocardiography in Pediatric Heart Disease. St. Louis, Mosby, 1990.*

    c. Configuration (saccular, fusiform, ectatic), size, number, and presence or absence of intraluminal or mural thrombi should be assessed. According to the new guidelines, aneurysms are classified as saccular (nearly equal axial and lateral diameters), fusiform (symmetric dilatation with gradual proximal and distal tapering), and ectatic (dilated without segmental aneurysm). "Giant" aneurysm is present when the diameter of the aneurysm is 8 mm or more. Figure 19–3 shows a large saccular aneurysm of the right coronary artery.

Clinical findings seen during the subacute phase and convalescent phase are not important in diagnosis or planning management but they are more or less useful in confirming the diagnosis at a later time.

Subacute Phase (11 to 25 Days after Onset)

1. Desquamation of the tips of the fingers and toes is characteristic.
2. Rash, fever, and lymphadenopathy disappear.
3. Significant cardiovascular changes, including coronary aneurysm, pericardial effusion, CHF, and myocardial infarction, occur in this phase. Approximately 20% of patients manifest coronary artery aneurysm on echo.
4. Thrombocytosis also occurs during this period, peaking at 2 weeks or more after the onset of the illness.

Convalescent Phase. This phase lasts until the elevated ESR and platelet count return to normal. Deep transverse grooves (Beau's lines) may appear across the fingernails and toenails.

DIAGNOSIS

In the absence of a specific diagnostic test or pathognomonic clinical feature, the diagnosis of Kawasaki disease relies on clinical criteria. Box 19–6 lists the principal clinical features that establish the diagnosis. In cases with less than full criteria for the disease (incomplete Kawasaki disease), other clinical and laboratory findings (as discussed earlier) may aid physicians in decision-making to initiate treatment. One could also consider the Harada score (see later) in the decision-making to initiate treatment.

1. Presence of fever of 5 or more days duration and at least four of the five principal criteria (see Box 19–6) are required to make the diagnosis of Kawasaki disease. More than 90% of patients have fever plus the first four of the five signs, but only about 50% of patients have lymphadenopathy.

2. However, patients with fever for 5 or more days and fewer than four criteria can be diagnosed as having Kawasaki disease when coronary artery abnormality is detected. Indeed, a substantial fraction of children with Kawasaki disease with coronary artery anomalies never meet the diagnostic criteria. However, coronary aneurysm rarely occurs before day 10 of Kawasaki disease. During this period, perivascular brightness or ectasia of the coronary artery, decreased LV systolic function, mild MR, or pericardial effusion may be present instead.

3. In the presence of four or more principal criteria plus fever, diagnosis of Kawasaki disease can be made on day 4 of illness rather than waiting until day 5 of illness. (However, there appears to be no advantage in giving intravenous immunoglobulin (IVIG) before 5 days of illness in preventing coronary artery aneurysm.)

4. Incomplete (preferable to "atypical") Kawasaki disease with two or three principal clinical features creates a management problem. Incomplete Kawasaki disease is more common in young infants than older children. Given the potential serious consequences of missing the diagnosis of Kawasaki disease in patients with incomplete manifestations of the principal clinical features, together with the efficiency and safety of early treatment with IVIG, physicians should not wait for full manifestations of the disease but should consider other clinical manifestations and laboratory findings in deciding whether or not to initiate treatment.

   a. When incomplete Kawasaki disease is suspected, some laboratory tests should be obtained because their results are similar to those found in complete cases.

      1). Abnormal acute phase reactants (CRP ≥ 3.0 mg/dL and ESR ≥ 40 mm/hr) are very helpful because they are similarly abnormal in incomplete cases.

      2). The following supplemental laboratory tests should also be obtained because they are frequently abnormal in incomplete cases (with their abnormal values shown in parentheses): serum albumin (3.0 g/dL), anemia for age, alanine aminotransferase (>50 or 60 U/L), platelets after 7 days ($\geq 450,000$/mm^3), white blood cell count ($\geq 15,000$/mm^3), and urine white cell (≥ 10 cells/high-power field).

      3). Patients with positive acute phase reactants plus three or more abnormal supplemental laboratory tests may be given treatment along with echo studies. Even if there are less than three abnormal laboratory tests, patients with abnormal echo findings qualify for treatment.

   b. Echo studies should also be obtained, especially in young infants with fever lasting longer than 7 days.

5. The definition of coronary artery abnormalities has changed since the original Japanese Ministry of Health criteria were devised. According to the original definition, a coronary artery is classified as abnormal (a) if the internal diameter is greater than 3 mm in children younger than 5 years or 4 mm in children 5 years of age or older, (b) if the internal diameter of a segment measures 1.5 times that of an adjacent segment, or (c) if the coronary artery lumen is irregular. New normative data are now available. Using the old criteria may result in underdiagnosis of coronary artery abnormalities.

   New normative data that are expressed according to the body surface area provide a more accurate assessment of the size of the proximal coronary artery segments (Table 19–3). A coronary dimension that is greater than +3 standard deviation (SD) in one of the three proximal segments (LMCA, LAD, and RCA) or one that is greater than +2.5 SD in two proximal segments is highly unusual in the normal population

Table 19–3. **Mean and Prediction Limits for 2 and 3 Standard Deviations for Major Coronary Artery Segments***

Segment	BSA (m²)	0.2	0.3	0.4	0.5	0.6	0.7	0.8	1.0	1.2	1.4	1.6	1.8	2.0
LAD[†]	Mean	1.2	1.4	1.6	1.8	1.9	2.0	2.2	2.3	2.5	2.7	2.8	2.9	3.0
	Mean + 2SD	1.5	1.8	2.1	2.3	2.5	2.7	2.8	3.0	3.3	3.5	3.7	4.0	4.2
	Mean + 3SD	1.7	2.0	2.3	2.5	2.8	3.0	3.2	3.4	3.8	4.0	4.3	4.5	4.7
RCA	Mean	1.3	1.4	1.6	1.7	1.8	2.0	2.1	2.3	2.5	2.7	2.8	3.0	3.2
	Mean + 2SD	1.9	2.1	2.3	2.4	2.6	2.7	2.8	3.1	3.4	3.6	3.8	4.0	4.3
	Mean + 3SD	2.2	2.4	2.6	2.8	3.0	3.1	3.3	3.5	3.8	4.1	4.3	4.5	4.8
LMCA	Mean	1.7	1.9	2.1	2.3	2.4	2.5	2.7	2.9	3.1	3.3	3.4	3.6	3.7
	Mean + 2SD	2.3	2.6	2.8	3.0	3.3	3.4	3.6	3.9	4.2	4.4	4.6	4.8	5.1
	Mean + 3SD	2.7	3.0	3.2	3.4	3.7	3.9	4.0	4.3	4.7	4.9	5.2	5.5	5.8

*Measurements are made from inner edge to inner edge. Values are rounded off to the nearest 0.1 mm.
[†]The dimension of LMCA should not be measured at orifice and immediate vicinity.
LAD, left anterior descending; LMCA, left main coronary artery; RCA, right coronary artery.
Values are from graphic data of Kurotobi S, Nagai T, Kawakami N, Sano T: Coronary diameter in normal infants, children and patients with Kawasaki disease. Pediatr Int 44:1–4, 2002.

(Kurotobi et al, 2002). A criterion of coronary artery dimension 1.5 times that of the adjacent segment is still useful. It is important that one measures the dimension of the LMCA at a point between the ostium and the first bifurcation of the artery. The LAD should be measured distal to and away from the bifurcation of the branch from the LMCA. The RCA should be measured in the relatively straight section of the artery just after the rightward turn from the initial anterior course of the artery.

6. The Harada score has been devised to predict increased risk of developing coronary aneurysm. According to this score, when assessed in the first 9 days of the illness, the presence of four of the following criteria indicates a high risk for future development of coronary artery aneurysm: (a) white cell count >12,000/mm³, (b) platelet count >350,000/mm³, (c) CRP >+3, (d) hematocrit <35%, (e) albumin <3.5 g/dL, (f) age 12 months or younger, and (g) male sex. These criteria have been adopted by the American Heart Association committee.

DIFFERENTIAL DIAGNOSIS

One must rule out diseases with similar manifestations through appropriate cultures and the use of laboratory tests (Box 19–7). Measles and group A β-hemolytic streptococcal infection most closely mimic Kawasaki disease. Children with Kawasaki disease are extremely irritable (often inconsolable). In addition, children with Kawasaki disease are less likely to have exudative conjunctivitis, pharyngitis, generalized lymphadenopathy, or discrete intraoral lesions and are more likely to have a perineal distribution of their rash. Other diseases with findings similar to Kawasaki disease, such as viral exanthems, drug reactions, juvenile rheumatoid arthritis, and Rocky Mountain spotted fever, require differentiation. Viral illness is more likely if acute phase reactants and platelet counts are normal after 7 days of the illness.

MANAGEMENT

No specific therapy is available. Two goals of therapy are reduction of inflammation within the coronary artery and in the myocardium and prevention of thrombosis by inhibition of platelet aggregation.

1. A high-dose (2 g/kg), single infusion (as a 10- to 12-hour infusion) of IVIG with aspirin (80 to 100 mg/kg per day), given within 10 days and if possible within

BOX 19–7	**DIFFERENTIAL DIAGNOSIS OF KAWASAKI DISEASE**

Viral infections (e.g., measles, adenovirus, enterovirus, Epstein-Barr virus)
Scarlet fever
Staphylococcal scalded skin syndrome
Toxic shock syndrome
Bacterial cervical lymphadenopathy
Drug hypersensitivity reaction
Stevens-Johnson syndrome
Juvenile rheumatoid arthritis
Rocky Mountain spotted fever
Leptospirosis
Mercury hypersensitivity reaction (acrodynia)

7 days of illness, is considered the treatment of choice. It is IVIG, not aspirin, that significantly reduces the prevalence of coronary artery abnormalities. Aspirin helps only to reduce thrombus formation; it does not reduce coronary artery aneurysm.

2. The efficacy of IVIG in reducing the prevalence of coronary artery abnormalities is well established. High-dose IVIG should be given because serum immunoglobulin G levels are inversely related to the development of coronary artery abnormalities, fever duration, and laboratory indices of acute inflammation. Two thirds of patients become afebrile by 24 hours after completion of IVIG infusion; 90% are afebrile by 48 hours. A repeated dose (2 g/kg) of IVIG is indicated in children with a persistent fever. IVIG given before 5 days of illness appeared no more likely to prevent coronary aneurysm but was associated with increased need for retreatment with gamma globulin for persistent or recrudescent fever. Gamma globulin should be given even after day 10 of illness if the patient has persistent fever, aneurysms, or ongoing systemic inflammation (by ESR or CRP). Measles and varicella immunization should be deferred for 11 months after a child receives high-dose IVIG.

3. Aspirin has anti-inflammatory effects at high doses (80 to 100 mg/kg/day) and an antiplatelet action at low doses (3 to 5 kg/day). The initial high dose of aspirin is reduced to 3 to 5 mg/kg/day in a single dose after the child has been afebrile for 48 to 72 hours. Other physicians continue high-dose aspirin until day 14 of illness and 48 to 72 hours or more after fever cessation. Aspirin is continued until the patient shows no evidence of coronary changes by 6 to 8 weeks after the onset of illness. For children who develop coronary abnormalities, aspirin may be continued indefinitely.

   Some Japanese authorities recommend the antiplatelet dose of aspirin from the onset because the high dose does not appear to reduce coronary aneurysm and it may inhibit production of prostacyclin (a compound with a potent vasodilating effect and a platelet aggregation inhibitory effect) and may result in increased frequency of hepatotoxicity, GI irritation and bleeding, and Reye's syndrome.

4. An earlier study, before IVIG was available, suggested that corticosteroids exert a detrimental effect with an increased incidence of coronary aneurysm. Concomitant use of corticosteroids has been reported to reduce the duration of fever and possibly the incidence of coronary aneurysm (Okada et al, 2003). However, the usefulness of steroids in the initial treatment of Kawasaki disease is not well established at this time.

5. For patients who continue to be febrile after IVIG (about 10% of patients), repeated IV gamma globulin (2 g/kg) is generally recommended. The use of corticosteroid therapy is restricted for patients who continue to be febrile despite two or more courses of IV gamma globulin.

6. In patients with a large coronary artery aneurysm, administration of abciximab, a platelet glycoprotein IIb/IIIa receptor inhibitor, was associated with greater regression of the aneurysm compared with patients who received only the

standard treatment (gamma globulin, aspirin) at 4 to 6 months follow-up (Williams et al, 2002).

7. In patients with coronary artery aneurysm, therapeutic regimens used depend on the severity of coronary involvement and include antiplatelet agents (aspirin, with or without dipyridamole [Persantine] or clopidogrel [Plavix]) and anticoagulant agents (oral warfarin or injectable low-molecular-weight heparin).

a. For mild and stable disease, low-dose aspirin may be appropriate.

b. With increasing severity and extent of coronary involvement, the combination of aspirin with other antiplatelet agents (e.g., dipyridamole, clopidogrel) may be more effective in suppressing platelet activation.

c. For giant aneurysm or the combination of stenosis and aneurysm, low-dose aspirin together with warfarin (with International Normalized Ratio [INR] maintained at 2.0 to 2.5) should be used.

NATURAL HISTORY

Kawasaki's disease is a self-limited disease for most patients. Cardiovascular involvement is the most serious complication.

1. Coronary aneurysm develops in 15% to 25% of untreated patients and is responsible for myocardial infarction (<5%) and mortality (1% to 5%). Significantly higher temperature (101.3°F [38.5°C] on days 9 to 12) and longer duration of fever (more than 14 days) appear to be risk factors for coronary aneurysm. Despite prompt treatment with high-dose IVIG, at least transient coronary artery abnormalities develop in 5% of the patients and giant aneurysm in 1%.

2. Angiographic resolution of aneurysm 1 to 2 years after the illness occurs in 50% to 67% of the patients, but these arteries do not dilate in response to exercise or coronary vasodilators. In some patients, stenosis, tortuosity, and thrombosis of the coronary arteries result. The resolution appears to be more likely to occur with a smaller aneurysm, age at onset younger than 1 year, fusiform rather than saccular aneurysm, and aneurysm located at a distal coronary segment.

3. More than 70% of myocardial infarctions occur in the first year after onset of the disease without warning symptoms or signs. Giant aneurysm (>8 mm) is associated with greater morbidity and mortality (because of thrombotic occlusion or stenotic obstruction and subsequent myocardial infarction).

4. If the coronary arteries remain normal throughout the first month after the onset, subsequent development of a new coronary lesion is extremely unusual.

LONG-TERM FOLLOW-UP

Serial cardiology follow-up is important for evaluation of the cardiac status. The recommendations of the Committee on Rheumatic Fever, Endocarditis, and Kawasaki Disease, American Heart Association (2004), are summarized in Table 19–4.

1. For children with no or transient coronary abnormalities, aspirin is discontinued after 6 to 8 weeks. No follow-up diagnostic tests are indicated. Only periodic counseling is recommended.

2. If there is coronary aneurysm, low-dose aspirin is continued indefinitely. With a large aneurysm, a combination of aspirin and warfarin is indicated.

3. Varying levels of activity restriction are indicated in patients who have a coronary artery aneurysm (see Table 19–4).

4. Echocardiography. In the absence of coronary artery abnormalities in the first 6 to 8 weeks, follow-up echoes are not indicated. If significant abnormalities of the coronary vessels, LV dysfunction, or valvular regurgitation is found, the echo should be repeated at 6- to 12-month intervals.

5. Exercise stress testing or myocardial perfusion evaluation is indicated in children with coronary artery aneurysms at 1- to 2-year intervals.

Table 19–4. **Follow-up Recommendations According to the Degree of Coronary Artery Involvement**

Risk Level	Pharmacologic Therapy	Physical Activity	Follow-up and Diagnostic Testing	Invasive Testing
I (no coronary artery changes at any stage of illness)	None beyond first 6–8 wk (aspirin for first 6–8 wk only)	No restrictions beyond first 6–8 wk	Cardiovascular risk assessment, counseling at 5-yr intervals	None recommended
II (transient coronary artery ectasia disappears within first 6–8 wk)	None beyond first 6–8 wk (aspirin for first 6–8 wk only)	No restrictions beyond initial 6–8 wk	Cardiovascular risk assessment and counseling at 3- to 5-yr intervals	None recommended
III (one small to medium coronary artery aneurysm/ major coronary artery)	Low dose aspirin (3–5 mg/kg/day), at least until aneurysm regression documented	For patients <11 yr, no restrictions beyond initial 6–8 wk Patients 11–20 yr old, physical activity guided by stress test or myocardial perfusion scan every 2 yr Contact or high-impact sports discouraged for patients taking antiplatelet agents	Annual cardiology follow-up with echocardiogram + ECG Cardiovascular risk assessment and counseling Stress test with myocardial perfusion scan every 2 yr in patients >10 yr	Angiography, if noninvasive test suggests ischemia
IV (≥one large or giant coronary artery aneurysms, or multiple or complex aneurysm in same coronary artery without obstruction)	Long-term aspirin (3–5 mg/kg/day) and warfarin (target: INR 2.0–2.5) or low-molecular-weight heparin (target: anti–factor Xa level 0.5–1.0 U/mL) should be combined in giant aneurysm	Contact or high-impact sports should be avoided because of risk of bleeding Other physical activity recommendations guided by annual stress test or myocardial perfusion evaluation	Cardiology follow-up with echocardiogram + ECG every 6 mo Annual stress test with myocardial perfusion evaluation For females of childbearing age, reproductive counseling is recommended	First angiography at 6–12 mo or sooner if clinically indicated Repeated angiography if noninvasive test, clinical, or laboratory findings suggest ischemia Elective repeated angiography under some circumstances (atypical anginal pain, inability to do stress testing, etc.)
V (coronary artery obstruction)	Long-term low-dose aspirin (3–5 mg/kg/day) Warfarin or low-molecular-weight heparin if giant aneurysm persists Consider use of β-blocker to reduce myocardial oxygen consumption	Contact or high-impact sports should be avoided because of risk of bleeding Other physical activity recommendations guided by stress test or myocardial perfusion scan	Cardiology follow-up with echocardiogram and ECG every 6 mo Annual stress test or myocardial perfusion scan For females of childbearing age, reproductive counseling is recommended	Angiography recommended to address therapeutic options of bypass grafting or catheter intervention

Modified from Newburger JW, Takahashi M, Gerber MA, et al: Diagnosis, treatment, and long-term management of Kawasaki disease: A statement for health professionals from the Committee on Rheumatic Fever, Endocarditis, and Kawasaki Disease, Council on Cardiovascular Disease in the Young, American Heart Association. Pediatrics 114:1708–1733, 2004.

6. Occasionally, coronary angiography may be indicated in infants with large aneurysms or stenosis, in patients with symptoms suggestive of ischemia, in patients with positive exercise tests or thallium studies, and/or in those with evidence of myocardial infarction.

7. Rarely, for patients with evidence of reversible ischemia from coronary artery stenosis (demonstrable on stress imaging tests), percutaneous intervention, such as balloon angioplasty, rotational atherectomy, stenting, or a combination of these procedures, may be indicated (Ishii et al, 2002). However, in a long-term follow-up, neoaneurysm formation or restenosis may occur. On rare occasions, coronary artery bypass surgery may be indicated. The internal mammary artery graft may be used for bypass surgery.

Lyme Carditis

PREVALENCE

Lyme carditis occurs in about 10% of patients with Lyme disease.

CAUSE AND PATHOLOGY

1. Lyme disease is the leading tick-borne illness in North America and Europe. The disease is endemic in three U.S. regions: the Northeast (most commonly in coastal areas from Maryland to northern Massachusetts), the upper Midwest (Wisconsin and Minnesota), and the Far West (California and Oregon). The disease has been reported from every part of the world, including most of the United States.

2. It is caused by the spirochete *Borrelia burgdorferi*, carried by hard-bodied ticks (e.g., *Ixodes dammini*). The spirochete initially produces a characteristic skin lesion (erythema chronicum migrans) and then spreads through the lymphatics and bloodstream and disseminates to other organs, including the heart and the central and peripheral nervous system.

3. The organism can be found in the heart and other parts of the body and is responsible for clinical symptoms and signs.

CLINICAL MANIFESTATIONS

1. Most cases are identified during the summer months, and a history of tick bites may be elicited.

2. Lyme disease can be divided into three stages.
   a. *Stage 1* (localized erythema migrans) begins 3 to 30 days after the tick bite with the onset of influenza-like symptoms (fever, headache, myalgia, arthralgias, malaise) and the characteristic rash, erythema chronicum migrans. The skin lesion, seen in 60% to 80% of patients at the site of the tick bite, begins as a macule or papule followed by progressive expansion of an erythematous ring over approximately 7 days. The ring may be as large as 15 cm with red borders and central clearing, most often appearing on the thigh, groin, or axilla. Erythema migrans lesions usually fade within 3 to 4 weeks, but they may recur.
   b. *Stage 2* (disseminated infection) starts 2 to 12 weeks after the tick bite, and neurologic (10% to 15%) and cardiac (10%) manifestations occur in this stage. The classic triad of Lyme neuroborreliosis includes aseptic meningitis, cranial nerve palsies (most commonly, unilateral or bilateral Bell's palsy), and peripheral radiculoneuropathy. The most common cardiac manifestation is fluctuating AV block (see later discussion), although myocarditis, pericarditis, and LV dysfunction can occur.
   c. *Stage 3* (persistent infection) manifests as large-joint arthritis weeks to years after stage 2 and is seen in about 50% of the patients not previously treated. In general, joint manifestation is self-limited but may recur in patients who do not receive appropriate antibiotic therapy.

3. Cardiac manifestations occur in about 10% of cases. They generally appear 4 to 8 weeks after the initial illness, but their appearance can vary from 4 days to 7 months.

The most common cardiac manifestation is varying degrees of AV block, occurring in up to 87% of cases. Over 95% of these patients show first-degree AV block at some time in their course. Up to 50% develop complete heart block, and some of them develop permanent heart block. First-degree AV block can change to complete heart block within minutes.

DIAGNOSIS

1. The diagnosis is suggested by the presence of the distinctive erythema chronicum migrans and other features of Lyme disease. A history of tick exposure (e.g., travel to an endemic area) and any of the manifestations of stages 2 and 3 are important clues to the disease. The presence of AV block alone is not specific for Lyme carditis; it can be caused by other infective agents, such as viral infections (coxsackievirus A and B, echovirus, mumps, polio), rickettsial infections, *Treponema pallidum*, *Yersinia enterocolitica*, toxoplasmosis, diphtheria, and Chagas' disease.

2. Although cultivation or visualization of *B. burgdorferi* is the most reliable technique to confirm the diagnosis, this test is rarely positive.

3. Enzyme-linked immunosorbent assays (ELISAs) are probably more accurate than indirect immunofluorescence assays. The diagnosis of Lyme disease is confirmed if there is a single titer greater than 1:256 or a fourfold increase in antibody titer over time and compatible clinical symptoms. A positive serologic test alone, in the absence of compatible clinical symptoms, should not be used indiscriminately to diagnose Lyme disease (or as the sole basis for administration of antibiotic therapy).

MANAGEMENT

1. Doxycycline (100 mg twice a day, orally, for 14 to 21 days) is the drug of choice for children older than 8 years. For children younger than 8 years, amoxicillin (25 to 50 mg/kg per day orally, divided into two doses, for 2 to 3 weeks) is the drug of choice. For patients allergic to penicillin, cefuroxime axetil is an alternative.

2. If antibiotic therapy is begun in stage 1, the duration of the skin lesion is shortened, and subsequent complications can be averted. Antibiotic treatment also improves cardiac and neurologic symptoms.

3. Heart block responds to antibiotic treatment, usually within 6 weeks, and has a good prognosis.

4. For high-level AV block, temporary pacing may be indicated (in up to one third of patients).

5. A Lyme disease vaccine (LYMErix, SmithKline Beecham) was licensed by the U.S. Food and Drug Administration for persons 15 to 70 years of age. The vaccine seems to be safe and effective, but its cost-effectiveness has yet to be determined. Other preventive measures such as avoiding tick-infested habitats and wearing protective clothing are important.

Postpericardiotomy Syndrome

Postpericardiotomy syndrome is a febrile illness with inflammatory reaction of the pericardium and pleura that develops after surgery involving pericardiotomy. It is believed to be an autoimmune response to damaged myocardium or pericardium or blood in the pericardial sac. There is a high titer of antiheart antibodies in patients who develop the syndrome, along with high antibody titers against adenovirus, coxsackievirus B1–6, and cytomegalovirus. Thus, it appears to be secondary to a recent or remote viral infection. The incidence is about 25% to 30% of patients who receive pericardiotomy. A nonsurgical example of this syndrome is seen after myocardial infarction (Dressler's syndrome) and traumatic hemopericardium.

CLINICAL MANIFESTATIONS

1. The onset of the syndrome is a few weeks to a few months (median 4 weeks) after cardiac surgery that involves pericardiotomy. It is rare in infants younger than 2 years.

2. The syndrome is characterized by fever and chest pain. Fever may be sustained or spike up to 104°F (40°C). Chest pain may be severe, caused by both pericarditis and pleuritis. Chest pain resulting from pericardial effusion radiates to the left side of the chest and shoulder and worsens in a supine position. Pleural pain worsens on deep inspiration. On physical examination, pericardial and pleural friction rubs and hepatomegaly are usually present. Tachycardia, tachypnea, rising venous pressure, and falling arterial pressure with a paradoxical pulse are signs of cardiac tamponade.

3. Chest x-ray films show an enlarged cardiac silhouette and pleural effusion, especially on the left. The ECG shows persistent ST-segment elevation and flat or inverted T waves in the limb leads and left precordial leads.

4. Echocardiography is the most reliable test in confirming the presence and amount of pericardial effusion and in evaluating evidence of cardiac tamponade.

5. Leukocytosis with a shift to the left and an elevated ESR are present. Acute phase reactant (ESR, CRP) levels are elevated.

6. Although the disease is self-limited, its duration is highly variable; the median duration is 2 to 3 weeks. Recurrences are common, appearing in 21% of patients.

MANAGEMENT

1. Bed rest is all that is needed for mild cases.

2. Nonsteroidal anti-inflammatory agents, such as ibuprofen or indomethacin, may be effective in most cases.

3. In severe cases, moderate doses of corticosteroids may be indicated for a few days if the diagnosis is secure and infection has been ruled out. A more prompt response is seen with steroid therapy, but a serious drawback is the tendency for the condition to rebound after withdrawal of the drug, with some patients becoming steroid bound.

4. Emergency pericardiocentesis may be required if signs of cardiac tamponade are present.

5. Diuretics may be used for pleural effusion.

6. Pericardiectomy may be necessary in patients with recurrent effusion.

Postperfusion Syndrome

Postperfusion syndrome, which occurs only after open-heart surgery using a pump oxygenator, is caused by cytomegalovirus infection. The virus may be transmitted to the patient from a viremia from healthy donors. The syndrome has almost disappeared because freshly drawn blood is no longer used, except in patients with severe cyanotic heart defects.

CLINICAL MANIFESTATIONS

1. The onset is 4 to 6 weeks after cardiac surgery using cardiopulmonary bypass.

2. The syndrome is characterized by the triad of fever, splenomegaly, and atypical lymphocytosis. Hepatomegaly is also common. Low-grade fever, with elevations to 100°F to 102°F (37.7°C to 38.8°C) occur. Malaise and anorexia are commonly present.

3. The fever and atypical lymphocytosis are short-term manifestations (lasting about 2 weeks), but splenomegaly usually lasts 3 to 4 weeks to 3 to 4 months. No recurrence has been reported.

4. The white blood cell count may be normal, but atypical lymphocytes are seen in the peripheral smears. Cytomegalovirus may be demonstrated in the urine, or a changing titer to the virus may be demonstrated in the serum.

MANAGEMENT

1. No specific treatment is available.
2. The syndrome is self-limited, lasting for a week to a few months.

Human Immunodeficiency Virus Infection

Infection with HIV has become a major pediatric health concern in the United States and around the world. The clinical manifestations of HIV infection are well known to primary care physicians, but the significance of cardiovascular manifestations (cardiomyopathy) is less well known.

CLINICAL MANIFESTATIONS

1. Initial symptoms may be subtle or nonspecific. Recurrent infections by opportunistic infective agents and by encapsulated organisms are common (occurring in 20%). GI candidiasis, periodontal disease, oral or esophageal ulcerations, and chronic or recurrent diarrhea with failure to thrive are frequent. Elevation of hepatic transaminases with or without cholestasis occasionally occurs. Anemia (occurring in 20% to 70%), leukopenia, neutropenia, and thrombocytopenia (occurring in 10% to 20%) may be seen. In contrast to those in adults, malignancies (non-Hodgkin's lymphoma, primary central nervous system lymphoma, and leiomyosarcoma) are infrequent in children (2% of cases).

2. Central nervous system involvement in perinatally infected children occurs in 40% to 90%, with a median age of 19 months. Progressive encephalitis is the most common form of central nervous system manifestation, with loss of motor development, cognitive deterioration, and acquired microcephaly. Imaging may show cerebral atrophy (in 85%), increased ventricular size, and basal ganglia calcifications.

3. In children, the prevalence of cardiovascular manifestations is about 20%, and these manifestations are importantly related to prognosis. HIV RNA transcripts have been found in the myocardium of patients with cardiomyopathy. The virus may infect the structure directly or may have an indirect role in the pathogenesis of myocardial manifestations. Coinfection with other viruses, such as Epstein-Barr virus and cytomegalovirus; malnutrition; and wasting may also contribute to the cardiac-related morbidity and mortality and the overall mortality.

    Common cardiovascular manifestations include cardiomyopathy, myocarditis, pericarditis, cardiac arrhythmias, and chronic CHF. The ECG and echo studies are helpful in detecting preclinical abnormalities of the cardiovascular system.
    a. Cardiac examination may reveal sinus tachycardia (in 64% of cases), gallop rhythm, tachypnea, and hepatosplenomegaly—all signs of CHF.
    b. Besides tachycardia, the ECG may show atrial and ventricular ectopic beats and second-degree AV block.
    c. Echo studies may demonstrate diminished LV contractility (in 26%), with some patients having dilated cardiomyopathy and others having hypertrophy of the LV. Pericardial effusions are frequent (26%), caused by opportunistic viral and bacterial infections, including mycobacteria. Occasionally, cardiac tamponade develops, which requires emergency pericardiocentesis. Calcification of cardiac valves also occurs. The incidence of these abnormalities is higher in vertically infected children than in an uninfected cohort from HIV-infected mothers.
    d. The presence of pericardial effusion correlates highly with pleural effusion and ascites. Thus, in children with pleural effusion or ascites, pericardial effusion and cardiac abnormalities should be suspected.

PROGNOSIS

The disease progresses more rapidly in children than in infected adults. Cardiac dysfunction is a predictor of a poor prognosis. In children, the 1-year mortality rate after the diagnosis of CHF is about 70%, and most children with CHF die within 2 years of the diagnosis. If cardiac abnormalities are diagnosed early, preventive and therapeutic strategies for progressive LV dysfunction can be applied.

MANAGEMENT

1. It has been shown that monthly IV infusion of immune globulin improves LV function in HIV-infected patients. This suggests that the LV dysfunction may be immunologically mediated.

2. An early study indicates that zidovudine neither worsens nor ameliorates progressive cardiac changes in HIV-infected patients.

3. Antibiotics are indicated when there is a bacterial infection of the pericardium or other structures.

4. Emergency pericardiocentesis may be required when tamponade is present.

5. If CHF develops, anticongestive measures, including diuretics, inotropic agents, and afterload-reducing agents, are indicated.

Chapter 20

Acute Rheumatic Fever

Prevalence

Acute rheumatic fever is relatively uncommon in the United States but is a common cause of heart disease in less developed countries. However, in the past few decades, new outbreaks have occurred, and new sporadic cases are being reported in the United States.

Causes

1. Acute rheumatic fever is believed to be an immunologic response that occurs as a delayed sequela of group A streptococcal infection of the pharynx but not of the skin. The attack rate of acute rheumatic fever after streptococcal infection varies with the severity of the infection, ranging from 0.3% to 3%.

2. Important predisposing factors include family history of rheumatic fever, low socioeconomic status (poverty, poor hygiene, medical deprivation), and age between 6 and 15 years (with a peak incidence at 8 years of age).

Pathology

1. The inflammatory lesion is found in many parts of the body, most notably in the heart, brain, joints, and skin.

2. Rheumatic carditis was considered to be pancarditis, with myocarditis being the most important element. It is now recognized that a valvular component may be as important as or much more important than myocardial and pericardial involvements. In rheumatic myocarditis, myocardial contractility is rarely impaired and the serum level of troponin is not elevated. It is not only the valve leaflets that are heavily involved with fibrinous vegetations on the coapting surfaces, the entire mitral valve apparatus is involved (with annular dilatation and stretching of chordae tendineae).

3. Valvular damage most frequently and most severely involves the mitral, less commonly the aortic, and rarely the tricuspid and pulmonary valves.

4. Aschoff bodies in the atrial myocardium are believed to be characteristic of rheumatic fever. These consist of inflammatory lesions associated with swelling, fragmentation of collagen fibers, and alterations in the staining characteristics of connective tissue, now believed to be necrotic myocardial cells.

Clinical Manifestations

Acute rheumatic fever is diagnosed by the use of revised Jones criteria (updated in 1993; see Box 20–1). The criteria are three groups of important clinical and laboratory findings: (1) five major manifestations, (2) four minor manifestations, and (3) supporting evidence of an antecedent group A streptococcal infection. These and other important clinical findings are presented here.

HISTORY

1. History of streptococcal pharyngitis, 1 to 5 weeks (average, 3 weeks) before the onset of symptoms, is common. The latent period may be as long as 2 to 6 months (average, 4 months) in cases of isolated chorea.
2. Pallor, malaise, easy fatigability, and other history, such as epistaxis (5% to 10%) and abdominal pain, may be present.

MAJOR MANIFESTATIONS

Arthritis. Arthritis, the most common manifestation of acute rheumatic fever (70% of cases), usually involves large joints (e.g., knees, ankles, elbows, wrists). Often more than one joint is involved, either simultaneously or in succession, with a characteristic migratory nature of the arthritis. Swelling, heat, redness, severe pain, tenderness, and limitation of motion are common. If the patient was given salicylate-containing analgesics, these signs of inflammation may be mild. The arthritis responds dramatically to salicylate therapy; if patients treated with salicylates (with documented therapeutic levels) do not improve in 48 hours, the diagnosis of acute rheumatic fever is probably incorrect.

BOX 20–1	**GUIDELINES FOR THE DIAGNOSIS OF INITIAL ATTACK OF RHEUMATIC FEVER**

MAJOR MANIFESTATIONS
Carditis
Polyarthritis
Chorea
Erythema marginatum
Subcutaneous nodule

MINOR MANIFESTATIONS

Clinical Findings
Arthralgia
Fever

Laboratory Findings
Elevated acute-phase reactants (erythrocyte sedimentation rate, C-reactive protein)
Prolonged PR interval

SUPPORTING EVIDENCE OF ANTECEDENT GROUP A STREPTOCOCCAL INFECTION
Positive throat culture or rapid streptococcal antigen test
Elevated or rising streptococcal antibody titer

If supported by evidence of preceding group A streptococcal infection, the presence of two major manifestations or of one major and two minor manifestations indicates a high probability of acute rheumatic fever.

Guidelines for the diagnosis of rheumatic fever. Jones Criteria, 1992 update. Special Writing Group of the Committee on Rheumatic Fever, Endocarditis, and Kawasaki Disease, Council on Cardiovascular Disease in the Young, American Heart Association. JAMA 268: 2069–2073, 1992.

Carditis. Carditis occurs in 50% of patients. Signs of carditis include some or all of the following.

1. Tachycardia (out of proportion to the degree of fever) is common; its absence makes the diagnosis of myocarditis unlikely.

2. A heart murmur of mitral regurgitation (MR) or aortic regurgitation (AR), or both, is almost always present. The American Heart Association's Jones criteria recommend not making the diagnosis of acute rheumatic carditis without audible murmurs of MR and/or AR, but this is debatable. Significant echo abnormalities may be present in the absence of heart murmur, and echo findings can determine the severity of cardiac enlargement, the presence and degree of MR and AR, and the presence of pericardial effusion more objectively. Inclusion of echo abnormalities may enhance correct diagnosis of acute rheumatic carditis (Vijayalakshmi et al, 2005). However, a hemodynamically insignificant echo finding of MR alone is considered not sufficient to diagnose myocarditis. Gross prolapse of the mitral valve or the presence of a posterolateral (not central) MR jet by color flow mapping may be significant. (With chronic rheumatic MR, fusion of the leaflets and chordae and contracture of these structures occur and the regurgitation jets tends to become more central.) Other abnormal echo findings may include pericardial effusion, increased left ventricular (LV) dimension, or impaired LV function.

3. Pericarditis (friction rub, pericardial effusion, chest pain, and ECG changes) may be present. Pericarditis does not occur without mitral valve involvement in rheumatic fever. Pericardial effusion is usually of small amount and almost never causes cardiac tamponade.

4. Cardiomegaly on chest x-ray films is indicative of the severity of rheumatic carditis (or valvulitis) or congestive heart failure (CHF).

5. Signs of CHF (gallop rhythm, distant heart sounds, cardiomegaly) are indications of severe cardiac dysfunction.

Erythema Marginatum. Erythema marginatum occurs in less than 10% of patients with acute rheumatic fever. The characteristic nonpruritic serpiginous or annular erythematous rashes are most prominent on the trunk and the inner proximal portions of the extremities; they are never seen on the face. The rashes are evanescent, disappearing on exposure to cold and reappearing after a hot shower or when the patient is covered with a warm blanket. They are seldom detected in air-conditioned rooms.

Subcutaneous Nodules. Subcutaneous nodules are found in 2% to 10% of patients, particularly in cases with recurrences; they are almost never present as a sole manifestation of rheumatic fever. They are hard, painless, nonpruritic, freely movable, swelling, and 0.2 to 2 cm in diameter. They are usually found symmetrically, singly or in clusters, on the extensor surfaces of both large and small joints, over the scalp, or along the spine. They are not transient, lasting for weeks, and have a significant association with carditis. Subcutaneous nodules are not exclusive to rheumatic fever. They occur in 10% of children with rheumatoid arthritis, and benign subcutaneous nodules have been described in children and adults. In adults, they occur with rheumatoid arthritis, systemic lupus erythematosus, and other diseases.

Sydenham's Chorea. Sydenham's chorea (St. Vitus' dance) is found in 15% of patients with acute rheumatic fever. It occurs more often in prepubertal girls (8 to 12 years) than in boys. It is a neuropsychiatric disorder consisting of both neurologic signs (choreic movement and hypotonia) and psychiatric signs (e.g., emotional lability, hyperactivity, separation anxiety, obsessions, and compulsions). It begins with emotional lability and personality changes. These are soon replaced (in 1 to 4 weeks) by the characteristic spontaneous, purposeless movement of chorea (which lasts 4 to 18 months), followed by motor weakness. The distractibility and inattentiveness outlast the choreic movements. The adventitious movements, weakness, and hypotonia continue for an average of 7 months (up to 17 months) before slowly waning in severity. Elevated titers of "antineuronal antibodies" recognizing basal ganglion tissues have been found in over 90% of patients. The levels of the antineuronal antibody titer are positively related to the severity of choreic movements. These findings suggest that chorea may be related to dysfunction of basal ganglia and cortical neuronal components.

MINOR MANIFESTATIONS

1. Arthralgia refers to joint pain without the objective changes of arthritis. It must not be considered a minor manifestation when arthritis is used as a major manifestation in making a diagnosis of rheumatic fever.

2. Fever (usually with a temperature of at least 102°F [38.8°C]) is present early in the course of untreated rheumatic fever.

3. In laboratory findings, elevated acute phase reactants (elevated C-reactive protein levels and elevated erythrocyte sedimentation rate) are objective evidence of an inflammatory process.

4. A prolonged PR interval on the ECG is neither specific for acute rheumatic fever nor an indication of active carditis.

EVIDENCE OF ANTECEDENT GROUP A STREPTOCOCCAL INFECTION

1. A history of sore throat or of scarlet fever unsubstantiated by laboratory data is not adequate evidence of recent group A streptococcal infection.

2. Positive throat cultures or rapid streptococcal antigen tests for group A streptococci are less reliable than antibody tests because they do not distinguish between recent infection and chronic pharyngeal carriage.

3. Streptococcal antibody tests are the most reliable laboratory evidence of antecedent streptococcal infection capable of producing acute rheumatic fever. The onset of the clinical manifestations of acute rheumatic fever coincides with the peak of the streptococcal antibody response.

   a. Antistreptolysin O (ASO) titer is well standardized and therefore is the most widely used test. It is elevated in 80% of patients with acute rheumatic fever and in 20% of normal individuals. Only 67% of patients with isolated chorea have an elevated ASO titer. ASO titers of at least 333 Todd units in children and 250 Todd units in adults are considered elevated. A single low ASO titer does not exclude acute rheumatic fever. If three antistreptococcal antibody tests (antistreptolysin O, antideoxyribonuclease B, and antihyaluronidase tests) are obtained, a titer for at least one antibody test is elevated in over 95% of patients.

   b. Antideoxyribonuclease B titers of 240 Todd units or greater in children and 120 Todd units or greater in adults are considered elevated.

   c. The Streptozyme test (Wampole Laboratories Cranbury, NJ), which detects antibodies, is a relatively simple slide agglutination test, but it is less standardized and less reproducible than the other antibody tests. It should not be used as a diagnostic test for evidence of antecedent group A streptococcal infection.

OTHER CLINICAL FEATURES

1. Abdominal pain, rapid sleeping heart rate, tachycardia out of proportion to fever, malaise, anemia, epistaxis, and precordial pain are relatively common but not specific.

2. A positive family history of rheumatic fever may also heighten the suspicion.

Diagnosis

1. The revised Jones criteria are used for the diagnosis of acute rheumatic fever (see Box 20–1). A diagnosis of acute rheumatic fever is highly probable when either two major manifestations or one major and two minor manifestations, plus evidence of antecedent streptococcal infection, are present. The absence of supporting evidence of a previous group A streptococcal infection makes the diagnosis doubtful (see later discussion for exceptions).

2. The following tips help in applying the Jones criteria:
   a. Two major manifestations are always stronger than one major plus two minor manifestations.
   b. Arthralgia or a prolonged PR interval cannot be used as a minor manifestation when using arthritis and carditis, respectively, as a major manifestation.
   c. The absence of evidence of an antecedent group A streptococcal infection is a warning that acute rheumatic fever is unlikely (except when chorea is present).
   d. The vibratory innocent (Still's) murmur is often misinterpreted as a murmur of MR and thereby is a frequent cause of misdiagnosis (or overdiagnosis) of acute rheumatic fever. The murmur of MR is a *regurgitant-type* systolic murmur (starting with the S1), but the innocent murmur is low pitched and an *ejection type*. A cardiology consultation during the acute phase minimizes the frequency of misdiagnosis.
   e. The possibility of the early suppression of full clinical manifestations should be sought during the history taking. Subtherapeutic doses of aspirin or salicylate-containing analgesics (e.g., Bufferin, Anacin) may suppress full manifestations.

3. Exceptions to the Jones criteria include the following three specific situations:
   a. Chorea may occur as the only manifestation of rheumatic fever.
   b. Indolent carditis may be the only manifestation in patients who come to medical attention months after the onset of rheumatic fever.
   c. Occasionally, patients with rheumatic fever recurrences may not fulfill the Jones criteria.

Differential Diagnosis

1. Juvenile rheumatoid arthritis is often misdiagnosed as acute rheumatic fever. The following findings suggest juvenile rheumatoid arthritis rather than acute rheumatic fever: involvement of peripheral small joints, symmetrical involvement of large joints without migratory arthritis, pallor of the involved joints, a more indolent course, no evidence of preceding streptococcal infection, and the absence of a prompt response to salicylate therapy within 24 to 48 hours.

2. Other collagen vascular diseases (systemic lupus erythematosus, mixed connective tissue disease); reactive arthritis, including poststreptococcal arthritis; serum sickness; and infectious arthritis (such as gonococcal) occasionally require differentiation.

3. Virus-associated acute arthritis (rubella, parvovirus, hepatitis B virus, herpesviruses, enteroviruses) is much more common in adults.

4. Hematologic disorders, such as sicklemia and leukemia, should be considered in the differential diagnosis.

Clinical Course

1. Only carditis can cause permanent cardiac damage. Signs of mild carditis disappear rapidly in weeks, but those of severe carditis may last for 2 to 6 months.

2. Arthritis subsides within a few days to several weeks, even without treatment, and does not cause permanent damage.

3. Chorea gradually subsides in 6 to 7 months or longer and usually does not cause permanent neurologic sequelae.

Management

1. When acute rheumatic fever is suggested by history and physical examination, one should obtain the following laboratory studies: complete blood count, acute phase reactants (erythrocyte sedimentation rate and C-reactive protein), throat culture,

ASO titer (and a second antibody titer, particularly with chorea), chest x-ray films, and ECG. Cardiology consultation is indicated to clarify whether there is cardiac involvement; two-dimensional echo and Doppler studies are usually performed at that time.

2. Benzathine penicillin G, 0.6 to 1.2 million units intramuscularly, is given to eradicate streptococci. This serves as the first dose of penicillin prophylaxis as well (see later discussion). In patients allergic to penicillin, erythromycin, 40 mg/kg per day in two to four doses for 10 days, may be substituted for penicillin.

3. Anti-inflammatory or suppressive therapy with salicylates or steroids must not be started until a definite diagnosis is made. Early suppressive therapy may interfere with a definite diagnosis of acute rheumatic fever by suppressing full development of joint manifestations and suppressing acute phase reactants.

4. When the diagnosis of acute rheumatic fever is confirmed, one must educate the patient and parents about the need to prevent subsequent streptococcal infection through continuous antibiotic prophylaxis. In patients with cardiac involvement, the need for prophylaxis against infective endocarditis should also be emphasized.

5. Bed rest of varying duration is recommended. The duration depends on the type and severity of the manifestations and may range from a week (for isolated arthritis) to several weeks for severe carditis. Bed rest is followed by a period of indoor ambulation of varying duration before the child is allowed to return to school. The erythrocyte sedimentation rate is a helpful guide to the rheumatic activity and therefore to the duration of restriction of activities. Full activity is allowed when the erythrocyte sedimentation rate has returned to normal, except in children with significant cardiac involvement. Table 20–1 is a general guide to the period of bed rest and indoor ambulation.

6. Therapy with anti-inflammatory agents should be started as soon as acute rheumatic fever has been diagnosed.
   a. For mild to moderate carditis, aspirin alone is recommended in a dose of 90 to 100 mg/kg per day in four to six divided doses. An adequate blood level of salicylates is 20 to 25 mg/100 mL. This dose is continued for 4 to 8 weeks, depending on the clinical response. After improvement, the therapy is withdrawn gradually over 4 to 6 weeks while monitoring acute phase reactants.
   b. For arthritis, aspirin therapy is continued for 2 weeks and gradually withdrawn over the following 2 to 3 weeks. Rapid resolution of joint symptoms with aspirin within 24 to 36 hours is supportive evidence of the arthritis of acute rheumatic fever.
   c. Prednisone (2 mg/kg per day in four divided doses for 2 to 6 weeks) is indicated only in cases of severe carditis (Table 20–2).

7. Treatment of CHF includes the following (also see Chapter 27):
   a. Complete bed rest with orthopneic position and moist, cool oxygen
   b. Prednisone for severe carditis of recent onset (see Table 20–2)
   c. Digoxin, used with caution, beginning with half the usual recommended dose, because certain patients with rheumatic carditis are supersensitive to digitalis (see Table 27–5)
   d. Furosemide, 1 mg/kg every 6 to 12 hours, if indicated

Table 20–1. **General Guidelines for Bed Rest and Indoor Ambulation**

	Arthritis Alone	**Mild Carditis***	**Moderate Carditis†**	**Severe Carditis‡**
Bed rest	1–2 wk	3–4 wk	4–6 wk	As long as congestive heart failure is present
Indoor ambulation	1–2 wk	3–4 wk	4–6 wk	2–3 mo

*Questionable cardiomegaly.
†Definite but mild cardiomegaly.
‡Marked cardiomegaly or heart failure.

Table 20–2. **Recommended Anti-inflammatory Agents**

	Arthritis Alone	Mild Carditis	Moderate Carditis	Severe Carditis
Prednisone	0	0	0	2–6 wk*
Aspirin	1–2 wk	3–4 wk[†]	6–8 wk	2–4 mo

*The dose of prednisone should be tapered and aspirin started during the final week.
[†]Aspirin may be reduced to 60 mg/kg/day after 2 weeks of therapy.
Dosages: Prednisone, 2 mg/kg/day, in four divided doses; aspirin, 100 mg/kg/day, in four to six divided doses.

8. Management of Sydenham's chorea:

 a. Reduce physical and emotional stress and use protective measures as indicated.

 b. Give benzathine penicillin G, 1.2 million units, initially for eradication of streptococcus and also every 28 days for prevention of recurrence, just as in patients with other rheumatic manifestations. Without the prophylaxis, about 25% of patients with isolated chorea (without carditis) develop rheumatic valvular heart disease in a 20-year follow-up.

 c. Anti-inflammatory agents are not needed in patients with isolated chorea.

 d. For severe cases, any of the following drugs may be used: phenobarbital (15 to 30 mg every 6 to 8 hours), haloperidol (starting at 0.5 mg and increasing every 8 hours to 2 mg every 8 hours), valproic acid, chlorpromazine (Thorazine), diazepam (Valium), or steroids.

 e. Results of plasma exchange (to remove antineuronal antibodies) and intravenous immune globulin therapy (to inactivate the effects of the antineuronal antibodies) are promising in decreasing the severity of chorea and they were better than prednisone (Garvey et al, 2005).

Prognosis

The presence or absence of permanent cardiac damage determines the prognosis. The development of residual heart disease is influenced by the following three factors:

1. Cardiac status at the start of treatment: The more severe the cardiac involvement at the time the patient is first seen, the greater the incidence of residual heart disease.

2. Recurrence of rheumatic fever: The severity of valvular involvement increases with each recurrence.

3. Regression of heart disease: Evidence of cardiac involvement at the first attack may disappear in 10% to 25% of patients 10 years after the initial attack. Valvular disease resolves more frequently when prophylaxis is followed.

Prevention

PRIMARY PREVENTION

Primary prevention of rheumatic fever is possible with a 10-day course of penicillin therapy for streptococcal pharyngitis. However, primary prevention is not possible in all patients because about 30% of the patients develop subclinical pharyngitis and therefore do not seek medical treatment. Another 30% of patients develop acute rheumatic fever without symptoms of streptococcal pharyngitis (30%).

SECONDARY PREVENTION

1. Who should receive prophylaxis?

Patients with documented histories of rheumatic fever, including those with isolated chorea and those without evidence of rheumatic heart disease, must receive prophylaxis.

2. For how long?

Ideally, patients should receive prophylaxis indefinitely. For patients who had acute rheumatic fever without carditis, the prophylaxis should continue for at least 5 years or until the person is 21 years of age, whichever is longer. For patients who are in a high-risk occupation (e.g., schoolteachers, physicians, nurses), prophylaxis should be continued for a longer period of time. The chance of recurrence is highest in the first 5 years after the acute rheumatic fever. If the patient had rheumatic carditis or residual valvular disease as a result of rheumatic fever, the duration of prophylaxis should be longer (Table 20–3).

3. What method of prophylaxis should be used?

The method of choice for secondary prevention is benzathine penicillin G, 1.2 million units given intramuscularly every 28 days (not once a month). Alternative methods, although not as effective, are the following:

1. Oral penicillin V, 250 mg, twice daily

2. Oral sulfadiazine 1 g or sulfisoxazole 0.5 g once daily

3. Oral erythromycin ethyl succinate, 250 mg, twice daily

Table 20–3. **Recommended Duration of Prophylaxis for Rheumatic Fever**

Category	Duration
Rheumatic fever without carditis	At least for 5 yr or until age 21 yr, whichever is longer
Rheumatic fever with carditis but without residual heart disease (no valvular disease)	At least for 10 yr or well into adulthood, whichever is longer
Rheumatic fever with carditis and residual heart disease (persistent valvular disease)	At least 10 yr since last episode and at least until age 40 yr; sometimes lifelong prophylaxis

Modified from Dajani A, Taubert K, Ferrieri P, et al: Treatment of acute streptococcal pharyngitis and prevention of rheumatic fever: A statement for health professionals: Committee on Rheumatic Fever, Endocarditis, and Kawasaki Disease of the Council on Cardiovascular Disease in the Young, The American Heart Association. Pediatrics 96:758–764, 1995.

Chapter 21

Valvular Heart Disease

Valvular heart diseases are either congenital or acquired in origin. Pathophysiology and clinical manifestations are similar for both entities and have been discussed in Chapter 10. Congenital stenoses of the aortic and pulmonary valves are discussed in depth in Chapter 13.

In this chapter, mitral stenosis (MS), mitral regurgitation, and aortic regurgitation (AR) of both congenital and acquired etiology are discussed, if they are isolated or the major lesion. Although the cause of mitral valve prolapse (MVP) is not entirely clear, it is discussed in this chapter because it involves a cardiac valve. Isolated congenital pulmonary regurgitation (PR), tricuspid regurgitation, and tricuspid stenosis of significance are exceedingly rare and therefore are not discussed. PR following TOF surgery is discussed under "Tetralogy of Fallot" in Chapter 14. Tricuspid regurgitation is most frequently seen with Ebstein's anomaly and is discussed under that condition.

Most acquired valvular heart diseases are of rheumatic etiology. They are, however, rare in the industrialized countries, although they still occur frequently in less developed countries. Among rheumatic heart diseases, mitral valve involvement occurs in about three fourths and aortic valve involvement in about one fourth of the cases. Stenosis and regurgitation of the same valve usually occur together. Isolated aortic stenosis (AS) of rheumatic origin without mitral valve involvement is extremely rare. Rheumatic involvement of the tricuspid and pulmonary valves almost never occurs.

Mitral Stenosis

PREVALENCE

Isolated congenital MS is very rare. It is usually associated with other anomalies such as Shone's complex. MS of rheumatic origin is rare in children (because it requires 5 to 10 years from the initial attack to develop the condition), but it is the most common valvular involvement in adult rheumatic patients in areas where rheumatic fever is still prevalent.

PATHOLOGY AND PATHOPHYSIOLOGY

1. Congenital MS is usually associated with obstruction at more than one level. The stenosis may be at the level of the valve leaflets (fusion of the leaflets), the papillary muscle (single papillary muscle seen with parachute mitral valve), the chordae (thickened and fused chordae seen in single papillary muscle), or the supravalvar region (supravalvar mitral ring), and it may be due to the hypoplasia of the valve ring itself (as seen with hypoplastic left heart syndrome).

2. In rheumatic MS, thickening of the leaflets and fusion of the commissures dominate the pathologic findings. Calcification with immobility of the valve results over time.

3. Regardless of the etiology, a significant MS results in the enlargement of the left atrium (LA), pulmonary venous hypertension, and pulmonary artery (PA) hypertension with resulting enlargement and hypertrophy of the right side of the heart.

4. In patients with severe pulmonary venous hypertension, pulmonary congestion and edema, fibrosis of the alveolar walls, hypertrophy of the pulmonary arterioles, and loss of lung compliance result.

CLINICAL MANIFESTATIONS

History

1. Patients with mild MS are asymptomatic.

2. In infants with severe MS, symptoms develop early in life with shortness of breath and failure to thrive.

3. Dyspnea with or without exertion is the most common symptom in older children. Orthopnea, nocturnal dyspnea, or palpitation is present in more severe cases.

Physical Examination (Fig. 21–1)

1. An increased right ventricular impulse is palpable along the left sternal border. Neck veins are distended if right-sided heart failure supervenes.

2. A loud S1 at the apex and a narrowly split S2 with accentuated P2 are audible if pulmonary hypertension is present. An opening snap (a short snapping sound accompanying the opening of the mitral valve) may be audible in rheumatic MS. A low-frequency mitral diastolic rumble is present at the apex (see Fig. 21–1). A crescendo presystolic murmur may be audible at the apex. Occasionally, a high-frequency diastolic murmur of PR (Graham Steell's murmur) is present at the upper left sternal border, but it is difficult to distinguish from AR.

Electrocardiography. Right axis deviation, left atrial hypertrophy (LAH), and right ventricular hypertrophy (RVH) (caused by pulmonary hypertension) are common. Atrial fibrillation is rare in children.

X-ray Studies

1. The LA and right ventricle (RV) are usually enlarged, and the main PA segment is usually prominent.

2. Lung fields show pulmonary venous congestion, interstitial edema shown as Kerley's B lines (dense, short, horizontal lines most commonly seen in the costophrenic angles), and redistribution of pulmonary blood flow with increased pulmonary vascularity to the upper lobes.

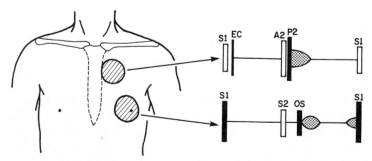

Figure 21–1. Cardiac findings of mitral stenosis. Abnormal sounds are shown in black and include a loud S1, an ejection click (EC), a loud S2, and an opening snap (OS). Also note the mid-diastolic rumble and presystolic murmur. The murmur of pulmonary regurgitation indicates long-standing pulmonary hypertension.

Echocardiography. Echo is the most accurate noninvasive tool for the detection of MS.

1. A two-dimensional echo study should define structural abnormalities of the valve, supravalvar region, chordae, and papillary muscles.

2. It shows a dilated LA. The main PA, RV, and right atrium (RA) are also dilated.

3. Doppler studies can estimate the pressure gradient and thus the severity of stenosis. A mean Doppler gradient of less than 4 to 5 mm Hg results from mild stenosis, 6 to 12 mm Hg is seen with moderate stenosis, and a mean gradient greater than 13 mm Hg is seen with severe stenosis. RV systolic pressure can be estimated from the tricuspid regurgitation jet velocity (by the Bernoulli equation), which may be elevated.

4. In patients with rheumatic MS, an M-mode echo may show a diminished E-to-F slope (reflecting a slow diastolic closure of the anterior mitral leaflet), anterior movement of the posterior leaflet during diastole, multiple echoes from thickened mitral leaflets, and large LA dimension.

NATURAL HISTORY

1. Infants with significant MS with failure to thrive require either balloon or surgical intervention.

2. Most children with mild MS are asymptomatic but become symptomatic with exertion.

3. Recurrence of rheumatic fever worsens the stenosis.

4. Atrial flutter or fibrillation and thromboembolism (related to the chronic atrial arrhythmias) are rare in children.

5. Subacute bacterial endocarditis (SBE) can occur, but it is rare.

6. Hemoptysis can develop from the rupture of small vessels in the bronchi as a result of long-standing pulmonary venous hypertension.

MANAGEMENT

Medical

1. Mild and moderate MS is managed with anticongestive measures (e.g., digoxin, diuretics).

2. Balloon dilatation of the valve should be considered in infants with failure to thrive and with repeated respiratory infections. It may delay surgical intervention. Balloon dilatation is an effective and safe option for children with rheumatic MS.

3. If atrial fibrillation develops, digoxin is the initial treatment to slow the AV conduction. Intravenous procainamide may be used for conversion to sinus rhythm in hemodynamically stable patients. For patients with chronic atrial fibrillation, anticoagulation with warfarin should be started 3 weeks before cardioversion to prevent systemic embolization of atrial thrombus. Anticoagulation is continued for 4 weeks after restoration of sinus rhythm (see Chapter 24 for further discussion). Quinidine may prevent recurrence.

4. Good dental hygiene and antibiotic prophylaxis against SBE are important.

5. Varying degrees of restriction of activity may be indicated.

6. Recurrence of rheumatic fever should be prevented with penicillin or sulfonamide (see Chapter 20).

Surgical

Indications. According to the ACC/AHA 2006 guidelines, the indications for mitral valve surgery for congenital MS in adolescents and young adults are as follows.

1. Surgery is indicated in patients with congenital MS who have symptoms (New York Heart Association [NYHA] functional class III or IV) and mean Doppler MV gradient greater than 10 mm Hg. (Symptoms may include angina, syncope, or dyspnea on exertion.)

2. Surgery is reasonable in mildly symptomatic patients with congenital MS (NYHA functional class I) and mean Doppler MV gradient greater than 10 mm Hg.

3. Surgery is reasonable in asymptomatic patients with PA pressure ≥ 50 mm Hg and mean MV gradient ≥10 mm Hg.

For infants and children with severe MS, the following indications may also apply.

1. Symptomatic infants or children with failure to gain weight, dyspnea on exertion, pulmonary edema, or paroxysmal dyspnea may be candidates for surgery (or balloon dilatation).

2. Failed balloon dilatation or severe MR resulting from the balloon procedure is an indication for surgery.

3. Recurrent atrial fibrillation, thromboembolic phenomenon, and hemoptysis may be indications for surgery in children.

Procedures and Mortality

1. Resection of a supravalvar mitral ring or splitting of thickened and fused chordae is an option depending on the nature of the lesion.

2. For rheumatic MS, if balloon dilatation is unsuccessful, closed or open mitral commissurotomy remains the procedure of choice for those with pliable mitral valves without calcification or MR. The operative mortality rate is less than 1%.

3. Mitral valve replacement. A prosthetic valve (Starr-Edwards, Björk-Shiley, St. Jude) is inserted either in the annulus or in a supra-annular position. The surgical mortality is 0 to 19%. All mechanical valves require anticoagulation with warfarin with its long-term risk, and reoperation may become necessary because of valve entrapment by pannus formation. The bioprostheses (porcine valve, heterograft valve) do not require anticoagulation therapy but require low-dose aspirin. Bioprostheses tend to deteriorate more rapidly because of calcific degeneration in children.

4. In patients with parachute mitral valve, creation of fenestration among the fused chordae may increase the effective orifice area and improve symptoms dramatically. MV replacement may occasionally be necessary but is especially problematic in patients with a hypoplastic mitral annulus, in whom an annulus-enlarging operation may be necessary.

5. Rarely, a valved conduit can be placed between the LA and the apex of the left ventricle.

Complications

1. Postoperative congestive heart failure (CHF) is the most common cause of early postoperative death.

2. Arterial embolization is a rare complication.

3. Bleeding diathesis is possible with anticoagulation therapy for an implanted prosthetic valve.

Postoperative Follow-up

1. Regular checkups every 6 to 12 months with echo and Doppler studies should be done for possible dysfunction of the repaired or replaced valve.

2. After replacement with a mechanical valve with no risk factors (which include atrial fibrillation, previous thromboembolism, and hypercoagulable state), warfarin is indicated to achieve an International Normalized Ratio (INR) of 2.5 to 3.5. Low-dose aspirin is also indicated. After replacement with a bioprosthesis and risk factors, warfarin is also indicated. When there are no risk factors after bioprosthesis placement, aspirin alone is indicated at 75 to 100 mg/day (see ACC/AHA 2006 guidelines).

3. Maintaining good dental hygiene and instituting SBE prophylaxis should be emphasized.

Mitral Regurgitation

PREVALENCE

MR is more common than MS. It is most often congenital and associated with AV canal defect. MR of rheumatic origin is rare, but it is the most common valvular involvement in children with rheumatic heart disease.

PATHOLOGY

1. Mitral valve regurgitation associated with AV canal occurs frequently through the cleft in the mitral valve. When the valve annulus is dilated from any causes that dilate the left ventricle (such as AR or dilated cardiomyopathy), central regurgitation occurs.
2. In rheumatic heart disease, mitral valve leaflets are shortened because of fibrosis, resulting in mitral regurgitation.
3. With increasing severity of MR, dilatation of the LA and left ventricle (LV) results, and the mitral valve ring may become dilated. Pulmonary hypertension may eventually develop as with MS.

CLINICAL MANIFESTATIONS

History

1. Patients are usually asymptomatic with mild MR.
2. Rarely, fatigue (caused by reduced forward cardiac output) and palpitation (caused by atrial fibrillation) develop.

Physical Examination (Fig. 21–2)

1. The jugular venous pulse is normal in the absence of CHF. A heaving, hyperdynamic apical impulse is palpable in severe MR.
2. The S1 is normal or diminished. The S2 may split widely as a result of shortening of the LV ejection and early closure of the aortic valve. The S3 is commonly present and loud. The hallmark of MR is a regurgitant systolic murmur starting with S1, grade 2 to 4/6, at the apex, with good transmission to the left axilla (best demonstrated in the left decubitus position). A short, low-frequency diastolic rumble may be present at the apex (see Fig. 21–2).

Electrocardiography

1. ECG is normal in mild cases.
2. Left ventricular hypertrophy (LVH) or LV dominance, with or without LAH, is usually present.
3. Atrial fibrillation is rare in children but often develops in adults.

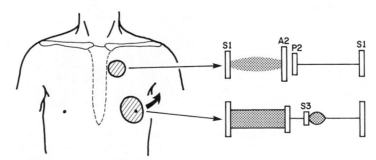

Figure 21–2. *Cardiac findings of mitral regurgitation. Arrow near the apex indicates the direction of radiation of the murmur toward the left axilla.*

X-ray Studies (Fig. 21–3)

1. The LA and LV are enlarged to varying degrees.
2. Pulmonary vascularity is usually within normal limits, but a pulmonary venous congestion pattern may develop if CHF supervenes.

Echocardiography

1. Two-dimensional echo shows dilated LA and LV; the degree of dilatation is related to the severity of MR.
2. Color flow mapping of the regurgitant jet into the LA and Doppler studies can assess the severity of the regurgitation.
3. The echocardiogram can distinguish eccentric regurgitation through the cleft mitral valve from central regurgitation (associated with annular dilatation).

NATURAL HISTORY

1. Patients are relatively stable for a long time with mild regurgitation.
2. Infective endocarditis is a rare complication.
3. LV failure and consequent pulmonary hypertension may occur in adult life.

MANAGEMENT

Medical

1. Preventive measures against SBE (see Chapter 19) and prophylaxis against recurrence of rheumatic fever (see Chapter 20) are important.
2. Activity need not be restricted in most mild cases.
3. Afterload-reducing agents are particularly useful in maintaining the forward cardiac output.
4. Anticongestive therapy (with diuretics and digoxin) is provided if CHF develops.
5. If atrial fibrillation develops (rare in children), digoxin is indicated to slow the ventricular response. For further discussion of the management of atrial fibrillation, see Chapter 24.

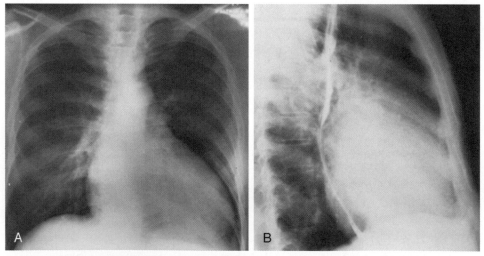

Figure 21–3. *Posteroanterior (**A**) and lateral (**B**) views of chest roentgenogram of a patient with moderately severe mitral regurgitation of rheumatic origin. The lateral view was obtained with barium swallow. The cardiothoracic ratio is increased (0.64), and the apex is displaced downward and laterally in the posteroanterior view. The lateral view shows an indentation of the barium-filled esophagus by an enlarged left atrium, and the left ventricle is displaced posteriorly.*

Surgical

Indications. The indications for valve repair surgery are not so stringent because surgery can significantly improve the regurgitation. Indications for valve surgery in adolescents and young adults with severe MR are as follows, according to the ACC/AHA 2006 guidelines. The following are noninvasive findings of *severe MR*: vena contracta width greater than 0.7 cm with large central MR jet (area greater than 40% of LA size) or with a wall-impinging jet of any size, swirling in LA, or enlargement of the LA and LV size.

1. Symptomatic patients with severe congenital MR with NYHA functional class III or IV (see earlier for noninvasive findings of severe MR)

2. Asymptomatic patients with severe congenital MR (see earlier) and LV systolic dysfunction (ejection fraction ≤0.6)

3. Surgery may be considered in patients with preserved LV function if the likelihood of successful repair without residual MR is great.

Some centers consider an LV diastolic dimension of 60 mm in adults an indication for mitral valve replacement. For children, intractable CHF, progressive cardiomegaly with symptoms, and pulmonary hypertension may be indications.

Procedures and Mortality. Mitral valve repair or replacement is performed under cardiopulmonary bypass.

1. Valve repair surgery is preferred over valve replacement, performed usually beyond infancy and during childhood. For cleft leak, repair of the cleft is performed. For central regurgitation with a dilated annulus, annuloplasty is performed by commissuroplasty (not using an annuloplasty ring, which restricts growth potential). Valve repair has a lower mortality rate (<1%), and anticoagulation is not necessary.

2. Valve replacement is rarely necessary for unrepairable regurgitation. Frequently used low-profile prostheses are the Björk-Shiley tilting disk and the St. Jude pyrolytic carbon valve. The surgical mortality rate is 2% to 7% for valve replacement. If a prosthetic valve is used, anticoagulation therapy must be continued.

Complications. Complications are similar to those listed for MS.

Postoperative Follow-up

1. Valve function (of either the repaired natural valve or the replacement valve) should be checked by echo and Doppler studies every 6 to 12 months.

2. After replacement with a mechanical valve with no risk factors, warfarin is indicated to achieve an INR of 2.5 to 3.5 along with low-dose aspirin. After replacement with a bioprosthesis with no risk factors, aspirin alone is indicated at the dose of 75 to 100 mg/day; when there are risk factors, warfarin is also indicated.

3. Maintaining good dental hygiene and instituting SBE prophylaxis should be emphasized.

Aortic Regurgitation

PREVALENCE

AR is more often congenital than rheumatic in origin. AR of rheumatic origin is almost always associated with mitral valve disease.

PATHOLOGY

1. Congenital causes of AR include the following:
   a. Congenital bicuspid aortic valve
   b. Following balloon dilatation of aortic valve
   c. Associated with ventricular septal defect (either subpulmonary or membranous)
   d. Secondary to subaortic stenosis
   e. In association with dilated aortic root (Marfan syndrome or Ehlers-Danlos syndrome)
2. Rarely, rheumatic heart disease is a cause of AR.

Clinical Manifestations

History

1. Patients with mild regurgitation are asymptomatic.

2. Exercise tolerance is reduced with more severe AR or CHF.

Physical Examination (Fig. 21–4)

1. With moderate or severe AR, the precordium may be hyperdynamic with a laterally displaced apical impulse. A diastolic thrill is occasionally present at the third left intercostal space. A wide pulse pressure and a bounding water-hammer pulse may be present with severe AR.

2. The heart sounds are normal with mild AR. The S1 is decreased in intensity with moderate to severe AR. The S2 may be normal or single. A high-pitched diastolic decrescendo murmur, best audible at the third or fourth left intercostal space, is the auscultatory hallmark. This murmur is more easily audible with the patient sitting and leaning forward. The longer the murmur, the more severe the regurgitation (see Fig. 21–4). A systolic murmur of varying intensity may be present at the second right intercostal space because of relative AS caused by an increased stroke volume. The combination of the diastolic and systolic murmurs gives rise to a to-and-fro murmur in patients with severe AR. A mid-diastolic mitral rumble (Austin Flint murmur) may be present at the apex when the AR is severe.

Electrocardiography. The ECG is normal in mild cases. In severe cases, LVH is usually present. LAH may be present in long-standing cases.

X-ray Studies. Cardiomegaly of varying degree involving the LV is present. A dilated ascending aorta and a prominent aortic knob are frequently present. Pulmonary venous congestion develops if LV failure supervenes.

Echocardiography. The LV dimension is increased, but the LA remains normal in size. The LV diastolic dimension is proportional to the severity of AR. Color flow and Doppler examination can aid in estimating the severity of the regurgitation. LV systolic dysfunction develops at a later stage in severe AR.

NATURAL HISTORY

1. Patients with mild to moderate AR remain asymptomatic for a long time, but when symptoms begin to develop, many patients deteriorate rapidly.

2. Anginal pain, CHF, and multiple premature ventricular contractions are unfavorable signs occurring with severe AR.

3. Infective endocarditis is a rare complication.

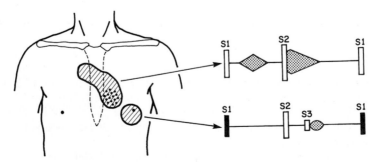

Figure 21–4. *Cardiac findings of aortic regurgitation. The S1 is abnormally soft (black bar). The predominant murmur is a high-pitched, diastolic decrescendo murmur at the third left intercostal space.*

MANAGEMENT

Medical

1. Good oral hygiene and antibiotic prophylaxis against SBE are important.

2. In case of a rheumatic cause, prophylaxis should be continued against the recurrence of rheumatic fever with penicillin or sulfonamides (see Chapter 20).

3. Activity need not be restricted in mild cases, but varying degrees of restriction are indicated in more severe cases. Aerobic exercise is a better form of exercise and weightlifting exercise should be discouraged.

4. When used on a long-term basis, the angiotensin-converting enzyme inhibitors have been shown to reduce (or even reverse) the dilatation and hypertrophy of the LV in children with AR but without CHF.

5. If CHF develops, digoxin, diuretics, and afterload-reducing agents may be beneficial, but the benefits are rarely maintained.

Surgical

Indications. A major clinical decision in AR is the timing of aortic valve replacement. Ideally, it should be performed before irreversible dilatation of the LV develops, but there is no reliable method of detecting that point. According to the ACC/AHA 2006 guidelines, the following are surgical indications in adolescent and adult patients with chronic severe AR. (Chronic severe AR is considered present when central jet width >86% left ventricular outflow tract or Doppler vena contracta width >0.6 cm is present.) Similar indications may apply for younger children.

1. Symptomatic patients (with angina, syncope, or dyspnea on exertion) with severe AR

2. Asymptomatic patients with LV systolic dysfunction (ejection fraction <0.5) on serial studies 1 to 3 months apart

3. Asymptomatic patients with progressive LV enlargement (end-diastolic dimension >mean + 4SD)

Procedure and Mortality. Aortic valve repair is favored over valve replacement whenever possible. Valve replacement does not incorporate growth potential, except for the Ross procedure. Surgery is performed under cardiopulmonary bypass. The mortality rate for valve repair is near zero and that for valve replacement is about 2% to 5%.

1. Valve repair may include repair of simple tears or valvuloplasty for prolapsed cusps, and so forth.

2. Valve replacement surgery.
   a. The antibiotic-sterilized aortic homograft has been widely used and appears to be the device of choice.
   b. The porcine heterograft has the risk of accelerated degeneration.
   c. The Björk-Shiley and St. Jude prostheses require anticoagulation therapy and are less suitable for young patients.

3. A pulmonary root autograft (Ross procedure) may be an attractive alternative to the conventional valve replacement surgery (see Fig. 13–10) in selected adolescents and young adults. In this procedure, the patient's own pulmonary valve and the adjacent PA are used to replace the diseased aortic valve and the adjacent aorta. The coronary arteries are detached from the aorta and implanted into the PA. The surgical mortality rate is near zero. This procedure does not require anticoagulant therapy, the autograft may last longer than a porcine bioprosthesis, and there is a growth potential for the autograft pulmonary valve.

Complications

1. Postoperative acute cardiac failure is the most common cause of death.

2. Thromboembolism, chronic hemolysis, and anticoagulant-induced hemorrhage may occur with a prosthetic valve.

3. Porcine valves tend to develop early calcification in children.

4. Prosthetic valve endocarditis is a rare complication.

Postoperative Follow-up

1. Regular follow-up of valve function should be done every 6 to 12 months by echo and Doppler studies.

2. Anticoagulation is needed after a prosthetic mechanical valve replacement. INR should be maintained between 2.5 and 3.5 for the first 3 months and 2.0 to 3.0 beyond that time. Low-dose aspirin (75 to 100 mg/day for adolescents) is indicated in addition to warfarin (ACC/AHA 2006 guidelines).

3. After aortic valve replacement with a bioprosthesis and no risk factors, aspirin (75 to 100 mg) is indicated, but warfarin is not indicated. When there are risk factors (which include atrial fibrillation, previous thromboembolism, LV dysfunction, and hypercoagulable state), warfarin is indicated to achieve an INR of 2.0 to 3.0 (ACC/AHA 2006 guidelines).

4. Following the Ross procedure, anticoagulation is not indicated.

5. The importance of good oral hygiene and antibiotic prophylaxis against SBE should be emphasized.

Mitral Valve Prolapse

PREVALENCE

The reported incidence of MVP of 2% to 5% in the pediatric population is probably an overestimate. The prevalence of MVP increases with age. This condition usually occurs in older children and adolescents (it is more common in adults) and has a female preponderance (male/female ratio of 1:2).

PATHOLOGY

1. MVP is primary in most cases and is due to an inherited abnormality (with an autosomal dominant mode of inheritance) of the mitral valve leaflets and their supporting chordae tendineae. Secondary cases of MVP can be caused by other conditions, including rupture or dysfunction of the papillary muscles related to myocardial infarction or ischemia, rupture of chordae tendineae related to infective endocarditis, or abnormal left ventricular wall motion associated with ischemia or primary myocardial disease. Secondary MVP is not discussed in this chapter.

2. In the primary form of MVP, thick and redundant mitral valve leaflets bulge into the mitral annulus (caused by myxomatous degeneration of the valve leaflets and/or the chordae). The posterior leaflet is more commonly and more severely affected than the anterior leaflet.

3. MVP is associated with several of the common heritable disorders of connective tissue, such as Marfan syndrome, Ehlers-Danlos syndrome, and Stickler's syndrome (and polycystic kidney disease in adults). Nearly all patients with Marfan syndrome have MVP.

4. A congenital heart defect is present in one third of patients with MVP. Secundum atrial septal defect is most common; ventricular septal defect and Ebstein's anomaly are found rarely.

CLINICAL MANIFESTATIONS

History

1. MVP is usually asymptomatic, but a history of nonexertional chest pain, palpitation, and, rarely, syncope may be elicited. Chest discomfort may be typical of anginal pain but more atypical in that it is not related to exertion and often consists of brief attacks or stabbing pain at the apex. Whether the chest pain is actually cardiac in origin (from papillary muscles) has not been fully determined,

but the discomfort could be secondary to abnormal tension on papillary muscle. Palpitation may be related to cardiac arrhythmias. Syncope or presyncope may be due to arrhythmias or a manifestation of an orthostatic phenomenon.

2. The patient occasionally has a family history of MVP.

Physical Examination (Fig. 21–5)

1. An asthenic build with a high incidence of thoracic skeletal anomalies (80%), including pectus excavatum (50%), straight back (20%), and scoliosis (10%), is common. (*Straight-back syndrome* is a condition in which the normal dorsal curvature of the spine is lost, resulting in a shortening of the chest's anteroposterior diameter.)

2. The midsystolic click with or without a late systolic murmur is the hallmark of this syndrome and is best audible at the apex (see Fig. 21–5). The presence or absence of the click and murmur, as well as their timing, varies from one examination to the next.

    a. The click and murmur may be brought out by held expiration, left decubitus position, sitting, standing, or leaning forward. They may disappear on inspiration.

    b. Various maneuvers can alter the timing of the click and the murmur:

    1). The click moves toward the S1 and the murmur lengthens with maneuvers that decrease the LV volume, such as standing, sitting, Valsalva's strain phase, tachycardia, and the administration of amyl nitrite.

    2). The click moves toward the S2 and the murmur shortens with maneuvers that increase the LV volume, such as squatting, hand grip exercise, Valsalva's release phase, bradycardia, and the administration of pressor agents or propranolol.

Electrocardiography

1. The ECG is usually normal but a superiorly directed T vector (with flat or inverted T waves in II, III, and aVF) occurs in 20% to 60% of patients (Fig. 21–6).

2. Arrhythmias are relatively uncommon and include supraventricular tachycardia, premature atrial contractions, and premature ventricular contractions.

3. First-degree atrioventricular block and RBBB are occasionally present.

4. The incidence of Wolff-Parkinson-White preexcitation or prolonged QT interval is higher in patients with MVP than in the general population.

5. LVH or LAH is rarely present.

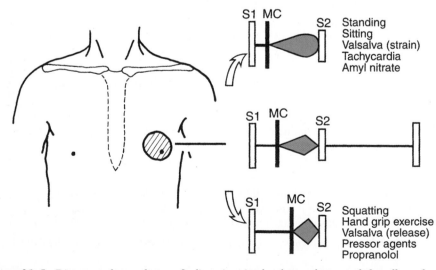

Figure 21–5. Diagram of auscultatory findings in mitral valve prolapse and the effect of various maneuvers on the timing of the midsystolic click (MC) and the murmur. The maneuvers that reduce ventricular volume enhance leaflet redundancy and move the click and murmur earlier in systole. An increase in left ventricular dimension has the opposite effect.

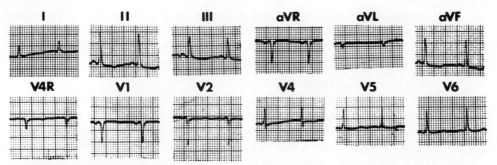

Figure 21–6. *Tracing from a 14-year-old girl with mitral valve prolapse. The T wave in aVF is inverted.*

X-ray Studies

1. X-ray films are unremarkable except for left atrial enlargement in patients with severe MR.
2. Thoracoskeletal abnormalities (e.g., straight back, pectus excavatum, scoliosis) may be present.

Echocardiography. Echo findings for adult patients with MVP have been established, but those for pediatric patients are not clearly defined.

1. Two-dimensional echo shows prolapse of the mitral valve leaflet(s) superior to the plane of the mitral valve. The parasternal long-axis view is most reliable. The superior displacement seen only on the apical four-chamber view is not diagnostic because more than 30% of preselected normal children show this finding. The "saddle-shaped" mitral valve ring explains the superior displacement of the mitral valve seen in normal people in the apical four-chamber view.
2. Some pediatric patients with characteristic body build and auscultatory findings of the condition do not show the adult echo criterion of MVP; they have only thickened mitral leaflets that show some posterosuperior displacement from their normal position, some even with mild MR. The reason may be that MVP is a progressive disease that shows the full manifestations only in adult life.
3. A large number of first-degree relatives of patients with MVP have echo findings of MVP.

NATURAL HISTORY

1. The majority of patients are asymptomatic, particularly during childhood.
2. Complications that are reported in adult patients, although rare in childhood, include sudden death (probably from ventricular arrhythmias), SBE, spontaneous rupture of chordae tendineae, progressive MR, CHF, arrhythmias, and conduction disturbances.

MANAGEMENT

1. Asymptomatic patients require no treatment or restriction of activity.
2. Antibiotic prophylaxis against bacterial endocarditis is recommended when MR is present by auscultation or by echo studies.
3. β-Adrenergic blockers (propranolol or atenolol) are often used in the following situations.
   a. Patients who are symptomatic (with palpitation, lightheadedness, dizziness, or syncope) secondary to ventricular arrhythmias. Symptomatic patients suspected to have arrhythmias should undergo ambulatory ECG monitoring or treadmill exercise testing, or both. Although β-blockers are the drug of choice, other drugs,

such as calcium blockers, quinidine, or procainamide, may prove to be effective in some patients.

    b. Patients with self-terminating episodes of SVT may also receive β-blockers.

    c. Patients with chest discomfort may also be treated with propranolol. (It is not relieved by nitroglycerin but may worsen.)

4. Reconstructive surgery or mitral valve replacement rarely may be indicated in patients with severe MR. MVP is the most common cause of isolated MR requiring surgical treatment in the United States.

Chapter 22

Cardiac Tumors

Prevalence

Cardiac tumors in the pediatric age group are extremely rare. A primary cardiac tumor was diagnosed in 0.001% to 0.003% of admissions at large children's referral centers. The male-to-female distribution is equal.

Pathology

1. The most common cardiac tumor in the pediatric age group is rhabdomyoma. In infants younger than 1 year, more than 75% of tumors are rhabdomyomas and teratomas. In children 1 to 15 years of age, 80% of cardiac tumors are rhabdomyomas, fibromas, and myxomas (Table 22–1). More than 90% of primary tumors are benign.

2. Primary malignant tumors are extremely rare in infants and children. Malignant teratoma, rhabdomyosarcoma, fibrosarcoma, and neurogenic sarcoma have been reported.

3. Secondary malignant tumors are also rare in children. Solid tumors and lymphosarcomas are the most common lesions. Persistent pericardial effusion, often blood-stained, is a common finding.

RHABDOMYOMA

Rhabdomyomas are by far the most frequent tumors in the pediatric age group, accounting for about half the cases of cardiac tumors. They are usually multiple, ranging in size from several millimeters to several centimeters. The most common location is in the ventricles, either in the ventricular septum or free wall, but they may rarely appear in the atrium. More than half the cases with multiple rhabdomyomas have tuberous sclerosis (e.g., with adenoma of the sebaceous glands, mental retardation, seizures). The tumors may produce symptoms of obstruction to blood flow, arrhythmias (usually ventricular tachycardia, occasionally supraventricular tachycardia), or sudden death. Cardiac rhabdomyomas are associated with a higher incidence of Wolff-Parkinson-White (WPW) preexcitation and may increase the risk for arrhythmias. (The tumor itself may be the cause of WPW syndrome.) Tumors regress in size or number or both in most patients younger than 4 years (but less so in older patients) (Nir et al, 1995). Spontaneous complete regression may occur. Surgical treatment is indicated only if the tumors produce obstruction or arrhythmias refractory to medical treatment; complete removal is not always possible.

FIBROMA

Cardiac fibromas usually occur as a single solid tumor, most commonly in the ventricular septum, although they may occur in the wall of any cardiac chamber. The size of

*Table 22–1. **Relative Incidence of Cardiac Tumors in Infants and Children***

Tumor	Incidence (%)
Infants (<12 mo) (total of 47 cases)	
Benign tumors (96%)	
Rhabdomyoma	60
Teratoma	19
Fibroma	13
Others	4
Malignant tumors (4%)	
Fibrosarcoma	2
Rhabdomyosarcoma	2
Children (1–15 yr) (total of 86 cases)	
Benign tumors (91%)	
Rhabdomyoma	41
Fibroma	14
Myxoma	14
Teratoma	13
Hemangioma	5
Others	5
Malignant tumors (9%)	
Malignant teratoma	5
Rhabdomyosarcoma	2
Others	2

*From a series of 444 primary tumors of the heart and pericardium in which 133 cases were from infants and children younger than 15 years.

Adapted from McAllister HA, Fenoglio JJ Jr: Tumors of the cardiovascular system. In Atlas of Tumor Pathology, 2nd series. Washington, DC, Armed Forces Institute of Pathology, 1978.

the tumor varies from several millimeters to several centimeters. Occasionally the tumor calcifies. The tumor may obstruct blood flow and disturb atrioventricular or ventricular conduction. In some cases, the tumor can be removed completely, but in others, the tumor intermingles with myocardial tissue so that complete resection is not possible.

TERATOMA

Teratomas contain elements from all three germ layers. Most of the tumors are intrapericardial and are attached to the root of the arterial pedicles in the base of the heart. Surgical excision is usually possible.

MYXOMA

Myxomas are the most common type of cardiac tumors in adults, accounting for about 30% of all primary cardiac tumors, but they are rare in infants and children. The majority of myxomas arise in the left atrium, 25% arise in the right atrium, and very few arise in the ventricles. Myxomas can produce hemodynamic disturbances, commonly interfering with mitral valve function or producing thromboembolic phenomena in the systemic circulation. With right atrial myxoma, similar effects on the tricuspid valve and thromboembolic phenomenon in the pulmonary circulation may be found. Rarely, patients may have symptoms while sitting and standing, but their symptoms improve when they lie down because of the intermittent protrusion of the tumor through the mitral valve. Surgical removal is usually successful.

Clinical Manifestations

1. Syncope or chest pain may be a presenting complaint. Sudden unexpected death may be the first manifestation. Rarely, symptoms vary with posture in cases of pedunculated tumors.

2. Clinical manifestations of cardiac tumors are often nonspecific and vary primarily with the location of the tumor.

    a. Tumors near cardiac valves may produce heart murmurs of stenosis or regurgitation of valves. So-called tumor plop may occur with a pedunculated and sessile tumor, such as a left atrial myxoma.

    b. Tumors involving the conduction tissue may manifest with arrhythmias or conduction disturbances.

    c. Intracavitary tumors may produce inflow or outflow obstruction, with clinical findings similar to those of mitral or semilunar valve stenosis or thromboembolic phenomenon.

    d. Involvement of the myocardium (mural tumors) may result in heart failure or cardiac arrhythmias.

    e. Pericardial tumors, which may signal malignancy, can produce pericardial effusion and cardiac tamponade or features simulating infective pericarditis.

3. Fragmentation of intracavitary tumors may lead to embolism of the pulmonary or systemic circulations.

4. Occasionally, for unknown reasons, fever and general malaise may manifest, especially with myxomas.

5. The ECG may show nonspecific ST-T changes, an infarct-like pattern, low-voltage QRS complexes, or preexcitation. Various arrhythmias and conduction disturbances have been reported.

6. Chest x-ray films occasionally may reveal altered contour of the heart, with or without changes in pulmonary vascular markings.

7. Echo and Doppler studies allow accurate determination of the presence, extent, and location of the tumor. These studies also determine the hemodynamic significance of the lesion. Cardiac tumors are usually found on routine echo studies when the diagnosis is not suspected, especially in small infants (Figs. 22–1 to 22–3).

    a. Multiple intraventricular tumors in infants and children most likely are rhabdomyomas (see Figs. 22–1 and 22–2).

    b. A solitary tumor of varying size, arising from the ventricular septum or the ventricular wall, is likely to be a fibroma (see Fig. 22–3).

    c. Left atrial tumors, especially when pedunculated, are usually myxomas (Fig. 22–4).

    d. An intrapericardial tumor arising near the great arteries most likely is a teratoma.

    e. Pericardial effusion suggests a secondary malignant tumor.

8. Abnormal laboratory findings, such as an elevated sedimentation rate, hypergammaglobulinemia, thrombocytosis or thrombocytopenia, polycythemia or anemia, and leukocytosis, have been reported.

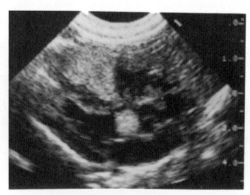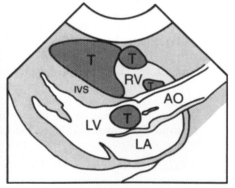

Figure 22–1. *Parasternal long-axis view showing multiple rhabdomyomas (T) in a newborn. There is a round, mobile mass in the left ventricular outflow tract, with resulting obstruction of the left ventricular outflow tract. One large and at least two other smaller tumor masses are imaged in the right ventricle (RV). The tumor in the left ventricular outflow tract was surgically removed because of the obstructive nature of the mass. AO, aorta; IVS, interventricular septum; LA, left atrium.*

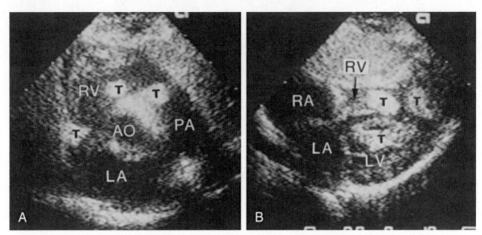

Figure 22–2. Parasternal short-axis view (**A**) and subcostal four-chamber view (**B**) showing multiple rhabdomyomas (T) in a newborn infant. AO, aorta; LA, left atrium; LV, left ventricle; PA, pulmonary artery; RA, right atrium; RV, right ventricle.

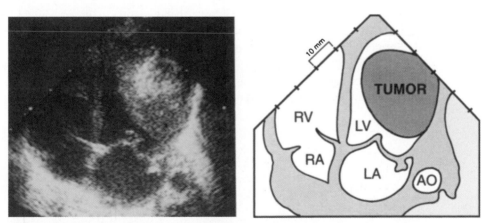

Figure 22–3. Apical four-chamber (apex-up) view showing a large solitary tumor in the left ventricular (LV) cavity in a newborn. The mass is attached to the LV free wall. Because of symptoms, a surgical attempt was made to remove the mass, but the infant died. Pathologic examination revealed the mass to be fibroma. AO, aorta; LA, left atrium; RA, right atrium; RV, right ventricle.

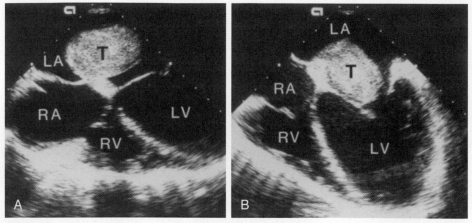

Figure 22–4. *Four-chamber view of the transverse plane of a transesophageal echo from a 54-year-old man with left atrial myxoma (T).* ***A****, A systolic freeze frame showing a large oval mass in the left atrium (LA). This mass is attached to the atrial septum. The primum atrial septum is also thickened.* ***B****, During diastole, the myxoma protrudes through the mitral valve. LV, left ventricle; RA, right atrium; RV, right ventricle.*

Management

Surgery is the only treatment for cardiac tumors that require intervention. Surgery is indicated in patients with symptoms of cardiac failure or ventricular arrhythmias refractory to medical treatment and in patients with inlet or outlet obstruction.

1. A successful complete resection of a fibroma is possible.

2. In asymptomatic patients with multiple rhabdomyomas, surgery should be delayed because of the possibility of spontaneous regression of the tumor.

3. Surgical removal is a standard procedure for myxomas and has a favorable outcome. The stalk of the tumor should be removed completely to prevent recurrence.

4. If myocardial involvement is extensive, surgical treatment is not possible. Cardiac transplantation may be an option in such cases.

Chapter 23

Cardiovascular Involvement in Systemic Diseases

Many collagen, neuromuscular, endocrine, and other systemic diseases may have important cardiovascular manifestations. The involvement of the cardiovascular system usually becomes evident when the diagnosis of the primary disease is well established, but occasionally cardiac manifestations may precede evidence of the basic disease. Cardiac manifestations of selected systemic diseases are briefly described here.

Mucopolysaccharidoses

The mucopolysaccharidoses are a diverse group of inherited metabolic disorders in which excessive amounts of glycosaminoglycans (previously called mucopolysaccharides) accumulate in various tissues, including the myocardium and coronary arteries. Stored glycosaminoglycans vary with different types and include dermatan sulfate, heparin sulfate, and keratan sulfate. Hurler (type IH), Hunter (II), Scheie (IS), Sanfilippo (III), and Morquio (IV) are well-known eponyms. A wide variety of clinical manifestations occur, including growth and mental retardation, skeletal abnormalities, clouded cornea, upper airway obstruction, and cardiac abnormalities. In most cases the cause of death is cardiorespiratory failure secondary to cardiac involvement and upper airway obstruction.

Echo studies show involvement of mitral and aortic valves (most frequently valve regurgitation) in more than 50% of the cases; about one fourth of the cases show cardiomyopathy. The prevalence of these abnormalities increases as the patient becomes older.

1. Mitral regurgitation is present in approximately 30% of the patients. It is more frequent in type IH (38%) than other types (24% in type II and 20% in type III). Thickening of the mitral valve is common.

2. Aortic regurgitation (AR) is present in about 15% of the cases, often with thickening of the valve. It is more common in type II (56%) and type IV (24%). Aortic stenosis is common in type IS.

3. Myocardial abnormalities, such as asymmetric septal hypertrophy, hypertrophic cardiomyopathy, dilated cardiomyopathy, and endocardial thickening, are present in about 25% of the cases.

4. Occasionally, systemic hypertension is present.

5. Rarely, myocardial infarction can occur.

Heart murmur may represent cardiac valve involvement. Chest x-ray films may show cardiomegaly in severe cases of valve regurgitation. The ECG may show a prolonged QT interval, right ventricular hypertrophy (RVH), left ventricular hypertrophy (LVH), or left atrial hypertrophy. Management depends on the abnormalities present.

Systemic Lupus Erythematosus

This chronic multisystem autoimmune disease can affect the cardiovascular system. The condition most commonly affects girls older than 8 years (78%), with a girls-to-boys ratio of 6.3:1.

The most common symptoms of lupus include constitutional complaints (fever, fatigue, anorexia, weight loss), joint pain and stiffness with or without swelling (commonly finger joints), skin rash (typical malar "butterfly" rash, seen only in 50%) and chest pain (from pleuritis or pericarditis). Evidence of renal involvement, hypertension, and Raynaud's phenomenon is also frequent. Chorea may be the sole presenting manifestation, requiring differentiation from rheumatic fever.

A positive antinuclear antibody (ANA) is present in over 95% of the cases, making it the most helpful initial screening test. However, a positive ANA test is not diagnostic of the disease, particularly if the titer is low. A positive ANA test is seen in other connective tissue diseases, such as juvenile rheumatoid arthritis (JRA) (but not in systemic-onset type), dermatomyositis, scleroderma, Sjögren's syndrome, and mixed connective tissue disease and also in some healthy children and adults. If the ANA test result is positive, further screening by a rheumatologist should be carried out.

Cardiovascular manifestations occur in about 30% to 40% of patients with lupus erythematosus, a higher rate than with other connective tissue diseases. Pathologically, varying degrees of immune-mediated changes occur in all layers of the heart: pericardium (patchy infiltration of inflammatory cells, fibrous adhesion), myocardium (mild to moderate acute and chronic inflammatory foci, perivasculitis of intramural arteries, increased interstitial connective tissue, myocardial cell atrophy), and cardiac valves (classic verrucous Libman-Sacks lesion).

1. Pericarditis with pericardial effusion is the most common manifestation (~25%) and is often asymptomatic. Tamponade is rare, and constrictive pericarditis is extremely rare.

2. Clinically evident myocarditis occurs in 2% to 25%, with resting tachycardia.

3. The classic verrucous endocarditis (Libman-Sacks) is found most commonly on the mitral valve, less commonly on the aortic valve, and rarely on the tricuspid and pulmonary valves. Echo studies show irregular vegetations 2 to 4 mm in diameter on the valve or subvalvular apparatus (seen in approximately 10%). Rarely, embolization of the vegetations can occur to a coronary or cerebral artery. Recent studies indicate that, instead of verrucous lesions, the mitral or aortic valve may exhibit diffuse thickening with or without regurgitation.

Anterior chest pain may occur with pericarditis. An apical systolic murmur of mitral regurgitation (MR) is frequently found, but pericardial friction rub is rarely audible. The ECG shows nonspecific ST-T changes, arrhythmias, or conduction disturbances. With pericarditis, T-wave inversion and ST-segment elevation may develop.

If active valvulitis is suspected, corticosteroid therapy may be warranted. Anticoagulation therapy should also be considered. Subacute bacterial endocarditis prophylaxis is indicated.

Rheumatoid Arthritis

Rheumatoid arthritis is an autoimmune disease in which the synovium is the principal target of inappropriate immune attack. Autopsy cases may exhibit multiple hemorrhages on parietal and visceral pericardial surfaces with dense fibrous adhesion. Myocardium may be hypertrophied with infiltration of inflammatory cells, and irregular nodular thickening may be seen on cardiac valves.

In clinical settings, the following cardiac manifestations may occur.

1. Pericarditis is the most common finding, occurring in about 50% of cases. Chest pain and friction rub signify pericarditis. It is most frequent in systemic-onset JRA, occasional in patients with polyarticular-onset JRA, and very rare in pauciarticular-onset JRA. Small pericardial effusion occurs without symptoms, but large effusion may cause symptoms. Cardiac tamponade rarely occurs. Constrictive pericarditis is extremely rare.

2. Myocarditis occurs infrequently (1% to 10%) in JRA but can lead to life-threatening congestive heart failure (CHF) and arrhythmias.

3. Rarely, MR and AR with thickening of these valves occur.

4. Occasionally, left ventricular (LV) systolic dysfunction (decreased ejection fraction and fractional shortening) with dilated LV is present. Diastolic dysfunction of abnormal relaxation form can be found.

5. ECG abnormalities occur in 20% of cases, with the most common findings being nonspecific ST-T changes. Rarely, involvement of the conduction system with heart block can occur.

6. On examination, tachycardia and nonspecific ejection systolic murmurs are commonly present. Occasionally, a regurgitant systolic murmur of MR may be audible.

Asymptomatic and mild pericarditis may be treated with nonsteroidal anti-inflammatory agents (such as naproxen 15 mg/kg/day in two divided doses). Symptomatic or severe pericarditis may require treatment with corticosteroids for 8 to 16 weeks. Prednisone 0.5 to 2 mg/kg/day for 1 week is gradually reduced by approximately 20%. Tamponade is treated with pericardiocentesis.

Friedreich's Ataxia

Friedreich's ataxia is inherited as an autosomal recessive trait. The onset of ataxia usually occurs before age 10 years and it progresses slowly, involving the lower extremities to a greater extent than the upper extremities. Explosive dysarthric speech and nystagmus are characteristic, but intelligence is preserved.

Hypertrophy of ventricles, especially the LV, is commonly found, but the endocardium and cardiac valves are usually not involved. Microscopically, diffuse interstitial fibrosis and fatty degeneration of the myocardium, with compensatory hypertrophy of the remaining cells, are frequently found. A varying degree of atheromatous involvement of the coronary arteries is common. CHF is the terminal event in 70% of patients.

Echo studies reveal evidence of cardiomyopathy in approximately 30% of the cases. Concentric hypertrophy of the LV is the most common finding. Asymmetric septal hypertrophy, systolic anterior motion of the mitral valve, or dilated cardiomyopathy may be present. Diastolic dysfunction of the LV may be present.

Cardiac symptoms (e.g., dyspnea, chest pain) are common, usually appearing in individuals with clear neurologic changes. Because of physical disability, cardiac problems may not be recognized until arrhythmias or signs of CHF develop. A systolic murmur may be audible at the upper left sternal border. ECG abnormalities are very common. The most common finding is the T-vector change in the limb leads or left precordial leads. Occasionally, LVH, RVH, abnormal Q waves, or short PR interval is found. Chest x-ray films are usually normal.

Treatments are the same as those described under different types of cardiomyopathy.

Muscular Dystrophy

Duchenne's muscular dystrophy is a sex-linked recessive disease. Involvement of the pelvic muscles leads to lordosis, waddling gait, protuberant abdomen, and difficulty rising. Becker's muscular dystrophy is the same fundamental disease as Duchenne's dystrophy, but it follows a milder and more protracted course. Significant cardiac involvement in the form of dilated cardiomyopathy is seen in both types of muscular dystrophy and manifests clinically during adolescence.

Cardiac enlargement, with occasional endocardial thickening of the LV and left atrium (LA), is found on gross examination. Fatty degeneration and lymphocytic infiltration are found on microscopic examination. Dystrophic changes in the papillary muscles may be evident, with MR or mitral valve prolapse (MVP). The coronary arteries, cardiac valves, and pericardium are normal.

Exertional dyspnea and tachypnea are common symptoms. The P2 may be loud if pulmonary hypertension is present. One may hear either a nonspecific systolic ejection murmur at the base or a regurgitant apical systolic murmur of MR. CHF is an ominous terminal sign.

ECG abnormalities occur in 90% of teenagers with Duchenne's type, and RVH and right bundle branch block are the most common abnormalities. Deep Q waves are frequently seen in the left precordial leads. Short PR interval is occasionally seen. T-vector changes may be seen in the limb leads or left precordial leads.

In early stages of the disease, only diastolic dysfunction (of reduced diastolic relaxation pattern) may be present. Systolic dysfunction appears later in the disease process. Echo features of MVP may be seen.

Treatment is the same as that described for dilated cardiomyopathy (see Chapter 18). Recent reports suggest that more aggressive treatment with angiotensin-converting enzyme (ACE) inhibitors (e.g., perindopril) and an added β-adrenergic blocker appear to lead to improved LV function and possible delay of progression of the disease. Although prospective treatment may be better (Duboc et al, 2005), they appear to improve LV function even if started after abnormal echo findings appear (Jefferies et al, 2005).

Myotonic Dystrophy

Myotonic muscular dystrophy is the second most common muscular dystrophy. This disease is characterized by myotonia (increased muscular irritability and contractility with decreased power of relaxation) combined with muscular weakness. This autosomal dominant disease causes dysfunction in multiple organ systems, including musculoskeletal, gastrointestinal, cardiovascular, endocrine, and immunologic systems.

In infancy, myotonic dystrophy arises with feeding difficulties. Later in life, developmental retardation, poor coordination, and muscle weakness are evident. During childhood, the trunk and proximal muscle groups are involved, and in late in life, the distal muscle groups, facial, and neck muscles are involved. "Hatchet" face is characteristic with open mouth, drooling, and expressionless face.

Cardiac abnormalities are frequent with involvement of the AV conduction and structural abnormalities. Fatty infiltration in the myocardium and fibrofatty degeneration in the sinus node and atrioventricular (AV) conduction system may be responsible for the manifestations.

1. The ECG may show first-degree AV block and intraventricular conduction delay. As disease progresses, second-degree and complete heart block may develop. In addition, atrial fibrillation and flutter, abnormal Q waves, and ventricular arrhythmias may develop. Sudden death is frequent, attributable to conduction abnormalities or arrhythmias, or both.

2. MVP may develop. A midsystolic click and nonspecific systolic ejection murmur may be present in children. In adults, MVP is frequently found.

3. LV systolic function is normal in most cases, but LV dysfunction appears with advancing age. Rarely, LV hypertrophy or left atrial dilatation and regional wall motion abnormality are seen.

Patients with symptoms or evidence of dysrhythmias should be considered for pacemaker treatment. LV dysfunction, if present, should be treated.

Marfan Syndrome

Marfan syndrome is a generalized connective tissue disease with clinical features involving skeletal, cardiovascular, and ocular systems. It is inherited as an autosomal dominant pattern with variable expressivity.

Clinically evident cardiovascular involvement occurs in over 50% of patients by the age of 21. Microscopic changes are probably present in almost all patients, even during infancy and childhood. A wide spectrum of cardiovascular abnormalities is seen in Marfan syndrome:

1. The common abnormalities include dilatation of the sinus of Valsalva, dilatation of the ascending aorta (with or without dissection or rupture), and AR. Microscopic examination of the proximal aorta (and the proximal coronary arteries) reveals disruption of the elastic media, with fragmentation and disorganization of the elastic fibers. Large accumulations of dermatan sulfate, heparan sulfate, and chondroitin sulfate have been reported in the media of the aorta.

2. Mitral valve abnormalities are equally common. The mitral valve and LA endocardium often undergo a fibromyxoid degeneration, resulting in MR and MVP.

3. Aneurysm of the pulmonary artery (PA) is less frequently seen.

4. Rarely, myocardial fibrosis and infarction, rupture of chordae tendineae, aneurysm of the abdominal aorta, and aneurysmal dilatation of the proximal coronary arteries have been reported.

In children and young adults, clinical findings of mitral valve involvement are more common than aortic lesions. Auscultatory findings of MR and MVP appear in more than 50% of patients (see Chapter 21). Rarely, the murmur of AR is audible. The S2 may be accentuated in many patients, especially in those with thin chest walls or dilated PAs. The ECG findings may include LVH; T-wave inversion in leads II, III, aVF, and left precordial leads; and first-degree AV block. Chest x-ray films may show cardiomegaly, either generalized or involving only the LV and LA, or a prominence of the ascending aorta, aortic knob, or the main PA segment.

Echo studies show an increased dimension of the aortic root with or without AR or "redundant" mitral valve or MVP with thickened valve leaflets and MR. Periodic examination of the aortic root dimension and the status of the mitral valve is required. Normal dimensions of the aortic root are shown in Table D–5, Appendix D. Differential diagnosis of aortic root dilatation includes aortic valve abnormalities (such as bicuspid aortic valve), other connective tissue disorders, hereditary aortic aneurysm, hypertension, and inflammatory aortic disease. As to the diagnosis of MVP in children, however, the adult criterion of MVP is met infrequently, probably because MVP is a progressive disease and a full manifestation of the disease does not occur until adulthood.

Early death in this syndrome is most commonly precipitated by aortic dissection, chronic AR, or severe MR. Early and improved surgery and the use of β-blockers have significantly increased the life expectancy of these patients.

1. β-Blockers (atenolol, propranolol) are effective in slowing the rate of aortic dilatation and reducing the development of aortic complications. Enalapril was found to reduce the rate of increase in the aortic root diameter (Yetman et al, 2005). Thus, β-blockers or ACE inhibitors, or both, should be administered to children when the aortic root size exceeds the upper limit of normal for age. The mean and 90% confidence limits of aortic root dimension are shown in Appendix D, Table D–5.

2. Surgery should be considered when the diameter increases significantly. However, there is controversy about what is considered significant enlargement for surgery. Some centers recommend surgery when the aortic root diameter is greater than 3.5 cm (Kim et al, 2005), others recommend surgery when the aortic root equals approximately twice the average measurement for that age group, and still others recommend surgery when the diameter reaches near 6.5 cm (Gott et al, 1999).

Valve-preserving surgery appears to be preferable to composite graft surgery, primarily to avoid the complications of anticoagulation.

3. Cardiac failure related to severe MR is treated with mitral valve repair or valve replacement.

Acute Glomerulonephritis

Significant myocardial damage is found in 10% of postmortem examinations. Clinically evident myocardial involvement is found in 30% to 40% of patients. Pulmonary edema, systemic venous congestion, and cardiomegaly are also common. Systemic hypertension, sometimes appearing with hypertensive encephalopathy, is a frequent manifestation and may be responsible for signs of CHF in some, but not all, patients. Although hypertension probably reflects fluid expansion (secondary to impaired salt and water excretion), peripheral resistance has been found to be elevated. Increased renin activity may be responsible for the latter.

Hyperthyroidism: Congenital and Acquired

The thyroid hormones increase oxygen consumption, stimulate protein synthesis and growth, and affect carbohydrates and lipid metabolism. On the cardiovascular system, the thyroid hormones (1) increase heart rate, cardiac contractility, and cardiac output; (2) increase systolic pressure and decrease diastolic pressure, with mean pressure unchanged; and (3) may increase myocardial sensitivity to catecholamines. Hyperthyroidism results from excess production of triiodothyronine (T_3), thyroxine (T_4), or both.

Congenital hyperthyroidism is most often caused by increased thyroid-stimulating immunoglobulin in infants of mothers who had Graves' disease during pregnancy. A newborn infant with congenital hyperthyroidism is often premature and usually has a goiter. The baby appears anxious, restless, alert, and irritable. The eyes are widely open and appear exophthalmic.

Juvenile hyperthyroidism is believed to be caused by thyroid-stimulating antibodies and is often associated with lymphocytic thyroiditis and other autoimmune disorders. The incidence of juvenile hyperthyroidism peaks during adolescence, with females affected more often than males. These children become hyperactive, irritable, and excitable. The thyroid gland is enlarged.

Both congenital hyperthyroidism and acquired hyperthyroidism manifest with tachycardia, full and bounding pulses, and increased systolic and pulse pressures. A nonspecific systolic murmur may be audible. Bruits may be audible over the enlarged thyroid in children but not in newborns. In severely affected patients, cardiac enlargement and cardiac failure may develop, requiring prompt recognition and treatment.

Chest x-ray films are usually normal but may show cardiomegaly and increased pulmonary vascularity, especially in the presence of heart failure. ECG abnormalities may include the following: sinus tachycardia, peaked P waves, various arrhythmias (supraventricular tachycardia, nodal rhythm), complete heart block, RVH, LVH, or biventricular hypertrophy, but arrhythmias are rare in acquired (juvenile) hyperthyroidism. Echo studies reveal a hyperkinetic state with increased fractional shortening.

In severely affected patients, a β-adrenergic blocker, such as propranolol, is indicated to reduce the effect of catecholamines. Treatment consists of oral administration of antithyroid drugs, propylthiouracil, or methimazole (Tapazole). Lugol solution 1 drop every 8 hours may be added in congenital hyperthyroidism. If CHF develops, treatment with anticongestive medications is indicated (see Chapter 27).

Hypothyroidism: Congenital and Acquired

Hypothyroidism results from deficient production of thyroid hormone or a defect in its receptor. The disorder may be manifest from birth or may be acquired.

Congenital hypothyroidism, or cretinism, is most often caused by a developmental defect of the thyroid gland. Hypothyroidism may not be apparent until 3 months of age. The typical picture includes a protuberant tongue, cool and mottled skin, subnormal temperature, carotenemia, and myxedema. Untreated children become mentally retarded and slow in physical development. In the congenital type, patent ductus arteriosus and pulmonary stenosis are frequently found.

The patient may have significant bradycardia, weak arterial pulse, hypotension, and nonpitting facial and peripheral edema. ECG abnormalities occur in over 90% of cases and consist of some or all of the following: (1) low QRS voltages, especially in the limb leads; (2) low T-wave amplitude, not affecting the T axis; (3) prolongation of PR and QT intervals; and (4) dome-shaped T wave with an absent ST segment ("mosque" sign) (Fig. 23–1). Echo studies may show cardiomegaly, pericardial effusion, hypertrophic cardiomyopathy, or asymmetric septal hypertrophy, in addition to congenital heart defects, if present. Sodium-L-thyroxine given orally is the treatment of choice.

Acquired (or juvenile) hypothyroidism most often results from lymphocytic thyroiditis (Hashimoto's disease or autoimmune thyroiditis). Hypothyroidism may result from subtotal or complete thyroidectomy or from protracted ingestion of goitrogens, iodides, or cobalt medications. Rarely, amiodarone can cause hypothyroidism. Serum levels of T_4 and T_3 are low or borderline.

The heart rate is relatively slow and the heart sounds may be soft. Weak arterial pulse and hypotension may be present. Myxedema may be present. There is increased occurrence of hypercholesterolemia. Echo studies frequently show pericardial effusion and asymmetric septal hypertrophy. The ECG, chest x-ray, and echo findings of juvenile hypothyroidism are the same as for congenital hypothyroidism. Treatment of hypothyroidism corrects the lipid abnormalities.

Sickle Cell Anemia

In sickle cell anemia, erythrocytes become rigid and "sickle," leading to capillary occlusion and sickle cell "crisis." The increased stroke volume of the heart compensates for anemia, and the heart gradually dilates and hypertrophies. Heart failure may be a late complication.

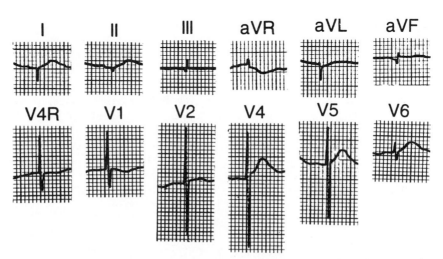

Figure 23–1. *Tracing from a 3-month-old infant with congenital hypothyroidism. Note low QRS voltages in the limb leads, relatively low T-wave amplitude, and dome-shaped T wave with an absent ST segment in V6.*

The arterial pulse is brisk, and the precordium is hyperactive. The diastolic pressure is low with a wide pulse pressure. An ejection systolic murmur is usually audible along the upper right and left sternal borders. Rarely, one may hear an apical rumble and a gallop rhythm. ECG abnormalities may include first-degree AV block, LVH, and nonspecific T-wave changes. Chest x-ray films show generalized cardiomegaly in nearly, but the ejection fraction and systolic time intervals are within normal limits.

Part VI

ARRHYTHMIAS AND ATRIOVENTRICULAR CONDUCTION DISTURBANCES

This part discusses cardiac arrhythmias, atrioventricular conduction disturbances, and cardiac pacemakers and implantable cardioverter-defibrillators in children.

Chapter 24

Cardiac Arrhythmias

The frequency and clinical significance of arrhythmias are different in children and in adults. Although arrhythmias are relatively infrequent in infants and children, the common practice of monitoring cardiac rhythm in children requires primary care physicians, emergency room physicians, and intensive care physicians to be able to recognize and manage basic arrhythmias.

The normal heart rate varies with age. The younger the child, the faster the heart rate. Therefore, the definitions of bradycardia (<60 beats/minute) and tachycardia (>100 beats/minute) used for adults do not apply to infants and children. *Tachycardia* is defined as a heart rate beyond the upper limit of normal for the patient's age, and *bradycardia is* defined as a heart rate slower than the lower limit of normal. Normal resting heart rates by age are presented in Table 24–1.

This chapter discusses basic arrhythmias according to the origin of their impulse. Each arrhythmia is described, along with its causes, significance, and treatment.

Rhythms Originating in the Sinus Node

All rhythms that originate in the sinoatrial (SA) node (sinus rhythm) have two important characteristics (Fig. 24–1). Both are required for a rhythm to be called sinus rhythm.

1. P waves precede each QRS complex with a regular PR interval. (The PR interval may be prolonged, as in first-degree atrioventricular [AV] block; thus, the rhythm is sinus with first-degree AV block.)

2. The P axis falls between 0 and +90 degrees, an often neglected criterion. This produces upright P waves in lead II and inverted P waves in aVR. (See Chapter 3 for a detailed discussion of sinus rhythm.)

REGULAR SINUS RHYTHM

Description. The rhythm is regular, and the rate is normal for age. The two characteristics of sinus rhythm described previously are present (see Fig. 24–1).

Table 24–1. **Normal Ranges of Resting Heart Rate**

Age	Mean (range)	Age	Mean (range)
Newborn	145 (90–180)	4 yr	108 (72–135)
6 mo	145 (106–185)	6 yr	100 (65–135)
1 yr	132 (105–170)	10 yr	90 (65–130)
2 yr	120 (90–150)	14 yr	85 (60–120)

From Davignon, A, Rautaharju P, Boisselle E, et al: Normal ECG standards for infants and children. Pediatr Cardiol 1:123–131, 1979–1980.

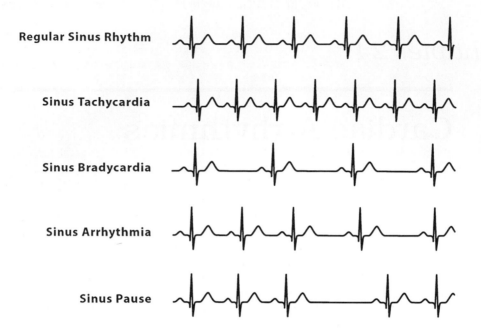

Figure 24–1. *Normal and abnormal rhythms originating in the sinoatrial node. (From Park MK, Guntheroth WG: How to Read Pediatric ECGs, 4th ed. Philadelphia, Mosby, 2006.)*

Significance. This *rhythm* is normal at any age.

Management. No treatment is required.

SINUS TACHYCARDIA

Description. Characteristics of sinus rhythm are present (see previous description). The rate is faster than the upper limit of normal for age (see Table 24–1). A rate greater than 140 beats/minute in children and greater than 170 beats/minute in infants may be significant. The heart rate is usually less than 200 beats/minute in sinus tachycardia (see Fig. 24–1).

Causes. Anxiety, fever, hypovolemia or circulatory shock, anemia, congestive heart failure (CHF), administration of catecholamines, thyrotoxicosis, and myocardial disease are possible causes.

Significance. Increased cardiac work is well tolerated by healthy myocardium.

Management. The underlying cause is treated.

SINUS BRADYCARDIA

Description. The characteristics of sinus rhythm are present (see previous description), but the heart rate is slower than the lower limit of normal for the age (see Table 24–1). A rate slower than 80 beats/minute in newborn infants and slower than 60 beats/minute in older children may be significant (see Fig. 24–1).

Causes. Sinus bradycardia may occur in normal individuals and trained athletes. It may occur with vagal stimulation, increased intracranial pressure, hypothyroidism, hypothermia, hypoxia, hyperkalemia, and administration of drugs such as digitalis and β-adrenergic blockers.

Significance. In some patients, marked bradycardia may not maintain normal cardiac output.

Management. The underlying cause is treated.

SINUS ARRHYTHMIA

Description. There is a phasic variation in the heart rate, increasing during inspiration and decreasing during expiration. The arrhythmia occurs with maintenance of characteristics of sinus rhythm (see Fig. 24–1).

Causes. This is a normal phenomenon and is due to phasic variation in the firing rate of cardiac autonomic nerves with the phases of respiration.

Significance. Sinus arrhythmia has no significance because it is a normal finding in children and a sign of good cardiac reserve.

Management. No treatment is indicated.

SINUS PAUSE

Description. In sinus pause, the sinus node pacemaker momentarily ceases activity, resulting in absence of the P wave and QRS complex for a relatively short time (see Fig. 24–1). *Sinus arrest* is of longer duration and usually results in an escape beat (see later discussion) by other pacemakers, such as the AV junctional or nodal tissue (junctional or nodal escape).

Causes. Increased vagal tone, hypoxia, digitalis toxicity, and sick sinus syndrome are possible causes.

Significance. Sinus pause usually has no hemodynamic significance but may reduce cardiac output.

Management. Treatment is rarely indicated except in sinus node dysfunction (or sick sinus syndrome) (see later discussion) and digitalis toxicity.

SINOATRIAL EXIT BLOCK

Description. A P wave is absent from the normally expected P wave, resulting in a long R-R interval. The duration of the pause is a multiple of the basic P-P interval. An impulse formed within the sinus node fails to depolarize the atria.

Causes. Excessive vagal stimulation, myocarditis or fibrosis involving the atrium, and drugs such as quinidine, procainamide, or digitalis may be causes.

Significance. It is usually transient and has no hemodynamic significance. Rarely, the patient may have syncope.

Management. The underlying cause is treated.

SINUS NODE DYSFUNCTION (SICK SINUS SYNDROME)

Description. In sinus node dysfunction, the sinus node fails to function as the dominant pacemaker of the heart or performs abnormally slowly, resulting in a variety of arrhythmias. These arrhythmias include profound sinus bradycardia, sinus pause or arrest, slow junctional escape beats, and ectopic atrial or nodal rhythm. Bradytachyarrhythmia occurs when bradycardia and tachycardia alternate. Bradycardia may originate in the sinus node, atria, AV junction, or ventricle, whereas tachycardia is usually caused by atrial flutter or fibrillation and less commonly caused by reentrant supraventricular tachycardia (SVT). When these arrhythmias are accompanied by symptoms such as dizziness or syncope, sinus node dysfunction is referred to as sick sinus syndrome.

Causes

1. Extensive cardiac surgery, particularly involving the atria (such as the Senning operation, Fontan procedure, or surgery for partial or total anomalous pulmonary venous return or endocardial cushion defect) is a possible cause.

2. Some cases of sick sinus syndrome are idiopathic, involving an otherwise normal heart without structural defect..

3. Rarely, myocarditis, pericarditis, or rheumatic fever is a cause.

4. CHD (e.g., sinus venosus atrial septal defect, Ebstein's anomaly).

5. Secondary to antiarrhythmic drugs (e.g., digitalis, propranolol, verapamil, quinidine).

6. Hypothyroidism.

Significance. Bradytachyarrhythmia is the most worrisome. Profound bradycardia after a period of tachycardia (overdrive suppression) can cause syncope and even death.

Management

1. Severe bradycardia is treated with intravenous (IV) atropine (0.04 mg/kg [IV] every 2 to 4 hours) or isoproterenol (0.05 to 0.5 µg/kg IV) or both.

2. Chronic medical treatment using drugs has not been uniformly successful, and it is not accepted as standard treatment of sinus node dysfunction. Agents used for treatment include fludrocortisone, atropine derivatives, adrenergic stimulatory drugs, theophylline, and ephedrine.

3. Antiarrhythmic drugs, such as propranolol or quinidine, may be given to suppress tachycardia, but they are often unsuccessful.

4. A transvenous temporary pacemaker is sometimes required.

5. Permanent pacemaker implantation is the treatment of choice in symptomatic patients, especially those with syncope. Atrial demand, dual-chambered demand or triggered, or ventricular demand pacemakers may be used (see Chapter 26).

Rhythms Originating in the Atrium

Rhythms that originate in the atrium (ectopic atrial rhythm) are characterized by the following (Fig. 24–2):

1. P waves have an unusual contour, which is caused by an abnormal P axis, and/or there is an abnormal number of P waves per QRS complex.

2. QRS complexes are usually of normal configuration, but occasional bizarre QRS complexes caused by aberrancy may occur (see later discussion).

PREMATURE ATRIAL CONTRACTION

Description. The QRS complex appears prematurely. The P wave may be upright in lead II when the ectopic focus is high in the atrium. The P wave is inverted when the ectopic focus is low in the atrium (so-called coronary sinus rhythm). The compensatory pause is incomplete; that is, the length of two cycles, including one premature beat, is less than the length of two normal cycles (see Fig. 24–2).

An occasional premature atrial contraction (PAC) is not followed by a QRS complex (i.e., a *nonconducted PAC*; see Fig. 24–2). A nonconducted PAC is differentiated from a second-degree AV block by the prematurity of the nonconducted P wave (P′ in Fig. 24–2). The P′ wave occurs earlier than the anticipated normal P wave, and the resulting P-P′ interval is shorter than the normal P-P interval for that individual. In second-degree AV block, the P wave that is not followed by the QRS complex occurs at the anticipated time, maintaining a regular P-P interval.

Causes. PAC appears in healthy children, including newborns. It may also appear after cardiac surgery and with digitalis toxicity.

Significance. PAC has no hemodynamic significance.

Management. Usually no treatment is indicated, except in cases of digitalis toxicity.

WANDERING ATRIAL PACEMAKER

Description. Wandering atrial pacemaker is characterized by *gradual* changes in the shape of P waves and PR intervals (see Fig. 24–2). The QRS complex is normal.

Causes. Wandering atrial pacemaker is seen in otherwise healthy children. It is the result of a gradual shift of the site of impulse formation in the atria through several cardiac cycles.

Significance. Wandering atrial pacemaker is a benign arrhythmia and has no clinical significance.

Management. No treatment is indicated.

ECTOPIC ATRIAL TACHYCARDIA

Description. There is a narrow QRS complex tachycardia (in the absence of aberrancy or preexisting bundle branch block) with visible P waves at an inappropriately rapid rate. The P axis is different from that of sinus rhythm. When the ectopic focus is near the sinus node, the P axis may be the same as in sinus rhythm. The usual heart rate

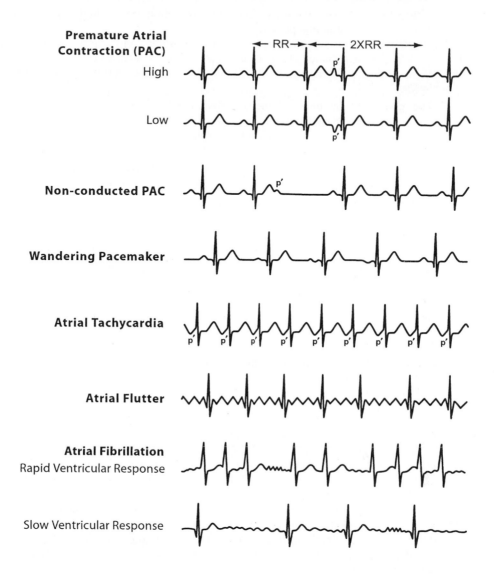

Figure 24–2. Arrhythmias originating in the atrium. (From Park MK, Guntheroth WG: How to Read Pediatric ECGs, 4th ed. Philadelphia, Mosby, 2006.)

in older children is between 110 and 160 beats/minute, but the tachycardia rate varies substantially during the course of a day, reaching 300 beats/minute with sympathetic stimuli. It represented 18% of SVT in one study. This arrhythmia is sometimes difficult to distinguish from the reentrant AV tachycardia, and thus it is included under "Supraventricular Tachycardia."

Causes. This arrhythmia is believed to be secondary to increased automaticity of nonsinus atrial focus or foci.

1. Most patients have a structurally normal heart (idiopathic).

2. Myocarditis, chronic cardiomyopathy, AV valve regurgitation, atrial dilatation, atrial tumors, and previous cardiac surgery involving atria (such as the Senning operation and Fontan procedure) may be the cause.

3. Occasionally, respiratory infections caused by mycoplasma or virus may trigger the arrhythmia.

Significance. CHF is common with chronic cases and there is a high association with tachycardia-induced cardiomyopathy.

Management. It is refractory to medical therapy and cardioversion. Drugs that are effective in reentrant atrial tachycardia (such as adenosine) do not terminate the tachycardia. Cardioversion is ineffective because the ectopic rhythm resumes immediately.

1. The goal may be to slow the ventricular rate rather than to try to convert the arrhythmia to sinus rhythm. Digoxin and β-blockers are equally effective in slowing the ventricular rate. IV amiodarone may achieve rate control relatively quickly.

2. Atrial pacing (e.g., esophageal, transvenous) to overdrive the atrial tachycardia to a point of consistent 2:1 AV block may lower the ventricular response rate.

3. Long-term oral medication is the mainstay of therapy in patients not undergoing radiofrequency ablation. Class IC (such as flecainide) and class III (such as amiodarone) antiarrhythmic agents are generally most effective (up to 75%).

4. Radiofrequency ablation may prove to be effective in nearly 90% of cases.

5. Surgical mapping and resection of the autonomic foci have been successful.

CHAOTIC (OR MULTIFOCAL) ATRIAL TACHYCARDIA

Description. This is an uncommon tachycardia characterized by three or more distinct P-wave morphologies. The P-P and R-R intervals are irregular with variable PR intervals. The arrhythmia may be misdiagnosed as atrial fibrillation.

Causes. Young infants with or without structural heart disease are affected; 30% to 50% have various cardiac anomalies.

Significance. The mechanism of this arrhythmia has been poorly defined. Heart failure may develop. Sudden death has been reported in up to 17% during therapy. Spontaneous resolution frequently occurs.

Management. Drugs that slow AV conduction (propranolol or digoxin) and those that decrease automaticity (such as class IA or IC or class III) may be useful. This arrhythmia is refractory to cardiac pacing, cardioversion, and adenosine.

ATRIAL FLUTTER

Description. The pacemaker lies in an ectopic focus, and "circus movement" in the atrium is the mechanism of this arrhythmia. Atrial flutter is characterized by an atrial rate (F wave with "sawtooth" configuration) of about 300 (range 240 to 360) beats/minute, a ventricular response with varying degrees of block (e.g., 2:1, 3:1, 4:1), and normal QRS complexes (see Fig. 24–2).

In children who have undergone atrial surgery with multiple suture lines (such as a Fontan operation), atrial flutter is secondary to a reentry mechanism within the atrial muscle (called *intra-atrial reentrant tachycardia*). In this situation, the atrial rates are commonly 250 beats/minute or slower

Causes. Atrial flutter usually suggests a significant cardiac pathology, although fetuses and neonates with atrial flutter frequently have a normal heart. Structural heart disease with dilated atria, acute infectious illness, myocarditis or pericarditis, previous surgery involving atria (the Senning procedure, Fontan operation, or atrial septal defect repair), digitalis toxicity, and thyrotoxicosis are possible causes.

Significance. The ventricular rate determines eventual cardiac output; a too-rapid ventricular rate may decrease cardiac output. Thrombus formation may lead to embolic events. Uncontrolled atrial flutter may precipitate heart failure. The flutter may be associated with syncope, presyncope, or chest pain.

Management. Management of atrial flutter is divided into acute conversion, chronic suppression of the arrhythmia, control of ventricular rate, prevention of recurrences, and refractory cases.

1. Acute situation:
   a. Adenosine does not convert the arrhythmia to sinus rhythm, although it may be helpful in confirming the diagnosis of atrial flutter by temporarily blocking AV conduction. An example is shown in Figure 24–4.
   b. Immediate synchronized DC cardioversion is the treatment of choice for atrial flutter of short duration, if the infant or child is in severe CHF.
   c. Temporary transvenous or transesophageal pacing may be used for the same purpose.
   d. In children, IV amiodarone (class III) or IV procainamide (class IA) may be effective.

2. For chronic cases: For long-standing atrial flutter or fibrillation (of 24 to 48 hours) or those with unknown duration, thrombus formation may lead to cerebral embolic events, especially when the atrial arrhythmia is terminated.
   a. It is essential to rule out atrial thrombi, preferably by echocardiography. Transesophageal echo may define atrial thrombi better than transthoracic echo.
   b. Anticoagulation with warfarin (with International Normalized Ratio between 2.0 and 3.0) is started and cardioversion delayed for 2 to 3 weeks. After conversion to sinus rhythm, anticoagulation is continued for an additional 3 to 4 weeks.

3. For rate control: For control of ventricular rate, calcium channel blockers appear to be the drug of choice. Propranolol may be equally effective. In the past, digoxin was popular for this purpose.

4. For prevention of recurrences: Class I and class III antiarrhythmic drugs have been shown to be successful in preventing recurrences in some cases. However, class IA drugs (procainamide, quinidine, disopyramide) also have anticholinergic effects that may produce faster conduction through the AV node, worsening the situation. Therefore, they should be used with drugs that offset the anticholinergic effect, such as digoxin, β-blockers, or diltiazem. Amiodarone and ibutilide (class III) have also been shown to be effective in treating atrial flutter.

5. For refractory cases: Antitachycardia pacing or radiofrequency ablation may be indicated for refractory cases.

ATRIAL FIBRILLATION

Description. Atrial fibrillation is less common than atrial flutter in children. The mechanism of this arrhythmia is circus movement, as in atrial flutter. Atrial fibrillation is characterized by an extremely fast atrial rate (f wave at a rate of 350 to 600 beats/minute) and an irregularly irregular ventricular response with normal QRS complexes (see Fig. 24–2).

Causes. Atrial fibrillation is usually associated with structural heart diseases with dilated atria, such as seen with rheumatic heart disease, Ebstein's anomaly, tricuspid atresia, atrial septal defect, AV valve regurgitation, or previous intra-atrial surgery. Thyrotoxicosis, pulmonary emboli, and pericarditis should be suspected in a previously normal child who develops atrial fibrillation.

Significance

1. The rapid ventricular rate, in addition to the loss of coordinated contraction of the atria and ventricles, decreases the cardiac output, as occurs in atrial tachycardia.

2. Atrial fibrillation usually suggests a significant cardiac pathology.

Management. Management for atrial fibrillation is similar to that described under atrial flutter (see previous discussion).

1. If atrial fibrillation has been present for more than 48 hours, anticoagulation with warfarin for 2 to 3 weeks is recommended to prevent systemic embolization of atrial thrombus, if the conversion can be delayed. Anticoagulation is continued for 3 to 4 weeks after the restoration of sinus rhythm. If cardioversion cannot be delayed, IV heparin should be started, and cardioversion performed when the activated partial thromboplastin time (aPTT) reaches 1.5 to 2.5 times control

(in 5 to 10 days), with subsequent oral anticoagulation with warfarin. An alternative to anticoagulation is transesophageal echo to rule out atrial thrombus.

2. Propranolol, verapamil, or digoxin may be used to slow the ventricular rate.

3. Class I antiarrhythmic agents (e.g., quinidine, procainamide, flecainide) and the class III agent amiodarone may be used.

4. In patients with chronic atrial fibrillations, anticoagulation with warfarin should be considered to reduce the incidence of thromboembolism. In chronic cases, rate control rather than conversion is increasingly used.

SUPRAVENTRICULAR TACHYCARDIA

Description. Three groups of tachycardia are included in SVT: atrial tachycardia (ectopic or nonreciprocating atrial tachycardia), nodal (or AV junctional) tachycardia, and AV reentrant (or reciprocating) tachycardia. The majority of SVTs are due to reciprocating AV tachycardia rather than rapid firing of a single focus in the atria (ectopic atrial tachycardia) or in the AV node (ectopic nodal tachycardia).

The heart rate is extremely rapid and regular (usually 240 ± 40 beats/minute). The P wave is usually invisible. When visible, the P wave has an abnormal P axis and either precedes or follows the QRS complex (see Fig. 24–2). The QRS duration is usually normal, but occasionally, aberrancy increases the QRS duration, making differentiation from ventricular tachycardia difficult (see later discussion).

AV reentrant (or *reciprocating) tachycardia* is not only the most common mechanism of SVT but also the most common tachyarrhythmia seen in the pediatric age group. This arrhythmia was formerly called *paroxysmal atrial tachycardia (PAT)* because the

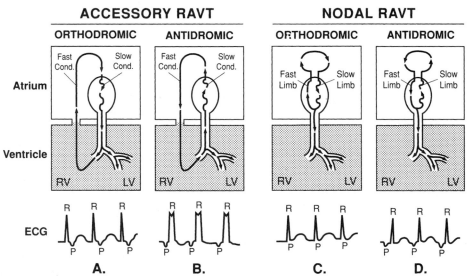

Figure 24–3. *Diagram showing the mechanism of reciprocating atrioventricular tachycardia (RAVT) in relation to ECG findings.* **A,** *Orthodromic accessory RAVT is the most common mechanism of supraventricular tachycardia in patients with Wolff-Parkinson-White syndrome. Antegrade conduction through the normal, slow AV node produces a normal QRS complex, and the retrograde conduction through the bypass tract creates inverted P waves after the QRS complex (with a short RP interval).* **B,** *In antidromic accessory RAVT, the antegrade conduction through the bypass tract produces a wide QRS complex. Retrograde P waves precede the wide QRS complex with a short PR interval (and a long RP interval).* **C,** *In orthodromic nodal RAVT (common form), the retrograde P waves are usually concealed in the QRS complex of normal duration. The ECG is similar to that of orthodromic accessory RAVT, and differentiation between these two is possible only when the tachyarrhythmia terminates by the presence of preexcitation in the accessory RAVT.* **D,** *In antidromic nodal RAVT (uncommon), narrow QRS complexes are preceded by retrograde P waves, with a short PR interval. The ECG is similar to that of ectopic atrial tachycardia. LV, left ventricle; RV, right ventricle. (From Park MK, Guntheroth WG: How to Read Pediatric ECGs, 4th ed. Philadelphia, Mosby, 2006.)*

onset and termination of this arrhythmia were characteristically abrupt. In SVT caused by reentry, two pathways are involved; at least one of these is the AV node, and the other is an accessory pathway. The accessory pathway may be an anatomically separate bypass tract, such as the bundle of Kent (which produces *accessory reciprocating AV tachycardia*; Fig. 24–3A and B), or only a functionally separate bypass tract, such as in a dual AV node pathway (which produces *nodal reciprocating AV tachycardia*; see Fig. 24–3C and D). Patients with accessory pathways frequently have Wolff-Parkinson-White (WPW) preexcitation.

Figure 24–3 shows the mechanism of reciprocating AV tachycardia in relation to ECG findings. If a PAC occurs, the prematurity of the extrasystole may find the accessory bundle refractory, but the AV node may conduct, producing a normal QRS complex; when the impulse reaches the bundle of Kent from the ventricular side, the bundle will have recovered and allows reentry into the atrium, producing a superiorly directed P wave that is difficult to detect. In turn, the cycle is maintained by reentry into the AV node, with a very fast heart rate. When there is an antegrade conduction through the AV node (slow pathway), the rhythm is called *orthodromic reciprocating AV tachycardia* (see Fig. 24–3A). Less common is a widened QRS complex with antegrade conduction into the ventricle through the accessory (fast) pathway and retrograde conduction through the (slower) AV node (*antidromic reciprocating* AV tachycardia; see Fig. 24–3B). A premature ventricular contraction (PVC) could initiate this arrhythmia if the recovery time of the two limbs is ideal for the initiation of the reentry.

Dual pathways in the AV node are more common than accessory bundles, at least as functional entities. For SVT to occur, the two pathways would have to have, at least temporarily, different conduction and recovery rates, creating the substrate for a reentry tachycardia. When the normal, slow pathway through the AV node is used in antegrade conduction to the bundle of His (*orthodromic*), the resulting QRS complex is normal with an abnormal P vector, but the latter is unrecognizable because it is superimposed on the QRS complex (see Fig. 24–3C). The resulting tachycardia could be the same as that seen with SVT associated with WPW syndrome. The two can be differentiated only after conversion from the SVT; after conversion, the patient with accessory bundle would have WPW preexcitation. In *antidromic* nodal reentrant AV tachycardia (see Fig. 24–3D), which is uncommon, the fast tract of the AV node transmits the antegrade impulse to the bundle of His, and the normal, slow pathway of the AV node transmits the impulse retrogradely. The resulting SVT demonstrates normal QRS duration, a short PR interval, and an inverted P wave.

Any type of AV block is incompatible with reentrant tachycardia; AV block would abruptly terminate the tachycardia, at least temporarily. This is the reason that adenosine, which transiently blocks AV conduction, works well for this type of arrhythmia.

Ectopic (or nonreciprocating) atrial tachycardia is a rare mechanism of SVT in which rapid firing of a single focus in the atrium is responsible for the tachycardia (see previous section). In ectopic atrial tachycardia, unlike reciprocating atrial tachycardia, the heart rate varies substantially during the course of a day, and second-degree AV block may develop. In reentrant tachycardia, second-degree AV block terminates the SVT.

Nodal ectopic tachycardia may superficially resemble atrial tachycardia because the P wave is buried in the T waves of the preceding beat and becomes invisible, but the rate of nodal tachycardia is relatively slower (120 to 200 beats/minute) than the rate of ectopic atrial tachycardia.

Causes

1. No heart disease is found in about half of patients. This idiopathic type of SVT occurs more commonly in young infants than in older children.

2. WPW preexcitation is present in 10% to 20% of cases, which is evident only after conversion to sinus rhythm.

3. Some congenital heart defects (e.g., Ebstein's anomaly, single ventricle, congenitally corrected transposition of the great arteries) are more susceptible to this arrhythmia.

4. SVT may occur following cardiac surgeries.

Significance

1. SVT may decrease cardiac output and result in CHF.

2. Many infants tolerate SVT well. If the tachycardia is sustained for 6 to 12 hours, signs of CHF usually develop.

3. Clinical manifestations of CHF include irritability, tachypnea, poor feeding, and pallor. When CHF develops, the infant's condition can deteriorate rapidly. Older children may complain of chest pain, palpitation, shortness of breath, lightheadedness, and fatigue. A pounding sensation in the neck (i.e., neck pulsation) is fairly unique to the reentrant type SVT and considered to be the result of cannon waves when the atrium contracts against a simultaneously contracting ventricle.

Management

1. Vagal stimulatory maneuvers (unilateral carotid sinus massage, gagging, pressure on an eyeball) may be effective in older children but are rarely effective in infants. Placing an ice-water bag on the face (for up to 10 seconds) is often effective in infants (by diving reflex). In children, a headstand often successfully interrupts the SVT.

2. Adenosine is considered the drug of choice. It has negative chronotropic, dromotropic, and inotropic actions with a very short duration of action (half-life <10 seconds) and minimal hemodynamic consequences. Adenosine is effective for almost all reciprocating SVT (in which the AV node forms part of the reentry circuit) and for both narrow- and wide-complex *regular* tachycardia. It is not effective for irregular tachycardia. It is not effective for nonreciprocating atrial tachycardia, atrial flutter or fibrillation, and ventricular tachycardia, but it has differential diagnostic ability. Its transient AV block may unmask atrial activities by slowing the ventricular rate and thus help to clarify the mechanism of certain supraventricular arrhythmias (Fig. 24–4).

    Adenosine is given by rapid IV bolus followed by a saline flush, starting at 50 µg/kg, increasing in increments of 50 µg/kg every 1 to 2 minutes. The usual effective dose is 100 to 150 µg/kg with maximum dose of 250 µg/kg.

3. If the infant is in severe CHF, emergency treatment is directed at immediate cardioversion. The initial dose of 0.5 joule/kg is increased in steps up to 2 joule/kg.

4. Esmolol, other β-adrenergic blockers, verapamil, and digoxin have also been used with some success. Intravenously administered propranolol has been commonly used to treat SVT in the presence of WPW syndrome. IV verapamil should be avoided in infants younger than 12 months because it may produce extreme bradycardia and hypotension in infants.

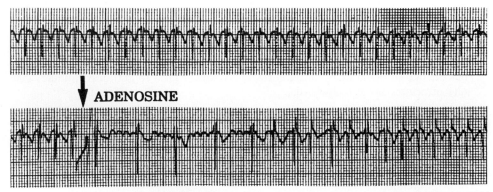

Figure 24–4. *Adenosine can uncover the mechanism of supraventricular tachycardia. A 3-month-old infant developed an extremely fast, narrow QRS complex tachycardia and a heart rate of 220 beats/minute after insertion of a central line through a jugular vein. Adenosine produced a transient atrioventricular block and unmasked very rapid atrial fibrillation waves (570 beats/minute).*

5. For postoperative atrial tachycardia (which requires rapid conversion), IV amiodarone may provide excellent results. The side effects may include hypotension, bradycardia, and decreased left ventricular (LV) function.

6. Overdrive suppression (by transesophageal pacing or by atrial pacing) may be effective in children who have been digitalized.

7. Radiofrequency catheter ablation or surgical interruption of accessory pathways should be considered if medical management fails or frequent recurrences occur. Radiofrequency ablation can be carried out with a high degree of success, a low complication rate, and a low recurrence rate.

Prevention of Recurrence of SVT

1. In infants without WPW preexcitation, oral propranolol for 12 months is effective. Verapamil can also be used but it should be used with caution in patients with poor LV function and in young infants.

2. In infants in CHF and ECG evidence of WPW preexcitation, one may start with digoxin (just to treat CHF), but digoxin should be switched to propranolol when the infant's heart failure improves.

3. In infants or children with WPW preexcitation on the ECG, propranolol or atenolol is used in the long-term management. In the presence of WPW preexcitation, digoxin or verapamil may increase the rate of antegrade conduction of the impulse through the accessory pathway and should be avoided.

Rhythms Originating in the Atrioventricular Node

Rhythms that originate in the AV node are characterized by the following findings (Fig. 24–5):

1. The P wave may be absent, or inverted P waves may follow the QRS complex.

2. The QRS complex is usually normal in duration and configuration.

Only the lower part (NH region) of the AV node has pacemaker ability. The upper (AN region) and middle (N region) parts do not function as pacemakers but delay the conduction of an impulse, either antegrade or retrograde.

NODAL PREMATURE BEATS

Description. A normal QRS complex occurs prematurely. P waves are usually absent, but inverted P waves may follow QRS complexes (see Fig. 24–5). The compensatory pause may be complete or incomplete.

Causes. Nodal premature beats are usually idiopathic in an otherwise normal heart; they may result from cardiac surgery and digitalis toxicity.

Significance. Nodal premature beats usually have no hemodynamic significance.

Management. Treatment is not indicated unless the cause is digitalis toxicity.

NODAL ESCAPE BEATS

Description. When the SA node impulse fails to reach the AV node, the NH region of the AV node initiates an impulse (nodal or junctional escape beat). The QRS complex occurs later than the anticipated normal beat. The P wave may be absent, or an inverted P wave follows the QRS complex (see Fig. 24–5). The duration and configuration of QRS complexes are normal.

Causes. Nodal escape beats may occur after cardiac surgery involving the atria (the Senning procedure or Fontan operation) or in otherwise healthy children.

Significance. Nodal escape beats have little hemodynamic significance.

Management. Generally no specific treatment is required.

NODAL OR JUNCTIONAL RHYTHM

Description. If the SA node consistently fails, the AV node may function as the main pacemaker of the heart, producing a relatively slow rate (40 to 60 beats/minute). Nodal rhythm is characterized by no P waves or inverted P waves after QRS complexes and normal QRS complexes with a rate of 40 to 60 beats/minute (see Fig. 24–5).

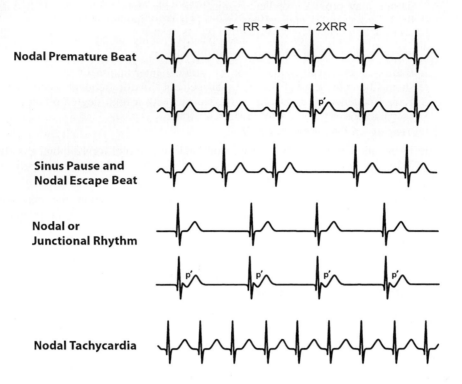

Figure 24–5. *Arrhythmias originating in the atrioventricular node. (From Park MK, Guntheroth WG: How to Read Pediatric ECGs, 4th ed. Philadelphia, Mosby, 2006.)*

Causes. Nodal or junctional rhythm may occur in an otherwise normal heart, with increased vagal tone (increased intracranial pressure, pharyngeal stimulation) and digitalis toxicity, or as a result of cardiac surgery. Rarely, it may be seen in children with polysplenia syndrome.

Significance. The slow heart rate may significantly decrease cardiac output and produce symptoms.

Management

1. Known causes such as digitalis toxicity should be treated.

2. No treatment is indicated if the patient is asymptomatic.

3. Atropine or electric pacing is indicated if the patient is symptomatic.

ACCELERATED NODAL RHYTHM

Description. When the patient has a normal sinus rate and AV conduction and the AV node (NH region) has enhanced automaticity and captures the pacemaker function at a faster rate (60 to 120 beats/minute), the rhythm is called *accelerated nodal (or AV junctional) rhythm*. Either P waves are absent or inverted P waves follow QRS complexes. The QRS complex is normal.

Causes. Accelerated nodal rhythm may be idiopathic, may result from digitalis toxicity or myocarditis, or may follow cardiac surgery.

Significance. Accelerated nodal rhythm has little hemodynamic significance.

Management. No treatment is necessary unless it is caused by digitalis toxicity.

NODAL TACHYCARDIA (JUNCTIONAL ECTOPIC TACHYCARDIA)

Description. The ventricular rate varies from 120 to 200 beats/minute. Either the P waves are absent or inverted P waves follow QRS complexes (see Fig. 24–5). The QRS complex is usually normal, but *aberration* may occur on rare occasions, as in atrial tachycardia. Nodal tachycardia is difficult to separate from atrial tachycardia. Therefore, both arrhythmias are grouped under SVT (see previous discussion).

Causes. The mechanism of the arrhythmia is suspected to be enhanced automaticity. It may occur as a congenital form without heart defect, with cardiac malformation (up to 50%), or postoperatively. Surgeries involving the atria (Fontan repair) or surgery for tetralogy of Fallot is a frequent cause of this arrhythmia.

Significance. The significance is similar to that of ectopic atrial tachycardia. CHF commonly develops and sudden death has been reported to occur.

Management. Digoxin, β-blockers, and calcium channel blockers are generally ineffective. Amiodarone has been the most successful drug, especially in postoperative patients. Cooling (to 31°C to 34°C) has been shown to be effective in postoperative patients.

Rhythms Originating in the Ventricle

Rhythms that originate in the ventricle (ventricular arrhythmias) are characterized by the following (Fig. 24–6):

1. Bizarre and wide QRS complexes.
2. T waves pointing in directions opposite to QRS complexes.
3. QRS complexes randomly related to P waves, if visible.

PREMATURE VENTRICULAR CONTRACTION

Description. A bizarre, wide QRS complex appears earlier than anticipated, and the T wave points in the opposite direction. A full compensatory pause usually appears; that is, the length of two cycles, including the premature beat, is the same as that of two normal cycles (see Fig. 24–6). The appearance of a full compensatory pause indicates that the sinus node is not prematurely discharged by the PVC. If the retrograde impulse discharges and resets the sinus node prematurely, it produces a pause that is not fully compensatory. PVCs may be classified into several types, depending on their interrelationship, similarities, timing, and coupling intervals.

Interrelationship

1. Ventricular *bigeminy* or *coupling*: Each abnormal QRS complex regularly alternates with a normal QRS complex.
2. Ventricular *trigeminy*: Each abnormal QRS complex regularly follows two normal QRS complexes.
3. *Couplets*: Two abnormal QRS complexes appear in sequence.

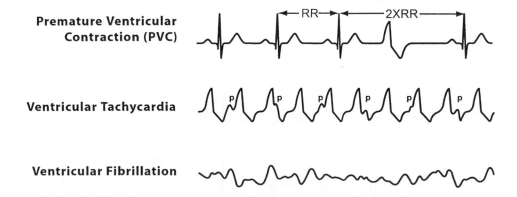

Figure 24–6. *Ventricular arrhythmias. (From Park MK, Guntheroth WG: How to Read Pediatric ECGs, 4th ed. Philadelphia, Mosby, 2006.)*

4. *Triplets.* Three abnormal QRS complexes appear in sequence. Three or more successive PVCs arbitrarily are termed *ventricular tachycardia.*

Similarities among PVCs. Depending on the similarities of the bizarre QRS complex, PVCs may be classified into the following types:

1. Uniform (monomorphic or unifocal) PVCs: Abnormal QRS complexes have the same configuration in a single lead. They are assumed to originate from a single focus.

2. Multiform (polymorphic or multifocal) PVCs: Abnormal QRS complexes have different configurations in a single lead. They are assumed to originate from different foci.

Timing in the Cardiac Cycle. Depending on their timing in the cardiac cycle, PVCs may be classified into several types (Fig. 24–7):

1. Interpolated PVC: The PVC appears between two conducted sinus beats. Sinus rhythm is not interrupted, and there is no compensatory pause after the PVC. The PR interval after the PVC is slightly increased (see Fig. 24–7B).

2. Early PVC: The PVC appears shortly after the normal T wave of the preceding beat. A compensatory pause may appear. If the sinus rate is slow and a retrograde atrial conduction prematurely discharges the sinus node, a noncompensatory pause results. Either a ventricular escape beat or a fusion beat resumes the cardiac cycle (see Fig. 24–7C and D).

3. Late PVC: The PVC appears slightly before the normal P wave of the next beat. A full compensatory pause results (see Fig. 24–7E).

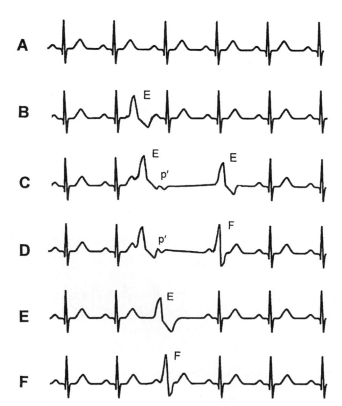

Figure 24–7. *Types of premature ventricular contractions (PVCs) according to timing in the cardiac cycle.* **A,** *Regular sinus rhythm.* **B,** *Interpolated PVC followed by a slightly prolonged PR interval.* **C,** *Early PVC, which results in a retrogradely conducted P wave (P′) with a less than full compensatory pause. The first postectopic beat is a ventricular escape beat (E).* **D,** *Early PVC with a retrogradely conducted P wave (P′) with a less than full compensatory pause. A ventricular fusion beat (F) resumes the cardiac cycle.* **E,** *Late PVC, which results in a full compensatory pause; presumably retrograde discharge of the sinus node did not occur.* **F,** *Ventricular fusion beat with a full compensatory pause.*

4. Fusion beats: The PVC occurs so late in the cardiac cycle that a normal sinus pacemaker impulse has already penetrated the AV node and started to depolarize the ventricle. The resulting QRS complex appears midway between the patient's normal conducted beat and the pure ectopic ventricular beat because it is produced partly by a normally conducted supraventricular impulse and partly by an ectopic ventricular impulse (see Fig. 24–7F). The presence of a "fusion" complex is a reliable sign of PVC and helps differentiate the ventricular tachycardia from a supraventricular arrhythmia with aberrant ventricular conduction (see later discussion).

Coupling Interval

Fixed Coupling. PVCs appear at a constant interval after the QRS complex of the previous cardiac cycle. This suggests ventricular *reentry* within the Purkinje system as the underlying mechanism. Most PVCs in children have a fixed coupling interval and a uniform left bundle branch block (LBBB) morphology.

Varying Coupling. When coupling intervals vary by more than 80 msec, the PVCs may result from parasystole. If the intervals between ectopic beats can be factored so that each interval is a multiple of a single basic interval (within 0.08 second), ventricular parasystole is diagnosed. (Ventricular parasystole consists of an impulse-forming focus in the ventricle that is independent of the sinus node–generated impulse and is protected from depolarization [entrance block] by sinus impulses.)

Causes

1. PVC may appear in otherwise healthy children. Up to 50% to 70% of normal children may show PVCs on 24-hour ambulatory ECGs.
2. A link has been found between LV false tendon and PVCs. False tendons are thin, chordal strands that extend from the ventricular septum to either the LV free wall or an LV papillary muscle; they are detectable by two-dimensional echo (Fig. 24–8). False tendons contain Purkinje fibers, which may be the source of the arrhythmia.

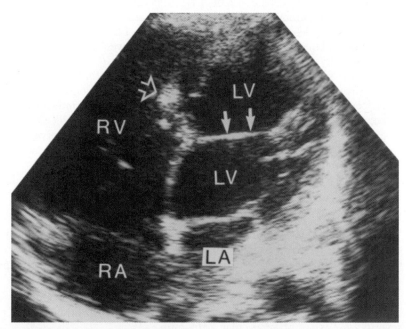

Figure 24–8. *Apical four-chamber view of echo showing a false tendon (solid arrows) in the left ventricle (LV) in a 13-year-old boy who had surgical repair of a ventricular septal defect (open arrow). This patient had a "twanging string" type of systolic murmur and occasional uniform premature ventricular contractions. LA, left atrium; RA, right atrium; RV, right ventricle.*

3. Myocarditis, myocardial injury or infarction, cardiomyopathy (dilated or hypertrophic), and cardiac tumors are possible causes.

4. Arrhythmogenic right ventricular dysplasia (RV cardiomyopathy) may be the cause in children with symptomatic tachycardia (see the section on primary myocardial disease in Chapter 18).

5. Long QT syndrome (see later section).

6. Congenital or acquired heart disease, preoperative or postoperative.

7. Drugs such as digitalis, catecholamines, theophylline, caffeine, amphetamines, and some anesthetic agents are possible causes.

8. Mitral valve prolapse (MVP) is a possible cause.

Significance

1. Occasional PVCs are benign in children, particularly if they are uniform and disappear or become less frequent with exercise.

2. PVCs are more significant if the following are true:
   a. They are associated with underlying heart disease (preoperative or postoperative status, MVP, cardiomyopathy).
   b. There is a history of syncope or a family history of sudden death.
   c. They are precipitated by, or become more frequent with, activity.
   d. They are multiform, particularly couplets.
   e. There are runs of PVCs with symptoms.
   f. There are incessant or frequent episodes of paroxysmal ventricular tachycardia (more likely myocardial tumors).

3. Ventricular parasystole does not appear to have any consequences in children.

Management

1. Some or all of the following tools are used in the investigation of PVCs and other ventricular arrhythmias.
   a. ECGs are used to detect corrected QT interval (QTc) prolongation, ST-T changes, and other abnormalities.
   b. Echo studies detect structural heart disease or functional abnormalities.
   c. 24-hour ambulatory ECG (Holter monitoring) or event recorder detects the frequency and severity of the arrhythmia.
   d. Exercise stress testing: Arrhythmias that are potentially related to exercise are significant and require documentation of the relationship. The induction or exacerbation of arrhythmia with exercise may be an indication of underlying heart disease. In children, PVCs characteristically are reduced or eliminated by exercise. Exercise may reveal prolongation of the QT interval, which may be normal on the routine ECG. A QTc interval greater than 0.44 second at 1 minute after cessation of exercise may be significant.
   e. Cardiac catheterization if arrhythmogenic RV dysplasia is suspected.
   f. Electrophysiologic studies and endomyocardial biopsy.

2. In children with otherwise normal hearts, occasional isolated uniform PVCs that are suppressed by exercise do not require extensive investigation or treatment. ECG, echo studies, and 24-hour Holter monitoring suffice.

3. Children with uniform PVCs, including ventricular bigeminy and trigeminy, do not need to be treated if the echo and exercise stress tests are normal.

4. Asymptomatic children with multiform PVCs and ventricular couplets should have 24-hour Holter monitoring, even if they have structurally normal hearts, to detect the severity and extent of ventricular arrhythmias.

5. All children with symptomatic ventricular arrhythmias and those with complex PVCs (multiform PVCs, ventricular couplets, unsustained ventricular tachycardia) should be treated.

a. β-Blockers (such as atenolol, 1 to 2 mg/kg orally in a single daily dose) are effective for cardiomyopathy and occasionally for RV dysplasia.

b. Other antiarrhythmic drugs, such as phenytoin sodium (Dilantin) and mexiletine, may be effective. Antiarrhythmic agents that prolong the QT interval, such as those of class IA (quinidine, procainamide), class IC (encainide, flecainide), and class III (amiodarone, bretylium), should be avoided (Box 24–1).

c. Frequent PVCs occasionally require treatment with an IV bolus of lidocaine (1 mg/kg per dose), followed by an IV drip of lidocaine (20 to 50 µg/kg per minute).

6. For patients with symptomatic ventricular arrhythmias or sustained ventricular tachycardia and seemingly normal hearts, cardiac catheterization may be indicated to investigate for RV dysplasia. Occasionally, invasive electrophysiologic studies and RV endomyocardial biopsy may be indicated.

7. Children with multiform PVCs and runs of PVCs (ventricular tachycardia) with or without symptoms need to be evaluated by an electrophysiologist.

BOX 24–1	ACQUIRED CAUSES OF QT PROLONGATION

DRUGS

Antibiotics—erythromycin, clarithromycin, telithromycin, azithromycin, trimethoprim-sulfamethoxazole

Antifungal agents—fluconazole, itraconazole, ketoconazole

Antiprotozoal agents—pentamidine isethionate

Antihistamines—astemizole, terfenadine (Seldane) (Seldane has been removed from the market for this reason)

Antidepressants—tricyclics such as imipramine (Tofranil), amitriptyline (Elavil), desipramine (Norpramin), and doxepin (Sinequan)

Antipsychotics—haloperidol, risperidone, phenothiazines such as thioridazine (Mellaril) and chlorpromazine (Thorazine)

Antiarrhythmic agents

Class 1A (sodium channel blockers)—quinidine, procainamide, disopyramide

Class III (prolong depolarization)—amiodarone (rare), bretylium, dofetilide, *N*-acetyl-procainamide, sotalol

Lipid-lowering agents—probucol

Antianginals—bepridil

Diuretics (through K loss)—furosemide (Lasix), ethacrynic acid (Edecrin)

Oral hypoglycemic agents—glibenclamide, glyburide

Organophosphate insecticides

Promotility agents—cisapride

Vasodilators—prenylamine

ELECTROLYTE DISTURBANCES

Hypokalemia—diuretics, hyperventilation

Hypocalcemia

Hypomagnesemia

UNDERLYING MEDICAL CONDITIONS

Bradycardia—complete atrioventricular block, severe bradycardia, sick sinus syndrome

Myocardial dysfunction—anthracycline cardiotoxicity, congestive heart failure, myocarditis, cardiac tumors

Endocrinopathy—hyperparathyroidism, hypothyroidism, pheochromocytoma

Neurologic—encephalitis, head trauma, stroke, subarachnoid hemorrhage

Nutritional—alcoholism, anorexia nervosa, starvation

A more exhaustive updated list of medications that can prolong the QTc interval is available at the University of Arizona Center for Education and Research on Therapeutics website (*www.torsades.org* or *www.qtdrugs.org*).

VENTRICULAR TACHYCARDIA

Description

1. Ventricular tachycardia (VT) is a series of three or more PVCs with a heart rate of 120 to 200 beats/minute. QRS complexes are wide and bizarre, with T waves pointing in opposite directions (see Fig. 24–6).

2. The onset may be paroxysmal (sudden) or nonparoxysmal. VT may be sustained (lasting more than 30 seconds) or unsustained (lasting less than 30 seconds). The QRS contour may be unchanging (uniform, monophasic) or may vary randomly (multiform, polymorphous, or pleomorphic).

3. Torsades de pointes (meaning "twisting of the points") is characterized by a paroxysm of VT during which there are progressive changes in the amplitude and polarity of QRS complexes separated by a narrow transition QRS complex. It is a distinct form of polymorphic VT, occurring in patients with marked QT prolongation.

4. Differentiating VT from SVT with aberrant conduction (see later discussion) is sometimes difficult. However, in children, almost all wide QRS tachycardias are VT. They should be treated as such until proved otherwise.

Causes

1. VT may occur in patients with structural heart diseases such as tetralogy of Fallot (TOF), aortic stenosis (AS), hypertrophic or dilated cardiomyopathy, or MVP.

2. Postoperative CHDs (such as TOF, TGA, or double-outlet right ventricle).

3. Myocarditis, pulmonary hypertension, arrhythmogenic RV dysplasia (in patients of southern European ancestry), Brugada syndrome (young men from Southeast Asia), Chagas' disease (trypanosomiasis, in South America), myocardial tumors, myocardial ischemia, and infarction are other possible causes of VT.

4. Metabolic causes include hypoxia, acidosis, hyperkalemia, hypokalemia, and hypomagnesemia.

5. Mechanical irritation—intraventricular catheter.

6. Pharmacologic or chemical causes include catecholamine infusion, digitalis toxicity, cocaine, and organophosphate insecticides. Most antiarrhythmic drugs (especially classes IA, IC, and III) are also proarrhythmic.

7. Torsades de pointes may be seen in patients with congenital long QT syndrome. Certain drugs that may prolong the QT interval include antiarrhythmic drugs, especially class IA (quinidine, procainamide), class IC (encainide, flecainide), and class III (amiodarone, bretylium); phenothiazines (chlorpromazine, thioridazine); tricyclic antidepressants (imipramine, desipramine); and certain antibiotics (erythromycin, trimethoprim-sulfamethoxazole) (see Box 24–1). Class II and IV antiarrhythmic agents do not prolong the QT interval.

8. VT may occur in healthy children who have a structurally and functionally normal heart. This group is discussed under a separate heading (see later).

Significance

1. VT may signify a serious myocardial pathology or dysfunction and can be a cause of sudden cardiac death.

2. With a fast heart rate, cardiac output may decrease notably, and the rhythm may deteriorate to ventricular fibrillation, in which effective cardiac output does not occur.

3. Most patients with arrhythmogenic RV dysplasia present with LBBB QRS pattern (because the tachycardia arises in the RV). Patients with Brugada syndrome (an autosomal dominant sodium channel defect) present with right bundle branch block (RBBB) and striking ST-segment elevation (in the right precordial leads).

4. Presenting symptoms may be dizziness, syncope, palpitation, or chest pain. Family history may be positive for ventricular arrhythmia or sudden death.

Management

1. Symptomatic VT must be treated promptly with synchronized DC cardioversion (0.5 to 1 joule/kg) if the patient is unconscious or has cardiovascular instability with clinical evidence of low cardiac output.

2. Rarely, if the patient is conscious, an IV bolus of lidocaine (1 mg/kg per dose over 1 to 2 minutes) followed by an IV drip of lidocaine (20 to 50 μg/kg per minute) may be effective. Lidocaine or procainamide is often initiated following cardioversion in an attempt to suppress reinitiation of the tachycardia.

3. The physician should search for reversible conditions contributing to the initiation and maintenance of VT (e.g., hypokalemia, hypoxemia) and correct the conditions, if possible.

4. IV amiodarone is used in patients with drug-refractory VT, particularly that seen in postoperative patients. The mechanism of action of amiodarone appears to be reduction of transmural heterogeneity of repolarization in the ventricular muscle.

5. Virtually all classes of antiarrhythmic agents have been used for various types of VT, including all class I and III drugs, with varying levels of success.

6. IV injection of magnesium sulfate is reportedly effective and safe treatment for torsades de pointes in adults (2 g in an IV bolus).

7. Recurrence may be prevented with administration of propranolol, atenolol, phenytoin sodium, or quinidine (see Appendix D for dosages). A combination of 24-hour Holter monitoring and treadmill exercise testing is the best noninvasive means of evaluating drug effectiveness. Complete pharmacologic suppression may not be achieved without serious complications. Therefore, controlling the rate to an asymptomatic level may be adequate.

8. Patients with long QT syndrome are treated with β-blockers, which alleviate symptoms in 75% to 80%. An implantable cardioverter-defibrillator (ICD) is sometimes recommended as initial therapy.

9. Some incessant VTs are amenable to surgical or radiofrequency ablation.

10. ICD has become the established standard for treating many, if not most, forms of VT, which are potentially lethal.

VENTRICULAR ARRHYTHMIAS IN CHILDREN WITH A NORMAL HEART

Although recurrent sustained VT usually signals an organic cause of the arrhythmia, some VTs are seen in healthy adolescents and young adults with a structurally and functionally normal heart. The prognosis is good. So-called right ventricular outflow tract VT and RBBB VT are examples of this group of VTs.

1. Right Ventricular Outflow Tract (RVOT) Ventricular Tachycardia.

This special form of VT seen in children with a structurally and functionally normal heart originates from the RV conal septum and thus has an inferior QRS axis and LBBB morphology (Fig. 24–9). This is usually benign tachycardia. It may manifest as PVCs, short runs, or salvos of VT, but many children are asymptomatic or minimally symptomatic. Exercise stress may not completely abolish the tachycardia. β-Blockers are sufficient for treatment. Verapamil and other agents may also prove to be effective. Radiofrequency ablation can be curative.

2. RBBB Ventricular Tachycardia (Belhassen's Tachycardia).

It appears to arise from the septal surface of the LV and is less common than RVOT ventricular tachycardia. It is characterized by RBBB morphology and superior QRS axis. It is sensitive to verapamil or adenosine. When it is refractory to medical therapy, radiofrequency ablation or surgery is effective. The long-term outcome is excellent.

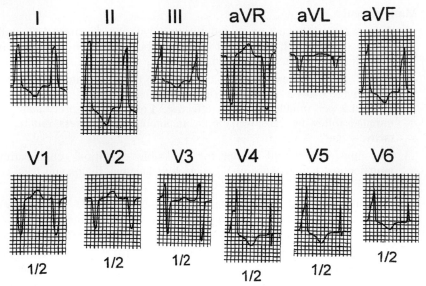

Figure 24–9. *A four-year old girl who is asymptomatic even with ventricular tachycardia with a heart rate of 160 beats per minute. The wide QRS complex has an inferior QRS axis (with positive R waves in leads II, III, and aVF). Spontaneous temporary interruption of ventricular tachycardia occurred while recording V4, V5, and V6 leads. The child was on atenolol.*

ABERRATION

When a supraventricular impulse prematurely reaches the AV node or bundle of His, it may find one bundle branch excitable and the other still refractory. Therefore, the resulting QRS complex resembles a bundle branch block pattern. The right bundle branch usually has a longer refractory period than the left bundle branch, producing QRS complexes similar to those of RBBB. The following features help in differentiating aberrant ventricular conduction from ectopic ventricular impulses:

1. An rsR′ pattern in V1 that resembles QRS complexes of RBBB suggests aberration. In ventricular ectopic beats, the QRS morphology is bizarre and does not resemble the classic form of RBBB or LBBB.

2. Occasional wide QRS complexes after P waves with regular PR intervals suggest an aberration.

3. The presence of a ventricular fusion complex (see previous discussion) is a reliable sign of ventricular ectopic rhythm.

VENTRICULAR FIBRILLATION

Description. Ventricular fibrillation is rare in the pediatric population. It is characterized by bizarre QRS complexes of varying sizes and configurations. The rate is rapid and irregular (see Fig. 24–6). The arrhythmia is maintained by multiple reentrant circuits because portions of the myocardium are depolarizing constantly.

Causes. All the causes listed for VT can cause ventricular fibrillation. Predisposing factors include electrolyte abnormalities, proarrhythmic medications, increased sympathetic activities or catecholamine infusion, hypoxia, or ischemia. Certain CHD (pre- and postoperative) and hereditary conditions are possible causes.

Abrupt ventricular fibrillation following blunt chest wall trauma that typically occurs in young participants in sports (notably ice hockey, lacrosse, baseball, and softball) can cause the arrhythmia (called commotio cordis).

Significance. Ventricular fibrillation is usually a degeneration of VT and is terminal arrhythmia because it results in ineffective circulation. Immediate resuscitation must be provided.

Management. Resuscitation from ventricular fibrillation is successful if performed in a timely fashion; the longer the myocardium is allowed to fibrillate, the more difficult is conversion to a sinus rhythm. Electric shocks (delivered in an asynchronous fashion) are aimed at depolarizing the myocardium to terminate fibrillating rhythm and allow an intrinsic cardiac pacemaker to resume control.

1. Acute care:
    a. Immediate cardiac and pulmonary resuscitation (CPR), providing ABC (airway, breathing, and circulation), airway management with 100% oxygen, and rhythm monitoring, is essential.
    b. Defibrillation with 2 joule/kg, 4 joule/kg, and 6 joule/kg if needed.
    c. Administration of epinephrine by the IV or intraosseous (IO) route, 0.01 mg/kg (1:10,000 solution, 0.1 mL/kg) or by endotracheal tube 0.1 mg/kg (1:1000 solution, 0.1 mL/kg).
    d. One should identify and treat causes, including metabolic environment (hypoxia, acidosis).
    e. One of the following antiarrhythmic agents may be used:
    Amiodarone 5 mg/kg bolus, IV/IO
    Lidocaine 1 mg/kg, IV/IO/ET (endotracheal)
    Magnesium sulfate 25 to 50 mg/kg, IV/IO (not to exceed 2 g) for torsades de pointes or hypomagnesemia

2. A child with susceptibility to ventricular fibrillation and those resuscitated from the arrhythmia should have a comprehensive pediatric electrophysiology evaluation.

3. ICDs are often indicated in patients who survived ventricular fibrillation. This device can be deployed through epicardial patch or transvenous lead placement.

Long QT Syndrome

Long QT syndrome (LQTS) is a disorder of myocardial repolarization characterized by a prolonged QT interval on the ECG and ventricular arrhythmias, usually torsades de pointes, that may result in sudden death. Patients with LQTS may present with complaints of syncope, seizures, or palpitation during exercise or with emotion. The first manifestation may be cardiac arrest.

The QT prolongation may be congenital or acquired.

1. Advances in molecular biology have revealed that ion channels that govern the electrical activity of the heart are defective in congenital LQTS. LQTS is caused by mutations of cardiac ion channel genes. Based on genetic background, six types of Romano-Ward syndrome and two types of Jervell and Lange-Nielsen syndrome are identified. Two additional syndromes (Andersen-Tawil syndrome and Timothy syndrome) are considered different subgroups. Table 24–2 lists molecular genotypes, frequency, chromosomes involved, mutant genes, and defective ionic channels according to subtypes of congenital LQTS.

2. Acquired prolongation of the QT interval can be caused by a number of drugs, electrolyte disturbances, and other underlying medical conditions (see Box 24–1). In the acquired type of LQTS, an ionic mechanism similar to that observed in congenital LQTS may be involved. Individuals who manifest acquired LQTS are believed to be genetically predisposed to the condition. This discussion is focused on congenital LQTS.

There are four groups of patients with congenital types of LQTS: patients with Jervell and Lange-Nielsen syndrome, patients with Romano-Ward syndrome, patients with a sporadic form of Romano-Ward syndrome, and patients with two new rare forms.

1. Jervell and Lange-Nielsen (1957) first described families in Norway in whom a long QT interval on the ECG was associated with congenital deafness, syncopal spells, and a family history of sudden death. This syndrome is transmitted in an autosomal recessive manner.

2. Romano-Ward syndrome, reported independently by Romano and colleagues in Italy (1963) and Ward in Ireland (1964), has all the features of Jervell and Lange-Nielsen

Table 24–2. **Congenital Causes of Long QT Syndrome**

Molecular Genotype	Frequency (%)	Chromosomes Involved	Mutant Genes	Defective Ionic Channel
Romano-Ward Syndrome (Autosomal Dominant)—with Normal Hearing				
LQT1	42	11p15.5	*KCNQ1/KVLQT1*	Potassium channel (I_{Ks})
LQT2	45	7q35-36	*KCNH2/HERG*	Potassium channel (I_{Kr})
LQT3	8	3p21-24	*SCN5A*	Sodium channel (I_{Na})
LQT4	?	4q25-27	*AKNB*	Na/Ca exchanger (I_{Na-Ca})
LQT5	3	21q22.2-22.2	*KCNE1/mink*	Potassium channel (I_{Ks})
LQT6	2	21q22.2-22.2	*KCNE2/MiRP1*	Potassium channel (I_{Ks})
Jervell and Lange-Nielsen Syndrome (Autosomal Recessive)—with Deafness				
JLN1	80	11p15.5	*KCNQ1/KVLQT1*	Potassium channel (I_{Ks})
JLN2	20	21q22.1-22.2	*KCNE1/mink*	Potassium channel (I_{Ks})
Andersen-Tawil Syndrome (Autosomal Dominant)				
ATS1	50	17q23	*KCNJ2*	Inward rectifier potassium channel (I_{K1})
Timothy Syndrome (Sporadic)				
TS1	?	1q42-q43	*CACNA1C*	Cardiac L-type calcium channel ($I_{ca.L}$)

Adapted from Collins KK, van Hare GF: Advances in congenital long QT syndrome. Curr Opin Pediatr 18:497–502, 2006.

syndrome but without deafness. This syndrome transmits in an autosomal dominant mode and is much more common than Jervell and Lange-Nielsen syndrome.

3. A significant number of individuals with Romano-Ward syndrome (with normal hearing) appear to represent sporadic cases, with a negative family history of the syndrome.

4. Two additional syndromes (Andersen-Tawil syndrome and Timothy syndrome) have been added recently (see Table 24–2). Andersen-Tawil syndrome is sometimes designated as LQT7, in which the QU interval, rather than the QT interval, is prolonged, along with muscle weakness (periodic paralysis), ventricular arrhythmias, and developmental abnormalities. Timothy syndrome is associated with webbed fingers and toes and long QT measurement.

PATHOPHYSIOLOGY

The QT interval on the ECG represents the duration of activation and recovery of the ventricular myocardium. Prolonged recovery from electrical excitation contributes to an increased likelihood of dispersion of refractoriness, when some parts of myocardium might be refractory to subsequent depolarization. Consequently, the wave of excitation may pursue a distinctive pathway around a focal point in the myocardium (circus reentry rhythm), leading to VT. Arrhythmic response in patients with LQTS can be precipitated by a variety of adrenergic stimuli, including exercise, emotion, loud noise, and swimming, but it may also occur without such preceding conditions.

CLINICAL MANIFESTATIONS

1. The family history is positive in about 60% of patients, and deafness is present in 5% of patients with the syndrome.

2. Presenting symptoms may be syncope (26%), seizure (10%), cardiac arrest (9%), presyncope, or palpitation (6%). The majority of these symptoms occur during exercise or with emotion. Symptoms of LQTS are related to ventricular arrhythmias and are usually manifested by the end of the second decade of life.

3. Syncope occurs in the setting of intense adrenergic arousal, intense emotion, and during or following rigorous exercise. Swimming appears to be a particular trigger among exercises. Abrupt auditory signals such as a loud doorbell, alarm clock, telephone, or security alarm can trigger symptoms.

4. The ECG shows the following.
   a. A prolonged QT interval with a QTc usually greater than 0.46 second (Fig. 24–10); the upper limit of normal is 0.44 second.
   b. Abnormal T-wave morphology (bifid, diphasic, or notched) is frequent.
   c. Bradycardia (20%), second-degree AV block, multiform PVCs, and monomorphic or polymorphic VT (10% to 20%) may be present. All these ECG findings are considered risk factors for sudden death.

5. Echocardiographic studies usually show a structurally and functionally normal heart.

6. A treadmill exercise test results in a highly significant prolongation of the QTc interval in response to exercise, with the maximal prolongation present after 1 to 2 minutes of recovery. Ventricular arrhythmias may develop during the test in up to 30% of patients.

7. Holter monitoring reveals prolongation of the QTc interval, major changes in the T-wave configuration (T-wave alternation), and ventricular arrhythmias. The QTc interval on Holter monitor may be longer than that recorded on a standard ECG (see later section).

DIAGNOSIS

The potential high risk of sudden death in undiagnosed and untreated patients requires a correct diagnosis so that proper and effective treatment can be instituted. Conversely, the diagnosis of this disease, which has a poor prognosis, should not be made lightly because it implies a lifelong commitment to treatment.

Any child who has a prolonged QTc ≥ 0.46 second or a compelling borderline QTc interval with symptoms, family history, unusual T waves (T wave alternans or notched T waves) should be carefully evaluated.

1. Accurate measurement of the QTc interval is necessary for the diagnosis of LQTS. A 12-lead ECG is the current screening tool for identification of LQTS. Because the

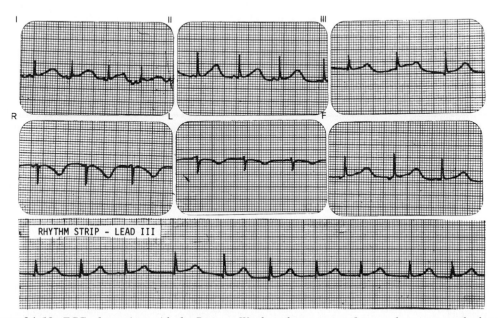

Figure 24–10. ECG of a patient with the Romano-Ward syndrome at age 6 years demonstrates the longest QTc interval (0.56 second). The precordial leads are not shown. Two negative P waves in aVF suggest a junctional mechanism. This child received 10 mg of propranolol four times a day until the age of 13, with complete cessation of syncopal attacks; the dose was smaller than the usual antiarrhythmic dose. There were seven cases of sudden death associated with syncopal attacks on the maternal side of the family. His mother (age 27) and sister (age 5) had moderate prolongation of QTc intervals but experienced no syncopal attacks.

onset of the QRS complex, the end of the T wave, or both may be difficult to define, the clinician cannot always obtain an accurate measurement of the QT interval.

a. Lead II is the preferred lead to measure the QT interval because a q wave is usually present in this lead, but precordial leads (V1, V3, or V5) may also be used because they provide better definition of T waves.

b. The QTc interval is calculated by using Bazett's formula (see Chapter 3). The QTc interval represents the QT interval normalized for a heart rate of 60 beats/minute.

c. The QTc interval varies with the R-R interval. The longest QTc interval follows the shortest R-R interval. In patients with sinus arrhythmia, the QT interval immediately following the shortest R-R interval should be used to calculate the QTc.

d. The QTc interval is longer during sleep; therefore, Holter monitoring may show the QTc interval to be 0.05 second longer than the interval on a standard ECG. Accordingly, comparison of the Holter with a standard ECG for the QTc interval may be inaccurate.

e. In patients with ventricular conduction disturbances such as bundle branch block, the QT interval may be prolonged secondary to the lengthening of the QRS duration, even in the absence of repolarization abnormalities. In such cases, the JT interval may be a more sensitive predictor of repolarization abnormalities than the QTc. The JT interval is measured from the J point (the junction of the S wave and the ST segment) to the end of the T wave. Rate correction is accomplished by the use of Bazett's formula (Berul et al, 1994). Normal JTc interval (mean ± SD) is 0.32 ± 0.02 second with the upper limit of normal 0.34 second in normal children and adolescents.

2. The diagnosis of LQTS is clear-cut when there is a marked prolongation of the QTc interval with a positive family history of the syndrome. However, many cases are at borderline, making it difficult to make or reject the diagnosis. Schwartz and colleagues refined the diagnostic criteria in 1993. A point system is used in the new criteria to distinguish the likelihood of a patient having the disease. The criteria take into account the ECG findings, clinical history, and family history and rank the findings by points based on the "importance" of the findings (Table 24–3). According to these criteria, the scoring of the probability of LQTS is done as follows.

≤1 point = low probability of LQTS

2 to 3 points = intermediate probability of LQTS

≥4 points = high probability of LQTS

*Table 24–3. **Schwartz Diagnostic Criteria for Long QT syndrome***

ECG Findings (in the Absence of Medications or Disorders Known to Prolong the QTc Interval)

QTc	
>480 msec	3
460–470 msec	2
450 (male) msec	1
Torsades de pointes	2
T-wave alternans	1
Notched T waves in three leads	1
Low heart rate for age (<2nd percentile)	0.5
Clinical History	
Syncope	
With stress	2
Without stress	1
Congenital deafness	0.5
Family History	
Family members with definite LQTS	1
Unexplained sudden cardiac death <30 yr	
among immediate family members	0.5

Adapted from Schwartz PJ, Moss AJ, Vincent GM, Crampton RS: Diagnostic criteria for the long QT syndrome: An update. Circulation 88:782–784, 1993.

3. Initial diagnostic strategy: Initially, five steps are considered in making the diagnosis of LQTS (modified from Seslar et al, 2006).
   a. History of presyncope, syncope, seizure, or palpitation and family history are carefully examined.
   b. Causes of acquired LQTS are excluded.
   c. ECG is examined for the QTc interval and morphology of the T waves. QT dispersion is calculated. ECGs are also obtained from immediate family members.
   d. The LQTS score is calculated (see Table 24–3) and the diagnostic possibility is graded as described previously.
   e. Patients with an LQTS score ≥4 or an abnormal exercise test are considered to have LQTS, and an LQTS score ≤1 is excluded from the diagnosis. Patients with an LQTS score of 2 or 3 are followed up for possible LQTS.

4. For borderline cases, additional testing, such as Holter monitoring, exercise testing, pharmacologic test, or electrophysiology study, may be performed, although they are not universally accepted tests.
   a. Holter monitoring may detect intermittent QT prolongation with changing heart rate (with QTc prolongation at a faster rate), bradyarrhythmia, macrovolt T-wave alternans, and T-wave notching. It may also detect VT. However, the results of Holter monitoring should be interpreted with caution because the standards for QTc on ambulatory monitoring are not established and tape speed may vary on the recording devices.
   b. Exercise testing. Some centers routinely perform exercise testing. In most children and young adults, the QT interval shortens with exercise and increased heart rate. However, in patients with LQTS, the QT interval may fail to shorten or may lengthen at higher heart rates and with exertion. A lack of appropriate shortening of the QTc duration and abnormal T-wave morphology are most often seen in LQTS patients.
   c. Epinephrine test. Continuous ECG monitoring during an infusion of IV epinephrine at escalating doses (0.025 to 0.3 μg/kg per minute), which usually shortens the QT interval in normal subjects. This test provides a good quality QT interval for accurate measurement, unlike exercise testing. The QTc was prolonged in all patients with LQT subgroups. The prolongation was greatest in patients with LQT1 (141 msec in LQT1 compared with 69 and 3 msec for LQT2 and LQT3).

5. Genetic testing may identify genotypes of the LQTS. Although it is not widely used in clinical practice at the present time, the testing will soon become available for clinical use.

MANAGEMENT

1. The known risk factors should be considered when making a treatment plan for the congenital type of LQTS.
   a. Risk factors for sudden death include:
      1) Bradycardia for age (sinus bradycardia, junctional escape rhythm, or second-degree AV block),
      2) An extremely long QTc interval (>0.55 second),
      3) Symptoms at presentation (syncope, seizure, cardiac arrest),
      4) Young age at presentation (<1 month), and
      5) Documented torsades de pointes or ventricular fibrillation.
   b. T-wave alternation (major changes in T-wave morphology) is a relative risk factor.
   c. Noncompliance with medication is an important risk factor for sudden death.

2. General measures:
   a. Physicians should be aware of the conditions and medications that prolong the QT interval (see Box 24–1).
   b. Physicians should avoid prescribing QT prolonging medications (and discontinue those medications if possible). Catecholamines and sympathomimetic drugs should

also be avoided if possible because they can potentially trigger torsades de pointes in patients with LQTS.

c. No competitive sports policy applies. This is particularly important in patients with LQS1. Physicians should also advise against swimming.

d. Patients should be educated about the importance of being compliant with their medication because noncompliance can result in sudden death.

Treatment of Congenital LQTS. For congenital LQTS, the initial treatment is aimed at interrupting sympathetic input to the myocardium with β-blockers. A surgical approach to interrupting sympathetic input to the heart (through left cardiac sympathetic denervation surgery) is no longer frequently used. Other therapies include permanent cardiac pacing and an ICD. The use of a specific ion channel blocking agent, when the mutations in the ion channel genes are known, is in the experimental stage.

1. *β-Blockers.* The present therapy of choice is treatment with β-blockers. The protective effect of β-blockers is related to their ability to reduce both syncope and sudden cardiac death. There is a consensus that all symptomatic children with LQTS should be treated with propranolol or other β-blockers (e.g., atenolol, metoprolol). All β-blockers appear to have similar effectiveness, but the QTc usually remains prolonged. Moderate doses of β-blockers may be better than larger doses because moderate doses lessen the trend toward bradycardia, a known risk factor for sudden death, especially in patients with sinus or AV node disorders. The addition of an IB antiarrhythmic agent (mexiletine) to β-blocker therapy may be helpful, especially in genotype LQT3.

   β-Blockers are effective in preventing cardiac events in approximately 70% of patients, and cardiac events continue to occur despite β-blocker therapy in the remaining 30% of patients. Even with treatment with β-blockers, sudden death can occur. More than 80% of cases of sudden death occur while patients are taking medications; some of these cases of sudden death are caused by noncompliance.

   Whether to start β-blockers in asymptomatic children with QTc prolongation has been controversial. Any patients who score 4 or greater in the Schwartz diagnostic criteria should be treated regardless of symptoms. However, it may be prudent to observe the asymptomatic children whose QTc intervals are at the borderline (0.46 to 0.47). Symptoms are more likely to occur in patients with QTc intervals greater than 0.48 second. In addition, β-blocker treatment may be dangerous to some patients with the syndrome because treatment tends to produce bradycardia, a known risk factor for sudden death. Definitive treatment of asymptomatic patients with congenital LQTS has been suggested by Schwartz (1997) in the following circumstances: newborns and infants, patients with sensorineuronal hearing loss, affected siblings with LQTS and sudden cardiac death, extremely long QTc (>0.60 second) or T-wave alternans, and to prevent the family's or patient's anxiety.

2. *Cardiac pacemakers.* Implantation of cardiac pacemakers (with continuous ventricular or dual chamber pacing) has been considered helpful because pacing eliminates arrhythmogenic bradycardia. Symptomatic bradycardia related to β-blockers may be considered an indication for elective pacing. In this situation, a maximally tolerated dose of β-blockers (e.g., atenolol 50 to 200 mg/day, metoprolol to 50 to 200 mg/day, propranolol 60 to 120 mg/day) may be used because the pacemaker is expected to prevent bradycardia from occurring. However, cardiac events have continued to occur in high-risk patients and pacing did not provide complete protection from sudden death, which occurred in 16% of patients, because the pacemaker lacks defibrillation capability. In view of the availability of the ICD, which can defibrillate as well as pace when bradycardia develops, cardiac pacemakers are likely to be used less often in patients with LQTS.

3. *Implantable cardioverter-defibrillator.* Implantation of a cardioverter-defibrillator appears to be the most effective therapy for high-risk patients, defined as those with aborted cardiac arrests or recurrent cardiac events despite conventional therapy (with β-blockers) and those with extremely prolonged QTc intervals (e.g., >0.60 second). A cardioverter-defibrillator is expected not only to prevent bradycardia but also to convert ventricular arrhythmias. The ICD has been shown to be safe and effective

in preventing sudden death in limited clinical experience with children. It is likely that the ICD will be used more frequently as clinical experience with this device accumulates. These patients should continue to receive β-blockers.

Complications are common with ICDs. These include infection, lead fracture and dislodgement, inappropriate discharge, psychiatric sequelae, and electrical storm. Alternatively, one could use a combination of β-blockers and pacemaker and/or stellectomy.

4. *Left cardiac sympathetic denervation.* Left cardiac sympathetic denervation is another method to reduce cardiac events in patients who continue to have symptoms by reducing sympathetic discharge. Because of the availability of other options, such as pacing and ICD, this procedure is rarely performed. The high thoracic left sympathectomy removes the lower part of the stellate ganglion along with the first four thoracic ganglia, with almost no risk for Homer's syndrome. Other denervation surgeries, such as left cervicothoracic sympathectomy, almost always result in Homer's syndrome and often provide inadequate cardiac sympathetic denervation. After a high thoracic sympathectomy, there is a dramatic reduction in the incidence of cardiac events, although sudden death still occurs (8%); the procedure has a 5-year survival rate of 94%. β-Blockers are usually continued after the surgical procedure.

5. *Targeted pharmacologic therapy.*
   a. The sodium channel blocker mexiletine was used in patients with mutations in the sodium channel gene *SCN5A (LQT3)* with significant shortening of the QTc. QTc shortening was observed only in patients with LQTc.
   b. Potassium supplementation might improve repolarization abnormalities in patients with LQT2 (with potassium channel abnormalities). Potassium supplementation in combination with spironolactone was associated with a significant reduction in QTc and some improvement in T-wave morphology.

6. *"Gene-specific" approach.* Gene or gene-specific therapy has not gained wide clinical application at this time.

Treatment of Acquired Long QT Syndrome. The management of acquired LQTS involves acute treatment of arrhythmias (with intravenous magnesium), discontinuation of any precipitating drug (see Box 24–1), and correction of any metabolic abnormalities (such as hypokalemia or hypomagnesemia).

An internet source with updated lists of drugs that prolong the QT interval is available at the University of Arizona Center for Education and Research on Therapeutics website (*www.torsades.org* or *www.qtdrugs.org*).

PROGNOSIS

LQTS is a serious disease, and treatment is at best only partially effective. The prognosis is very poor in untreated patients, with annual mortality as high as 20% and 10-year mortality of 50%. β-Blockers may reduce mortality to some extent, but they do not completely protect patients from sudden death. The ICD appears promising in improving prognosis.

Short QT Syndrome

Recently, a familial short QT interval has been reported to be a cause of sudden death. Short QT syndrome is characterized by a very short QTc (≤300 msec); symptoms of palpitation, dizziness, or syncope; and family history of sudden death. The cause of death is believed to be ventricular fibrillation. This syndrome is transmitted in an autosomal dominant manner. Treatment plans similar to those described for LQTS should apply.

Brugada Syndrome

This rare condition is considerably more common among young men in Southeast Asia. It is also known as "sudden unexpected death syndrome." Mutations in the sodium channel appear to be the cause of the condition, at least in 20% of sufferers. The ECG is abnormal but without demonstrable structural abnormalities of the heart. The ECG typically shows RBBB with J point elevation and concave ST elevation. The patient may present with complaints of blackout or palpitations. There may be a family history of sudden death. Cardiac examination is usually normal.

Diagnosis is suspected on the basis of the ECG appearance, which may not always be present. The condition can carry a poor prognosis, particularly in those who are symptomatic; there is at least a 10% death rate per year. No antiarrhythmic drugs, including β-blockers, appear to reduce the risk of death in these patients. It is therefore standard practice at present to use an ICD to protect most patients.

Chapter 25

Disturbances of Atrioventricular Conduction

Atrioventricular (AV) block is a disturbance in conduction between the normal sinus impulse and the eventual ventricular response. The block is assigned to one of three classes, depending on the severity of the conduction disturbance. First-degree AV block is a simple prolongation of the PR interval, but all P waves are conducted to the ventricle. In second-degree AV block, some atrial impulses are not conducted into the ventricle. In third-degree AV block (or complete heart block), none of the atrial impulses is conducted into the ventricle (Fig. 25–1).

First-Degree Atrioventricular Block

Description. The PR interval is prolonged beyond the upper limits of normal for the patient's age and heart rate (see Table 3–2 and Fig. 25–1). The PR interval includes time required for depolarization of atrial myocardium, the delay of conduction in the AV node, and conduction through the bundle of His to the time of the onset of ventricular depolarization. The abnormal delay in conduction usually occurs at the level of the AV node.

Causes. First-degree AV block can appear in otherwise healthy children and young adults, particularly in athletes. Other causes include congenital heart diseases (such as endocardial cushion defect, atrial septal defect, Ebstein's anomaly), infectious disease, inflammatory conditions (rheumatic fever), cardiac surgery, and certain drugs (such as digitalis, calcium channel blockers).

Significance. First-degree AV block does not produce hemodynamic disturbance. It sometimes progresses to a more advanced AV block.

Management. No treatment is indicated, except when the block is caused by digitalis toxicity (see Chapter 30).

Second-Degree Atrioventricular Block

Some, but not all, P waves are followed by a QRS complex (dropped beats). There are three types: Mobitz type I (Wenckebach phenomenon), Mobitz type II, and two-to-one (or higher) AV block.

MOBITZ TYPE I

Description. The PR interval becomes progressively prolonged until one QRS complex is dropped completely (see Fig. 25–1).

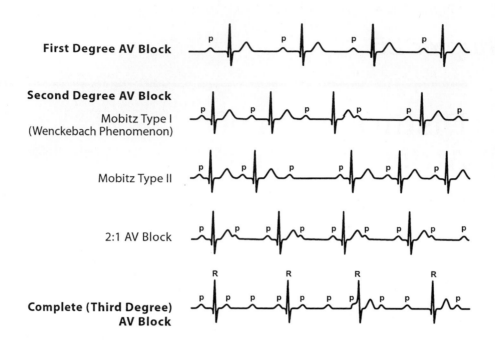

Figure 25–1. *Atrioventricular (AV) block. (From Park MK, Guntheroth WG: How to Read Pediatric ECGs, 4th ed. Philadelphia, Mosby, 2006.)*

Causes. Mobitz type I AV block appears in otherwise healthy children. Other causes include myocarditis, cardiomyopathy, myocardial infarction, congenital heart defect, cardiac surgery, and digitalis toxicity.

Significance. The block is at the level of the AV node. It usually does not progress to complete heart block. It occurs in individuals with vagal dominance.

Management. The underlying causes are treated.

MOBITZ TYPE II

Description. The AV conduction is "all or none." AV conduction is either normal or completely blocked (see Fig. 25–1).

Causes. Causes are the same as for Mobitz type I.

Significance. The block is at the level of the bundle of His. It is more serious than type I block because it may progress to complete heart block, resulting in Stokes-Adams attack.

Management. The underlying causes are treated. Prophylactic pacemaker therapy may be indicated.

TWO-TO-ONE (OR HIGHER) ATRIOVENTRICULAR BLOCK

Description. A QRS complex follows every second, third, or fourth P wave, resulting in 2:1, 3:1, or 4:1 AV block (see Fig. 25–1).

Causes. Causes are similar to those of other second-degree AV blocks.

Significance. The block is usually at the bundle of His, alone or in combination with the AV nodal block. It may occasionally progress to complete heart block.

Management. The underlying causes are treated. Electrophysiologic studies may be necessary to determine the level of the block. Pacemaker therapy is occasionally necessary.

Third-Degree Atrioventricular Block

Description. In third-degree AV block (complete heart block), atrial and ventricular activities are entirely independent of each other (see Fig. 25–1).

1. The P waves are regular (regular P-P interval), with a rate comparable to the normal heart rate for the patient's age. The QRS complexes are also regular (regular R-R interval), with a rate much slower than the P rate.

2. In congenital complete heart block, the duration of the QRS complex is normal because the pacemaker for the ventricular complex is at a level higher than the bifurcation of the bundle of His. The ventricular rate is faster (50 to 80 beats/minute) than that in the acquired type, and the ventricular rate is somewhat variable in response to varying physiologic conditions.

3. In surgically induced or acquired (after myocardial infarction) complete heart block, the QRS duration is prolonged because the pacemaker for the ventricular complex is at a level below the bifurcation of the bundle of His. The ventricular rate is in the range of 40 to 50 beats/minute (idioventricular rhythm) and the ventricular rate is relatively fixed.

Causes

Congenital Type. Causes are an isolated anomaly (without associated structural heart defect), structural heart disease such as congenitally corrected transposition of the great arteries, or maternal diseases such as systemic lupus erythematosus, Sjögren's syndrome, or other connective tissue disease.

Acquired Type. Cardiac surgery is the most common cause of acquired complete heart block in children. Other rare causes include severe myocarditis. Lyme carditis, acute rheumatic fever, mumps, diphtheria, cardiomyopathies, tumors in the conduction system, overdoses of certain drugs, and myocardial infarction. These causes produce either temporary or permanent heart block.

Significance

1. Congestive heart failure (CHF) may develop in infancy, particularly when there are associated congenital heart defects.

2. Patients with isolated congenital heart block who survive infancy are usually asymptomatic and achieve normal growth and development for 5 to 10 years. Chest x-ray films may show cardiomegaly.

3. Syncopal attacks (Stokes-Adams attacks) may occur with a heart rate below 40 to 45 beats/minute. A sudden onset of acquired heart block may result in death unless treatment maintains the heart rate in the acceptable range.

Management

1. Atropine or isoproterenol is indicated in symptomatic children and adults until temporary ventricular pacing is secured.

2. A temporary transvenous ventricular pacemaker is indicated in patients with heart block, or it may be given prophylactically in patients who might develop heart block.

3. No treatment is required for children with asymptomatic congenital complete heart block with acceptable rate, narrow QRS complex, and normal ventricular function.

4. Pacemaker therapy is indicated in patients with congenital heart block:

   a. If the patient is symptomatic or develops CHF. Dizziness or lightheadedness may be an early warning sign of the need for a pacemaker.
   b. If an infant has a ventricular rate less than 50 to 55 beats/minute or if the infant has a congenital heart defect with a ventricular rate less than 70 beats/minute.
   c. If the patient has a wide QRS escape rhythm, complex ventricular ectopy, or ventricular dysfunction.

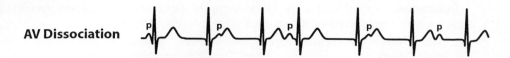

AV Dissociation

Figure 25–2. *Diagram of atrioventricular (AV) dissociation owing to either marked slowing of the sinus node or acceleration of the AV node. The fourth complex is conducted, changing the rhythm (called "interference"). All of the other complexes originate in the AV node, where there is higher automaticity than usual.*

5. A permanent artificial ventricular pacemaker is indicated in patients with surgically induced heart block that is not expected to resolve or persists at least 7 days after cardiac surgery.

6. A variety of problems may arise after a pacemaker is placed in children. Stress placed on the lead system by the linear growth of the child, fracture of the lead system in a physically active child, electrode malfunction (scarring of the myocardium around the electrode, especially in infants), and the limited life span of the pulse generator require follow-up of children with artificial pacemakers.

Atrioventricular Dissociation

AV dissociation should not be confused with third-degree AV block. AV dissociation results from a marked slowing of the sinus node or atrial bradycardia or acceleration of the AV node. In AV dissociation the atrial rate is slower than the ventricular rate, whereas in complete heart block the ventricular rate is usually slower than the atrial rate. In AV dissociation an atrial impulse may conduct to the AV node if it comes at the right time (Fig. 25–2). The conducted beats can be recognized by their relative prematurity.

Chapter 26

Cardiac Pacemakers and Implantable Cardioverter-Defibrillators in Children

A pacemaker is a device that delivers battery-supplied electrical stimuli over leads to electrodes that are in contact with the heart. It primarily treats bradycardia. An implantable cardioverter-defibrillator (ICD) is a multiprogrammable antiarrhythmic device for treating ventricular tachycardia and ventricular fibrillation. The ICD also possesses pacemaking capability to treat bradycardia. The electrical leads are either placed directly over the epicardium or inserted transvenously into the cardiac chambers. Electronic circuitry regulates the timing and characteristics of the stimuli. The power source is usually a lithium-iodine battery.

Physicians encounter an increasing number of children with either temporary or permanent pacemakers. Basic knowledge about the pacemaker and the pacemaker rhythm strip is essential in taking care of these children. This chapter presents examples of ECG rhythm strips from children with various types of pacemakers and elementary information regarding pacemaker and ICD therapy in children.

ECGs of Artificial Cardiac Pacemakers

The need to recognize rhythm strips of artificial pacemakers has increased in recent years, especially in intensive care and emergency room settings. The position and number of the pacemaker spikes on the ECG rhythm strip are used to recognize different types of pacemakers. Thus, a pacemaker may be classified as a ventricular pacemaker, atrial pacemaker, or P-wave–triggered ventricular pacemaker.

1. When the pacemaker stimulates the atrium, the resulting P wave demonstrates an abnormal P axis.

2. When the pacemaker stimulates the ventricle, wide QRS complexes result.

3. The ventricle that is stimulated (or the ventricle on which the pacemaker electrode is placed) can be identified by the morphology of the QRS complexes. With the pacing electrode on the right ventricle, the QRS complex resembles a left bundle branch block (LBBB) pattern; with the pacemaker placed on the left ventricle, a right bundle branch block (RBBB) pattern results.

VENTRICULAR PACEMAKER (VENTRICULAR SENSING AND PACING)

This mode of pacing is recognized by vertical pacemaker spikes that initiate ventricular depolarization with wide QRS complexes (Fig. 26–1A). The electronic spike has no fixed relationship with atrial activity (P wave). The pacemaker rate may be fixed (as in Fig. 26–1A),

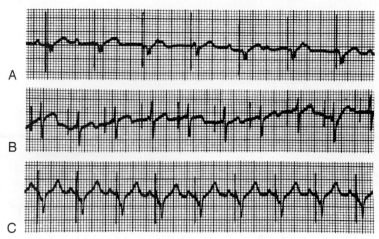

Figure 26–1. *Examples of some artificial pacemakers.* ***A,*** *Fixed-rate ventricular pacemaker. Note the regular rate of the electronic spikes with no relationship to the P waves.* ***B,*** *Atrial pacemaker. This tracing is from a 2-year-old child in whom extreme, symptomatic bradycardia developed following the Mustard operation.* ***C,*** *P-wave–triggered pacemaker. This tracing is from a child in whom surgically induced complete heart block developed after repair of tetralogy of Fallot. Note that, in the figure, the electronic spikes are either tall or short, but all are of shorter duration. (From Park MK, Guntheroth WG: How to Read Pediatric ECGs, 4th ed. Philadelphia, Mosby, 2006.)*

or it may be on a demand (or standby) mode in which the pacemaker fires only after a long pause between the patient's own ventricular beats.

ATRIAL PACEMAKER (ATRIAL SENSING AND PACING)

The atrial pacemaker is recognized by a pacemaker spike followed by an atrial complex; when atrioventricular (AV) conduction is normal, a QRS complex of normal duration follows (see Fig. 26–1B). This type of pacemaker is indicated in patients with sinus node dysfunction with bradycardia. When the patient has high-degree or complete AV block in addition to sinus node dysfunction, an additional ventricular pacemaker may be required (AV sequential pacemaker, not illustrated in Fig. 26–1). The AV sequential pacemaker is recognized by two sets of electronic spikes—one before the P wave and another before the wide QRS complex.

P-WAVE–TRIGGERED VENTRICULAR PACEMAKER (ATRIAL SENSING, VENTRICULAR PACING)

This pacemaker may be recognized by pacemaker spikes that follow the patient's own P waves at regular PR intervals and with wide QRS complexes (see Fig. 26–1C). The patient's own P waves are sensed and trigger a ventricular pacemaker after an electronically preset PR interval. This type of pacemaker is the most physiologic and is indicated when the patient has advanced AV block but a normal sinus mechanism. Advantages of this type of pacemaker are that the heart rate varies with physiologic need and the atrial contraction contributes to ventricular filling and improves cardiac output.

Pacemaker Therapy in Children

Remarkable technologic advances have been made in pacemaker design and function. Surgical corrections of cardiac defects and their late sequelae have increased the need for pacemaker therapy in children. New permanent pacemakers (physiologic pacemakers) are capable of closely mimicking normal cardiac rhythm, and most of them are small enough to be implanted in an infant.

INDICATIONS

The indications for permanent pacemaker implantation in children are continually evolving as the reliability of pacing systems improves and clinical experience increases. Box 26–1 lists conditions for which pacemaker therapy is or is not indicated, based on the 2002 joint recommendations of the American College of Cardiology, American Heart Association, and the North American Society for Pacing and Electrophysiology (ACC/AHA/NASPE). In the guidelines, class I conditions are those for which there is general agreement that the device will be beneficial and class II conditions are those for which there is ambivalence regarding whether the device will be beneficial. Class IIa conditions are those for which the weight of evidence or opinion is in favor of usefulness or efficacy, and class IIb conditions are those for which usefulness or efficacy is less well established. Class III conditions are those for which there is agreement that the device will not be useful.

In general, pediatric conditions that require pacemaker implantation fit into one of four categories: (1) symptomatic bradycardia (with symptoms of syncope, dizziness, exercise intolerance, or congestive heart failure), (2) congenital AV block, (3) surgical or acquired advanced second- or third-degree AV block, and (4) recurrent bradycardia-tachycardia. Bradycardia is the most common and noncontroversial indication for permanent pacemaker therapy in both children and adults. In children, significant bradycardia with syncope or near syncope results most commonly from surgery involving the atria (e.g., the Senning operation for transposition of the great arteries, surgery for atrial septal defect or total anomalous pulmonary venous return, and the Fontan operation for functional single ventricle). Another noncontroversial indication is surgically acquired heart block that lasts more than 2 weeks after surgery. The risk of death from surgically acquired heart block is as high as 35% in unpaced patients. Most children with congenital heart block, especially those with additional structural heart defects, require pacemaker therapy.

Temporary pacing is indicated for (1) patients with advanced second-degree or complete heart block secondary to overdose of certain drugs, myocarditis, or myocardial infarction and (2) certain patients immediately after cardiac surgery.

TYPES OF PACING DEVICES

The North American Society of Pacing and Electrophysiology and the British Pacing and Electrophysiology Group devised a generic letter code to describe the types and functions of pacemakers, and it was updated in 2002 (Table 26–1). The first three letters are used exclusively for antibradyarrhythmia functions.

1. The letter in the first position identifies the chamber paced (O, none; A, atrium; V, ventricle, D, dual chamber or both A and V).
2. The second is the chamber sensed (O, none; A, atrium; V, ventricle; D, dual).
3. The third letter corresponds to the response of the pacemaker to an intrinsic cardiac event (O, none; I, inhibited; T, triggered; D, dual [I + T]).
4. The fourth letter indicates both programmability and rate modulation.
5. The fifth position of the code is used to indicate whether multisite pacing is present.

Some examples of the first three letters (and their indications) are as follows.

1. A VOO device provides ventricular pacing, no sensing, and no response to an intrinsic cardiac event. This type of pacemaker is commonly used for emergency pacing.
2. An AOO device provides atrial pacing with no sensing.
3. A VVI device is ventricle stimulated and ventricle sensed; it inhibits paced output if endogenous ventricular activity occurs (thus preventing competition with native QRS activity). This type is commonly used for episodic AV block or bradycardia in small infants.
4. An AAI device paces and senses the atrium and is inhibited by the patient's own atrial activity. This type is commonly used in sinus node dysfunction with intact AV conduction.

BOX 26–1	**INDICATIONS FOR PERMANENT PACING IN CHILDREN AND ADOLESCENTS**

CLASS I (DEVICE WILL BE BENEFICIAL)

1. Advanced second- or third-degree atrioventricular (AV) block associated with symptomatic bradycardia, ventricular dysfunction, or low cardiac output.

2. Sinus node dysfunction with symptoms during age-appropriate bradycardia. The definition of bradycardia varies with patient's age and expected heart rate.

3. Postoperative advanced second- or third-degree AV block that is not expected to resolve or persists at least 7 days after cardiac surgery.

4. Congenital third-degree AV block with a wide QRS escape rhythm, complex ventricular ectopy, or ventricular dysfunction.

5. Congenital third-degree AV block in an infant with a ventricular rate <50 to 55 beats/minute or with congenital heart disease and a ventricular rate <70 beats/minute.

6. Sustained pause-dependent ventricular tachycardia, with or without prolonged QT, in which the efficacy of pacing is thoroughly documented.

CLASS IIA (AMBIVALENT BUT IN FAVOR OF USEFULNESS OR EFFICACY)

1. Bradycardia-tachycardia syndrome with the need for long-term antiarrhythmic treatment other than digitalis.

2. Congenital third-degree AV block beyond the first year of life with an average heart rate <50 beats/minute, abrupt pauses in ventricular rate that are two to three times the basic cycle length, or associated with symptoms due to chronotropic incompetence.

3. Long QT syndrome with 2:1 AV block or third-degree AV block.

4. Asymptomatic sinus bradycardia in the child with complex congenital heart disease with resting heart rate <40 beats/minute or pauses in the ventricular rate >3 seconds.

5. Patients with congenital heart disease and impaired hemodynamics due to sinus bradycardia or loss of AV synchrony.

CLASS IIB (AMBIVALENT, USEFULNESS OR EFFICACY LESS WELL ESTABLISHED)

1. Transient postoperative third-degree AV block that reverts to sinus rhythm with residual bifascicular block.

2. Congenital third-degree AV block in the asymptomatic infant, child, adolescent, or young adult with an acceptable rate, narrow QRS complex, and normal ventricular function.

3. Asymptomatic sinus bradycardia in the adolescent with congenital heart disease with resting heart rate <40 beats/minute or pauses in the ventricular rate >3 seconds.

4. Neuromuscular diseases with any degree of AV block (including first-degree AV block), with or without symptoms, because there may be unpredictable progression of AV conduction disease.

CLASS III (DEVICE WILL NOT BE BENEFICIAL)

1. Transient postoperative AV block with return of normal AV conduction.

2. Asymptomatic postoperative bifascicular block with or without first-degree AV block.

3. Asymptomatic type I second-degree AV block.

4. Asymptomatic sinus bradycardia in the adolescent with the longest RR interval <3 seconds and minimum heart rate >40 beats/minute.

Adapted from Gregoratos G, Abrams J, Epstein AE, et al: ACC/AHA/NASPE 2002 guideline update for implantation of cardiac pacemakers and antiarrhythmia devices. Circulation 106:2145–2161, 2002.

Table 26–1. **Revised NASPE/BPEG Generic Code for Antibradycardia Pacing**

I: Chamber(s) Paced	II: Chamber(s) Sensed	III: Response to Sensing	IV: Programmability, Rate Modulation	V: Antiarrhythmia Function
O, None	O, None	O, None	O, None	O, None
A, Atrium	A, Atrium	T, Triggered	R, Rate modulation	A, Atrium
V, Ventricle	V, Ventricle	I, Inhibited		V, Ventricle
D, Dual (A + V)	D, Dual (A + V)	D, Dual (T + I)		D, Dual (A + V)

NASPE, North American Society of Pacing and Electrophysiology; BPEG, British Pacing and Electrophysiology Group.
Adapted from Bernstein AD, Daubert AC, Fletcher RD, et al, and the NASPE/BPEG: The revised NASPE/BPEG generic code for antibradycardia, adaptive-rate, and multisite pacing. Pacing Clin Electrophysiol 25:260–264, 2002.

5. A DDD device is a dual-chamber pacemaker that is capable of pacing either chamber, sensing activity in either chamber, and either triggering or inhibiting paced output (with resulting AV synchrony). This type is used in AV block where AV synchrony is important.

6. A DVI device paces both the atrium and ventricle, sensing the ventricle only, and ventricular sensing inhibits atrial and ventricular pacing. This type allows AV synchrony and is commonly used in patients with atrial arrhythmias.

SELECTION OF PACING MODE

The pacemaker choice is based on several factors, including the presence or absence of underlying cardiac disease, the size of the patient, and the relevant hemodynamic factors (including the need for atrial contribution in cardiac output).

1. A patient who has sinus node dysfunction but intact AV node function may receive a single-chamber atrial pacemaker or ventricular pacemaker if AV synchrony is not necessary.

2. In patients with AV block, if AV synchrony is not necessary, a single-chamber ventricular pacing device may be implanted.

3. If the sinus node and AV node are both dysfunctional, a dual-chamber device is implanted.

Rate-adaptive pacemakers have the ability to increase the pacing rate through sensors that monitor physiologic processes such as activity (activity sensing with vibration detection by piezoelectric crystal or accelerometer) and minute ventilation.

BATTERY, LEADS, AND ROUTE

Lithium anode batteries are used almost exclusively. The most widely used type of lithium battery is the lithium iodide. Battery longevity depends on several factors, such as battery size, stimulation frequency, and output per stimulation. Battery life varies from 3 years for a dual-chamber pacemaker used in a small child to 15 years for a large single-chamber device needed infrequently.

There are two types of leads: unipolar and bipolar. The unipolar lead (in which the tip of the lead is the negative pole and the pacemaker itself is the positive pole) has the advantages of a smaller size and a larger sensing circuit, which amplifies low-voltage P waves. The bipolar lead (which possesses a tip electrode [−] and a ring electrode [+] near the end of the pacing catheter) can screen pectoral muscle "noise," has a lower likelihood of external muscle stimulation, and can function even if the pacemaker is out of contact with the body.

Historically, epicardial pacing was more common in children, but transvenous implantation is the method of choice. With improved technology, generators and leads have become smaller and more advanced, allowing transvenous pacing systems in small children. In general, the transvenous route is a reasonable approach for children weighing at least 10 kg, although others have reported successful transvenous pacing in neonates without complications. Transvenous implantation is performed on the side contralateral to the dominant hand. Transvenous implantation has several advantages over epicardial implantation: Both atrial and ventricular capture thresholds are generally lower, and pacing problems are significantly fewer than with epicardial implantation. Epicardial implantation is performed through a xyphoid approach and is chosen when transvenous implantation is precluded, when the patient is a neonate or a small infant (<10 kg), and when the transvenous approach is not possible (after the Fontan operation or superior vena cava obstruction).

Implantable Cardioverter-Defibrillator Therapy

An ICD is used in patients at risk for recurrent, sustained ventricular tachycardia (VT) or fibrillation. The efficacy of ICD therapy in saving lives of patients at high risk of sudden death has been shown convincingly. Multiple studies have shown the ICD to be superior to antiarrhythmic drug therapy in patients with a history of life-threatening ventricular tachyarrhythmias (i.e., VT or fibrillations).

All ICDs also have a built-in pacemaker. Pacing may be necessary for bradycardia, which may follow an electrical shock delivered by the ICD. The pacemaker also allows correction of certain tachycardias by overdrive suppression.

The ICD automatically detects, recognizes, and treats tachyarrhythmias and brady-arrhythmias using tiered therapy (i.e., bradycardia pacing, overdrive tachycardia pacing, low-energy cardioversion, high-energy shock defibrillation). It also offers a host of other sophisticated functions (such as storage of detected arrhythmic events and the ability to do "noninvasive" electrophysiologic testing). ICDs can discharge voltages ranging from less than 1 V for pacing to 750 V for defibrillation.

The ICD is implanted beneath the skin over the left chest (for right-handed persons) pectoralis muscle, and the leads are connected to the ICD. Virtually all ICD systems are implanted transvenously. The longevity of the ICD depends on the frequency of shock delivery, the degree of pacemaker dependence, and other programmable options, but most are expected to last from 5 to 10 years.

The most common problem with the ICD is inappropriate shocks, which are usually the result of detection of a supraventricular tachycardia, most commonly atrial fibrillation. In adult patients, inappropriate shock has been reported in up to 20% of patients within the first year and 40% by 2 years after implantation, causing pain and anxiety generated by this complication.

INDICATIONS

Indications for ICD implantation include patients with life-threatening arrhythmias; aborted sudden death; family history of the same disease that can cause sudden death; those with dilated and hypertrophic cardiomyopathy, especially when unexplained fainting episodes have occurred; and other conditions that may increase the risk for sudden arrhythmic death. The ICD is usually recommended as initial therapy in patients who present with sustained VT or resuscitated cardiac arrest. Box 26–2 lists indications for ICD therapy according to the 2002 ACC/AHA/NASPE guideline.

Fewer than 1% of all ICD implantations are performed in pediatric patients.

1. The two most common indications for ICD implantation in children are hypertrophic cardiomyopathy and long QT syndrome.

2. Other potential indications include idiopathic dilated cardiomyopathy, Brugada syndrome, and arrhythmogenic right ventricular dysplasia/cardiomyopathy.

3. A family history of sudden death may influence the decision to use an ICD in a pediatric patient.

4. Some postoperative congenital heart diseases such as tetralogy of Fallot and transposition of the great arteries are rare indications for ICD implantation.

5. ICD may also be considered as a bridge to orthotopic heart transplantation in pediatric patients, given the longer time to donor procurement in pediatric patients.

BOX 26–2	INDICATIONS FOR IMPLANTABLE CARDIOVERTER-DEFIBRILLATOR THERAPY

CLASS I (DEVICE WILL BE BENEFICIAL)

1. Cardiac arrest due to ventricular fibrillation (VF) or ventricular tachycardia (VT) not due to a transient or reversible cause.

2. Spontaneous sustained VT in association with structural heart disease.

3. Syncope of undetermined origin with clinically relevant, hemodynamically significant sustained VT or VF induced at electrophysiologic study when drug therapy is ineffective, not tolerated, or not preferred.

4. Nonsustained VT in patients with coronary disease, prior myocardial infarction (MI), LV dysfunction, and inducible VF or sustained VT at electrophysiologic study that is not suppressible by a class I antiarrhythmic drug.

5. Spontaneous sustained VT in patients who do not have structural heart disease that is not amenable to other treatments.

CLASS IIA (AMBIVALENT BUT IN FAVOR OF USEFULNESS OR EFFICACY)

1. Patients with LV ejection fraction of 30% or less, at least 1 month after myocardial infarction and 3 months after coronary artery revascularization surgery.

CLASS IIB (AMBIVALENT, USEFULNESS OR EFFICACY LESS WELL ESTABLISHED)

1. Cardiac arrest presumed to be due to VF when electrophysiologic testing is precluded by other medical conditions.

2. Severe symptoms (e.g., syncope) attributable to ventricular tachyarrhythmias in patients awaiting cardiac transplantation.

3. Familial or inherited conditions with a high risk for life-threatening ventricular tachyarrhythmias such as long-QT syndrome or hypertrophic cardiomyopathy.

4. Nonsustained VT with coronary artery disease, prior MI, LV dysfunction, and inducible sustained VT or VF at electrophysiologic study.

5. Recurrent syncope of undetermined etiology in the presence of ventricular dysfunction and inducible ventricular arrhythmias at electrophysiologic study when other causes of syncope have been excluded.

6. Syncope of unexplained etiology or family history of unexplained sudden cardiac death in association with typical or atypical right bundle branch block and ST-segment elevations (Brugada syndrome).

7. Syncope in patients with advanced structural heart disease in which thorough invasive and noninvasive investigation has failed to define a cause.

CLASS III (DEVICE WILL NOT BE BENEFICIAL)

1. Syncope of undetermined cause in a patient without inducible ventricular tachyarrhythmias and without structural heart disease.

2. Incessant VT or VF.

3. VF or VT resulting from arrhythmias amenable to surgical or catheter ablation; for example, atrial arrhythmias associated with the Wolff-Parkinson-White syndrome, right ventricular outflow tract VT, idiopathic left ventricular tachycardia, or fascicular VT.

4. Ventricular tachyarrhythmias due to a transient or reversible disorder (e.g., acute myocardial infarction, electrolyte imbalance, drugs, or trauma) when correction of the disorder is considered feasible and likely to substantially reduce the risk of recurrent arrhythmia.

5. Significant psychiatric illness that may be aggravated by device implantation or may preclude systematic follow-up.

6. Terminal illnesses with projected life expectancy less than 6 months.

Continued

BOX 26–2	**INDICATIONS FOR IMPLANTABLE CARDIOVERTER-DEFIBRILLATOR THERAPY—cont'd**

CLASS III (DEVICE WILL NOT BE BENEFICIAL)—cont'd

7. Patients with coronary artery disease with LV dysfunction and prolonged QRS duration in the absence of spontaneous or inducible sustained or nonsustained VT who are undergoing coronary bypass surgery.

8. NYHA class IV drug-refractory congestive heart failure in patients who are not candidates for cardiac transplantation.

Adapted from Gregoratos G, Abrams J, Epstein AE, et al: ACC/AHA/NASPE 2002 guideline update for implantation of cardiac pacemakers and antiarrhythmia devices. Circulation 106:2145–2161, 2002.

LIVING WITH A PACEMAKER OR IMPLANTABLE CARDIOVERTER-DEFIBRILLATOR

Electromagnetic interference (EMI) can cause malfunction of the pacemaker or ICD by rate alteration, sensing abnormalities, reprogramming, and other functions, which may result in malfunction of the device or even damage to the pulse generator. EMI is defined as any signal—biologic or nonbiologic—that is within a frequency spectrum detectable by the sensing circuitry of the pacemaker or ICD.

The patients should be well educated to avoid situations that may cause malfunction or damages to the device. EMI can occur within or outside the hospital. Patients with pacemakers should wear a medical identification bracelet or necklace to show that they have the pacemaker in case of emergency. The following lists some common situations that may or may not affect pacemakers or ICDs.

1. Most home appliances do *not* interfere with the pacemaker signal.
   a. Kitchen appliances (microwave ovens, blenders, toaster ovens, electric knives)
   b. Television, stereos, FM and AM radios, ham radios, and CB radios
   c. Electric blanket, heating pads
   d. Electric shavers, hair dryers, curling irons
   e. Garage door openers, electric gardening trimmers
   f. Computers, copying and fax machines
   g. Properly grounded shop tools (except power generator or arc welding equipment)

2. The patient must use caution in the following situations.
   a. Security detectors at airports and government buildings such as courthouses. The patient should not stay near the electronic article surveillance (EAS) system longer than is necessary and should not lean against the system.
   b. Cellular phones; one should not carry a cell phone in the breast pocket when the ICD is implanted in the left upper chest. Keep the cell phone at least 6 inches away from the ICD. When talking on the cell phone, hold it on the opposite side of the body from the ICD
   c. Avoid working with, holding, or carrying magnets near the pacemaker.
   d. Turn off large motors such as car or boat motors when working on them. Do not use a chain saw.
   e. Avoid industrial welding equipment. Most welding equipment used for "hobby" welding should not cause any significant problem.
   f. Avoid high-tension wires, radar installations, smelting furnaces, electric steel furnaces, and other high-current industrial equipment.
   g. Abstain from diathermy (the use of heat to treat muscles).
   h. Contact sports are not recommended for children with a pacemaker or ICD.

3. Hospital sources of potentially significant EMI are as follows.
   a. Electrocautery during surgical procedures. Notify the surgeon or dentist so that electrocautery will not be used to control bleeding. ICD therapy should be deactivated

before surgery and reinitiated after surgery by a qualified professional. Alternatively, a magnet can be placed over the pacemaker throughout the procedure.

b. For cardioversion or defibrillation. Paddles should be placed in the anteroposterior position, keeping the paddles at least 4 inches from the pulse generator. A qualified pacemaker programmer should be available.

c. Magnetic resonance imaging is considered a relative contraindication in patients with a pacemaker or ICD.

FOLLOW-UP FOR PACEMAKER AND IMPLANTABLE CARDIOVERTER-DEFIBRILLATOR

Patients with pacemakers and ICDs must be followed on a regular schedule. Many of the same considerations are relevant to both pacemaker and ICD follow-up.

Some physicians prefer regular office assessment, others prefer transtelephonic follow-up, and still others prefer a combination of the two techniques. The frequency of clinic follow-up varies, but a popular schedule is twice in the first 6 months after implantation and then once every 12 months for single-chamber pacemakers. For dual-chamber pacemakers, twice in the first 6 months, then once every 6 months is popular. Monthly transtelephonic pacing system evaluation is simple, convenient, and relatively inexpensive, allowing follow-up with fewer cardiology office visits.

Transtelephonic assessment includes (1) collection of a nonmagnet ECG strip, (2) collection of an ECG strip with magnet applied to the pacemaker, and (3) measurement of magnet rate and pulse duration (pulse duration on both atrial and ventricular channels for a dual-chamber pacemaker).

During an office visit, the clinical status of the patient is assessed and the same information as described for transtelephonic assessment should be collected. Once a year, appropriateness of the rate response should be checked for rate-adaptive pacing devices.

For an ICD follow-up, the following specific information is collected and assessed. Many caregivers follow up every 3 to 6 months for the first 3 to 4 years, after which follow-up frequency increases.

1. History—specific emphasis on awareness of delivered therapy and any tachycardia events
2. Device interrogation
3. Assessment of battery status and charge time
4. Retrieval and assessment of stored diagnostic data, such as the cycle length or rate of the detected tachyarrhythmias and ECGs of detected arrhythmias
5. Periodic radiographic assessment
6. Periodic arrhythmia induction in the electrophysiology laboratory to assess defibrillation threshold and efficacy

Part VII

SPECIAL PROBLEMS

This part explores common pediatric cardiac problems not discussed in previous chapters. The topics include congestive heart failure, systemic hypertension, pulmonary hypertension, child with chest pain, syncope, palpitation, dyslipidemia and other cardiovascular risk factors, athletes with cardiac problems, and cardiac transplantation.

Chapter 27

Congestive Heart Failure

Definition

Congestive heart failure (CHF) is a clinical syndrome in which the heart is unable to pump enough blood to the body to meet its needs, to dispose of systemic or pulmonary venous return adequately, or a combination of the two.

Causes

The heart failure syndrome may arise from diverse causes. Common causes of CHF are volume or pressure overload, or both, caused by congenital or acquired heart disease and myocardial diseases. Tachyarrhythmias and heart block can also cause heart failure at any age. By far the most common causes of CHF in infancy are congenital heart diseases (CHDs). Beyond infancy, myocardial dysfunctions of various etiologies are important causes of CHF. Among the rare causes of CHF are metabolic and endocrine disorders, anemia, pulmonary diseases, collagen vascular diseases, systemic or pulmonary hypertension, neuromuscular disorders, and drugs such as anthracyclines.

CONGENITAL HEART DISEASE

Volume overload lesions such as ventricular septal defect (VSD), patent ductus arteriosus (PDA), and endocardial cushion defect (ECD) are the most common causes of CHF in the first 6 months of life. In infancy, the time of the onset of CHF varies predictably with the type of defect. Table 27–1 list commons defects according to the age at which CHF develops. When looking at the table, the following should also be noted.

1. Children with tetralogy of Fallot (TOF) do not develop CHF unless they have received a large aorta–to–pulmonary artery (PA) shunt procedure, for example, too large a Gore-Tex interposition shunt (modified Blalock-Taussig shunt).
2. Atrial septal defect (ASD) rarely causes CHF in the pediatric age group, although it causes CHF in adulthood.
3. Large left-to-right shunt lesions, such as VSD and PDA, do not cause CHF before 6 to 8 weeks of age because the pulmonary vascular resistance does not fall low enough to cause a large left-to-right shunt until this age. The onset of CHF resulting from these left-to-right shunt lesions may be earlier in premature infants (within the first month) because of an earlier fall in the pulmonary vascular resistance in these infants.

Table 27–1. **Causes of Congestive Heart Failure Resulting from Congenital Heart Disease**

Age of Onset	Cause

At birth	HLHS
	Volume overload lesions:
	    Severe tricuspid or pulmonary insufficiency
	    Large systemic arteriovenous fistula

First wk	TGA
	PDA in small premature infants
	HLHS (with more favorable anatomy)
	TAPVR, particularly those with pulmonary venous obstruction
	Others:
	    Systemic arteriovenous fistula
	    Critical AS or PS

1–4 wk	COA with associated anomalies Critical AS Large left-to-right shunt lesions (VSD, PDA) in premature infants All other lesions previously listed
4–6 wk	Some left-to-right shunt lesions such as ECD
6 wk–4 mo	Large VSD Large PDA Others such as anomalous left coronary artery from the PA

AS, aortic stenosis; COA, coarctation of the aorta; ECD, endocardial cushion defect; HLHS, hypoplastic left heart syndrome; PA, pulmonary artery; PDA, patent ductus arteriosus; PS, pulmonary stenosis; TAPVR, total anomalous pulmonary venous return; TGA, transposition of the great arteries; VSD, ventricular septal defect.

ACQUIRED HEART DISEASE

Acquired heart disease of various causes can lead to CHF. With acquired heart disease, the age at onset of CHF is not as predictable as with CHD, but the following generalities apply:

1. Endocardial fibroelastosis, a rare primary myocardial disease, causes CHF in infancy; 90% of cases occur in the first 8 months of life.

2. Viral myocarditis tends to be more common in small children older than 1 year. It occurs occasionally in the newborn period, with a fulminating clinical course with poor prognosis.

3. Myocarditis associated with Kawasaki disease is seen in children 1 to 4 years of age.

4. Acute rheumatic carditis is an occasional cause of CHF that occurs primarily in school-age children.

5. Rheumatic valvular heart diseases, usually volume overload lesions such as mitral regurgitation (MR) or aortic regurgitation (AR), cause CHF in older children and adults. These diseases are uncommon in industrialized countries.

6. Dilated cardiomyopathy may cause CHF at any age during childhood and adolescence. The cause of the majority of dilated cardiomyopathy is idiopathic, but it may be caused by infectious, endocrine, or metabolic disorders or autoimmune diseases or may follow antineoplastic treatment (e.g., anthracycline).

7. Doxorubicin cardiomyopathy may manifest months to years after the completion of chemotherapy for malignancies in children.

8. Cardiomyopathies associated with muscular dystrophy and Friedreich's ataxia may cause CHF in older children and adolescents.

9. Patients who received surgery for some types of CHD (such as a Fontan operation, surgery for TOF, transposition of the great arteries, and other cyanotic defects) may remain in or develop CHF.

MISCELLANEOUS CAUSES

Miscellaneous causes of CHF include the following:

1. Metabolic abnormalities (severe hypoxia and acidosis, as well as hypoglycemia and hypocalcemia) can cause CHF in newborns.

2. Endocrinopathy such as hyperthyroidism can cause CHF.

3. Supraventricular tachycardia (SVT) causes CHF in early infancy.

4. Complete heart block associated with structural heart defects causes CHF in the newborn period or early infancy.

5. Severe anemia may be a cause of CHF at any age. Hydrops fetalis may be a cause of CHF in the newborn period and severe sicklemia at a later age.

6. Bronchopulmonary dysplasia seen in premature infants causes predominantly right-sided heart failure in the first few months of life.

7. Primary carnitine deficiency (plasma membrane carnitine transport defect) causes progressive cardiomyopathy with or without skeletal muscle weakness that begins at 2 to 4 years of age.

8. Acute cor pulmonale caused by acute airway obstruction (such as seen with large tonsils) can cause CHF at any age but most commonly during early childhood.

9. Acute systemic hypertension, as seen in acute postinfectious glomerulonephritis, causes CHF in school-age children. Fluid retention with poor renal function is important as the cause of hypertension in this condition.

Pathophysiology of Congestive Heart Failure

According to the Frank-Starling law, as the ventricular end-diastolic volume (or preload) increases, the healthy heart increases cardiac output until a maximum is reached and cardiac output can no longer be augmented (see Fig. 27–1). When the left ventricular (LV) end-diastolic pressure reaches a certain point, pulmonary congestion develops with pulmonary congestive symptoms (tachypnea and dyspnea). Congestive symptoms occur even with normally functioning myocardium if the end-diastolic pressure is greatly increased, such as with infusion of a large amount of fluid or blood. An increase in the stroke volume is also achieved in the failing heart when the preload is increased, but the failing heart does not achieve the same level of maximal cardiac output as the normal heart, and congestive symptoms (dyspnea and hepatomegaly) result.

The increased stroke volume results in increased wall tension, which in turn increases oxygen consumption. Increase in the wall tension is also seen in dilated ventricular cavity, according to the Laplace law.

$$\text{Wall stress} = \text{pressure} \times \text{radius}/2 \times \text{wall thickness}$$

The Laplace law, although an oversimplification, emphasizes two points:

1. The bigger the left ventricle and the greater the radius, the greater the wall stress.

2. At any given radius (LV size), the greater the pressure developed in the LV, the greater the wall stress.

In heart failure, cardiac hypertrophy (with increased wall thickness) develops to balance the increased pressure and keep the wall stress unchanged, and reduction of heart size decreases wall stress and improves cardiac output or LV function.

Among many compensatory responses to the failing heart is the activation of two important neurohormonal mechanisms: the sympathetic nervous system and the renin-angiotensin-aldosterone system. Although these responses are an attempt to preserve cardiovascular homeostasis and thus are beneficial initially, chronic stimulation of these systems may be deleterious in the natural history of myocardial dysfunction.

1. One major compensatory mechanism for increasing cardiac output is an increase in sympathetic tone, secondary to increased adrenal secretion of circulating epinephrine and increased neural release of norepinephrine. The initial beneficial effects

of adrenergic stimulation include increased heart rate and myocardial contractility with resulting increase in cardiac output. However, chronic adrenergic stimulation eventually leads to adverse myocardial effects, including increased afterload, hypermetabolism, arrhythmogenesis, and direct myocardial toxicity.

   a. Catecholamines are toxic to cardiac muscle, perhaps by producing calcium overload or by inhibiting the synthesis of contractile proteins.

   b. High catecholamine levels decrease the density of β-adrenergic receptors on the surface of the myocardial cell, which may be the major cause of functional loss of the catecholamine-mediated positive inotropic response.

   In clinical settings, the reduction of adrenergic stimulation by the use of β-adrenergic blockers has resulted in clinical improvement in patients with dilated cardiomyopathy, in whom increased levels of catecholamines have been shown to be present.

2. The reduced blood flow to the kidneys in patients with CHF causes a marked increase in renin output, and this in turn causes the formation of angiotensin II. Angiotensin II leads to further increase in reabsorption of both water and salt from the renal tubules. Angiotensin II may cause a trophic response in vascular smooth muscle (with vasoconstriction) and myocardial hypertrophy. Angiotensin II also promotes myocardial fibrosis. Thus, although the hypertrophic response is adaptive by attempting to restore wall stress to normal, angiotensin II plays a maladaptive role in CHF by initiating fibrosis and altering ventricular compliance.

   Thus, reasons for using β-adrenergic blockers and angiotensin-converting enzyme (ACE) inhibitors in the treatment of CHF are to block the maladaptive role of the adrenergic and renin-angiotensin-aldosterone systems.

Diagnosis

The diagnosis of CHF relies on several sources of clinical findings, including history, physical examination, chest x-ray films, and echocardiographic studies. No single test is specific for CHF. In addition to physical findings discussed subsequently, cardiomegaly on a chest film is nearly a prerequisite sign of CHF. An ECG is perhaps the least important test for the diagnosis of CHF, although it may help identify the cause of heart failure. Echocardiographic studies are the most helpful noninvasive studies; they confirm the diagnosis of heart failure and estimate the severity of heart failure. They may also help identify the cause of heart failure.

Plasma levels of natriuretic peptides, atrial natriuretic peptide (ANP) and B-type natriuretic peptide (BNP), are increased in most adult patients with heart failure. They are important markers of heart failure and may help distinguish dyspnea caused by heart failure and pulmonary disease in adult patients. ANP is stored mainly in the right atrium and is released when the atrial distending pressure increases. BNP is stored in ventricular myocardium and appears to be released when the ventricular filling pressure increases. Both peptides exhibit vasodilating effects and natriuretic effects on the kidneys and counteract the water-retaining effects of the renin-angiotensin-aldosterone system. The plasma levels of these peptides are elevated in the newborn and in the first weeks of life but decrease to the levels observed in normal adults. Increased levels of BNT and the N-terminal segment of its prohormone (NT-ProBNT) have been reported in most children with either pressure or volume overload cardiac lesions compared with the levels seen in normal children (Nir et al, 2005). However, the usefulness of the levels of these peptides appears limited because an appropriate reference range has not been established. The levels of these peptides are different depending on the commercial testing kits used.

HISTORY

1. Poor feeding of recent onset, tachypnea that worsens during feeding, poor weight gain, and cold sweat on the forehead suggest CHF in infants.

2. Older children may complain of shortness of breath, especially with activities, early fatigability, puffy eyelids, or swollen feet.

PHYSICAL EXAMINATION

Physical findings of CHF may be classified as follows, depending on their pathophysiologic mechanisms. The more common findings are in italics.

1. The following are found as compensatory responses to impaired cardiac function:
   a. *Tachycardia*, *gallop rhythm*, and weak and thready pulses are common.
   b. *Cardiomegaly* is almost always present. Chest x-ray films are more reliable than physical examination in demonstrating cardiomegaly.
   c. There are signs of increased sympathetic discharges (e.g., *growth failure*, *perspiration*, cold and wet skin).

2. Pulmonary venous congestion (from left-sided failure) results in the following manifestations:
   a. *Tachypnea* is common and is an early manifestation of CHF in infants.
   b. Dyspnea on exertion (equivalent to poor feeding in small infants) is common in children.
   c. Orthopnea may be seen in older children.
   d. Wheezing and pulmonary crackles are occasionally audible.

3. Systemic venous congestion (related to right-sided failure) results in the following:
   a. Hepatomegaly is common but it is not always indicative of CHF. A large liver may be palpable in conditions that cause hyperinflated lungs (asthma, bronchiolitis, during hypoxic spells) and in infiltrative liver disease. Conversely, the absence of hepatomegaly does not rule out CHF; hepatomegaly may be absent in (early) left-sided failure.
   b. Puffy eyelids are common in infants.
   c. Distended neck veins and ankle edema, which are common in adults, are not seen in infants.
   d. Splenomegaly is not indicative of CHF; it usually indicates infection.

X-RAY STUDIES

The presence of cardiomegaly should be demonstrated by chest x-ray films. The absence of cardiomegaly almost rules out the diagnosis of CHF. The only exception to this rule arises when the pulmonary venous return is obstructed; in such cases, the lung parenchyma shows pulmonary edema or venous congestions.

ELECTROCARDIOGRAPHY

ECGs help determine the type of heart defect causing heart failure but are not helpful in deciding whether CHF is present.

ECHOCARDIOGRAPHY

Echo studies may confirm enlargement of ventricular chambers and impaired LV systolic function (decreased fractional shortening or ejection fraction) as well as impaired diastolic function by the use of Doppler techniques. A more important role of echo may be due to its ability to determine the cause of CHF. Echo is also helpful in serial evaluation of the efficacy of therapy.

CARDIAC CATHETERIZATION

Endomyocardial biopsy obtained during cardiac catheterization offers a new approach to specific diagnosis of the cause of CHF, such as inflammatory disease, infectious process, or metabolic disorder. When viral myocarditis is suspected, the polymerase chain reaction provides a means of isolating the offending viral agent from biopsy specimens. In a patient with dilated cardiomyopathy, evaluation of biopsy specimens, including genetic analysis, may provide data permitting the diagnosis of specific metabolic causes, such as carnitine deficiency.

Management

The treatment of CHF consists of (1) elimination of the underlying causes, (2) treatment of the precipitating or contributing causes (e.g., infection, anemia, arrhythmias, fever), and (3) control of the heart failure state. Eliminating the underlying causes is the most desirable approach whenever possible. Surgical correction of congenital heart defects is such an approach. Every patient with CHF should receive maximal medical treatment, but continuing with long-term anticongestive measures is unwise when the heart defect can be safely repaired through surgery. The heart failure state is controlled by the use of multiple drugs, including inotropic agents, diuretics, and afterload-reducing agents, along with general supportive measures.

TREATMENT OF UNDERLYING CAUSES OR CONTRIBUTING FACTORS

1. When surgically feasible, treatment of underlying congenital heart defects and valvular heart disease is the best approach for complete cure.

2. If hypertension is the underlying cause of CHF, antihypertensive treatment should be given.

3. If arrhythmias or advanced heart block is the cause of or a factor contributing to heart failure, antiarrhythmic agents or cardiac pacemaker therapy is indicated.

4. If hyperthyroidism is the cause of heart failure, this condition should be treated.

5. Fever should be controlled with antipyretics.

6. When there is a concomitant infection, it should be treated with appropriate antibiotics.

7. For anemia, packed cell transfusion is given to raise the hematocrit to 35% or higher.

GENERAL MEASURES

General support to improve congestive symptoms and nutritional support are important.

1. A "cardiac chair" or "infant seat" is used to keep infants in a semiupright position to relieve respiratory distress.

2. Oxygen (40% to 50%) with humidity is administered to infants with respiratory distress if pulse oximetry indicates compromise of blood oxygenation.

3. Adequate calories and fluid should be provided to permit appropriate weight gain. Infants in CHF need significantly higher caloric intakes than recommended for average children. The required caloric intake may be as high as 150 to 160 kcal/kg/day for infants in CHF. Compounding this problem is that these infants typically cannot take in needed calories even for normal growth owing to tachypnea, increased work of breathing, diminished strength of sucking, and difficulty with coordination of sucking and swallowing.
   a. Increasing caloric density of feeding may be required, and it may be accomplished with fortification of feeding (Table 27–2).
   b. Frequent small feedings are better tolerated than large feedings in infants.

Table 27–2. **Increasing Caloric Density of Feedings**

---

1. Human milk fortifier (Enfamil, Mead Johnson), 1 packet per 25 mL of breast milk = 24 kcal/oz
2. Formula concentration to 24 kcal/oz by:
   a. 1 cup powdered formula + 3 cups water or
   b. 4 oz ready-to-feed + ½ scoop powdered formula
3. Supplementation of formula to 26–30 kcal/oz is accomplished in the following manner.
   a. Fat modular products
      1). Medium-chain triglycerides (MCT) oil (Mead Johnson), 8 kcal/mL
      2). Microlipid (safflower oil emulsion, Mead Johnson), 4.5 kcal/mL
   b. Low-osmolality polymers
      1). Polycose (Ross), 23 kcal/tablespoon
      2). Moducal (Mead Johnson), 30 kcal/tablespoon
4. PediaSure (Ross), 30 kcal/oz ready-to-feed (for children over 1 yr of age)

From Wright GE, Rochini AP: Primary and general care of the child with congenital heart disease. ACC Curr J Rev Mar/Apr:89–93, 2002.

c. If oral feedings are not well tolerated, intermittent or continuous nasogastric (NG) feeding is indicated. To promote normal development of oral-motor function, infants may be allowed to take calorie-dense oral feeds throughout the day and then be given continuous NG feeds overnight.

d. Salt restriction in the form of a low-salt formula and severe fluid restriction are not indicated in infants. Use of diuretics has replaced these measures.

e. Parents should be taught proper feeding techniques.

4. In older children, salt restriction (<0.5 g/day) and avoidance of salty snacks (chips, pretzels) and table salt are recommended. Bed rest remains an important component of management. The availability of a television screen and computer games for entertainment ensures bed rest in older children.

5. If respiratory failure accompanies cardiac failure, intubation and positive-pressure ventilation are occasionally required. Respiratory failure usually signifies that surgical intervention will be needed for CHDs when the patient is stabilized.

6. Daily weight measurement is essential in hospitalized patients.

DRUG THERAPY

Three major classes of drugs are commonly used in the treatment of CHF in children: inotropic agents, diuretics, and afterload-reducing agents. Rapid-acting inotropic agents (dopamine, dobutamine) are used in critically or acutely ill infants and children. Diuretics are usually used with inotropic agents. Afterload-reducing agents, such as ACE inhibitors, have gained popularity because they can increase cardiac output without increasing myocardial oxygen consumption. Recently, low-dose β-adrenergic blockade has been added to the treatment of dilated cardiomyopathy with encouraging results.

Diuretics. Diuretics remain the principal therapeutic agent to control pulmonary and systemic venous congestion. Diuretics reduce preload and improve congestive symptoms but do not improve cardiac output or myocardial contractility (Fig. 27–1). Patients with mild CHF may improve rapidly after a dose of fast-acting diuretics, such as ethacrynic acid or furosemide, even before digitalization. Table 27–3 shows dosages of commonly available diuretic preparations. There are three main classes of diuretics that are commercially available.

1. Thiazide diuretics (e.g., chlorothiazide, hydrochlorothiazide), which act at the proximal and distal tubules, are no longer popular.

2. Rapid-acting diuretics, such as furosemide and ethacrynic acid, are the drugs of choice. They act primarily at the loop of Henle ("loop diuretics").

3. Aldosterone antagonists (such as spironolactone) act on the distal tubule to inhibit sodium-potassium exchange. The serum aldosterone level is significantly increased in patients with persistent CHF, contributing to fluid and salt retention. Patients with an increased level of circulating aldosterone have a diminished response to diuretic agents because aldosterone increases tubular reabsorption of sodium and water at a site distal to the sites of action of other diuretic agents (thiazides or furosemide). These drugs have value in preventing hypokalemia produced by other diuretics and thus are used in conjunction with a loop diuretic. However, when ACE inhibitors are used, spironolactone should be discontinued to avoid hyperkalemia.

Side Effects of Diuretic Therapy. Diuretic therapy alters the serum electrolytes and acid-base equilibrium.

1. Hypokalemia is a common problem with diuretic therapy, except when used with spironolactone. It is more profound with potent loop diuretics. Hypokalemia may increase the likelihood of digitalis toxicity.

2. Hypochloremic alkalosis may result because the loss of chloride ions is greater than the loss of sodium ions through the kidneys, with a resultant increase in bicarbonate levels. Alkalosis also predisposes to digitalis toxicity.

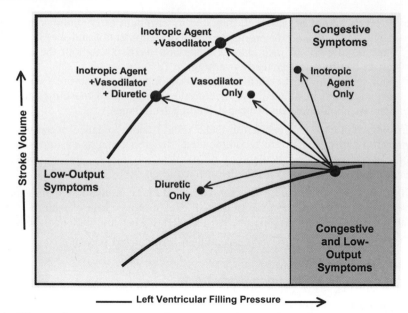

Figure 27–1. *Effects of anticongestive medications on the Frank-Starling relationship for ventricular function. In persons with a normal heart, cardiac output increases as a function of ventricular filling pressure (upper curve). In patients with heart failure, the normal relationship between cardiac output (or stroke volume) and filling pressure (preload) is shifted lower and to the right such that a low-output state and congestive symptoms may coincide. Congestive symptoms (dyspnea, tachypnea) may appear even in a normal heart if the filling pressure reaches a certain point. At one extreme, the addition of a pure inotropic agent, such as digoxin, primarily increases the stroke volume with minimal impact on filling pressure (so that the patient may still have congestive symptoms). Conversely, the addition of a diuretic primarily decreases the filling pressure (with improved congestive symptoms) but without improving cardiac output. Clinically, it is common to use multiple classes of agents (usually a combination of inotropic agents, diuretics, and vasodilators) to produce both increased cardiac output and decreased filling pressure. (Adapted from Cohn JN, Franciosa JS: Vasodilator therapy of cardiac failure [first of two parts]. N Engl J Med 297:27–31, 1977.)*

Rapidly Acting Inotropic Agents. In critically ill infants with CHF, in those with renal dysfunction (such as infants with coarctation of the aorta), or in postoperative cardiac patients with heart failure, rapidly acting catecholamines with a short duration of action are preferable to digoxin. This class of agents includes dopamine, dobutamine, isoproterenol, and epinephrine. These agents possess inotropic and vasodilator actions and thus are useful in acute situations. Inotropic agents increase the contractile property

*Table 27–3. **Diuretic Agents and Dosages***

Preparation	Route	Dosage
Thiazide Diuretics		
Chlorothiazide (Diuril)	Oral	20–40 mg/kg/day in 2–3 divided doses
Hydrochlorothiazide (HydroDIURIL)	Oral	2–4 mg/kg/day in 2–3 divided doses
Loop Diuretics		
Furosemide (Lasix)	IV	1 mg/kg/dose
	Oral	2–3 mg/kg/day in 2–3 divided doses
Ethacrynic acid (Edecrin)	IV	1 mg/kg/dose
	Oral	2–3 mg/kg/day in 2–3 divided doses
Aldosterone Antagonist		
Spironolactone (Aldactone)	Oral	1–3 mg/kg/day in 2–3 divided doses

of the myocardium toward the normal curve (see Fig. 27–1). There is an added beneficial effect when an inotropic agent has vasodilating action as in dopamine. Dobutamine has less chronotropic effects than dopamine. Dopamine in high doses causes α-receptor stimulation with vasoconstriction and reduction of renal blood flow. Dosages for intravenous drip of these catecholamines are suggested in Table 27–4.

Amrinone is a noncatecholamine agent that exerts its inotropic effect and vasodilator effects by inhibiting phosphodiesterase. Thrombocytopenia is a side effect; the drug should be discontinued if the platelet count falls below 150,000/mm^3. Amrinone is useful in patients with severe CHF (dilated cardiomyopathy) who have received prolonged treatment with β-stimulants (see Appendix E, Table E–2 for dosage).

Digitalis Glycosides

Dosage of Digoxin. Digoxin is the most commonly used digitalis preparation in pediatric patients. Inotropic agents increase the cardiac output (or contractile state of the myocardium), resulting in an upward and leftward shift of the ventricular function curve relating cardiac output to filling volume of pressure (see Fig. 27–1). When inotropic agents are used with a vasodilator or a diuretic, a much greater improvement is seen both in the contractile state and in congestive symptoms than when a single class of agent is used (see Fig. 27–1).

Use of digoxin in infants with large left-to-right shunt lesions (such as large VSD) is controversial because ventricular contractility is normal in this situation. However, studies have shown that digoxin improves symptoms in these infants, perhaps because of other actions of digoxin. Digoxin also has parasympathomimetic action with slowing of heart rate and inhibition of atrioventricular (AV) conduction. Digoxin is a diuretic agent as well. Therefore, most cardiologists favor the use of digoxin in infants with CHF from large-shunt lesions.

The total digitalizing dose and maintenance dosage of digoxin by oral and intravenous routes are shown in Table 27–5. A high dose may be needed in treating SVT, in which the goal of treatment is to delay AV conduction. The maintenance dose is more closely related to the serum digoxin level than the digitalizing dose, which is given to build a sufficient body store of the drug and to shorten the time required to reach the pharmacokinetic steady state.

The pediatric dosage of digoxin is much larger than the adult dosage on the basis of body weight. Pharmacokinetic studies indicate that infants and children require a larger dose of digoxin than adults to attain comparable serum levels, primarily because of a larger volume of distribution and, less important, more rapid renal clearance, including tubular secretion. The volume of distribution of digoxin is 7.5 L/kg in neonates, 16 L/kg in infants and children, and 4 L/kg in adults.

How to Digitalize. Loading doses of the total digitalizing dose are given over 12 to 18 hours, followed by maintenance doses. This results in a pharmacokinetic steady state in 3 to 5 days. The intravenous route is preferred over the oral route, particularly when

Table 27–4. Suggested Starting Dosages of Catecholamines

Drug	Dosage and Route	Side Effects
Epinephrine (Adrenalin)	0.1–1 µg/kg/min IV	Hypertension, arrhythmias
Isoproterenol (Isuprel)	0.1–0.5 µg/kg/min IV	Peripheral and pulmonary vasodilatation
Dobutamine (Dobutrex)	2–8 µg/kg/min IV	Less tachycardia than with dopamine, vasodilatation, arrhythmias
Dopamine (Intropin)	5–10 µg/kg/min IV	Tachycardia, arrhythmias, hypertension or hypotension Dose-related cardiovascular effects (µg/kg/min): Renal vasodilatation: 2–5 Inotropic: 5–8 Tachycardia: >8 Mild vasoconstriction: >10 Vasoconstriction: 15–20

Table 27–5. **Oral Digoxin Dosage for Congestive Heart Failure**

Age	Total Digitalizing Dose (μg/kg)	Maintenance Dose* (μg/kg/day)
Prematures	20	5
Newborns	30	8
<2 yr	40–50	10–12
>2 yr	30–40	8–10

*The maintenance dose is 25% of the total digitalizing dose in two divided doses. The IV dose is 75% of the oral dose.
Adapted from Park MK: The use of digoxin in infants and children with specific emphasis on dosage. J Pediatr 108:871–877, 1986.

dealing with infants in severe heart failure. The intramuscular route is not recommended because absorption of the drug from the injection site is unreliable. When an infant is in mild heart failure, the maintenance dose may be administered orally without loading doses; this results in a steady state in 5 to 8 days.

The following is a suggested step-by-step method of digitalization:

1. Obtain a baseline ECG (rhythm and PR interval) and baseline levels of serum electrolytes. Changes in ECG rhythm and PR interval are important signs of digitalis toxicity (see later discussion). Hypokalemia and hypercalcemia predispose to digitalis toxicity.

2. Calculate the total digitalizing dose (see Table 27–5).

3. Give one half the total digitalizing dose immediately, followed by one fourth and then the final one fourth of the total digitalizing dose at 6- to 8-hour intervals.

4. Start the maintenance dose 12 hours after the final total digitalizing dose. Obtaining an ECG strip before starting the maintenance dose is advised.

Monitoring for Digitalis Toxicity by ECG. Digitalis toxicity is best detected by monitoring with ECGs, not serum digoxin levels, during the first 3 to 5 days after digitalization. Box 27–1 lists ECG signs of digitalis effects and toxicity. In general, the digitalis

BOX 27–1	ECG CHANGES ASSOCIATED WITH DIGITALIS

EFFECTS

Shortening of QTc, the earliest sign of digitalis effect
Sagging ST segment and diminished amplitude of T wave (the T vector does not change)
Slowing of heart rate

TOXICITY

Prolongation of PR interval: sometimes a prolonged PR interval is seen in children without digitalis, making a baseline ECG mandatory; the prolongation may progress to second-degree AV block
    Profound sinus bradycardia or sinoatrial block
    Supraventricular arrhythmias, such as atrial or nodal ectopic beats and tachycardias (particularly if accompanied by AV block), which are more common than ventricular arrhythmias in children
    Ventricular arrhythmias such as ventricular bigeminy and trigeminy, which are extremely rare in children, although they are common in adults with digitalis toxicity; isolated premature ventricular contractions, which are not uncommon in children, are a sign of toxicity

effect is confined to *ventricular repolarization*, whereas toxicity involves disturbances in the *formation and conduction of the impulse*. One should assume that any arrhythmia or conduction disturbance occurring *with* digitalis is *caused by* digitalis until proved otherwise.

Serum Digoxin Levels. Therapeutic ranges of serum digoxin levels for treating CHF are 0.8 to 2 ng/mL. Levels obtained during the first 3 to 5 days after digitalization tend to be higher than those obtained when the pharmacokinetic steady state is reached. Blood for serum digoxin levels should be drawn at least 6 hours after the last dose or just before a scheduled dose; samples obtained earlier than 6 hours after the last dose give a falsely elevated level.

Determining serum digoxin levels frequently and using those levels for therapeutic goals are neither justified nor practical; occasional determination of the levels is adequate. Determination of the serum digoxin levels is useful in evaluating possible toxicity (see later section), determining the patient's compliance, and detecting abnormalities in absorption and excretion, and is mandatory in managing accidental overdoses.

Serum digoxin levels may be elevated when digoxin is administered concomitantly with other drugs such as quinidine, verapamil, amiodarone, β-blockers, tetracycline, and erythromycin. Lower serum levels have been noted with rifampin, kaolin-pectin, neomycin, and cholestyramine.

Digitalis Toxicity. Digitalis toxicity may result during treatment with digoxin or from an accidental overdose of digoxin. With the relatively low dosage recommended in Table 27–5, digitalis toxicity is unlikely to develop. However, one should beware of possible digitalis toxicity in every child receiving digitalis preparations. Patients with conditions listed in Box 27–2 are more likely to develop toxicity. The diagnosis of digitalis toxicity is a clinical decision and is usually based on the following clinical and laboratory findings:

1. The patient has a history of accidental ingestion.

2. Noncardiac symptoms appear in digitalized children: anorexia, nausea, vomiting, diarrhea, restlessness, drowsiness, fatigue, and visual disturbances in older children.

3. Heart failure worsens.

BOX 27–2	**FACTORS THAT MAY PREDISPOSE TO DIGITALIS TOXICITY**

HIGH SERUM DIGOXIN LEVEL

High-dose requirement, as in treatment of certain arrhythmias
Decreased renal excretion
    Premature infants
    Renal disease
Hypothyroidism
Drug interaction (e.g., quinidine, verapamil, amiodarone)

INCREASED SENSITIVITY OF MYOCARDIUM (WITHOUT HIGH SERUM DIGOXIN LEVEL)

Status of myocardium
    Myocardial ischemia
    Myocarditis (rheumatic, viral)
Systemic changes
    Electrolyte imbalance (hypokalemia, hypercalcemia)
    Hypoxia
    Alkalosis
    Adrenergic stimuli or catecholamines
    Immediate postoperative period after heart surgery under cardiopulmonary bypass

4. ECG signs are probably more reliable and appear early (see Box 27–1).

5. An elevated serum level of digoxin (>2 mg/mL) is likely to be associated with toxicity in a child if the clinical findings suggest digitalis toxicity.

Afterload-Reducing Agents. Vasoconstriction that occurs as a compensatory response to reduced cardiac output seen in CHF may be deleterious to the failing ventricle. Vasoconstriction is produced by a rise in sympathetic tone and circulating catecholamines and an increase in the activity of the renin-angiotensin system. Reducing afterload tends to augment the stroke volume without a great change in the contractile state of the heart and therefore without increasing myocardial oxygen consumption (see Fig. 27–1). When a vasodilator is used with an inotropic agent, the degree of improvement in the inotropic state as well as in congestive symptoms is much greater than when a vasodilator alone is used. Combined use of an inotropic agent, a vasodilator, and a diuretic produces most improvement in both inotropic state and congestive symptoms (see Fig. 27–1).

Afterload-reducing agents now occupy a prominent role in the treatment of infants with CHF secondary to large left-to-right shunt lesions (e.g., VSD, AV canal, PDA). Infants with large left-to-right shunts have been shown to benefit from captopril and hydralazine. Beneficial effects of afterload-reducing agents are also seen in dilated cardiomyopathy, doxorubicin(Adriamycin)-induced cardiomyopathy, myocardial ischemia, postoperative cardiac status, severe MR or AR, and systemic hypertension. These agents are usually used in conjunction with digitalis glycosides and diuretics for a maximal benefit.

Afterload-reducing agents may be divided into three groups based on the site of action: arteriolar vasodilators, venodilators, and mixed vasodilators. Dosages of these agents are presented in Table 27–6.

1. Arteriolar vasodilators (hydralazine) augment cardiac output by acting primarily on the arteriolar bed, with resulting reduction of the afterload. Hydralazine is often administered with propranolol because it activates the baroreceptor reflex, with resulting tachycardia.

2. Venodilators (nitroglycerin, isosorbide dinitrate) act primarily by dilating systemic veins and redistributing blood from the pulmonary to the systemic circuit (with a resulting decrease in pulmonary symptoms). Venodilators are most beneficial in patients with pulmonary congestion but may have adverse effects when preload has been restored to normal by diuretics or sodium restriction.

3. Mixed vasodilators include ACE inhibitors (captopril, enalapril), nitroprusside, and prazosin. These agents act on both arteriolar and venous beds. ACE inhibitors are

*Table 27–6. **Dosages of Vasodilators***

Drug	Route and Dosage	Comments
Hydralazine (Apresoline)	IV: 0.1–0.2 mg/kg/dose, every 4–6 hr (maximum 2 mg/kg every 6 hr)	May cause tachycardia; may be used with propranolol
	Oral: 0.75–3 mg/kg/day, in 2–4 doses (maximum 200 mg/day)	May cause gastrointestinal symptoms, neutropenia, and lupus-like syndrome
Nitroglycerin	IV: 0.5–2 μg/kg/min (maximum 6 μg/kg/min)	Start with small dose and titrate based on effects
Captopril (Capoten)	Oral: Newborn: 0.1–0.4 mg/kg/dose, 1–4 times a day	May cause hypotension, dizziness, neutropenia, and proteinuria
	Infant: 0.5–6 mg/kg/day, 1–4 times a day	Dose should be reduced in patients with
	Child: 12.5 mg/dose, 1–2 times a day	impaired renal function
Enalapril (Vasotec)	Oral: 0.1 mg/kg, once or twice daily	Patient may develop hypotension, dizziness, or syncope
Nitroprusside (Nipride)	IV: 0.5–8 μg/kg/min	May cause thiocyanate or cyanide toxicity (e.g., fatigue, nausea, disorientation), hepatic dysfunction, or light sensitivity
Prazosin (Minipress)	Oral: first dose, 5 μg/kg; increase to 25–150 μg/kg/day in 4 doses	Has fewer side effects than hydralazine; orthostatic hypotension or tachyphylaxis may develop

popular in children with chronic severe CHF, whereas sodium nitroprusside is used primarily in acute situations such as following cardiac surgery under cardiopulmonary bypass, especially in patients who had pulmonary hypertension and those with postoperative rises in PA pressure. When nitroprusside is used, blood pressure must be monitored continuously. ACE inhibitors reduce systemic vascular resistance by inhibiting angiotensin II generation and augmenting production of bradykinin.

OTHER DRUGS

β-Adrenergic Blockers. As with their beneficial effects reported in adult patients with dilated cardiomyopathy, β-adrenergic blockers have been shown to be beneficial in some pediatric patients with chronic CHF who were symptomatic despite being treated with standard anticongestive drugs (digoxin, diuretics, ACE inhibitors). Recent evidence suggests that the adrenergic overstimulation often seen in patients with chronic CHF may have detrimental effects on the hemodynamics of heart failure by inducing myocyte injury and necrosis rather than being a compensatory mechanism, as traditionally thought. β-Adrenergic blockers should not be given to those with decompensated heart failure. They should be deferred until reestablishment of good fluid balance and stable blood pressure and should be started with a small dose and gradually increased.

Carvedilol, a nonselective β-adrenergic blocker with additional α_1-antagonist activities, when added to standard medical therapy for CHF, has been shown to be beneficial in children with dilated cardiomyopathy (Bruns et al, 2001). The patients included in the study were those with idiopathic dilated cardiomyopathy, chemotherapy-induced cardiomyopathy, postmyocarditis myopathy, and muscular dystrophy and those who had chronic heart failure following surgeries for congenital heart defects (such as a Fontan or Senning operation). The initial dose was 0.09 mg/kg twice daily and the dose was increased gradually to 0.36 and 0.75 mg/kg as tolerated, up to the maximum adult dose of 50 mg/day. Side effects of the drug include dizziness, hypotension, and headache (also see Dilated Cardiomyopathy).

Metoprolol was added to standard anticongestive medicines in patients with chronic CHF from dilated cardiomyopathy. Metoprolol increased LV fractional shortening and ejection fraction and improved symptoms. The starting dose was 0.1 to 0.2 mg/kg per dose twice a day and was slowly increased over a period of weeks to 1.1 mg/kg/day (range 0.5 to 2.3 mg/kg/day) (Shaddy et al, 1999). The improvement in the LV fractional shortening appears slightly better with carvedilol than with metoprolol.

Beneficial effects of propranolol added to conventional treatment for CHF were reported in a small number of infants with large left-to-right shunts and severe CHF in whom conventional therapy had failed. Propranolol (1.6 mg/kg/day) decreased respiratory and heart rates and improved symptoms of CHF. Plasma renin, aldosterone, and norepinephrine levels also decreased significantly.

Carnitine. Carnitine, which is an essential cofactor for transport of long-chain fatty acids into mitochondria for oxidation, has been shown to be beneficial in some cases of cardiomyopathy, especially those with suggestive evidence of disorders of metabolism (Helton et al, 2000). Most of these patients had dilated cardiomyopathy. The dosage of L-carnitine was 50 to 100 mg/kg/day, given twice or three times a day orally (maximum daily dose 3 g). It improved myocardial function, reduced cardiomegaly, and improved muscle weakness. Animal studies suggest potential protective and therapeutic effects on doxorubicin-induced cardiomyopathy in rats.

SURGICAL MANAGEMENT

If medical treatment with the previously mentioned regimens does not improve CHF caused by congenital heart defects within a few weeks to months, one should consider either palliative or corrective cardiac surgery for the underlying cardiac defect when technically feasible.

Cardiac transplantation is an option for a patient with progressively deteriorating cardiomyopathy despite maximal medical treatment.

Chapter 28

Systemic Hypertension

Definition

For adults, the Seventh Report of the Joint National Committee on Prevention, Detection, Evaluation, and Treatment of High Blood Pressure (Chobanian et al, 2003) has recommended the following classification. A blood pressure (BP) level of 120/80 mm Hg, previously considered normal, is now classified as prehypertension and levels lower than 120/80 are now considered normal. Hypertension is further classified as stage 1 and stage 2 depending on the level of abnormalities (Table 28–1).

In children, hypertension is defined statistically because BP levels vary with age and gender and because outcome-based data are not available for this population. The Fourth Report of the National High Blood Pressure Education Program (NHBPEP) Working Group on High Blood Pressure in Children and Adolescents (2004) has recommended the following definitions (also see Table 28–1).

1. *Hypertension* is defined as systolic and/or diastolic pressure levels that are greater than the 95th percentile for age and gender on at least three occasions. As with adults, adolescents with BP levels ≥120/80 mm Hg are considered hypertensive even if they are less than the 95th percentile.

2. *Prehypertension* is defined as an average systolic and/or diastolic pressure between the 90th and 95th percentiles for age and gender.

Table 28–1. **Classification of Blood Pressure for Adults and Children**

BP Classification	Adults		Children and Adolescents*
	Systolic BP	**Diastolic BP**	
Normal	<120	<80	<90th percentile
Prehypertension	120–139	80–89	90th–95th percentile
Stage 1 hypertension	140–159	90–99	95th–99th percentile
Stage 2 hypertension	≥160	≥100	≥5 mm Hg + 99th percentile value

BP, blood pressure.

*Pediatric classification is according to the Fourth Report on the Diagnosis, Evaluation, and Treatment of High Blood Pressure in Children and Adolescents. Pediatrics 111:555–576, 2004.

Adapted from Chobanian AV, Bakris GL, Black HR, et al: The Seventh Report of the Joint National Committee on Prevention, Detection, Evaluation, and Treatment of High Blood Pressure: The JNC 7 report. JAMA 289:2560–2572, 2003.

3. When the BP reading is above the 95th percentile, one could further classify the hypertension into stages 1 and 2 as follows:

   a. Stage 1 hypertension is present when BP readings are between the 95th and 99th percentiles.

   b. Stage 2 hypertension is present when BP readings are 5 mm Hg or more above the 99th percentile values.

4. *"White-coat hypertension"* is present when BP readings in health care facilities are greater than the 95th percentile but are normotensive outside a clinical setting.

A prerequisite for the pediatric definitions is the availability of reliable normative BP standards, but there are no such normal standards. The BP tables recommended by the Working Group of the NHBPEP are not acceptable standards because they are statistically and logically unsound and not evidence-based, besides being impractical (see "Blood Pressure Measurement" in Chapter 2 for further discussion).

Normative Blood Pressure Standards

Many well-conducted epidemiologic studies have provided data on the normal distribution of BP levels in children determined by the auscultatory method. A comparison of these observations reveals a wide variation in BP values. The differences between the highest and lowest mean BP levels (Fig. 28–1) as well as differences in the "95th percentile systolic pressure" among these national studies are as much as 30 mm Hg for certain age groups. The implications of this are profound. For example, a child who is considered to have borderline hypertension based on one set of normative values may be in the hypertensive range based on other normative values.

The main reason for this discrepancy is probably the methodology used, such as the selection of the occluding cuff, the position of the patient (supine or sitting), the number of measurements made (single or multiple), and the choice of diastolic signal (phase 4 or 5 Korotkoff sounds). The width of the BP cuff for children has traditionally been based on the length of the upper arm, which is scientifically unsound. Even though the physical principle of using an occluding cuff was well established almost 100 years ago, two National Institutes of Health task forces (1977 and 1987) have recommended unscientific methods and thereby delayed the establishment of scientifically correct normative BP standards for children for several decades.

For adults, the BP cuff width has been based on the circumference of the arm since the American Heart Association recommendation of 1951. With this cuff selection method, indirect systolic pressure readings have been shown to correlate well with direct arterial pressure measurements. More recently, for children, two national committees, the American Heart Association and the Working Group of the NHBPEP (1996 and 2004), correctly recommended that the cuff width be 40% to 50% of the arm circumference. The NHBEP Working Group has recommended Korotkoff phase 5 (K5) as the diastolic signal, which is debatable. Earlier studies and national committees had recommended K4 as the diastolic pressure for children up to 12 years of age and K5 for children 13 years of age or older. In addition, the normative BP standards recommended by the Working Groups of NHBPEP (2004) are not acceptable for several reasons (Park, 2005). This aspect has been discussed in some detail under "Blood Pressure Measurement" in Chapter 2. Acceptable normative BP standards should have been developed by currently acceptable methodology.

1. For the auscultatory method, normative BP standards derived from the San Antonio Children's Blood Pressure Study shown in Chapter 2 (and in Tables B–3 and B–4, Appendix B) are the best alternative standards available at this time.

2. For the oscillometric method, normative BP standards from the San Antonio Study are available (Park et al, 2005).

   Readers should be aware that BP readings obtained by some models such as Dinamap Monitor model 8100 are not interchangeable with those obtained by the auscultatory method because Dinamap readings were on average 10 mm Hg higher

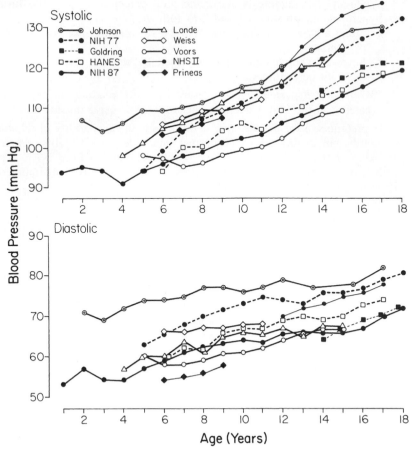

Figure 28–1. *Comparison of normative blood pressure levels reported by various epidemiologic studies. Mean (or 50th percentile) values of indirect blood pressure measurements of boys from 10 large epidemiologic surveys are shown for comparison. When racial differences are present, values for white children have been illustrated. Selection of the occluding cuff and diastolic signals varies from study to study. Note that a difference of more than 20 mm Hg exists between the highest and the lowest values for certain age groups for both systolic and diastolic pressures. Similar differences are present for 95th percentile values.*

for the systolic pressure and 5 mm Hg higher for the diastolic pressure than values obtained by the auscultatory method.

a. Dinamap-specific normative BP data for children 5 to 17 years old are presented in Tables B–6 and B–7, Appendix B.

b. Normative oscillometric BP levels for neonates and small children in the first 5 years of life are presented in Table 2–4 (and more detailed data in Table B–5, Appendix B). These normative oscillometric BP data were obtained in an office setting using the currently recommended cuff selection method, and the values are averages of three readings.

Causes

Hypertension is classified into two general types: essential (or primary) hypertension, in which a specific cause cannot be identified, and secondary hypertension, in which a cause can be identified (Box 28–1). The incidence of essential hypertension in children and adolescents is not known. However, more than 90% of secondary hypertension in nonobese children is caused by three conditions: renal parenchymal disease, renal artery disease, and coarctation of the aorta (COA). The most common cause of hypertension appears to be overweight: about 10% to 30% of overweight children are reported to have high BP. With the prevalence of obesity increased, overweight and obesity may be the most common cause of pediatric hypertension.

Table 28–2 lists the common causes of hypertension by age group in children. In general, the younger the child and the more severe the hypertension, the more likely that an underlying cause can be identified.

Diagnosis and Workup

Diagnosis of hypertension relies on accurate BP measurement and comparing the reading with reliable BP standards. If an abnormal reading was a single reading, two additional measurements should be made. If the reading is still high, a repeated set of three readings at the end of the office visit may help identify children with white-coat hypertension. Even if these readings are still high, the diagnosis of hypertension should not be made until one confirms persistently elevated BP levels at least on three consecutive office visits. Multiple BP readings outside health care facilities, such as those taken by school nurses, may be helpful in ruling out white-coat hypertension as well as in deciding whether to treat hypertension.

Careful evaluation of the history, physical findings, and laboratory tests usually points to the cause of hypertension. Evaluation of the hypertensive child should include assessment of additional risk factors. Currently recognized cardiovascular risk factors include the following:

1. Family history of premature coronary artery disease, cerebrovascular accident, or occlusive peripheral vascular disease (with onset before age 55 for men and 65 for women in parents or grandparents)

2. Hypercholesterolemia

3. Low levels of high-density lipoproteinuria (<40 mg/100 mL)

4. Cigarette smoking

5. Diabetes mellitus

6. Physical inactivity

Many children with mild hypertension are asymptomatic, and hypertension is diagnosed through routine BP measurement, highlighting the importance of accurate measurement of BP. Children with acute severe hypertension may be symptomatic (headache, dizziness, nausea and vomiting, irritability, personality changes). Occasionally, neurologic manifestations, congestive heart failure, renal dysfunction, and stroke may be the presenting symptoms. A prompt referral to an appropriate subspecialist should be made if the patient is symptomatic, has neurologic manifestations, or has stage 2 hypertension.

HISTORY

The past and present medical history and the family history are gathered.

Past and Current History

1. Neonatal: use of umbilical artery catheters or bronchopulmonary dysplasia

2. Cardiovascular: history of COA or surgery for it; history of palpitation, headache, and excessive sweating (excessive catecholamine levels)

3. Renal: history of obstructive uropathies, urinary tract infection, and radiation, trauma, or surgery to the kidney area

4. Endocrine: weakness and muscle cramps (hypokalemia seen with hyperaldosteronism)

5. Medications: corticosteroids, amphetamines, antiasthmatic drugs, cold medications, oral contraceptives, nephrotoxic antibiotics, cyclosporin, cocaine use; also, ingestion of large quantity of licorice

6. Habits: smoking

BOX 28–1	CAUSES OF SECONDARY HYPERTENSION

RENAL

Renal parenchymal disease
    Glomerulonephritis, acute and chronic
    Pyelonephritis, acute and chronic
    Congenital anomalies (polycystic or dysplastic kidneys)
    Obstructive uropathies (hydronephrosis)
    Hemolytic-uremic syndrome
    Collagen disease (periarteritis, lupus)
    Renal damage from nephrotoxic medications, trauma, or radiation
Renovascular disease
    Renal artery disorders (e.g., stenosis, polyarteritis, thrombosis)
    Renal vein thrombosis

CARDIOVASCULAR

Coarctation of the aorta
Conditions with large stroke volume (patent ductus arteriosus, aortic insufficiency, systemic arteriovenous fistula, complete heart block) (these conditions cause only systolic hypertension)

ENDOCRINE

Hyperthyroidism (systolic hypertension)
Excessive catecholamine levels
    Pheochromocytoma
    Neuroblastoma
Adrenal dysfunction
    Congenital adrenal hyperplasia
        11-β-Hydroxylase deficiency
        17-Hydroxylase deficiency
    Cushing's syndrome
    Hyperaldosteronism
        Primary
            Conn's syndrome
            Idiopathic nodular hyperplasia
            Dexamethasone-suppressible hyperaldosteronism
        Secondary
            Renovascular hypertension
            Renin-producing tumor (juxtaglomerular cell tumor)
Hyperparathyroidism (and hypercalcemia)

NEUROGENIC

Increased intracranial pressure (any cause, especially tumors, infections, trauma)
Poliomyelitis
Guillain-Barré syndrome
Dysautonomia (Riley-Day syndrome)

DRUGS AND CHEMICALS

Sympathomimetic drugs (nose drops, cough medications, cold preparations, theophylline)
Amphetamines
Steroids
Nonsteroidal anti-inflammatory drugs
Oral contraceptives
Heavy-metal poisoning (mercury, lead)
Cocaine, acute or chronic use
Cyclosporine

MISCELLANEOUS

Hypervolemia and hypernatremia
Stevens-Johnson syndrome
Bronchopulmonary dysplasia (newborns)

Table 28–2. **Common Causes of Chronic Sustained Hypertension**

Age Group	Causes
Newborns	Renal artery thrombosis, renal artery stenosis, congenital renal malformation, COA, bronchopulmonary dysplasia
<6 yr	Renal parenchymal disease, COA, renal artery stenosis
6–10 yr	Renal artery stenosis, renal parenchymal disease, primary hypertension
>10 yr	Primary hypertension, renal parenchymal disease

COA, coarctation of the aorta.
Adapted from Report of the Second Task Force on Blood Pressure Control in Children. Pediatrics 79:1–25, 1987.

Family History

1. Essential hypertension, atherosclerotic heart disease, and stroke
2. Familial or hereditary renal disease (polycystic kidney, cystinuria, familial nephritis)

PHYSICAL EXAMINATION

1. Accurate measurement of BP is essential.
2. Complete physical examination is also essential, with emphasis on delayed growth (renal disease), bounding peripheral pulse (patent ductus arteriosus or aortic regurgitation), weak or absent femoral pulses or BP differential between the arms and legs (COA), abdominal bruits (renovascular), and tenderness over the kidney (renal infection).
3. Children's weight status, including body mass index percentile, should be obtained because overweight is a common cause of hypertension.

ROUTINE LABORATORY TESTS

Initial laboratory tests should be directed toward detecting renal parenchymal disease, renovascular disease, and COA and therefore should include urinalysis; urine culture; serum electrolyte, blood urea nitrogen, creatinine, and uric acid levels; ECG; chest x-ray studies; and possibly echo (Table 28–3). Uric acid level has been reported to be directly correlated with systolic and diastolic BP levels, raising the possibility that it might have a role in the pathogenesis of primary (essential) hypertension (Feig et al, 2003). A serum uric acid level greater than 5.5 mg/dL was found in 89% of subjects with primary hypertension, 30% of children with secondary hypertension, and no subjects with white-coat hypertension and normal control subjects. When overweight is the likely cause of hypertension, metabolic aspects of risk factors should be checked.

SPECIALIZED STUDIES

More specialized studies may be indicated for the detection of rare causes of secondary hypertension: excretory urography, plasma renin activity, aldosterone levels in serum and urine, 24-hour urine collection for catecholamine levels (norepinephrine, epinephrine) and their metabolites (vanillylmandelic acid levels), renal vein renin, and abdominal aortogram.

Table 28–3 summarizes the applicability of routine and specialized tests in identifying the cause of secondary hypertension. The decision to undertake special tests and procedures depends on availability of and familiarity with the procedure, severity of hypertension, age of the patient, and history and physical findings suggestive of a certain cause. For example, children younger than 10 years with sustained hypertension require extensive evaluation because identifiable and potentially curable causes are more likely to be found. Adolescents with mild hypertension and a positive family history of essential hypertension are more likely to have essential hypertension, and extensive studies are not indicated.

In patients suspected of having renal pathology, renal sonography provides a comparison of kidney sizes and a view of the anatomy of the collecting system. A radionuclide scan is helpful in distinguishing variation in perfusion or scarring of the two kidneys. Renal Doppler ultrasound and angiography may demonstrate lesions in the main arteries or in the segmental branches.

Table 28–3. **Routine and Special Laboratory Tests and Their Significance**

Laboratory Test	Significance
Urinalysis, urine culture, blood urea nitrogen, creatinine, uric acid	Renal parenchymal disease
Serum electrolytes (hypokalemia)	Hyperaldosteronism (primary or secondary) Adrenogenital syndrome Renin-producing tumors
ECG, chest x-ray studies, and possibly echocardiography	Cardiac cause of hypertension; also baseline function
Intravenous pyelogram (or ultrasonography, radionuclide studies, computed tomography, or magnetic resonance imaging of the kidneys)	Renal parenchymal disease Renovascular hypertension Tumors (neuroblastoma, Wilms' tumor)
Plasma renin activity (peripheral)	High-renin hypertension (renovascular hypertension, renin-producing tumors, some Cushing's syndrome, some essential hypertension) Low-renin hypertension (adrenogenital syndrome, primary hyperaldosteronism)
24-hr urine collection for 17-ketosteroid and 17-hydroxycorticosteroids	Cushing's syndrome Adrenogenital syndrome
24-hr urine collection for catecholamine levels and vanillylmandelic acid	Pheochromocytoma Neuroblastoma
Aldosterone	Hyperaldosteronism (primary or secondary) Renovascular hypertension Renin-producing tumors
Renal vein plasma renin activity	Unilateral renal parenchymal disease Renovascular hypertension
Abdominal aortogram	Renovascular hypertension Abdominal coarctation of the aorta Unilateral renal parenchymal disease Pheochromocytoma
Intra-arterial digital subtraction angiography	Renovascular hypertension

Management

ESSENTIAL HYPERTENSION

Nonpharmacologic Intervention. Nonpharmacologic intervention should be started as an initial treatment. Counseling should encourage weight reduction, if indicated; low-salt (and potassium-rich) foods; regular aerobic exercise; and avoidance of smoking and oral contraceptives.

Pharmacologic Intervention. Drug therapy is not recommended initially. Drugs are used when a nonpharmacologic approach has not been found to be effective, in part because possible adverse effects of long-term drug therapy on growing children have not been evaluated adequately and because many antihypertensive agents have side effects.

Indications. Although there are no clear guidelines for identifying those who should be treated with antihypertensive drugs, the following are generally considered indications for initiating drug therapy in hypertensive children:

1. Severe symptomatic hypertension, which should be treated with intravenous (IV) antihypertensive medications

2. Significant secondary hypertension, such as that due to renovascular and reno-parenchymal diseases

3. Hypertensive target organ damage

4. Family history of early complications of hypertension

5. Diabetes (types 1 and 2)

6. Child who has dyslipidemia and other coronary artery risk factors

7. Persistent hypertension despite nonpharmacologic measures

The most reliable end-organ damage at this time is the presence of left ventricular hypertrophy (LVH) evidenced by echo studies. However, echocardiographic measurements of LV mass have important limitations and normal values vary from study to study. There are also disagreements about how the values should be indexed: by height, by body surface area, or by the 2.7 power of height in meters. According to one study (Daniels et al, 1988), an LV mass of more than 99.8 g/m or 103 g/m^2 in males 6 to 23 years old indicates LVH. For females the comparable values were 81 g/m or 84.2 g/m^2. Therefore, the thickness of the LV wall measured by M-mode echo could be used instead.

The *choice of drug* for initial antihypertensive therapy resides in the preference of the responsible physician. In adults, most studies found that moderate doses of all classes of drugs provided similar efficacy. Some diuretics and β-adrenergic blockers have a long history of safety and efficacy based on clinical experience, and they remain appropriate for pediatric use. Similarly, some newer antihypertensive agents such as angiotensin-converting enzyme (ACE) inhibitors, calcium channel blockers, and angiotensin receptor blockers appear to be safe and effective.

A popular approach is to initiate therapy with a small dose of a single antihypertensive drug, either a thiazide diuretic or an adrenergic inhibitor, and then proceed to a full dose, if necessary. If the first drug is not effective, a second drug may be added to, or substituted for, the first drug, starting with a small dose and proceeding to a full dose. In many situations, however, more than one drug is needed to control elevated BP. Therefore, a combination of a low-dose thiazide diuretic and the appropriate second choice may logically be used at the onset of therapy. Single daily dosing improves adherence to the medication. Long-acting preparations are available within each class of antihypertensive drugs. If the BP still remains elevated with the combination of two drugs, a third drug, such as an ACE inhibitor or calcium channel blocker, may be added to the regimen. At this point, the possibility of secondary hypertension should be reconsidered. Table 28–4 shows the dosages of commonly used antihypertensive drugs for children.

Specific classes of antihypertensive drugs should be used preferentially in certain children with specific underlying or concurrent medical conditions (Table 28–5). It should be noted that the preferred class of drugs based on race is not very well established and is based on relatively weak studies. There are also differences in recommendations across the Atlantic Ocean as to the drug of choice for initial antihypertensive therapy. Unlike the U.S. national hypertension guidelines, the British National Institute for Health and Clinical Excellence and the British Hypertension Society (Sever, 2006) have recommended against using beta blockers, with or without diuretics, primarily because of their high diabetogenic properties; instead, they recommend ACE inhibitors (or angiotensin II blockers) in younger patients and calcium channel blockers or diuretics for older patients and black patients of any age.

Classes of Antihypertensive Drugs

Diuretics. Diuretics are the cornerstone of antihypertensive drug therapy, except in patients with renal failure. Their action is related initially to a decrease in extracellular and plasma volume and later to a decline in peripheral resistance. The thiazide diuretics (hydrochlorothiazide and chlorthalidone) are most commonly used. An important side effect of diuretic therapy in children is hypokalemia, occasionally requiring potassium supplementation in the diet or potassium salt. One should check serum electrolytes initially and periodically. Diuretics may increase glucose, insulin, and cholesterol levels. Potassium-sparing diuretics (spironolactone, triamterene) may cause hyperkalemia, especially if given with ACE inhibitors or angiotensin receptor blockers.

Adrenergic Inhibitors. Propranolol (Inderal), a β-adrenergic blocker, acts at three important locations: on the juxtaglomerular apparatus of the kidney to suppress the renin-angiotensin system, on the central vasomotor center to decrease systemic vascular resistance, and on the myocardium to suppress contractility. One can judge the adequacy of β-adrenergic blockade by noting the suppression of the increase in heart rate when the patient stands up after a few minutes of recumbency. β-Adrenergic blockers should not be used in insulin-dependent diabetics. Propranolol is contraindicated in patients with asthma. Atenolol (Tenormin) has the advantage of being a longer-acting β-blocker, requiring only a single daily dose.

Angiotensin-Converting Enzyme Inhibitors. Captopril is an ACE inhibitor widely used in the treatment of pediatric hypertension. Enalapril and lisinopril are newer, long-acting ACE inhibitors that have also been shown to be effective in children with hypertension.

Table 28–4. Oral Dosages of Select Antihypertensive Drugs for Children

Drugs	Initial Dose	Times/Day
Diuretics		
Hydrochlorothiazide (HydroDIURIL)	1 mg/kg/day (Max 3 mg/kg/day up to 50 mg/day)	1
Chlorthalidone	0.3 mg/kg/day (Max 2 mg/kg/day up to 50 mg/day)	1
Furosemide (Lasix)	0.5–2 mg/kg/dose (Max 6 mg/kg/day)	1–2
Spironolactone (Aldactone)	1 mg/kg/day (Max 3.3 mg/kg/day up to 100 mg/day	1–2
Triamterene (Dyrenium)	1–2 mg/kg/day (Max 3–4 mg/kg/day up to 300 mg/day)	2
Adrenergic Inhibitors		
Propranolol (Inderal)	1–2 mg/kg/day (Max 4 mg/kg/day up to 640 mg/day)	2–3
Metoprolol (Lopressor)	1–2 mg/kg/day (Max 6 mg/kg/day up to 200 mg/day)	2
Atenolol (Tenormin)	0.5–1 mg/kg/day (Max 2 mg/kg/day up to 100 mg/day)	1–2
Angiotensin-Converting Enzyme Inhibitors		
Captopril (Capoten)	0.3–0.5 mg/kg/dose (Max 6 mg/kg/day)	3
Enalapril (Vasotec)	0.08 mg/kg/day up to 5 mg/day (Max 0.6 mg/kg/day up to 40 mg/day)	1–2
Lisinopril (Zestril, Prinivil)	0.07 mg/kg/day up to 5 mg/day (Max 0.6 mg/kg/day up to 40 mg/day)	1
Angiotensin Receptor Blocker		
Losartan (Cozaar)	0.7 mg/kg/day up to 50 mg/day (Max 1.4 mg/kg/day up to 100 mg/day)	1
Calcium Channel Blockers		
Amlodipine (Norvasc)	6–17 yr: 2.5–5 mg/day	1
Isradipine (DynaCirc)	0.15–0.2 mg/kg/day (Max 0.8 mg/kg/day up to 20 mg/day	3–4
Extended-release nifedipine (Adalat, Procardia)	0.25–0.5 mg/kg/day (Max 3 mg/kg/day up to 120 mg/day)	1–2
Vasodilators, Direct Acting		
Hydralazine (Apresoline)	0.75 mg/kg/day (Max 7.5 mg/kg/day up to 200 mg/day)	4
Minoxidil (Loniten)	>12 yr: 5 mg/day (Max 100 mg/day)	1–3

Adopted from The Fourth Report on the Diagnosis, Evaluation, and Treatment of High Blood Pressure in Children and Adolescents. Pediatrics 114:555–576, 2004.

A diuretic clearly enhances the effectiveness of ACE inhibitors. Side effects of ACE inhibitors include rash, loss of taste, and leukopenia. Occasional side effects include cough and angioedema. If cough appears, an angiotensin receptor blocker may be used. ACE inhibitors are contraindicated in pregnancy. Serum electrolytes and creatinine should be checked for hyperkalemia and azotemia.

Angiotensin receptor blockers are a new class of antihypertensive agents that act by displacing angiotensin II from its receptor, antagonizing all of angiotensin's known effects with a resulting decrease in peripheral resistance. Cough is not a side effect, although angioedema can occur.

Calcium Channel Blockers. Calcium channel blockers are being used increasingly in the treatment of adult hypertension. They have had limited use in the pediatric age group. Nifedipine has the greatest peripheral vasodilatory action, with little effect on cardiac automaticity, conduction, or contractility. Concomitant dietary sodium restriction or the use of a diuretic agent may not be necessary because calcium antagonists cause natriuresis

Table 28–5. **Preferences and Contraindications for the Use of Antihypertensive Drugs**

Class of Drugs	Preferred (Indications)	Contraindicated
Diuretics	Systolic hypertension Asthmatics Blacks?	Gout
β-Adrenergic blockers	Migraine Hyperdynamic hypertension (with rapid pulse rates) Hyperthyroidism Nonblacks?	Diabetes Asthmatics
ACE inhibitors or angiotensin receptor blockers	Diabetes Other nephropathy or proteinuria Nonblacks?	Pregnancy Bilateral renal artery stenosis, or hyperkalemia
Calcium channel blockers	Migraine Blacks?	Heart block

ACE, angiotensin-converting enzyme.
From Kaplan NM: Systemic hypertension: Therapy. In Zipea DP, Libby P, Bonow RO, Braunwald E (eds): Braunwald's Heart Disease, 7th ed. Philadelphia, Elsevier Saunders, 2005, and The Fourth Report on the Diagnosis, Evaluation, and Treatment of High Blood Pressure in Children and Adolescents, Pediatrics 114:555–576, 2004.

by producing renal vasodilatation. The safety and efficacy of amlodipine (Norvasc) have been reported for children with various forms of hypertension (Flynn et al, 2004). Occasional side effects include headache, flushing, and local ankle edema.

Vasodilators. Hydralazine (Apresoline), a direct-acting vasodilator, is popular in the treatment of hypertension in children. When used alone, it produces side effects related to increased cardiac output (flushing, headache, tachycardia, palpitation) and salt retention. Therefore, the concomitant use of a β-adrenergic blocker and a diuretic is recommended. Hydralazine can cause lupus-like syndrome. Minoxidil, a less commonly used vasodilator, can cause hypertrichosis when used on chronic basis.

SECONDARY HYPERTENSION

Treatment of secondary hypertension should be aimed at removing the cause of hypertension whenever possible. Table 28–6 lists curable causes of systemic hypertension.

Cardiovascular Causes. Surgical or catheter interventional correction is indicated for COA and other cardiovascular causes of hypertension.

Renal Parenchymal Disease. In nephritis, medical management should be instituted to lower BP in the same manner as discussed for essential hypertension. Salt restriction, avoidance of excessive fluid intake, and antihypertensive drug therapy can control hypertension caused by most renal parenchymal diseases. Concomitant antibiotic therapy for infectious processes and general supportive measures may be indicated, depending on the nature of the renal disease. If hypertension is difficult to control and the disease is unilateral, unilateral nephrectomy may be considered.

Table 28–6. **Curable Forms of Hypertension**

Organ/System	Diseases/Conditions
Renal	Unilateral kidney disease (pyelonephritis, hydronephrosis, traumatic damage, radiation nephritis, hypoplastic kidney) Wilms' and other kidney tumors
Cardiovascular	Coarctation of the aorta Renal artery abnormalities (e.g., stenosis, aneurysm, fibromuscular dysplasia, thrombosis)
Adrenal	Pheochromocytoma and neuroblastoma Adrenogenital syndrome Cushing's syndrome Primary aldosteronism
Miscellaneous	Glucocorticoid therapy Oral contraceptives

Surgical Treatment. Renovascular disease may be cured by successful surgery, such as reconstruction of a stenotic renal artery, autotransplantation, or unilateral nephrectomy. Hypertension caused by tumors that secrete vasoactive substances, such as pheochromocytoma, neuroblastoma, and juxtaglomerular cell tumor, are treated primarily by surgery.

FOLLOW-UP EVALUATION

Follow-up examinations should include ongoing monitoring of BP levels, target organ damage, periodic serum electrolyte determination in children treated with ACE inhibitors or diuretics, counseling regarding other cardiovascular risk factors, and adherence to a newly adopted healthy lifestyle.

The *goal of the treatment* is reduction of BP to less than the 95th percentile for children with uncomplicated primary hypertension without hypertensive end-organ damage. For children with chronic renal disease, diabetes, or hypertensive target organ damage, the goal is reduction of BP to less than the 90th percentile.

A *"step-down" therapy* or cessation of therapy may be considered in selected patients who have uncomplicated primary hypertension that is well under control, especially overweight children who successfully lose weight. Such patients require ongoing follow-up of their BP levels and nonpharmacologic treatment.

Hypertensive Crisis

In hypertensive crisis, BP is rapidly rising or a high BP level is associated with neurologic manifestations, heart failure, or pulmonary edema.

Hypertensive crisis may be loosely divided into the following subgroups:

1. Hypertensive emergencies: situations in which immediate reduction of BP (within minutes) is needed, usually with parenteral therapy.

2. Hypertensive urgencies: situations in which reduction of BP is needed within hours, usually with oral agents.

3. Accelerated malignant hypertension: situations in which papilledema, hemorrhage, and exudate are associated with a markedly elevated BP; the diastolic pressure is usually greater than 140 mm Hg.

4. Hypertensive encephalopathy: situations in which markedly elevated BP is associated with severe headache and various alterations in consciousness. Hypertensive encephalopathy may be seen in a previously normotensive patient who suddenly becomes hypertensive, such as children with acute glomerulonephritis or young women with eclampsia. Chronically hypertensive patients less commonly develop encephalopathy and only at much higher pressures.

Aggressive parenteral administration of antihypertensive drugs is indicated to lower BP.

1. Labetalol (α- and β-blocker) 0.2 to 2 mg/kg/hour IV drip; diazoxide (Hyperstat), 3 to 5 mg/kg as an IV bolus; or nitroprusside (Nipride), 1 to 3 μg/kg per minute as an IV drip, is the treatment of choice.

2. If hypertension is less severe, hydralazine (Apresoline), 0.15 mg/kg intravenously or intramuscularly, may be used. The onset of action is 10 minutes after an IV dose and 20 to 30 minutes after an intramuscular dose. The dose may be repeated at 4- to 6-hour intervals. Nifedipine, 0.2 to 0.5 mg/kg (maximum, 10 mg), may be given orally every 4 to 6 hours in severe cases.

3. A rapid-acting diuretic, such as furosemide (1 mg/kg), is given intravenously to initiate diuresis.

4. Because fluid balance must be controlled carefully, intake is limited to urine output plus insensible loss.

5. Seizures may be treated with slow IV infusion of diazepam (Valium), 0.2 mg/kg, or another anticonvulsant medication.

6. When a hypertensive crisis is under control, oral medications replace the parenteral medications (see Table 28–5 for oral dosages of antihypertensive drugs).

Chapter 29

Pulmonary Hypertension

Definition

When measured directly in the cardiac catheterization laboratory, the normal pulmonary artery (PA) systolic pressure of children and adults is ≤30 mm Hg and the mean PA pressure is ≤25 mm Hg at sea level. A diagnosis of pulmonary hypertension can be made when the mean PA pressure is >25 mm Hg in a resting individual at sea level. The PA pressure is higher at high elevations.

The noninvasive Doppler method, however, often overestimates the PA pressure and may even suggest PA hypertension in people who are normal. Using tricuspid regurgitation jet velocity and the modified Bernoulli equation, with right atrial pressure assumed to be 10 mm Hg, the mean PA systolic pressure (±SD) was found to be 28.3 ± 4.9 mm Hg (range 15 to 57 mm Hg) in infants and adults, higher values than previously reported using invasive methods (McQuillan et al, 2001). The estimated upper 95% limit for PA systolic pressure was 37.2 mm Hg. (This results from a tricuspid regurgitation jet velocity of 2.7 m/second in the absence of pulmonary stenosis.) Thus, a Doppler-estimated PA systolic pressure of 36 to 40 mm Hg has been assumed as a cutoff value for mild PA hypertension.

There is a wide range of severity in pulmonary hypertension; in some, it reaches or surpasses the systemic pressure. The status of pulmonary hypertension also varies; in some, it is static, and in others, it is dynamic.

Causes

Pulmonary hypertension is a group of conditions with multiple causes rather than a single one. Pathogenesis and management differ among entities. Box 29–1 lists, according to pathogenesis, conditions that cause pulmonary hypertension of a temporary or permanent, acute or chronic nature.

The causes of pulmonary hypertension can be grouped into the following five. Some oversimplification is inevitable in dividing this diverse group into five categories.

1. Increased pulmonary blood flow (PBF) seen in congenital heart diseases (CHDs) with large left-to-right shunts (hyperkinetic pulmonary hypertension)

2. Alveolar hypoxia

3. Increased pulmonary venous pressure

4. Primary pulmonary vascular disease

5. Other diseases that involve pulmonary parenchyma or pulmonary vasculature

The term *cor pulmonale* describes right ventricular hypertrophy (RVH) and/or dilatation secondary to pulmonary hypertension, which is caused by diseases of the pulmonary

---

BOX 29–1	CAUSES OF PULMONARY HYPERTENSION

1. Large left-to-right shunt lesions (hyperkinetic pulmonary hypertension): ventricular septal defect, patent ductus arteriosus, endocardial cushion defect

2. Alveolar hypoxia

   a. Pulmonary parenchymal disease

      1) Extensive pneumonia

      2) Hypoplasia of lungs (primary or secondary, such as that seen in diaphragmatic hernia)

      3) Bronchopulmonary dysplasia

      4) Interstitial lung disease (Hamman-Rich syndrome)

      5) Wilson-Mikity syndrome

   b. Airway obstruction

      1) Upper airway obstruction (large tonsils, macroglossia, micrognathia, laryngotracheomalacia, sleep-disordered breathing)

      2) Lower airway obstruction (bronchial asthma, cystic fibrosis)

   c. Inadequate ventilatory drive (central nervous system diseases, obesity hypoventilation syndrome)

   d. Disorders of chest wall or respiratory muscles

      1) Kyphoscoliosis

      2) Weakening or paralysis of skeletal muscle

   e. High altitude (in certain hyperreactors)

3. Pulmonary venous hypertension: mitral stenosis, cor triatriatum, total anomalous pulmonary venous return with obstruction, chronic left heart failure, left-sided obstructive lesions (aortic stenosis, coarctation of the aorta). Rarely, congenital pulmonary vein stenosis causes incurable pulmonary hypertension.

4. Primary pulmonary vascular disease

   a. Persistent pulmonary hypertension of the newborn

   b. Primary pulmonary hypertension—rare, fatal form of pulmonary hypertension with obscure cause

5. Other diseases that involve pulmonary parenchyma or pulmonary vasculature

   a. Thromboembolism: ventriculoatrial shunt for hydrocephalus, sickle cell anemia, thrombophlebitis

   b. Connective tissue disease: scleroderma, systemic lupus erythematosus, mixed connective tissue disease, dermatomyositis, rheumatoid arthritis

   c. Disorders directly affecting the pulmonary vasculature: schistosomiasis, sarcoidosis, histiocytosis X

   d. Portal hypertension, human immunodeficiency virus infection

---

parenchyma or pulmonary vasculature (including pulmonary veins). It does not include nonpulmonary causes of right ventricular (RV) dysfunction, such as seen with mitral stenosis (MS) or left ventricular (LV) failure.

Physiology

The basics of the physiology of pulmonary circulation and pulmonary vascular responses are summarized here for a quick review.

1. Pulmonary vascular resistance (PVR) is primarily determined by the cross-sectional area of small muscular arteries and arterioles. With stenosis of the pulmonary arteries

and hypoplastic lungs, PVR increases. Other determinants of PVR include blood viscosity, total mass of the lungs, stenosis of the blood vessels, and extramural compression on the vessels. Normal PVR is 1 Wood unit (or 67 ± 23 [SD] dyne-sec/cm^{-5}), which is one tenth of systemic vascular resistance.

2. With exercise, a large increase in PBF is accomplished by only a small increase in PA pressure. The increase in the left atrial (LA) pressure appears to account for most of the increase in PA pressure.

3. The endothelial cells and lung tissues normally synthesize and/or activate certain vasoactive hormones and inactivate others. Balance among the vasoactive substances maintains normal vascular tone. Normally, balanced release of nitric oxide (a vasodilator) and endothelin (a vasoconstrictor) by endothelial cells is a key factor in the regulation of the pulmonary vascular tone.

    a. ET_1, the dominant isoform of endothelin, is a potent vasoconstrictor.

    b. Nitric oxide (NO), synthesized in the vascular endothelium, is a vasodilator.

    c. Prostaglandins (PGs) are synthesized, metabolized, and released by lung tissues. PGI_2 and PGE_1 are vasodilators, whereas $PGF_{2\alpha}$ and PGA_2 are vasoconstrictors.

    d. Serotonin is a vasoconstrictor that promotes smooth muscle cell hypertrophy. Serotonin stimulates release of NO in normal endothelial cells but is unable to stimulate NO release when endothelial dysfunction is present.

    e. Angiotensin II, a potent vasoconstrictor, is activated from angiotensin I in the lungs by angiotensin-converting enzyme.

4. Under certain conditions, PVR changes in the following manner.

    a. In hypoxia-induced vasoconstriction, NO production is reduced and endothelin production is increased. Endothelin receptor antagonists reduce hypoxic pulmonary vasoconstriction. Alveolar oxygen tension is the major physiologic determinant of pulmonary arteriolar tone.

    b. Acidosis significantly increases PVR, acting synergistically with hypoxia.

    c. The α- and β-adrenoceptors produce vasoconstriction and vasodilation, respectively. α-Adrenergic blockers (such as phentolamine, tolazoline) lower PVR.

    d. High altitude (with low alveolar oxygen tension) is associated with pulmonary vasoconstriction (and pulmonary hypertension) of varying degrees. There is a large species and individual variation in the reactivity of the pulmonary arteries to low alveolar oxygen tension.

Pathogenesis

Pressure (P) is related to both flow (F) and vascular resistance (R), as shown in the following formula:

$$P = F \times R$$

An increase in flow, vascular resistance, or both can result in pulmonary hypertension. Regardless of its cause, pulmonary hypertension eventually involves constriction of the pulmonary arterioles, resulting in an increase in PVR and hypertrophy of the RV.

The normally thin RV cannot sustain sudden pressure loads over 40 to 50 mm Hg. Thus, acute right-sided heart failure may develop in any condition in which PVR increases abruptly. However, if pulmonary hypertension develops slowly, the RV hypertrophies and it can tolerate mild pulmonary hypertension (with a systolic pressure of about 50 mm Hg) without producing clinical problems. If another burden such as superimposed lung disease, alveolar hypoxia, or acidosis is added to a mildly hypertrophied RV, requiring generation of higher pressures approximating systemic arterial pressure, the RV may fail. Pathogenesis of pulmonary hypertension is discussed according to the (first four) general categories of causes because they are distinctly different from each other.

HYPERKINETIC PULMONARY HYPERTENSION

Pulmonary hypertension associated with large left-to-right shunt lesions, such as ventricular septal defect (VSD) and patent ductus arteriosus (PDA), is called *hyperkinetic pulmonary hypertension*. It is the result of an increase in PBF, a direct transmission of the systemic pressure to the PA, and an increase in PVR by compensatory pulmonary vasoconstriction. If no vasoconstriction occurs, the increase in PBF is much larger and an intractable congestive heart failure (CHF) results. Defects in the vasodilation machinery of the endothelial cell, such as overproduction of vasoconstrictor elements, have been implicated in this form of pulmonary hypertension. Hyperkinetic pulmonary hypertension is usually reversible if the cause is eliminated before permanent changes occur in the pulmonary arterioles (see later section).

If large left-to-right shunt lesions (such as VSD, PDA, complete atrioventricular canal) are left untreated, irreversible changes take place in the pulmonary vascular bed, with severe pulmonary hypertension and cyanosis because of a reversal of the left-to-right shunt. This stage is called Eisenmenger's syndrome or pulmonary vascular obstructive disease (PVOD). Surgical correction is not possible at this stage. The time of onset of PVOD varies, ranging from infancy to adulthood, but the majority of patients develop PVOD during late childhood or early adolescence. It develops even later in patients with atrial septal defect. Many patients with transposition of the great arteries begin to develop PVOD within the first year of life for reasons not entirely clear. Children with Down syndrome with large left-to-right shunt lesions tend to develop PVOD much earlier than normal children with similar lesions.

ALVEOLAR HYPOXIA

An acute or chronic reduction in the oxygen tension (Po_2) in the alveolar capillary region (alveolar hypoxia) elicits a strong pulmonary vasoconstrictor response, which may be augmented by acidosis. Hypoxia in the alveolar space elicits a much stronger vasoconstrictor effect than a low Po_2 in the PA.

The exact mechanism of the pulmonary vasoconstrictor response to alveolar hypoxia is not completely understood, but studies in animals and humans suggest that endothelin and NO, the two important vascular endothelium–released vasoactive substances, are the strongest candidates responsible for the response. Normally, balanced releases of NO and endothelin by endothelial cells regulate the pulmonary circulation. A reduction in NO production occurs in chronically hypoxic animals, whereas prolonged inhalation of NO attenuates hypoxic pulmonary vasoconstriction and vascular remodeling (proliferation) in these animals. Conversely, plasma levels of endothelin-1 are increased in association with hypoxia in humans. Endothelin receptor antagonists have been demonstrated to reduce hypoxic pulmonary vasoconstriction and vascular remodeling in animals. A number of other growth factors (including platelet-derived growth factors and vascular endothelial growth factor) also mediate pulmonary vascular remodeling in response to hypoxia.

Alveolar hypoxia may be an important basic mechanism of many forms of pulmonary hypertension, including that seen in pulmonary parenchymal disease, airway obstruction, inadequate ventilatory drive (central nervous system diseases), disorders of chest wall or respiratory muscles, and high altitude. Even a small area of affected lung may produce vasoconstriction throughout the lungs, possibly through a circulating humoral agent.

PULMONARY VENOUS HYPERTENSION

Increased pressure in the pulmonary veins produces reflex vasoconstriction of the pulmonary arterioles, raising PA pressure to maintain a high enough pressure gradient between the PA and the pulmonary vein. This pressure gradient maintains a constant forward flow in the pulmonary circulation. There is a marked individual variation in the degree of reactive pulmonary arteriolar vasoconstriction. For example, when the pulmonary venous pressure is elevated in excess of 25 mm Hg from MS, marked reactive pulmonary hypertension occurs in less than one third of patients. The mechanism for the vasoconstriction is not entirely clear, but a neuronal component may be present. Moreover, an elevated pulmonary venous pressure may also narrow or close small airways, resulting in alveolar hypoxia, which may contribute to the vasoconstriction. MS, total anomalous pulmonary venous return (TAPVR) with obstruction (of pulmonary venous return to the LA), and chronic left-sided heart failure are examples of this entity.

Pulmonary hypertension with increased pulmonary venous pressure is usually reversible when the cause is eliminated, with the exception of congenital pulmonary vein stenosis, for which no curative surgery is available.

PRIMARY PULMONARY VASCULAR DISEASE

Primary pulmonary hypertension is characterized by progressive, irreversible vascular changes similar to those seen in Eisenmenger's syndrome but without intracardiac lesions. There is a decrease in the cross-sectional area of the pulmonary vascular bed caused by pathologic changes in the vascular tissue itself, thromboembolism, platelet aggregation, or a combination of these. This condition is extremely rare in pediatric patients; it is a condition of adulthood and is more prevalent in women. A familial form of the disease has been reported worldwide in approximately 6% of the cases with primary pulmonary hypertension. It has a poor prognosis.

The pathogenesis of primary pulmonary hypertension is not fully understood, but endothelial dysfunction of the pulmonary vascular bed and enhanced platelet activities may be important factors. In normal pulmonary vascular bed, the endothelial cells modulate the tone of vascular smooth muscles (by synthesizing prostacyclin, nitric oxide, and endothelin); control the potential proliferation of smooth muscle cells; and interact with platelets to release anticlotting factors in the blood to maintain a nonthrombotic state (by releasing prostacyclin, an inhibitor of platelet function). These delicate functions are themselves influenced by factors such as shear stress, hypoxia, and tissue metabolism.

The striking features of the pulmonary vasculature in patients with primary pulmonary hypertension are marked intimal proliferation (and in some vessels with complete vascular occlusion) and in situ thrombosis of the small pulmonary arteries with intraluminal thrombin deposition. Interactions among endothelin, growth factors, platelets, and the vascular wall may play a fundamental role in the pathologic processes seen in this condition. Endothelin is overproduced in pulmonary hypertension, and this excess endothelin is associated with not only vasoconstriction but also cell proliferation, inflammation, medial hypertrophy, and fibrosis. Two receptors, ET_A and ET_B receptors, are known. Endothelium receptor antagonists (such as bosentan) produce vasodilation.

OTHER DISEASE STATES

Pulmonary hypertension associated with other disease states has pathophysiologies similar to those described in the preceding four categories, singly or in combination.

Pathology

Regardless of the initial events that lead to PA hypertension, elevated PA pressure eventually induces varying severity of anatomic changes in the pulmonary vessels.

1. Hyperkinetic pulmonary hypertension is the result of congenital heart defects with left-to-right shunts. Heath and Edwards classified the changes into six grades (Fig. 29–1). Grade I consists of hypertrophy of the medial wall of the small muscular arteries; grade II, hyperplasia of the intima; and grade III, hyperplasia and fibrosis of the intima with narrowing of the vascular lumen. Changes up to grade III are considered reversible if the cause is eliminated. In grade IV, dilatation and so-called plexiform lesion of the muscular pulmonary arteries and arterioles are present. Grade V changes include complex plexiform, angiomatous, and cavernous lesions and hyalinization of intimal fibrosis. Grade VI is characterized by the presence of necrotizing arteritis. The advanced changes seen in grades IV through VI are considered irreversible, and they augment the hypertension and sustain it even when the original stimulus is removed. Thus, the presence of irreversible pulmonary vascular changes precludes surgical repair of congenital heart defects.

2. The progressive vascular changes that occur in primary pulmonary hypertension are identical to those that occur with congenital heart defects.

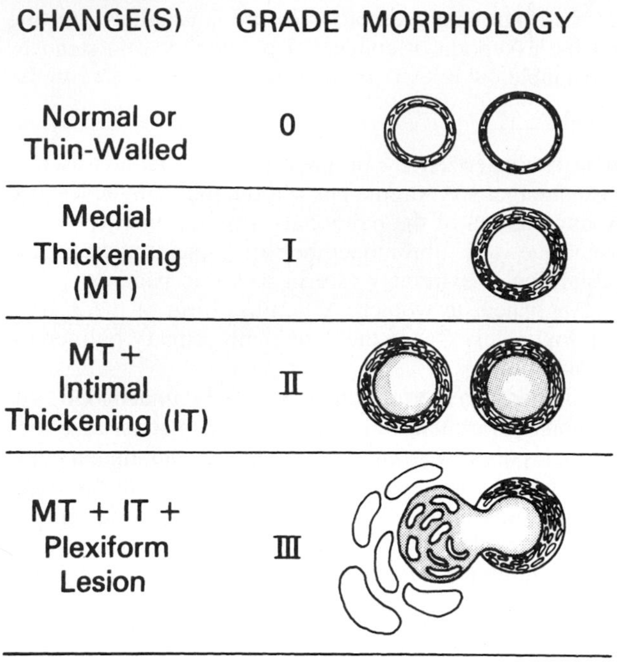

CHANGE(S)   GRADE   MORPHOLOGY

CHANGE(S)	GRADE	MORPHOLOGY
Normal or Thin-Walled	0	
Medial Thickening (MT)	I	
MT + Intimal Thickening (IT)	II	
MT + IT + Plexiform Lesion	III	

Figure 29–1. Heath-Edwards grading of the morphologic changes in the pulmonary arteries of patients with pulmonary hypertension (see text). (From Roberts WC: Congenital Heart Disease in Adults. Philadelphia, FA Davis, 1979.)

3. With pulmonary venous hypertension, the pulmonary arteries may show severe medial hypertrophy and intimal fibrosis. However, the changes are limited to grades I through III of the Heath and Edwards classification, and they are often reversible when the cause is eliminated.

Pathophysiology

1. If severe pulmonary hypertension develops suddenly in the presence of an unprepared (nonhypertrophied) RV, right-sided heart failure develops. Examples of this include infants who develop acute upper airway obstruction and adult patients who develop massive pulmonary thromboembolism.

2. With chronic pulmonary hypertension, gradual hypertrophy and dilatation of the RV develop. The RV pressure rises gradually with accompanying RV hypertrophy, and the PA pressure may exceed the systemic pressure.

3. A decrease in cardiac output may result from at least two mechanisms:
   a. A volume and pressure overload of the RV impairs cardiac function, primarily by impaired coronary perfusion of the hypertrophied and dilated RV and decreased LV function. The LV dysfunction results from the dramatic leftward shift of the interventricular septum caused by the increasing RV volume. The dilated RV also alters LV structures and decreases the compliance of the LV, resulting in an increase in both LV end-diastolic pressure and LA pressure and thus worsening pulmonary vasoconstriction.
   b. A sudden increase in PVR may decrease pulmonary venous return to the LA, with resulting hypotension in the absence of a right-to-left intracardiac shunt.

4. Pulmonary edema can occur without elevation of LA pressure. Direct disruption of the walls of the small arterioles proximal to the hypoxically constricted arterioles may be responsible (a mechanism similar to that proposed for high-altitude pulmonary edema). The disruption is more likely if there is no hypertrophy of the smooth muscles in the media of these vessels.

5. Deterioration of arterial blood gas levels occurs. Hypoxemia, acidosis, and occasionally hypercapnia may result from pulmonary venous congestion or edema, compression of small airways, or intracardiac shunts, which may worsen pulmonary hypertension.

Clinical Manifestations

Regardless of the cause, clinical manifestations of pulmonary hypertension are similar when significant hypertension exists.

History

1. Exertional dyspnea and fatigue are the earliest and most frequent complaints. Some patients may have histories of headache.

2. Syncope, presyncope, or chest pain also occurs on exertion, which generally represents more advanced disease with a fixed cardiac output.

3. History of a heart defect or CHF in infancy is present in most cases of Eisenmenger's syndrome.

4. Patients with underlying lung disease may also complain of frequent episodes of cough or wheezing.

5. Hemoptysis (associated with pulmonary infarction secondary to thrombosis) is a late and sometimes fatal development.

Physical Examination

1. Cyanosis with or without clubbing may be present. The neck veins are distended, with a prominent *a* wave.

2. An RV lift or tap (on the left parasternal area) occurs on palpation.

3. There is a single S2, or it splits narrowly; the P2 is loud. An ejection click and an early diastolic decrescendo murmur of pulmonary regurgitation (PR) are usually present along the mid-left sternal border. A holosystolic murmur of tricuspid regurgitation (TR) may be audible at the lower left sternal border.

4. Signs of right-sided heart failure (e.g., hepatomegaly, ankle edema) may be present.

5. Arrhythmias occur in the late stage.

6. Patients with associated illness often have clinical findings of that disease.

Electrocardiography

1. Right axis deviation (RAD) and RVH with or without "strain" are seen with severe pulmonary hypertension.

2. Right atrial hypertrophy (RAH) is frequently seen late.

X-ray Studies

1. The heart size is normal or only slightly enlarged with or without RA enlargement. Cardiomegaly appears when CHF supervenes.

2. A prominent PA segment and dilated hilar vessels with clear lung fields are characteristic.

3. With acute exacerbation, pulmonary edema may be seen.

Echocardiography

Echo usually demonstrates the following.

1. Enlargement of the RA and RV, with normal or small LV dimensions.

2. Thickened interventricular septum and abnormal septal motion (as a result of the RV pressure overload).

3. Thickened RV free wall and RV dysfunction are difficult to demonstrate and quantitate.

Semiquantitative estimation of PA pressures can be obtained using various methods such as M-mode or two-dimensional echo and Doppler examination. It should be noted, however, that the Doppler-estimated PA pressure and that measured in the cardiac catheterization laboratory are not interchangeable (as discussed earlier in this chapter). These noninvasive methods of estimating the severity of pulmonary hypertension are presented in the following.

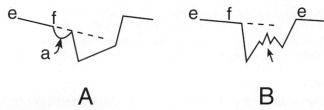

A   B

Figure 29–2. M-mode echo of the pulmonary valve in pulmonary hypertension. **A,** Normal M-mode echo. **B,** Pulmonary hypertension demonstrating an absent a wave, diminished or negative EF slope, and midsystolic notch or flutter (arrow).

1. *Abnormal valve motion on M-mode echo*: An absent or diminished *a* wave, a reduced EF slope, and a midsystolic closure (notching) indicate pulmonary hypertension (Fig. 29–2). However, these abnormalities are not always present, and a false-positive result occurs rarely.

2. *Two-dimensional echo*: With an elevated RV pressure, the interventricular septum shifts toward the LV and appears flattened at the end of systole. An inspection of the septal curvature at the end of systole provides an estimate of the RV systolic pressure (Fig. 29–3).

3. Doppler echo:
   a. Peak TR velocity determined by continuous-wave Doppler is used to estimate the *systolic* pressure in the PA. The simplified Bernoulli equation ($\Delta P = 4V^2$) is used

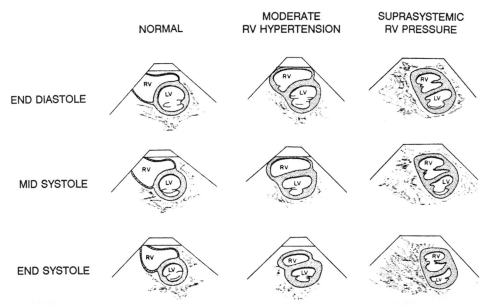

Figure 29–3. Parasternal short-axis stop frames of interventricular septal configurations of normal patients and patients with right ventricular (RV) hypertension. The top row represents the end-diastolic frames, the middle row represents the midsystolic frames, and the bottom row represents the end-systolic frames. In normal children (left column), the typical rounded configuration of the interventricular septum is demonstrated throughout the cardiac cycle. In moderate pulmonary hypertension (middle column), the interventricular septum becomes progressively flattened from the end of diastole to the end of systole. When RV pressure is suprasystemic (right column), the interventricular septum is flattened at the end of diastole; at the end of systole, it reverses its curvature to become convex toward the left ventricle. (Modified from King ME, Braun H, Goldblatt A, et al: Interventricular septal configuration as a predictor of right ventricular systolic hypertension in children: A cross-sectional echocardiographic study. Circulation 68:68–75, 1983.)

to estimate a systolic pressure drop across the tricuspid valve; a normal central venous pressure of 10 mm Hg is added to the result to estimate PA *systolic* pressure. (Note that the normal Doppler-derived values are different from those obtained by invasive methods; the upper limit of normal PA systolic pressure is 36 to 40 mm Hg by Doppler method.) In the absence of pulmonary stenosis, the systolic pressure in the RV equals that in the PA.

b. With a shunt lesion, such as VSD, PDA, or systemic-to-PA shunt, the peak systolic velocity across the shunt can be used to estimate systolic pressure in the RV or PA. The systolic pressure in the LV (which is equal to the aortic pressure) estimated by systolic pressure in the arm, minus the systolic pressure drop across the VSD or PDA, estimates RV and PA systolic pressures, respectively. Note that the systolic pressure in the arm is a little higher (5 to 10 mm Hg) than the LV systolic pressure because of the peripheral amplification of systolic pressure; see Chapter 2.

c. The end-diastolic velocity of PR can be used to estimate the *diastolic* pressure in the PA. The end-diastolic (not early diastolic) velocity is measured and entered into the modified Bernoulli equation, and a normal central venous pressure of 10 mm Hg is added.

Other Imaging Studies

1. Radionuclide ventriculography may provide information regarding RV function.

2. A lung perfusion scan may reveal a relatively normal perfusion pattern or diffuse, patch perfusion abnormalities.

3. A pulmonary function test may reveal a reduced vital capacity or hyperreactivity of the bronchial tress (which can be misdiagnosed as asthma).

4. Computed tomography can be used to determine the presence and severity of pulmonary hypertension based on the diameter of the main PA.

Exercise Testing. A symptom-limited exercise, such as the 6-minute walk test, has been found to be useful in the evaluation of adult patients with pulmonary hypertension (see "Stress Testing" in Chapter 6 for the 6-minute walk test). At this time, reference values for healthy children and adolescents are not available but the test is useful for following disease progression or measuring the response to medical interventions.

Natural History

1. Pulmonary hypertension secondary to the upper airway obstruction is usually reversible when the cause is eliminated.

2. Chronic conditions that produce alveolar hypoxia have a relatively poor prognosis. Pulmonary hypertension of variable degree persists with right-sided heart failure. Superimposed pulmonary infection may be an exacerbating factor.

3. Pulmonary hypertension with large left-to-right shunt lesions (hyperkinetic type) or associated with pulmonary venous hypertension improves or disappears after surgical repair of the cause, if treatment of the condition is possible and performed early.

4. Primary pulmonary hypertension is progressive and has a fatal outcome, usually 2 to 3 years after the onset of symptoms.

5. Pulmonary hypertension associated with Eisenmenger's syndrome, collagen disease, and chronic thromboembolism is usually irreversible and has a poor prognosis but may be stable for two to three decades.

6. Right-sided heart failure is common in the late stage.

7. Chest pain, hemoptysis, and syncope are ominous signs.

8. Atrial and ventricular arrhythmias also occur late.

9. The two most frequent causes of death are progressive RV failure and sudden death (probably secondary to arrhythmias).

10. Cerebrovascular accident from paradoxical embolization is a rare complication.

Diagnosis

1. The history and physical findings suggest pulmonary hypertension.
2. Noninvasive tools (ECG, chest x-ray films, and echo) are used to detect pulmonary hypertension. Collectively, they are reasonably accurate in assessing severity. There is a possibility of overestimating the severity of pulmonary hypertension by the Doppler method, and higher normal values of PA pressure are obtained by this method.
3. Cardiac catheterization demonstrates the presence and severity of pulmonary hypertension. Whether the elevated PVR is due to active vasoconstriction ("responders") or to permanent changes in the pulmonary arterioles ("nonresponders") may be assessed by the use of tolazoline (Priscoline, α-adrenoceptor blocker) or the administration of oxygen during cardiac catheterization. Intravenous adenosine or epoprostenol (prostacyclin) or inhaled nitric oxide can also be used for the same purpose.
4. Characteristic angiographic findings of advanced pulmonary hypertension secondary to CHD include sparseness of arborization, abrupt tapering of small arteries, and reduced background capillary filling.
5. Lung biopsies have been used in an attempt to evaluate the "operability" of patients with pulmonary hypertension and CHD. Unfortunately, pulmonary vascular changes are not uniformly distributed and the biopsy findings correlated poorly with the natural history of the disease or the operability. Hemodynamic data appear to predict survival better than biopsy findings.

Management

Most cases of pulmonary hypertension are difficult to treat and impossible to reverse unless the cause can be eliminated. The primary emphasis must be on the prevention and elimination of causes whenever possible; once PVOD is established, reversal of the condition is usually not possible.

1. Measures to remove or treat the underlying cause include the following.
   a. Timely corrective surgery for congenital defects, such as large-shunt VSD, endocardial cushion defect, or PDA, before obstructive anatomic changes occur in the pulmonary vessels.
   b. Tonsillectomy and adenoidectomy when the cause of pulmonary hypertension is the upper airway obstruction.
   c. Treatment of underlying diseases, such as cystic fibrosis, asthma, pneumonia, or bronchopulmonary dysplasia.
2. General measures are aimed at preventing further elevation of PA pressure or treating its complications.
   a. Avoidance or limitation of strenuous exertion, isometric activities (weightlifting), trips to high altitudes, and possibly flights on commercial aircraft.
   b. Oxygen supplementation is provided as needed.
   c. Avoidance of vasoconstrictor drugs, including decongestants with α-adrenergic properties.
   d. Patients should be strongly advised to avoid pregnancy. Pregnancy increases circulating blood volume and oxygen consumption, may increase the risk of pulmonary embolism from deep vein thrombosis or amniotic fluid, and may cause syncope and cardiac arrest. Oral contraceptives worsen pulmonary hypertension (surgical contraception is preferred).
   e. CHF is treated with chronic administration of digoxin and diuretics and a low-salt diet. Digoxin may improve RV contractility against the elevated afterload and is also useful if there is coexisting LV dysfunction. Diuretics provide marked benefit in symptom relief by reducing intravascular volume, hepatic congestion, and pulmonary congestion.

f. Cardiac arrhythmias are treated.

g. Partial erythropheresis is performed for polycythemia and headache.

h. Annual flu shots are recommended.

i. The use of nitroglycerin for anginal pain is avoided because it may worsen the pain.

3. Anticoagulation.

a. Anticoagulation with warfarin (Coumadin) is widely recommended in patients with thromboembolic disease and may be beneficial in those with pulmonary hypertension from other causes, with significant improvement in survival. An International Normalized Ratio (INR) of 2.0 to 2.5 is the goal of therapy. Unlike the approach for patients with a prosthetic mechanical heart valve, concomitant use of aspirin is not recommended because it may increase effects of warfarin.

b. Some recommend antiplatelet drugs (aspirin) instead of warfarin to prevent microembolism in the pulmonary circulation.

4. *For responders.* The following pulmonary vasodilators are used in patients without fixed PVR. Most of the experiences are based on adult trials. Vasodilator drugs are not always salutary because they may decrease the systemic vascular resistance more than the PVR. Vasodilators should not be used without testing first in the catheterization laboratory.

a. Nifedipine, a calcium channel blocking agent, is one of the oldest drugs used, with beneficial effects seen in 40% of children with primary pulmonary hypertension who have shown vasodilator responses during cardiac catheterization. The oral dose of nifedipine is 0.2 mg/kg every 8 hours. Calcium channel blockers could worsen the underlying pulmonary hypertension because of their negative inotropic effects and their reflex sympathetic stimulation. Hypotension is a side effect of the medication. In adults, only very large doses (not the conventional dose) of the agent were shown to be salutary, making it mandatory to evaluate the effects non-invasively.

b. Prostacyclins, by continuous intravenous infusion, have been shown to improve quality of life and survival in patients with primary hypertension, Eisenmenger's syndrome, or chronic lung disease. Epoprostenol is administered through a central venous line and delivered by an ambulatory infusion system. (The starting dose of epoprostenol was 2 ng/kg/minute, with increments of 2 ng/kg/minute every 15 minutes, until desired effects appeared; the average final dose was 9 to 11 ng/kg/minute.) Thrombosis, pump malfunction (with rebound pulmonary hypertension), flushing, headache, nausea, diarrhea, and jaw discomfort are reported complications and side effects. Several prostacyclin analogues have been used in adults and can be administered intravenously (treprostinil), by inhalation (iloprost), or orally (beraprost).

c. Endothelin receptor antagonists, bosentan and sitaxsentan, are new oral therapeutic agents that have been used in both primary pulmonary hypertension and Eisenmenger's syndrome.

1). Bosentan, a nonselective endothelin receptor blocker, given orally in a dose of 125 mg twice a day for 16 weeks, has resulted in a significant improvement in the level of exercise capability in adult patients. Similarly beneficial effects have been reported in pediatric patients. In children with primary pulmonary hypertension or Eisenmenger's syndrome, oral bosentan in a dose of 31.25 mg twice a day for children less than 20 kg, 62.5 mg twice a day for children 20 to 40 kg, and 125 mg twice a day for children more than 40 kg (with or without concomitant IV prostacyclin therapy) for a medial duration of 14 months resulted in a significant functional improvement in about 50% of the cases (Barst et al, 2003; Rosenzweig et al, 2005; Maiya et al, 2006). A rare side effect of the drug is increased liver enzyme.

2). Sitaxsentan, a selective endothelin-A receptor antagonist, given orally once daily at a dose of 100 mg (for mostly adult patients and children older than 12 years) resulted in improved exercise capacity after 18 weeks of treatment

(Barst et al, 2006). Elevation of aspartate aminotransferase (AST) and alanine aminotransferase (ALT) was a rare side effect.

d. Sildenafil, a phosphodiesterase inhibitor, given orally, has been shown to be a potent and selective pulmonary vasodilator with efficacy equal to that of inhaled NO in adult patients. A small pediatric study with sildenafil for 12 months resulted in improvement in hemodynamics and exercise capacity in children with primary pulmonary hypertension and secondary pulmonary hypertension from CHDs. The dosage used was 0.25 to 1 mg/kg four times daily, starting with the lower dose (Humpl et al, 2005).

e. Nitric oxide inhalation is effective in lowering PA pressure in adult respiratory distress syndrome, primary pulmonary hypertension, and persistent pulmonary hypertension of the newborn. Nitric oxide can be administered only by inhalation because it is inactivated by hemoglobin.

f. In addition to the preceding vasodilators, inotropic agents (e.g., digoxin, dopamine) are often helpful in lowering PA pressure. Improved oxygenation by intubation and ventilatory support may lower PA pressure. Hyperventilation-induced respiratory alkalosis may produce pulmonary vasodilatation.

5. *For nonresponders.* The following measures can be used in patients with fixed PVR and severe pulmonary hypertension, including primary pulmonary hypertension.

a. Nitric oxide inhalation and continuous intravenous or possibly nebulized prostacyclin (PGI_2) may provide selective pulmonary vasodilatation.

b. Atrial septectomy (by either catheter or surgery) improves survival rates and abolishes syncope by providing a right-to-left atrial shunt and thereby helping to maintain cardiac output.

c. Lung transplantation. It was believed initially that, because of severe RV dysfunction, heart-lung transplantation was the only option. However, bilateral or single lung transplantation has been shown to reduce PVR and improve RV function. Bilateral lung transplantation is preferred at most centers because of a greater pulmonary vascular reserve, but some centers prefer single lung transplantation because of its simpler surgical technique and shorter waiting time for organ procurement.

Two examples of pulmonary hypertension seen in the neonate, bronchopulmonary dysplasia and diaphragmatic hernia, are briefly discussed next.

Bronchopulmonary Dysplasia

Bronchopulmonary dysplasia (BPD) develops in about 50% of premature infants with birth weights of 500 to 750 g and about 10% of premature infants weighing less than 1500 g who were mechanically ventilated.

PATHOPHYSIOLOGY

1. BPD results from the prolonged mechanical ventilation and high inspired oxygen concentration that are required to treat severe respiratory distress syndrome (RDS) in premature infants.

2. BPD results in chronic pulmonary hypertension, with gradual dilatation and hypertrophy of the RV. The RV pressure varies but may reach the level of systemic pressure, and RV failure may develop with a reduction of cardiac output if there is an inadequate right-to-left atrial shunt. If there is an adequate right-to-left intracardiac shunt, arterial desaturation results.

CLINICAL MANIFESTATIONS

1. A history of premature birth and severe RDS requiring administration of oxygen at a concentration greater than 60% and mechanical ventilation with high airway pressure is present.

2. The patient has retraction of the chest walls and pulmonary crackles. Some neonates have systemic hypertension (the mechanisms of which are not clear), with echo evidence of LV wall hypertrophy. Cardiac examination is usually unremarkable except

for an occasional nonspecific ejection systolic murmur or soft regurgitant systolic murmur of TR. The liver is often enlarged.

3. Chest x-ray films may reveal diffuse bilateral haziness, sometimes with lacy densities, areas of hyperinflation, increased anteroposterior diameter of the chest, and occasional pectus excavatum. The heart may be of normal size but is frequently enlarged.

4. Echo findings include the following:
   a. The RV is dilated, but RV wall thickness is within normal limits (2 to 5 mm).
   b. The LV posterior wall is thickened (7 to 10 mm) in over 80% of infants; this may account for pulmonary edema and systemic hypertension.

MANAGEMENT

1. Diuretic therapy decreases airway resistance and improves lung compliance but usually does not affect gas exchange. One of the following may be used.
   a. Hydrochlorothiazide, 2 mg/kg every 12 hours, is administered with or without spironolactone, 1.5 mg/kg every 12 hours.
   b. Furosemide, 1 mg/kg every 12 hours, is administered every other day.

2. Digoxin may be tried, but its beneficial effects are uncertain. Because of intermittent disturbances in serum potassium levels, digoxin may be dangerous.

3. Home oxygen inhalation decreases PA pressures and promotes weight gain.

4. Sufficient calories, protein, and vitamins for growth and tissue repair are important. Daily sodium intake should be limited to 1 to 2 mEq/kg of body weight.

PROGNOSIS

1. At least 15% of severely affected infants die in the first year. Most surviving infants are asymptomatic by 2 years, and signs and symptoms of lung disease are rare after 5 years. This is the result of continuous generation of new alveolar-vascular units until the age of 2 years.

2. Even years later, some patients have abnormalities of respiratory function and in their exercise tolerance test results.

Diaphragmatic Hernia

Diaphragmatic hernia is almost always associated with a varying degree of pulmonary hypertension. Pulmonary hypertension is the result of hypoplasia of the lungs, which results from some abdominal organs having been displaced into the thorax and compressed on the developing lungs during fetal life. Severity of lung hypoplasia and pulmonary hypertension are important determinants of survival in these neonates. Respiratory distress of newborns with diaphragmatic hernia is the result of these pathologic changes.

PATHOLOGY

1. Defects are more common on the left (70% to 85%).

2. Some degree of pulmonary hypoplasia is always present. Both lungs are small compared with those of age- and weight-matched controls, with the affected side of the lung more severely hypoplastic. There is a decrease in the number of alveoli and bronchial generations. The total cross-sectional area of pulmonary vasculature is reduced with a marked increase in muscular layer of the arterioles.

3. Associated anomalies are present in 20% to 30% and include central nervous system lesions, esophageal atresia, omphalocele, cardiovascular lesions, and malrotation of the intestine.

4. Association with other syndromes has been described, including trisomy 21 and other lethal syndromes (such as trisomy 13 and trisomy 18).

CLINICAL MANIFESTATIONS

1. Severe respiratory distress within the first hours of life is common.
2. Chest x-ray study is usually diagnostic. The lateral view frequently demonstrates the intestine passing through the posterior portion of the diaphragm.

MANAGEMENT

Diaphragmatic hernia was once considered a surgical emergency. However, recognition of the role of pulmonary hypoplasia and pulmonary hypertension in survival has led to a policy of delayed repair.

1. Initially, sedation, paralysis, and modest hyperventilation may be attempted. Volume resuscitation, dopamine, and bicarbonate (to keep pH >7.5) may also be helpful. If the infant stabilizes and demonstrates stable PVR without a significant right-to-left atrial shunt, surgery is performed at 24 to 72 hours of age.
2. If stabilization is not possible or a significant right-to-left shunt occurs, infants require extracorporeal membrane oxygenation (ECMO) support. Vasoactive agents, nitric oxide, and dipyridamole (antiplatelet agent) may be given. The duration of ECMO for these neonates is much longer (7 to 14 days and sometimes up to 4 weeks) than for those with RDS.
3. The timing of the repair on ECMO is controversial; some centers prefer early repair to allow a greater duration of postrepair ECMO, whereas others delay repair until the infant has demonstrated the ability to tolerate weaning from ECMO.
4. Doppler-estimated PA pressure at the time of repair appears to be directly related to survival. All patients who had normal PA pressure survived. All patients who had systemic or suprasystemic PA pressure died. Seventy-five percent of the patients who had an intermediate reduction in PA pressure survived (Dillon et al, 2004).

Chapter 30

Child with Chest Pain

A complaint of chest pain is frequently encountered in children in the office and emergency room. Although chest pain does not indicate serious disease of the heart or other systems in most pediatric patients, in a society with a high prevalence of atherosclerotic cardiovascular disease, it can be alarming to the child and parents. Physicians should be aware of the differential diagnosis of chest pain in children and should make every effort to find a specific cause before making a referral to a specialist or reassuring the child and the parents of the benign nature of the complaint. Making a routine referral to a cardiologist is not always a good idea; it may increase the family's concern and may result in a prolonged and expensive cardiac evaluation.

Causes and Prevalence

Chest pain occurs in children of all ages and equally in male and female patients, with an average age of presentation at 13 years. Table 30–1 lists the frequency of the causes of chest pain in children according to organ systems. According to several reports, the three most common causes of chest pain in children are costochondritis, a pathologic condition of the chest wall (trauma or muscle strain), and respiratory diseases, especially those associated with coughing (see Table 30–1). These three conditions account for 45% to 65% of cases of chest pain in children. Costochondritis is more common in females. Box 30–1 is a partial list of *possible* causes of noncardiac and cardiac chest pain in children. Although the differential diagnosis of chest pain in children is exhaustive, chest pain in children is least likely to be cardiac in origin, occurring in 0% to 4% of children with chest pain. Psychogenic causes are less likely to be found in children younger than 12 years; they are more likely to be found in females older than 12 years.

Clinical Manifestations

IDIOPATHIC CHEST PAIN

No cause can be found in 12% to 85% of patients, even after a moderately extensive investigation. In many children with chronic chest pain, an organic cause is less likely to be found. In some of these children, chest pain resolves spontaneously, and some of them are eventually referred for specialty evaluations.

NONCARDIAC CAUSES OF CHEST PAIN

Most cases of pediatric chest pain originate in organ systems other than the cardiovascular system. Identifiable noncardiac causes of chest pain are found in 56% to 86% of reported cases. Causes of chest pain are found most often in the thorax and respiratory system.

BOX 30–1	SELECTED CAUSES OF CHEST PAIN

NONCARDIAC CAUSES

Musculoskeletal

Costochondritis
Trauma to chest wall (from sports, fights, or accident)
Muscle strains (pectoral, shoulder, or back muscles)
Overused chest wall muscle (from coughing)
Abnormalities of the rib cage or thoracic spine
Tietze's syndrome
Slipping rib syndrome
Precordial catch (Texidor's twinge or stitch in the side)

Respiratory

Reactive airway disease (exercise-induced asthma)
Pneumonia (viral, bacterial, mycobacterial, fungal, or parasitic)
Pleural irritation (pleural effusion)
Pneumothorax or pneumomediastinum
Pleurodynia (devil's grip)
Pulmonary embolism
Foreign bodies in the airway

Gastrointestinal

Gastroesophageal reflux
Peptic ulcer disease
Esophagitis
Gastritis
Esophageal diverticulum
Hiatal hernia
Foreign bodies (such as coins)
Cholecystitis
Pancreatitis

Psychogenic

Life stressor (death in family, family discord, divorce, failure in school, nonacceptance
   from peers, or sexual molestation)
Hyperventilation
Conversion symptoms
Somatization disorder
Depression
Bulimia nervosa (esophagitis, esophageal tear)

Miscellaneous

Sickle cell disease (vaso-occlusive crisis)
Mastalgia
Herpes zoster

CARDIAC CAUSES

Ischemic Ventricular Dysfunction

Structural abnormalities of the heart (severe AS or PS, hypertrophic obstructive
   cardiomyopathy, Eisenmenger's syndrome)
Mitral valve prolapse
Coronary artery abnormalities (previous Kawasaki disease, congenital anomaly, coronary
   heart disease, hypertension, sickle cell disease)
Cocaine abuse
Aortic dissection and aortic aneurysm (Turner's, Marfan, and Noonan's syndromes)

Inflammatory Conditions

Pericarditis (viral, bacterial, or rheumatic)
Postpericardiotomy syndrome
Myocarditis (acute or chronic)
Kawasaki disease

Arrhythmias (and Palpitations)

Supraventricular tachycardia
Frequent PVCs or ventricular tachycardia (possible)

Table 30–1. Relative Frequency of Causes of Chest Pain in Children

Idiopathic	12%–85%
Musculoskeletal	15%–43%
Respiratory	12%–21%
Psychogenic	5%–17%
Gastrointestinal	4%–7%
Others	4%–21%
Cardiac	0%–4%

Modified from Kocis KC: Chest pain in pediatrics. Pediatr Clin North Am 46:189–203, 1999.

Costochondritis. Costochondritis causes chest pain in 9% to 22% of children with such pain. It is more common in girls than boys. It is characterized by mild to moderate anterior chest pain, usually unilateral but occasionally bilateral. The pain may be preceded by exercise, an upper respiratory infection, or physical activity. A specific position may also cause the pain. The pain may radiate to the remainder of the chest, back, and abdomen; it may be exaggerated by breathing; and it may persist for several months. Physical examination is diagnostic; the clinician finds a reproducible tenderness on palpation over the chondrosternal or costochondral junction. It is a benign condition.

Tietze's syndrome is a rare form of costochondritis characterized by a large, tender, fusiform (spindle-shaped), nonsuppurative swelling at the chondrosternal junction. It usually affects the upper ribs, particularly the second and third junctions.

Musculoskeletal. Musculoskeletal chest pain is also common in children. The pain is caused by strains of the pectoral, shoulder, or back muscles after exercise; overuse of chest wall muscle for coughing; or trauma to the chest wall from sports, fights, or accidents. A history of vigorous exercise, weightlifting, or direct trauma to the chest and the presence of tenderness of the chest wall or muscles clearly indicate muscle strain or trauma. Abnormalities of the rib cage or thoracic spine can cause mild, chronic chest pain in children.

Respiratory. Respiratory problems are responsible for about 10% to 20% of cases of pediatric chest pain, which may result from lung pathology, pleural irritation, or pneumothorax. A history of severe cough, with tenderness of intercostal or abdominal muscles, is usually present. The presence of crackles, wheezing, tachypnea, retraction, or fever on examination suggests a respiratory cause of chest pain. Pleural effusion may cause pain that is worsened by deep inspiration. Chest x-ray examination may confirm the diagnosis of pleural effusion, pneumonia, or pneumothorax.

Exercise-Induced Asthma. The prevalence of exercise-induced asthma is probably underestimated. Exercise triggers bronchospasm in up to 80% of individuals with asthma. The response of the asthmatic patient to exercise is quite characteristic. Running for 1 to 2 minutes often causes bronchodilatation in patients with asthma, but strenuous exercise for 3 to 8 minutes causes bronchoconstriction in virtually all asthmatic subjects, especially when the heart rate rises to 180 beats/minute. Symptoms range from mild to severe and may include coughing, wheezing, dyspnea, and chest congestion, constriction, or pain. Patients also complain of limited endurance during exercise. Environmental factors such as cold temperature, pollens, and air pollution as well as viral respiratory infection can worsen exercise-induced asthma. Diagnosis is made by the exercise-induced bronchospasm provocation test, which has been described under "Stress Testing" in Chapter 6.

Gastrointestinal

1. Some gastrointestinal disorders, including gastroesophageal reflux (GER), may arise as chest pain in children. The onset and relief of pain in relation to eating and diet may help clarify the diagnosis. The incidence of GER is higher in patients with Down syndrome, cerebral palsy, and other causes of developmental delay.

2. Esophagitis resulting from GER should be suspected in a child who complains of burning substernal pain that worsens with a reclining posture or abdominal pressure or that worsens after certain foods are eaten.

3. Young children sometimes ingest foreign bodies, such as coins, which lodge in the upper esophagus, or they may ingest caustic substances that burn the entire esophagus. In such cases, the history makes the diagnosis obvious.

4. Cholecystitis arises with postprandial pain referred to the right upper quadrant of the abdomen and part of the chest.

Psychogenic. Psychogenic disturbances account for 5% to 17% of cases and are more likely to be seen in female adolescents. Often a recent stressful situation parallels the onset of the chest pain: a death or separation in the family, a serious illness, a disability, a recent move, failure in school, or sexual molestation. However, a psychological cause of chest pain should not be lightly assigned without a thorough history taking and a follow-up evaluation. Psychological or psychiatric consultation may reveal conversion symptoms, a somatization disorder, or even depression.

Miscellaneous

1. The precordial catch (Texidor's twinge or stitch in the side), a one-sided chest pain, lasts a few seconds or minutes and is associated with bending or slouching. The cause is unclear, but the pain is relieved by straightening and taking a few shallow breaths or one deep breath. The pain may recur frequently or remain absent for months.

2. Slipping rib syndrome results from excess mobility of the 8th to 10th ribs, which do not directly insert into the sternum.

3. Some male and female adolescents complain of chest pain caused by breast masses (*mastalgia*). These tender masses may be cysts (in postpubertal girls) or may be part of normal breast development in pubertal boys and girls.

4. *Pleurodynia* (devil's grip), an unusual cause of chest pain caused by coxsackievirus infection, is characterized by sudden episodes of sharp pain in the chest or abdomen.

5. *Herpes zoster* is another unusual cause of chest pain.

6. *Spontaneous pneumothorax* and *pneumomediastinum* are serious but rare respiratory causes of acute chest pain in children; children with asthma, cystic fibrosis, or Marfan syndrome are at risk. Inhalation of cocaine can provoke pneumomediastinum and pneumothorax with subcutaneous emphysema.

7. *Pulmonary embolism*, although extremely rare in children, has been reported in female adolescents who use oral contraceptives or have had elective abortions. It has also been reported in male adolescents with recent trauma of the lower extremities and in children with shunted hydrocephalus. It may occur in children with hypercoagulation syndromes. Affected patients usually have dyspnea, pleuritic pain, fever, cough, and hemoptysis.

8. *Hyperventilation* can produce chest discomfort and is often associated with paresthesia and lightheadedness.

CARDIOVASCULAR CAUSES OF CHEST PAIN

Cardiovascular disease is identified as the cause of pediatric chest pain in 0% to 4% of cases. Cardiac chest pain may be caused by ischemic ventricular dysfunction, pericardial or myocardial inflammatory processes, or arrhythmias. A typical *anginal pain* is located in the precordial or substernal area and radiates to the neck, jaw, either or both arms, back, or abdomen. The patient describes the pain as a deep, heavy pressure; the feeling of choking; or a squeezing sensation. Exercise, cold stress, emotional upset, or a large meal typically precipitates anginal pain. Table 30–2 summarizes important clinical findings of cardiac causes of chest pain in children.

Ischemic Myocardial Dysfunction

Congenital Heart Defects. Severe obstructive lesions, such as aortic stenosis (AS), subaortic stenosis, severe pulmonary stenosis (PS), and pulmonary vascular obstructive disease (Eisenmenger's syndrome), may cause chest pain. Mild stenotic lesions do not cause ischemic chest pain. Chest pain from severe obstructive lesions results from increased myocardial oxygen demands from tachycardia and increased pressure work by the ventricle. Therefore, the pain is usually associated with exercise and is a typical anginal pain, as previously discussed. Cardiac examination often reveals a loud heart murmur best audible at the upper right or left sternal border, usually with a thrill. The ECG usually shows ventricular hypertrophy with or without "strain" pattern. Chest x-ray

*Table 30–2. **Important Clinical Findings of Cardiac Causes of Chest Pain***

Condition	History	Physical Findings	ECG	Chest X-ray Film
Severe AS	Hx of CHD (+)	Loud (> grade 3/6 SEM at URSB with radiation to neck)	LVH with or without strain	Prominent ascending aorta and aortic knob
Severe PS	Hx of CHD (+)	Loud (grade >3/6) SEM at ULSB	RVH with or without strain	Prominent PA segment
HOCM	Positive FH in one third of cases	Variable heart murmurs Brisk brachial pulses (±)	LVH Deep Q/small R or QS pattern in LPLs	Mild cardiomegaly with globular-shaped heart
MVP	Positive FH (±)	Midsystolic click with or without late systolic murmur Thin body build Thoracic skeletal anomalies (80%)	Inverted T waves in aVF (±)	Normal heart size Straight back (±) Narrow AP diameter (±)
Eisenmenger's syndrome	Hx of CHD (+)	Cyanosis and clubbing RV impulse Loud and single S2 Soft or no heart murmur	RVH	Markedly prominent PA with normal heart size
Anomalous origin of left coronary artery	Recurrent episodes of distress in early infancy	Soft or no heart murmur	Anterolateral MI	Moderate to marked cardiomegaly
Sequelae of Kawasaki or other coronary artery diseases	Hx of Kawasaki disease (±) Typical exercise-related anginal pain	Usually negative Continuous murmur in coronary fistula	ST-segment elevation (±) Old MI pattern (±)	Normal heart size or mild cardiomegaly
Cocaine abuse	Hx of substance abuse (±) Nonspecific heart murmur (±)	Hypertension	ST-segment elevation (±)	Normal heart size in acute cases
Pericarditis and myocarditis	Hx of URI (±) Sharp chest pain	Friction rub Muffled heart sounds Nonspecific heart murmur (±)	Low QRS voltages ST-segment shift Arrhythmias (±)	Cardiomegaly of varying degree
Postpericardiotomy syndrome	Hx of recent heart surgery, pain, and dyspnea	Muffled heart sounds (±) Friction rub	Persistent ST-segment elevation	Cardiomegaly of varying degree
Arrhythmias (and palpitation)	Hx of WPW syndrome (±) FH of long QT syndrome (±)	May be negative Irregular rhythm (±)	Arrhythmias (±) WPW preexcitation (±) Long QTc syndrome (>0.46 sec)	Normal heart size

AP, anteroposterior; AS, aortic stenosis; CHD, congenital heart disease; FH, family history; HOCM, hypertrophic obstructive cardiomyopathy; Hx, history; LPLs, left precordial leads; LVH, left ventricular hypertrophy; MI, myocardial infarction; MVP, mitral valve prolapse; PA, pulmonary artery; PS, pulmonary stenosis; RV, right ventricle; RVH, right ventricular hypertrophy; SEM, systolic ejection murmur; ULSB, upper left sternal border; URI, upper respiratory infection; URSB, upper right sternal border; WPW, Wolff-Parkinson-White; (+), positive; (±), may be present.

films may be abnormal in patients with AS and PS with a prominent ascending aorta and main pulmonary artery trunk, respectively. Chest films are definitely abnormal in patients with Eisenmenger's syndrome, with a marked prominence of the main pulmonary artery segment. Echocardiography and Doppler studies permit accurate diagnosis of the type and severity of the obstructive lesion. An exercise ECG may aid in the functional assessment of severity.

Mitral Valve Prolapse. Chest pain associated with mitral valve prolapse (MVP) has been reported in about 20% of patients with the condition. The pain is usually a vague, nonexertional pain of short duration, located at the apex, without a constant relationship to effort or emotion. The pain is presumed to result from papillary muscle or left ventricular endomyocardial ischemia, but there is increasing doubt about the causal relationship between chest pain and MVP in children. Occasionally, supraventricular or ventricular arrhythmias may result in cardiac symptoms, including chest discomfort. Thoracoskeletal deformities commonly occur in these children and may cause chest pain. Nearly all patients with Marfan syndrome have MVP.

Cardiac examination reveals a midsystolic click with or without a late systolic murmur. The ECG may show T-wave inversion in the inferior leads. Two-dimensional echo findings of MVP in adults are well established, but diagnostic echo findings of MVP have not been established in children (see Chapter 21).

Cardiomyopathy. Hypertrophic and dilated cardiomyopathy can cause chest pain from ischemia, with or without exercise, or from rhythm disturbances. Cardiac examination reveals no diagnostic findings, but the ECG or chest x-ray films are abnormal, leading to further studies. Echo studies are diagnostic of the condition (see Chapter 18).

Coronary Artery Disease. Coronary artery anomalies rarely cause chest pain. They include rare cases of anomalous origin of the left coronary artery from the pulmonary artery (usually symptomatic during early infancy), single coronary artery, coronary artery fistula, aneurysm or stenosis of the coronary arteries as a result of Kawasaki disease, or coronary insufficiency secondary to previous cardiac surgery involving the coronary arteries or the vicinity of these arteries.

The pain caused by coronary artery abnormalities is typical of anginal pain. Cardiac examination may be normal or may reveal a heart murmur (systolic murmur of mitral regurgitation or continuous murmur of fistulas). The ECG may show myocardial ischemia (ST-segment elevation) or old myocardial infarction. Chest x-ray films may reveal abnormalities suggestive of these conditions. An abnormal exercise ECG further indicates myocardial ischemia. Although echo can be helpful, coronary angiography is usually indicated for the definitive diagnosis.

Cocaine Abuse. Even children with normal hearts are at risk for ischemia and myocardial infarction if cocaine is used. Cocaine blocks the reuptake of norepinephrine in the central nervous system and peripheral sympathetic nerves. An increase in the sympathetic output and circulating level of catecholamines causes coronary vasoconstriction. Cocaine also induces the activation of platelets in some patients and causes increased production of endothelin and decreased production of nitric oxide. The resulting increase in heart rate and blood pressure, increase in myocardial oxygen consumption, possible increase in platelet activation, and myocardial electrical abnormalities may collectively produce anginal pain, infarction, arrhythmias, or sudden death. History and drug screening help physicians in the diagnosis of cocaine-induced chest pain.

Aortic Dissection or Aortic Aneurysm. Aortic dissection or aortic aneurysm rarely causes chest pain. Children with Turner's, Marfan, and Noonan's syndromes are at risk.

Pericardial or Myocardial Disease

Pericarditis. Irritation of the pericardium may result from inflammatory pericardial disease; pericarditis may have a viral, bacterial, or rheumatic origin. In a child who had recent open-heart surgery, the cause of the pain may be postpericardiotomy syndrome. Older children with pericarditis may complain of a sharp, stabbing precordial pain that worsens when lying down and improves after sitting and leaning forward. Examination may reveal distant heart sounds, neck vein distention, friction rub, and paradoxical pulse. The ECG may reveal low QRS voltages and ST-T changes, and chest x-ray films may show varying degrees of cardiac enlargement and changes in the cardiac silhouette. Diagnosis of pericardial effusion with or without tamponade can be accurately made by echo examination.

Myocarditis. Acute myocarditis often involves the pericardium to a certain extent and can cause chest pain. Examination may reveal fever, respiratory distress, distant heart sounds, neck vein distention, and friction rub. Chest x-ray films and the ECG may suggest the correct diagnosis, which can be confirmed by echo examination (see Chapter 19).

Arrhythmias. Chest pain may result from a variety of arrhythmias, especially with sustained tachycardia resulting in myocardial ischemia. Even without ischemia, children may consider palpitation or forceful heartbeats as chest pain. When chest pain is associated with dizziness and palpitation, a resting ECG and a 24-hour ambulatory ECG using a Holter monitor should be obtained. Alternatively, an event recorder with a telephone transmission device may be used to relay the ECG while the patient experiences symptoms.

Diagnostic Approach

The first goral of evaluating children with a complaint of chest pain is to rule out a cardiac cause of chest pain, which is usually the main concern to the child and parents, and to look for three common causes of chest pain—costochondritis, musculoskeletal causes, and respiratory diseases—which account for 45% to 65% of chest pain in children.

A thorough history taking and careful physical examination suffice to rule out cardiac causes of chest pain and often find a specific cause of the pain. In order to rule out cardiac causes of chest pain, physicians need at least chest x-ray films and an ECG. (Cardiologists, in addition, obtain an echocardiogram to accomplish the same.) Cardiac causes of chest pain can be ruled out by nonexertional nature of pain, negative cardiac examination, and normal results of other investigations. Finding a specific, benign, or noncardiac cause of pain strengthens the diagnosis of noncardiac chest pain. Even if physicians cannot find a specific cause of chest pain, most patients and parents are relieved and satisfied to learn that the heart is not the cause of chest pain.

HISTORY OF PRESENT ILLNESS

The initial history should be directed at determining the nature of the pain, in terms of the duration, intensity, frequency, location, and points of radiation. An important aspect of the history is whether the chest pain occurred during or after heavy physical activities or occurred at rest or while sitting in class. It is important to remember that ischemic cardiac chest pain is associated with exertion and is described as a pressure or squeezing sensation, not a sharp pain. Associated symptoms, concurrent or precipitating events, and relieving factors may help clarify the origin of the pain.

The following are some examples of questions to ask.

1. What seems to bring on the pain (e.g., exercise, eating, trauma, emotional stress)?
2. Do you get the same type of pain while you watch TV or sit in class?
3. What is the pain like (e.g., sharp, pressure sensation, squeezing)?
4. What are the location (e.g., specific point, localized or diffuse), severity, radiation, and duration (seconds, minutes) of the pain?
5. Does the pain get worse with deep breathing? (If so, the pain may be caused by pleural irritation or chest wall pathology.) Does the pain improve with certain body positions? (This is sometimes seen with pericarditis.)
6. Does the pain have any relationship with your meals?
7. How often and how long have you had similar pain (frequency and chronicity)?
8. Have you been hurt while playing, or have you used your arms excessively for any reason?
9. Are there any associated symptoms, such as cough, fever, syncope, dizziness, or palpitation?
10. What treatments for the pain have already been tried?

PAST AND FAMILY HISTORIES

After gaining some idea about the nature of the pain, the clinician should focus on important past and family histories. Examples of questions are as follows.

1. Are there any known medical conditions (e.g., congenital or acquired heart disease, cardiac surgery, infection, asthma)?
2. Is the child taking medicines, such as asthma medicines or birth control pills?
3. Has there been recent heart disease, chest pain, or a cardiac death in the family?
4. Does any disease run in the family?
5. What is the patient or family member concerned about?
6. Has the child been exposed to drugs (cocaine) or cigarettes?

PHYSICAL EXAMINATION

1. A careful general physical examination should be performed before the focus turns to the chest. The clinician should note whether the child is in severe distress from pain, is in emotional stress, or is hyperventilating.

2. The skin and extremities should be examined for trauma or chronic disease. Bruising elsewhere on the body may indicate chest trauma that cannot be seen.

3. The abdomen should be carefully examined because it may be the source of pain referred to the chest.

4. The chest should be carefully inspected for trauma or asymmetry. The chest wall should be palpated for signs of tenderness or subcutaneous air. Special attention should be paid to the possibility of costochondritis as the cause of chest pain, which is a quite common identifiable cause of the pain. Physicians should use the soft part of the terminal phalanx of a middle finger to palpate each costochondral *and* chondrosternal junction, not the palm of a hand; using the latter method may frequently miss the diagnosis. Pectoralis muscles and shoulder muscles should be examined for tenderness, which may be caused by excessive weightlifting or other work requiring the use of these muscles.

5. The heart and lungs should be auscultated for arrhythmias, heart murmurs, rubs, muffled heart sounds, gallop rhythm, crackles, wheezes, or decreased breath sounds.

6. Finally, the child's psychological state should be assessed.

OTHER INVESTIGATIONS

If the three common causes or other identifiable causes of chest pain are not found by physical examination, the clinician should obtain chest x-ray films and an ECG and direct attention to the cardiac causes of chest pain listed in Table 30–2, which summarizes important history, physical findings, and abnormalities of chest x-ray films and ECGs for cardiac causes of chest pain.

1. Cardiac examination is to detect a pathologic heart murmur. One must be careful not to interpret commonly occurring innocent murmurs as pathologic.

2. Chest x-ray films should be evaluated for pulmonary pathology, cardiac size and silhouette, and pulmonary vascularity.

3. A resting 12-lead ECG should be evaluated for cardiac arrhythmias, hypertrophy, conduction disturbances (including Wolff-Parkinson-White preexcitation), abnormal T and Q waves, and an abnormal QT interval.

If the family history is negative for hereditary heart disease (such as long QT syndrome, cardiomyopathies, unexpected sudden death), if the past history is negative for heart disease or Kawasaki's disease, if the cardiac examination is unremarkable, and if the ECG and chest x-ray films are normal, the chest pain is not likely to be of cardiac origin. At this point, the clinician can reassure the patient and family of the probable benign nature of the chest pain. If any of the preceding aspects is positive, a formal cardiac consultation may be indicated. Echocardiographic studies are usually obtained by cardiologists.

If a cardiac cause and the three common causes of chest pain are not found, the pain is probably due to a condition in other systems, such as the gastrointestinal or respiratory system, including psychogenic or idiopathic origin. Simple follow-up may clarify the cause. Drug screening for cocaine may be worthwhile in adolescents who have acute, severe chest pain and distress with an unclear cause.

REFERRAL TO CARDIOLOGISTS

The following are some of the indications for referral to a cardiologist for cardiac evaluation:

1. When history reveals that chest pain is triggered or worsened by physical activities, the pain suggests anginal pain, or chest pain is accompanied by other symptoms such as palpitation, dizziness, or syncope.

2. When there are abnormal findings in the cardiac examination or when abnormalities occur in the chest x-ray films or ECG, cardiology referral is clearly indicated. The examiner's ability to recognize common innocent heart murmurs minimizes the frequency of such referrals.

3. When there is a positive family history for cardiomyopathy, long QT syndrome, sudden unexpected death, or other hereditary diseases commonly associated with cardiac abnormalities.

4. High levels of anxiety in the family and patient and a chronic, recurring nature of the pain are also important reasons for referral to a cardiologist.

Management

When a specific cause of chest pain is identified, treatment is directed at correcting or improving the cause.

1. Costochondritis can be treated by reassurance and occasionally by nonsteroidal anti-inflammatory agents (such as ibuprofen) or acetaminophen. Ibuprofen is better than acetaminophen because the former is an anti-inflammatory agent and the latter is only analgesic.

2. Most musculoskeletal and nonorganic causes of chest pain can be treated with rest, acetaminophen, or nonsteroidal anti-inflammatory agents.

3. If respiratory causes of chest pain are found, treatment is directed at those causes. Referral to a pulmonologist should be considered.

4. Exercise-induced asthma is most effectively prevented by inhalation of a β_2-agonist immediately before exercise. Inhaled albuterol usually affords protection for 4 hours. Other antiasthmatic agents have been reported to be effective as well. Use of a muffler or cold weather mask to warm and humidify air before inhalation is also effective.

5. If gastritis, GER, or peptic ulcer disease is suspected, trials of antacids, hydrogen ion blockers, or a prokinetic agent (such as metoclopramide [Reglan]) are helpful therapeutically (as well as diagnostically).

6. If serious cardiac anomalies, arrhythmias, or exercise-induced asthma is diagnosed, a referral is made to the cardiology or pulmonary service. Cardiac evaluation requires further specialized studies such as echo, an exercise stress test, Holter monitoring, event recorder, or even cardiac catheterization. Depending on the cause, treatment may be surgical or medical.

7. If organic causes of chest pain are not found and a psychogenic etiology is suspected, psychological consultation may be considered.

8. The correct therapy of acute cocaine toxicity has not been established. Calcium channel blockers (nifedipine, nitrendipine), β-adrenergic blockers, nitrates, and thrombolytic agents have resulted in varying levels of success. The use of β-blockers is controversial; they may worsen coronary blood flow.

Chapter 31

Syncope

Prevalence

The prevalence of syncope and near syncope in children is unknown, but it is estimated that as many as 15% of children and adolescents have a syncopal event between the ages of 8 and 18 years. The incidence may be as high as 3% of emergency room visits in some areas. Before age 6 years, syncope is unusual except in the setting of seizure disorders, breath holding, and cardiac arrhythmias.

Definition

Syncope is a transient loss of consciousness and muscle tone that result from inadequate cerebral perfusion. Presyncope is the feeling that one is about to pass out but remains conscious with a transient loss of postural tone. The most common prodromal symptom is dizziness. Dizziness is a nonspecific symptom that may include vertigo, presyncope, and lightheadedness. The patient may say "my head is spinning" or "the room is whirling" to describe vertigo (a manifestation of vestibular disorder). Lightheadedness often accompanies hyperventilation and is frequently associated with psychological distress, including anxiety, depression, and panic attacks. Any of these complaints could represent a serious cardiac condition that could cause sudden death.

Causes

The normal function of the brain depends on a constant supply of oxygen and glucose. Significant alterations in the supply of oxygen and glucose may result in a transient loss or near loss of consciousness. The differential diagnosis of syncope is rather broad. It may be due to noncardiac causes (usually autonomic dysfunction), cardiac conditions, neuropsychiatric conditions, and metabolic disorders. Box 31–1 lists possible causes of syncope.

In contrast to adults, in whom most cases of syncope are caused by cardiac problems, in children and adolescents, most incidents of syncope are benign, resulting from vasovagal episodes (probably the most common cause), orthostatic intolerance syndromes, hyperventilation, and breath holding. However, the primary purpose of the evaluation of patients with syncope is to determine whether the patient is at increased risk for death.

Athletic adolescents may experience syncope or presyncope during or after strenuous physical activities. However, although serious cardiac problems may be the cause of the exercise-related syncope, it is usually secondary to a combination of venous pooling

BOX 31–1	CAUSES OF SYNCOPE

AUTONOMIC (NONCARDIAC)

Orthostatic intolerance group
  Vasovagal syncope (also known as simple, neurocardiogenic, or neurally mediated syncope)
  Orthostatic (postural) hypotension (dysautonomia)
  Postural orthostatic tachycardia syndrome (POTS)
Exercise-related syncope (see further discussion in text)
Situational syncope
  Breath holding
  Cough, micturition, defecation, etc.
  Carotid sinus hypersensitivity
Excess vagal tone

CARDIAC

Arrhythmia

  Tachycardia: SVT, atrial flutter/fibrillation, ventricular tachycardia (seen with long
    QT syndrome, arrhythmogenic RV dysplasia)
  Bradycardias: Sinus bradycardia, asystole, complete heart block, pacemaker malfunction

Obstructive Lesions

  Outflow obstruction: AS, PS, hypertrophic cardiomyopathy, pulmonary hypertension
  Inflow obstruction: MS, tamponade, constrictive pericarditis, atrial myxoma

Myocardial Dysfunction

  Coronary artery anomalies, hypertrophic cardiomyopathy, dilated cardiomyopathy;
    MVP, arrhythmogenic RV dysplasia

NEUROPSYCHIATRIC

  Hyperventilation
  Seizure
  Migraine
  Tumors
  Hysterical

METABOLIC

  Hypoglycemia
  Electrolyte disorders
  Anorexia nervosa
  Drugs/toxins

AS, aortic stenosis; MS, mitral stenosis; MVP, mitral valve prolapse; PS, pulmonary stenosis; RV, right ventricular; SVT, supraventricular tachycardia.

and dehydration associated with athletic activities. Secondary hyperventilation (with hypocapnia) from exertional activities may contribute to this form of syncope.

In this chapter, only circulatory causes of syncope are discussed in some detail. Discussion of the metabolic and neuropsychiatric causes of syncope is beyond the scope of this book.

NONCARDIAC CAUSES OF SYNCOPE

Orthostatic Intolerance

Orthostatic intolerance encompasses disorders of blood flow, heart rate, and blood pressure (BP) regulation that are most easily demonstrable during orthostatic stress, yet are present in all positions. Improved understanding of changes in these parameters is the result of the recently popularized head-up tilt test. Three easily definable entities of orthostatic intolerance are vasovagal syncope, orthostatic hypotension, and postural orthostatic tachycardia syndrome (POTS).

Vasovagal Syncope

Vasovagal syncope (also called simple fainting or neurocardiogenic or neurally mediated syncope) is the most common type of syncope in otherwise healthy children and adolescents. This syncope is uncommon before 10 to 12 years of age but quite prevalent in adolescent girls. It is characterized by a prodrome (warning symptoms and signs) lasting a few seconds to a minute; the prodrome may include dizziness, nausea, pallor, diaphoresis, palpitation, blurred vision, headache, and/or hyperventilation. The prodrome is followed by loss of consciousness and muscle tone. The patient usually falls without injury, the unconsciousness does not last more than a minute, and the patient gradually awakens. The syncope may occur after rising in the morning or in association with prolonged standing, anxiety or fright, pain, blood drawing or the sight of blood, fasting, hot and humid conditions, or crowded places. It may occur following prolonged exercise (if it is stopped suddenly).

Pathophysiology of vasovagal syncope is not completely understood. The following is a popular hypothesis (although dismissed by some). In normal individuals, an erect posture without movement shifts blood to the lower extremities and causes a decrease in venous return, thus decreasing stroke volume and BP. This reduced filling of the ventricle places less stretch on the mechanoreceptor (i.e., C fibers) and causes a decrease in afferent neural output to the brain stem, reflecting hypotension. This decline in neural traffic from the mechanoreceptors and decreased arterial pressure elicit an increase in sympathetic output, resulting in an increase in heart rate and peripheral vasoconstriction to restore BP to the normal range. Thus, the normal responses to the assumption of an upright posture are a reduced cardiac output (by 25%), an increase in heart rate, an unchanged or slightly diminished systolic pressure (Fig. 31–1), and an increase in diastolic pressure to ensure coronary artery perfusion. Cerebral blood flow decreases by approximately 6% with cerebrovascular autoregulation functioning near its maximal limit.

In susceptible individuals, however, a sudden decrease in venous return to the ventricle produces a large increase in the force of ventricular contraction; this causes activation of the left ventricular mechanoreceptors, which normally respond only to stretch.

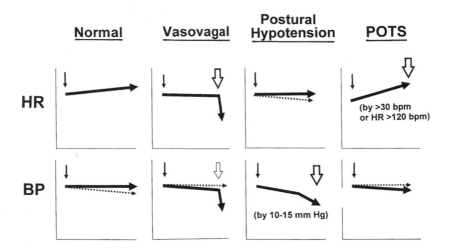

Figure 31–1. *Schematic drawing of changes in heart rate and blood pressure observed during the head-up tilt test.* Thin arrows *mark the start of orthostatic stress.* Large unfilled arrows *indicate appearance of symptoms with changes seen in heart rate and blood pressure. In normal individuals, the heart rate increases slightly with no change or a slight reduction in blood pressure. In patients with vasovagal syncope, both the heart rate and blood pressure drop precipitously with appearance of symptoms. Postural hypotension is characterized by a drop in blood pressure by 10 to 15 mm Hg as symptoms appear. In POTS, heart rate increases significantly by more than 30 beats/minute (or the heart rate is 120 beats/minute or higher) with development of symptoms. BP, blood pressure; HR, heart rate; POTS, postural orthostatic tachycardia syndrome.*

The resulting paroxysmal increase in neural traffic to the brain stem somehow mimics the conditions seen in hypertension and thereby produces a paradoxical withdrawal of sympathetic activity with subsequent peripheral vasodilatation, hypotension, and brady-cardia (see Fig. 31–1). Characteristically, the reduction of BP and especially the heart rate is severe enough to decrease cerebral perfusion and produce loss of consciousness. The finding that patients who have received cardiac transplants retain the ability to faint implies that the ventricular receptor theory cannot explain all vasovagal syncope.

History is most important in establishing the diagnosis of vasovagal syncope. Tilt testing of various protocols is useful in diagnosing vasovagal syncope, but it has not been well standardized and its specificity and reproducibility are questionable.

Placing the patient in a supine position until the circulatory crisis resolves may be all that is indicated. If the patient feels the prodrome to a faint, he or she should be told to lie down with the feet raised above the chest; this usually aborts the syncope. Success in preventing syncope has been reported with medications, such as fludrocorti-sone (Florinef), β-blockers, pseudoephedrine, and others (see "Treatment" section later).

Orthostatic Hypotension (Dysautonomia)

The normal response to standing is reflex arterial and venous constriction and a slight increase in heart rate. In orthostatic hypotension, the normal adrenergic vasoconstriction of the arterioles and veins in the upright position is absent or inadequate, resulting in hypotension without a reflex increase in heart rate (see Fig. 31–1). In contrast to the prodrome seen with vasovagal syncope, in orthostatic hypotension, patients experience only lightheadedness. Orthostatic hypotension is usually related to medication (see later) or dehydration, but it can be precipitated by prolonged bed rest, prolonged standing, and conditions that decrease the circulating blood volume (e.g., bleeding, dehydration). Drugs that interfere with the sympathetic vasomotor response (e.g., calcium channel blockers, antihypertensive drugs, vasodilators, phenothiazines) and diuretics may exacerbate ortho-static hypotension. Dysautonomia may also be seen during an acute infectious disease or in peripheral neuropathies such as Guillain-Barré syndrome.

In patients suspected of having orthostatic hypotension, BPs should be measured in the supine and standing positions. The American Autonomic Society has defined ortho-static hypotension as a persistent fall in systolic/diastolic pressure of more than 20/10 mm Hg within 3 minutes of assuming the upright position without moving the arms or legs, with no increase in the heart rate but without fainting. Patients with ortho-static hypotension also have a positive tilt test but do not display the autonomic nervous system signs of vasovagal syncope, such as pallor, diaphoresis, and hyperventilation.

The same management as given for vasovagal syncope is sometimes successful. Elastic stockings, a high-salt diet, sympathomimetic amines, and corticosteroids have been used with varying degrees of success. The patient should be told to move to an upright position slowly.

Postural Orthostatic Tachycardia Syndrome

This new syndrome, most often observed in young women, is a form of autonomic neu-ropathy that predominantly affects the lower extremities. Venous pooling associated with assuming a standing position leads to a reduced venous return and a resulting increase in sympathetic discharge with a significant degree of tachycardia. These patients mani-fest an orthostatic intolerance with presenting complaints of chronic fatigue, exercise intolerance, palpitation, lightheadedness, nausea, and recurrent near syncope (and some-times syncope). The findings may be related to *chronic fatigue syndrome*, and the patients may be misdiagnosed as having panic attacks or chronic anxiety. The general physical examination is often unrevealing.

For the diagnosis of POTS, heart rate and BP are measured in the supine, sitting, and standing positions. POTS is defined as the development of orthostatic symptoms that are associated with at least a 30 beats/minute increase in heart rate (or a heart rate of ≥120 beats/minute) that occurs within the first 10 minutes of standing or upright tilt. An exaggerated increase in heart rate is often accompanied by hypotension in associa-tion with the symptoms described previously (see Fig. 31–1). Occasional patients develop swelling of the dependent lower extremities with purplish discoloration of the dorsum of the foot and ankle. Tilt table testing is often useful as a standardized measure of response to postural change. Some patients may exhibit an exaggerated response to isoproterenol.

The same management approaches as for vasovagal syncope are used with varying levels of success. One should check whether any medications the patient is taking could be contributing to the problem (such as vasodilators, tricyclic antidepressants, monoamine oxidase inhibitors, or alcohol). The patient is advised to avoid extreme heat and dehydration and to increase salt and fluid intake. Pharmacologic agents such as fludrocortisone, midodrine (a peripheral vasoconstrictor, at the dose of 5 to 10 mg three times a day), or venlafaxine (a selective serotonin reuptake inhibitor) are useful in many patients.

Exercise-Related Syncope

Sudden unconsciousness that occurs during or after strenuous physical activities or sports may signal an organic cause such as cardiopulmonary diseases. However, in most cases, exercise-related syncope is not an indicator of serious underlying cardiopulmonary or metabolic disease. It is more often due to a combination of venous pooling in vasodilated leg muscles, inadequate hydration, and high ambient temperature. Hyperventilation with hypocapnia (with tingling or numbness of extremities) secondary to strenuous activities may also cause syncope. To prevent venous pooling, athletes should keep moving after running competitions.

Rare Causes of Syncope

Micturition syncope is a rare form of orthostatic hypotension. In this condition, rapid bladder decompression results in decreased total peripheral vascular resistance with splanchnic stasis and reduced venous return to the heart, resulting in postural hypotension.

Cough syncope follows paroxysmal nocturnal coughing in asthmatic children. The patient's face become plethoric and cyanotic, and the child perspires, becomes agitated, and is frightened. Loss of consciousness is associated with muscle contractions lasting for several seconds. Urinary incontinence is frequent. Consciousness is regained within a few minutes. Paroxysmal coughing produces a marked increase in intrapleural pressure with a reduced venous return and reduced cardiac output, resulting in altered cerebral blood flow and loss of consciousness. Treatment is aimed at preventing bronchoconstriction with aggressive asthma treatment plans.

CARDIAC CAUSES OF SYNCOPE

Cardiac causes of syncope may include obstructive lesions, myocardial dysfunction, and arrhythmias, including long QT syndrome. A cardiac cause of syncope is suggested by the occurrence of syncope even in the recumbent position, syncope provoked by exercise, chest pain associated with syncope, a history of unoperated or operated heart disease, or a family history of sudden death.

Obstructive Lesions

Patients with severe obstructive lesions such as aortic stenosis (AS), pulmonary stenosis (PS), or hypertrophic obstructive cardiomyopathy (HOCM), as well as those with pulmonary hypertension, may have syncope. Peripheral vasodilatation secondary to exercise is not accompanied by an adequate increase in cardiac output because of the obstructive lesion, which results in diminished perfusion to the brain. Exercise often precipitates syncope associated with these conditions. Patients may also complain of chest pain, dyspnea, and palpitation.

Obstructive lesions and pulmonary hypertension can be diagnosed by careful physical examination, ECG, chest x-ray studies, and echo. Surgery is indicated for most of these conditions, with the exception of irreversible forms of pulmonary hypertension.

Myocardial Dysfunction

Although rare, myocardial ischemia or infarction secondary to congenital anomalies of the coronary arteries or acquired disease of the coronary arteries (such as Kawasaki disease or atherosclerotic heart disease) may cause syncope. Patients with dilated cardio-myopathy may have episodes of syncope associated with self-terminating episodes of ventricular tachycardia, which can lead to cardiac arrest. Syncope is a major risk factor for subsequent sudden cardiac death in hypertrophic cardiomyopathy, particularly if it is repetitive and occurs with exertion. Patients with arrhythmogenic right ventricular (RV) dysplasia often develop ventricular tachycardia.

Arrhythmias

Either extreme tachycardia or bradycardia can decrease cardiac output and lower the cerebral blood flow below the critical level, causing syncope. Commonly encountered rhythm disturbances include supraventricular tachycardia (SVT), ventricular tachycardia, sick sinus syndrome, and complete heart block. Simple bradycardia is usually well tolerated in children, but the combination of tachycardia followed by bradycardia (overdrive suppression) is more likely to produce syncope. Arrhythmias may occur with or without structural heart defects.

No Identifiable Structural Defects. Syncope from arrhythmias in children with struc-turally normal hearts may be seen in the following conditions.

1. Long QT syndrome is characterized by syncope caused by ventricular arrhythmias, prolongation of the QT interval on the ECG, and occasionally a family history of sudden death. Congenital deafness is also a component of Jervell and Lange-Nielsen syndrome but not that of Romano-Ward syndrome.

2. Wolff-Parkinson-White (WPW) preexcitation may cause SVT.

3. RV dysplasia (RV cardiomyopathy) is a rare anomaly of the myocardium and is associated with repeated episodes of ventricular tachycardia (see Chapter 18).

4. Brugada syndrome is a rare cause of sudden death by ventricular arrhythmias, seen mostly in Southeast Asian men. The ECG typically shows right bundle branch block with J-point elevation and concave ST elevation in V1.

Structural Heart Defects. The following congenital and acquired heart conditions, unoperated or operated, are associated with arrhythmias that may result in syncope.

1. Preoperative congenital heart diseases (CHDs), such as Ebstein's anomaly, mitral stenosis (MS), or mitral regurgitation (MR), and congenitally corrected transposi-tion of the great arteries (L-TGA) may cause arrhythmias.

2. Postoperative CHDs may cause arrhythmias, especially after repairs of tetralogy of Fallot (TOF) and TGA and after the Fontan operation. These children may have sinus node dysfunction (sick sinus syndrome), SVT or ventricular tachycardia, or complete heart block.

3. Dilated cardiomyopathy can cause sinus bradycardia, SVT, or ventricular tachycardia.

4. Hypertrophic cardiomyopathy is a rare cause of ventricular tachycardia and syncope.

5. Mitral valve prolapse (MVP) is an extremely rare cause of ventricular tachycardia.

Evaluation of a Child with Syncope

The goal of the evaluation of a patient with syncope is to identify high-risk patients with underlying heart disease, which may include ECG abnormalities (such as seen in long QT syndrome, WPW preexcitation, Brugada syndrome), cardiomyopathy (hyper-trophic or dilated), or structural heart diseases. The evaluation of pediatric patients with syncope may extend to other family members when a genetic condition is suspected or identified.

History. Because physical examinations of patients are almost always normal long after the event, accurate history taking is most important in determining a cost-effective diagnostic workup for each patient. Sometimes, a complete history cannot be obtained owing to amnesia about the event, but witness accounts are useful. The following are some important aspects of history taking.

1. About the syncopal event.
    a. The time of the day.
       Syncope occurring after rising in the morning suggests vasovagal syncope. Hypoglycemia is a very rare cause of syncope.
    b. The patient's position (supine, standing, or sitting).
       Syncope while sitting or recumbent suggests arrhythmias or seizures.
       Syncope after standing for some time suggests orthostatic intolerance group including vasovagal syncope.
    c. Relationship to exercise.
       Syncope occurring during exercise suggest arrhythmias.
       Syncope occurring immediately after cessation of physical activities suggests venous pooling in the leg (with reduced venous return and cardiac output). Vigorousness and duration of the activity, relative hydration status, and ambient temperature are important.
    d. Associated symptoms are sometimes helpful in suspecting the cause of syncope.
       Palpitation or racing heart rate suggests tachycardia or arrhythmias.
       Chest pain suggests possible myocardial ischemia (e.g., obstructive lesions, cardiomyopathy, carditis).
       Shortness of breath or tingling or numbness of extremities suggests hyperventilation.
       Nausea, epigastric discomfort, and diaphoresis suggest vasovagal syncope.
       Headache or visual changes suggest vasovagal syncope.
    e. The duration of syncope.
       Syncopal duration less than 1 minute suggests vasovagal syncope, hyperventilation, or syncope related to another orthostatic mechanism.
       A longer duration of syncope suggests convulsive disorders, migraine, or arrhythmias.
    f. The patient's appearance during and immediately following the episode.
       Pallor indicates hypotension.
       Abnormal movement or posturing, confusion, focal neurologic signs, amnesia, or muscle soreness suggests the possibility of seizure.

2. Past history of cardiac, endocrine, neurologic, or psychological disorders may suggest a disorder in that system.

3. Medication history, including prescribed, over-the-counter, and recreational drugs, should be checked.

4. Family history should include:
    a. Coronary heart disease risk factors, including history of myocardial infarction in family members younger than 30 years.
    b. Cardiac arrhythmia, CHD, cardiomyopathies, long QT syndrome, seizures, metabolic and psychological disorders.
    c. Positive family history of fainting is common in patients with vasovagal syncope.

5. Social history is important in assessing whether there is a possibility of substance abuse, pregnancy, or factors leading to a conversion reaction.

Physical Examination. Although the results of the physical examination are usually normal, a complete physical examination should always be performed, focusing on the patient's cardiac and neurologic status.

1. If orthostatic intolerance group is suspected, the heart rate and BP should be measured repeatedly while the patient is supine and after standing without moving for up to 10 minutes.

2. Careful auscultation is carried out to detect a heart murmur or an abnormally loud second heart sound.

3. Neurologic examination should include a funduscopic examination, test for Romberg's sign, gait evaluation, deep tendon reflexes, and cerebellar function.

Diagnostic Studies. History and physical examinations guide practitioners in choosing the diagnostic tests that apply to a given syncopal patient. A cardiology consultation should be obtained if there is a heart murmur, a family history of sudden death or cardiomyopathy, or an abnormal ECG finding.

1. Serum glucose and electrolytes are of limited value because the patients are seen hours or days after the episode.

2. In suspected cases of arrhythmia as the cause of syncope, the physician must document a causal relationship between arrhythmias and symptoms by ECG recording or an exercise stress test, or both. Some equivocal cases in which arrhythmias and symptoms are not causally related may require electrophysiologic studies.

   a. All patients presenting with syncope should have an ECG. The ECG should be inspected for heart rate (bradycardia), arrhythmias, WPW preexcitation, heart block, and long QTc interval as well as abnormalities suggestive of cardiomyopathies and myocarditis.

   b. Ambulatory ECG monitoring: A correlation between patients' symptoms and a diagnostic arrhythmia confirms the arrhythmic cause of syncope. Symptoms without arrhythmia probably exclude an arrhythmic cause of syncope.

      1). The Holter monitor usually records ECG for up to 24 hours.

      2). The external loop recorders with extended monitoring (usually for a month) may increase the diagnostic yield.

      3). The implantable loop recorder (implanted in the left pectoral region) is a device that can be used to record ECGs for a period much longer than 1 month.

   c. Exercise stress test. If the syncopal event is associated with exercise, a treadmill exercise stress test should also be performed, with full ECG and BP monitoring (see Chapter 6).

   d. Cardiac catheterization and electrophysiologic testing may be indicated in some equivocal cases. Because of the low yield of electrophysiologic testing in patients without underlying heart disease, this test is not routinely recommended in such cases.

3. Echocardiographic studies. Echo studies identify structural abnormalities that can cause chest pain. Identifiable structural causes include severe obstructive CHDs (such as AS, PS, HOCM), possible pulmonary hypertension, certain CHDs (Ebstein's anomaly, mitral stenosis or regurgitation, L-TGA), and the status of postoperative CHDs (such as TOF, TGA, Fontan operation).

4. Head-up tilt table test. If patients with positional syncope have autonomic symptoms (such as pallor, diaphoresis, or hyperventilation), tilt table testing is useful (see subsequent section for full discussion).

5. Neurologic consultation. Patients exhibiting prolonged loss of consciousness, seizure activity, and a postictal phase with lethargy or confusion should be referred for neurologic consultation and electroencephalography. Without the preceding history, the reported positive yield of electroencephalography or imaging studies is very low.

Head-up Tilt Table Test. The goal of tilt table testing is to provoke patients' symptoms exactly during an orthostatic stress while closely monitoring them, with demonstration of the cardiac rhythm and rate and BP responses associated with symptoms. Orthostatic stress is created by a tilting table with patients placed in an upright position to obtain the necessary pooling of blood to the lower extremities.

Patients lie supine on an electric tilt table and have an intravenous line established. ECG monitoring and automated BP measurements are performed. Some laboratories perform an autonomic challenge test, which includes deep breathing to accentuate sinus arrhythmia, carotid massage (not done in adults, especially elderly people), Valsalva maneuver, and the application of ice to the face to induce the diving reflex. Patients are then tilted into the 60- to 80-degree head-up position for a period of up to 30 minutes. These patients remain upright, with recording of BP every 1 or 2 minutes and continuous heart rate and rhythm monitoring. If a patient becomes symptomatic or the 30-minute time elapses, the tilt table is immediately returned to the supine position.

If the tilt test alone is not positive, the procedure is repeated with an infusion of isoproterenol, starting at 0.02 µg/kg per minute and increasing to 1 µg/kg per minute for 15 minutes. The use of isoproterenol in the evaluation of patients with vasovagal syncope remains somewhat controversial. Some believe that responses to isoproterenol are nonspecific.

Positive responses commonly include lightheadedness, dizziness, nausea, visual changes, and frank syncope. Sinus bradycardia, junctional bradycardia, and asystole for as long as 30 seconds are common. Hypotension is generally manifested by systolic BPs of less than 70 mm Hg, with frequently immeasurable diastolic pressures. Returning these patients to the supine position produces resolution of symptoms rapidly, with a return of normal sinus rhythm, usually with a reactive tachycardia. Patients frequently comment that they "had a spell" and that they feel tired and weak.

Several distinct abnormal patterns have been identified following head-up tilt table tests (see Fig. 31–1).

1. Vasovagal: an abrupt decrease in BP, usually with bradycardia

2. Dysautonomia (or postural hypotension): a gradual decrease in BP leading to syncope

3. POTS: an excessive heart rate increase to maintain an adequate BP to prevent syncope

Following a positive tilt test, many laboratories begin a therapeutic trial of a short-acting β-blocker, such as an esmolol infusion, and repeat the tilt test. If these patients do not become symptomatic during this tilt test, an oral β-blocker is prescribed (see subsequent discussion). If these patients are again symptomatic, they are tested with a phenylephrine infusion with a repeated tilt table test. Finally, patients are tested with a bolus of 1 L normal saline. If they remain asymptomatic during the test, these patients are treated with volume expansion therapy using a mineralocorticoid (Florinef) and salt supplementation (see later).

There are, however, serious questions about the sensitivity, specificity, diagnostic yield, and day-to-day reproducibility of the tilt test, although many cardiology laboratories use a tilt table test not only to establish a diagnosis but also to select therapy. In adults, the overall reproducibility of syncope by the tilt test is disappointingly low (62%), which causes doubt about the specificity of the test for diagnosis and the validity of evaluating the effect of oral drug treatment by a repeated tilt test. About 25% of adolescents with no prior fainting history fainted during the tilt test. Moreover, among habitual fainters, 25% to 30% did not faint during the test on a given day.

Treatment

Ideally, the cause of the syncopal event determines the appropriate therapy. However, the same preventive measures are used for all in the orthostatic intolerance group. Beginning the therapy empirically without performing a head-up tilt table test is not unreasonable. Success in preventing syncope has been reported with the following medications.

1. Orthostatic intolerance syndromes
   a. Increased salt and fluid intake is encouraged but rarely effective.
   b. Elastic support hose (waist high) are useful in some patients (with postural hypotension).
   c. Fludrocortisone (Floricef), a mineralocorticoid, can be given in a low dosage (0.1 mg by mouth once or twice a day; adult dose around 0.2 mg/day) with increased salt intake or a salt tablet (1 g daily). Average preadolescents or adolescents commonly gain 1 kg or 2 kg water weight into their circulating volume within 2 or 3 weeks. The increased vascular volume allows these patients to maintain cerebral BP despite the normal episodic parasympathetically mediated venodilation.
   d. β-Blocker therapy is used commonly, especially in adolescents and young adults, to modify the feedback loop. Atenolol (1 to 1.2 mg/kg/day by mouth, maximum

dose 2 mg/kg/day) and metoprolol (1.5 mg/kg/day given by mouth in two or three doses) are most commonly used.

e. α-Agonist therapy using pseudoephedrine or an ephedrine-theophylline combination (Marax) stimulates the heart rate and increases the peripheral vascular tone, preventing reflex bradycardia and vasodilation. Pseudoephedrine, 60 mg, given orally twice a day, has been reported to be beneficial in some older children and adolescents.

f. The efficacy of serotonin agonists (sertraline [Zoloft]) has also been described in the treatment of patients with refractory syncope.

2. Primary cardiac arrhythmias arising as syncopal events may require antiarrhythmic medications. Most arrhythmias respond to antiarrhythmic therapy. Long QT syndrome is treated with β-blockers, pacemakers, or an implantable cardioverter-defibrillator (see Chapter 24). Propranolol or other antiarrhythmic drugs may be indicated in patients with symptomatic MVP syndrome. Occasionally, catheter ablation may be indicated (such as in WPW syndrome causing frequent SVT).

3. Beneficial effects of an implanted pacemaker for vasovagal syncope have been reported by some investigators but not by others. In a double-blind randomized trial in adult patients, recurrent syncope still occurred; even though the pacemaker maintained heart rate, BP dropped, and symptoms still occurred (Connolly et al, 2003).

Differential Diagnosis

A thorough history taking usually directs the physician to the correct diagnosis and thereby reduces the number of unnecessary tests.

Epilepsy. Patients with epilepsy may have incontinence, marked confusion in the postictal state, and abnormal electroencephalograms (EEGs). Patients are rigid rather than limp and may have sustained injuries. Patients do not experience the prodromal symptoms of syncope (e.g., dizziness, pallor, palpitation, diaphoresis). The duration of unconsciousness is longer than that typically seen with syncope (<1 minute).

Hypoglycemia. Hypoglycemia has characteristics similar to those of syncope, such as pallor, perspiration, abdominal discomfort, lightheadedness, confusion, unconsciousness, and possible subsequent occurrence of seizures. However, hypoglycemic attacks differ from syncope in that the onset and recovery occur more gradually, they do not occur during or shortly after meals, and the presyncopal symptoms do not improve in the supine position.

Hyperventilation. Hyperventilation is believed to produce hypocapnia, resulting in intense cerebral vasoconstriction, and causes syncope. A recent study, however, demonstrated that hyperventilation alone is not sufficient to cause syncope, suggesting that it may also have a psychological component. A typical spell usually begins with an apprehensive feeling and deep sighing respirations that the patient rarely notices. The patient often experiences air hunger, shortness of breathing, chest tightness, abdominal discomfort, palpitations, dizziness, numbness or tingling of the face and extremities, and rarely loss of consciousness. It is often associated with emotional disturbances. The supine position may help the patient relax and may stop the anxiety-hyperventilation cycle. The syncopal episode can be reproduced in the office when the patient hyperventilates.

Hysteria. Syncope resulting from hysteria is not associated with injury and occurs only in the presence of an audience. A teenager may be able to give an accurate presyncopal history, but during these attacks, he or she does not experience the pallor and hypotension that characterize true syncope. The attacks may last longer (up to an hour) than a brief syncopal spell. Episodes usually occur in an emotionally charged setting and are rare before 10 years of age. Spells are not consistently related to postural changes and are not improved by the supine position.

Chapter 32

Palpitation

Definition and Description

1. Palpitation is an unpleasant subjective awareness of one's own heartbeats. This usually occurs as a sensation in the chest of rapid, irregular, or unusually strong heartbeats.
2. The patient describes it as pounding, jumping, racing, irregularity of the heartbeat, a "flip flopping" or "rapid fluttering" in the chest, or pounding in the neck. Palpitation can be felt in the chest, throat, or neck. The pulse rate may become faster than normal. Rarely, slow heart rates may cause palpitation.
3. The term "palpitation" is used so loosely that specific questions must be asked to determine the exact nature of the symptom.

Causes

Palpitation is one of the most common cardiac symptoms encountered in medical practice, but it poorly corresponds to demonstrable abnormalities. Many palpitations are not serious. However, palpitation may indicate the possible presence of serious cardiac arrhythmias.

Box 32–1 lists causes of palpitation. A high percentage of patients with palpitation have no etiology that can be established. Occasionally, a psychogenic or psychiatric cause for their symptoms can be suspected. Certain drugs and substances can be identified as a cause of palpitation. Caffeine, a common stimulant, is found in many foods and drinks, such as coffee, tea, hot cocoa, soda, chocolate, and some medicines. Most energy drinks (such as Venom, Whoop Ass, Red Bull, Adrenaline Rush), which are the latest popular fad in youth culture, contain large doses of caffeine and other legal stimulants including ephedrine, guarana, taurine, and ginseng. Some medical conditions, such as hyperthyroidism, anemia, and hypoglycemia, may be the cause of palpitation. Although relatively rare, cardiac arrhythmias and structural heart disease should be looked into as a cause of palpitation. However, most palpitations are not accompanied by arrhythmias and most arrhythmias are not perceived and reported as palpitations. Some adult patients with palpitations have panic disorder or panic attack. Panic attack and arrhythmias may be difficult to distinguish clinically because both may arise as palpitations, shortness of breath, and lightheadedness.

Evaluation

History. In a child who is old enough to provide a detailed history, careful history taking often suggests possible causes. Palpitation usually occurs without other symptoms.

BOX 32–1	CAUSES OF PALPITATION

NORMAL PHYSIOLOGIC EVENT

Exercise, excitement, fever

PSYCHOLOGENIC OR PSYCHIATRIC

Fear, anger, stress, anxiety disorders, panic attack, or panic disorder

CERTAIN DRUGS AND SUBSTANCES

Stimulants—caffeine (coffee, tea, soda, chocolate), some energy drinks, smoking

Over-the-counter drugs—decongestants, diet pills, etc.

Drugs that cause tachycardia—catecholamines, theophylline, hydralazine, minoxidil, cocaine

Drugs that cause bradycardia—β-blockers; antihypertensive drugs, calcium channel blockers

Drugs that cause arrhythmias—antiarrhythmics (some of which are proarrhythmic), tricyclic antidepressants, phenothiazines

CERTAIN MEDICAL CONDITIONS

Anemia

Hyperthyroidism

Hypoglycemia

Hyperventilation

Poor physical condition

HEART DISEASES

Certain congenital heart defects that are susceptible to arrhythmias or that result in poor physical condition

Following surgeries for CHD—Fontan connection, Senning operation

Mitral valve prolapse

Hypertrophic cardiomyopathy

Dilated cardiomyopathy

Valvular disease—aortic stenosis

Cardiac tumors or infiltrative diseases

CARDIAC ARRHYTHMIAS

Tachycardia

Bradycardia

Premature atrial contractions

Premature ventricular contractions

Supraventricular tachycardias

Ventricular tachycardias

Atrial fibrillation

Wolff-Parkinson-White preexcitation

Sick sinus syndrome

However, the presence of additional symptoms such as dizziness, fainting, nausea, sweating, chest pain, and shortness of breath, may be more significant.

1. The nature and onset of palpitation may suggest causes.
   a. Isolated "jumps" or "skips" suggest premature beats.
   b. Sudden start and stop of rapid heartbeat or a pounding of the chest suggest supraventricular tachycardia (SVT). Some children appear sweaty or pale with SVT.
   c. A gradual onset and cessation of palpitation suggest sinus tachycardia or anxiety state.
   d. When the rate is known to be normal and the rhythm is regular, anxiety state is the cause.
   e. Palpitation characterized by slow heart rate may be due to atrioventricular (AV) block or sinus node dysfunction.

2. Relationship to exertion:
   a. A history of palpitation during strenuous physical activity may be a normal phenomenon (related to sinus tachycardia), although it could be due to exercise-induced arrhythmias.
   b. Nonexertional palpitation may suggest atrial flutter or fibrillation, febrile state, thyrotoxicosis, hypoglycemia, or anxiety state.
   c. A rapidly developing palpitation, although not abrupt, unrelated to exertion or excitement, may occur with hypoglycemia or tumor of adrenal medulla.
   d. Palpitation on standing suggests postural hypotension (or orthostatic intolerance).

3. Associated symptoms.
   a. Symptoms of dizziness or fainting associated with palpitation may indicate ventricular tachycardia.
   b. The presence of other symptoms, such as chest pain, sweating, nausea, or shortness of breath, may be more significant and may increase the likelihood of identifiable causes of palpitation.

4. Personal and family history may help identify the cause.
   a. Ask about eating and drinking habits, such as sodas, coffee, tea, hot cocoa, and chocolates, which contain caffeine.
   b. Ask if the patient is taking energy drinks.
   c. Ask about prescription and over-the-counter medications that could cause palpitation.
   d. Ask about medical or heart conditions that may cause tachycardia or palpitation (listed in Box 32–1).
   e. Ask about family history of syncope, sudden death, or arrhythmias.

Physical Examination

1. Most children with palpitation have normal physical examinations, except for those with hyperthyroidism.

2. Cardiac examination may reveal findings of mitral valve prolapse, obstructive lesions, or possibly cardiomyopathy.

Recording of ECG Rhythm

1. Routine ECG during office visit: check for prolonged QTc interval, delta waves (Wolff-Parkinson-White preexcitation), or AV block.

2. When palpitation occurs frequently, especially when associated with symptoms, 24-hour Holter monitoring is usually most helpful in making the diagnosis of the rhythm. This may clarify the diagnosis and secure management plans. Some children actually complain of palpitation during sinus tachycardia.

3. When palpitation occurs infrequently, long-term event monitor recording (up to 30 days) is indicated. With infrequent palpitations that are fairly long-lasting, handheld or patient-activated event recorders are indicated. However, with infrequent short-lasting palpitation, external loop recorders are indicated.

4. An implantable loop recorder (inserted under the skin at about the second rib on the left front of the chest) can be used to monitor for a period longer than 1 month.

5. If there is a high suspicion of ventricular tachycardia, sometimes electrophysiologic studies may be indicated.

6. If the symptoms occur during exercise, an exercise stress test may be helpful in making the diagnosis.

Laboratory Studies. When other medical conditions are suspected as a cause of palpitation, full blood count (for anemia), electrolytes, blood glucose, and thyroid function testing may be indicated.

Management

1. If the rhythm recorded on 24-hour Holter monitoring shows sinus tachycardia during the complaint of palpitation, all one has to do is to reassure the parent and child of the normal, benign nature of palpitation. Some parents are unaware of the fact that children's heart rates are faster than adults' heart rates and that children's heartbeats are easily palpable when they place their palms over the child's chest.

2. For isolated premature atrial contractions or premature ventricular contractions, nothing needs to be done except avoidance of stimulants such as caffeine, excessive amounts of sodas, or energy drinks. If they are so frequent that they are a hindrance to normal daily living, a β-blocker could be tried.

3. When a significant cardiac arrhythmia or an AV conduction disturbance is the suspected cause of palpitation, further evaluation and therapy are guided by recommendations discussed in Chapters 24 and 25.

4. Examination of all medications that the patient is taking may be helpful in the diagnosis and in modifying the dosage or schedule or changing to other medications.

5. If palpitation is associated with symptoms, such as fainting, dizziness, chest pain, pallor, or diaphoresis, further evaluation is guided as described in Chapters 30 and 31.

Chapter 33

Dyslipidemia and Other Cardiovascular Risk Factors

The primary purpose of this chapter is to raise physicians' attention to the emerging importance of practicing medicine for the prevention of future cardiovascular disease (and type 2 diabetes) during childhood.

Standard cardiovascular risk factors are often associated with obesity, which has shown a rapid increase in recent decades. Obesity is now known to be an independent risk factor for cardiovascular disease and diabetes. When these risk factors for heart disease and diabetes occur in clusters in the same individual, the condition is known as the metabolic syndrome. The combination of risk factors predisposes individuals to the development of coronary artery disease (CAD) and type 2 diabetes. Management of patients with the metabolic syndrome requires a comprehensive approach to the problem complex rather than treating only one condition.

This chapter discusses the following topics in the order listed:

1. Evidence of childhood onset of atherosclerotic heart disease

2. Identification of standard cardiovascular risk factors and the diagnosis of metabolic syndrome in children

3. In-depth discussion of dyslipidemia in children, including its diagnosis and treatment

4. Diagnosis and principles of management of childhood obesity

5. Strategies for smoke cessation

6. The summary table of the American Heart Association guidelines on practice of pediatric preventive cardiology

Hypertension, another cardiovascular risk factor, is discussed in Chapter 28.

Childhood Onset of Coronary Artery Disease

Atherosclerotic cardiovascular disease (CVD) is a major cause of morbidity and mortality and is responsible for more than 50% of all the deaths in the United States and other Western countries. Atherosclerotic lesions start to develop in early childhood and progress to irreversible lesions in adolescence and adulthood. The strongest evidence of childhood onset of CAD comes from the Bogalusa Heart Study (Berenson et al, 1998) and the Pathological Determinants of Atherosclerosis in Youth (PDAY) Research Group (Strong et al, 1995; McGill et al, 2002). Autopsy studies of the aorta and coronary arteries in youth after unexpected deaths in the Bogalusa Heart Study and in the study by the PDAY Research Group have found that atherosclerosis originates in childhood, with a rapid increase in the prevalence of coronary pathology during adolescence and young adulthood. These studies found that fatty streak, the earliest lesion of the atherosclerosis, occurred by 5 to 8 years of age and fibrous plaque, the advanced lesion, appeared in the coronary arteries in subjects in their late teens. Fibrous plaque was found in over 30% of 16- to 20-year-olds, and the prevalence of the lesion reached nearly 70% by age 26 to 39. These studies also confirmed that the extent of pathologic changes in the aorta and coronary arteries increased with age and the number of known cardiovascular risk factors that the individual had at the time of death.

Cardiovascular Risk Factors and the Metabolic Syndrome

Box 33–1 lists major risk factors for CVD, according to the Third Report of the National Cholesterol Education Program (NCEP) (2002).

Cardiovascular risk factors include positive family history of coronary heart disease, smoking, high levels of cholesterol, hypertension, being overweight, and diabetic or prediabetic states. These risk factors are all associated with an increased prevalence and extent of atherosclerosis (as discussed earlier). Obtaining a history of these cardiovascular risk factors should be a routine process in the practice of medicine.

A family history of premature CAD in first-degree relatives (parents and siblings) has been found to be the single best predictor of risk for adults. For children, however, family history includes the first- *and* second-degree relatives (including parents, siblings, grandparents, or blood-related aunts and uncles) who have or had CAD before age 55 for males and before age 65 for females. The reason that the second-degree relatives are included in family history for children is that some children's parents are too young to have developed clinical CAD when their children are examined.

The relationship between obesity and CAD has been a subject of some dispute for many years. For example, data from the Seven Counties Study (1984) and the massive autopsy study called the Geographic Pathology of Atherosclerosis (1986) revealed little or a weak correlation between body weight and incidence of coronary heart disease. However, multivariate analysis of Framingham data (Hubert et al, 1983) strongly suggests that most of the relationship between body weight and CAD risk is mediated through the standard, major risk factors (listed in Box 33–1).

More recent studies have shown that obesity is a risk factor for CAD independent of the standard risk factors, probably through the emerging risk factors. The emerging risk factors, which are commonly found in obese persons, include atherogenic dyslipidemia (also known as the "lipid triad," consisting of raised level of triglycerides and small low-density lipoprotein [LDL] particles and low levels of high-density lipoprotein [HDL]

BOX 33–1	MAJOR RISK FACTORS FOR CORONARY HEART DISEASE

Family history of premature coronary heart disease, cerebrovascular or occlusive peripheral vascular disease (with onset before age 55 years for men and 65 years for women in parents or grandparents)
    Cigarette smoking
    Hypercholesterolemia
    Hypertension (blood pressure >140/90 or taking antihypertensive medication)
    Low levels of high-density lipoprotein (<40 mg/100 mL)
    Diabetes mellitus (as a coronary heart disease risk equivalent)

    Adapted from Summary of the Third Report of the National Cholesterol Education Program (NCEP) Expert Panel on Detection, Education, and Treatment of High Blood Cholesterol in Adults (Adult Treatment Panel III) final report. Circulation 106:3143–3421, 2002.

cholesterol), insulin resistance (hyperinsulinemia), a proinflammatory state (elevation of serum high-sensitivity C-reactive protein), and a prothrombotic state (increased amount of plasminogen activator inhibitor 1). The cluster of these risk factors occurring in one person is known as the metabolic syndrome. In metabolic syndrome, LDL cholesterol levels may not be elevated but apoprotein B (apoB) and small LDL particles are elevated; the smallest particle in the LDL fraction is known to have the greatest atherogenicity. This syndrome occurs more commonly in individuals with abdominal (visceral) obesity, although there are exceptions, especially in individuals from Asia. With increasing adiposity, the lipid triad becomes more pronounced. Hispanics and South Asians seem to be particularly susceptible to the syndrome. Black men have a lower frequency of the syndrome than white men, probably because of a lower prevalence of atherogenic dyslipidemia.

Clinically identifiable components of the metabolic syndrome for adults are listed in Box 33–2. The presence of at least three of the risk factors is required to make the diagnosis of the metabolic syndrome in adults. Evidence has supported that waist circumference (reflecting visceral adiposity) is a better predictor of CVD than body mass index (BMI). Other components of metabolic syndrome, such as proinflammatory and prothrombotic states, are not routinely measured in clinical practice. C-reactive protein ≥3 mg/L may be significant in adults.

Interestingly, however, the PDAY Research Group (McGill et al, 2002) reported that the relationship between obesity and the severity of coronary atherosclerosis is present only in males; the relationship was very weak for young women, except those with a thick panniculus adiposus. It appears that body fat distribution may be important; men are more likely to have abdominal obesity than women, who tend to have gluteal adiposity. The exact mechanism for the role of visceral adiposity is not completely understood, but it has been assumed that obese adipose tissue releases an excess of fatty acids and cytokines that induce insulin resistance.

A direct association between obesity and insulin resistance also exists in children. Cook and coworkers have proposed a pediatric definition of the metabolic syndrome (Box 33–3). The prevalence of the metabolic syndrome in adolescents has been shown to be about 4%, but it increases to 30% to 50% in overweight adolescents (Singh, 2006). As in adults, the presence of at least three of the risk factors is required to make the diagnosis of the metabolic syndrome in children. Also as in adults, waist circumference is preferable to BMI for children. Ethnicity- and gender-specific waist circumference percentiles are now available for children from the Third National Health and Nutrition Examination Survey (NHANES III) (Fernandez et al, 2004) (see Tables C–1 through C–3, Appendix C). There are significant differences in waist circumference according to ethnicity and gender. In general, Mexican American boys and girls have higher waist

---

BOX 33–2	CLINICAL IDENTIFICATION OF THE METABOLIC SYNDROME IN ADULTS

1. Abdominal obesity: Men, waist circumference ≥40 inches (102 cm); women, waist circumference ≥35 inches (88 cm)

2. Elevated triglycerides ≥150 mg/dL

3. Reduced HDL cholesterol: Men <40 mg/dL; women <50 mg/dL

4. Hypertension: 130/85 mm Hg or greater

5. Elevated fasting glucose: ≥100 mg/dL

The presence of at least three of the preceding abnormalities constitutes metabolic syndrome.

From Cook S, Weizman M, Auinger P, et al: Prevalence of a metabolic syndrome phenotype in adolescents: Findings from the third National Health and Nutrition Examination Survey, 1988–1994. Arch Pediatr Adolsc Med 157:821–827, 2003.

BOX 33–3	**PROPOSED DEFINITION OF THE METABOLIC SYNDROME IN ADOLESCENTS**

1. Triglycerides ≥110 mg/dL

2. HDL cholesterol ≤40 mg/dL

3. Waist circumference ≥90th percentile or body mass index (BMI) ≥95th percentile

4. Fasting glucose ≥110 mg/dL

5. Systolic blood pressure ≥90th percentile for age and gender

The presence of at least three of the preceding abnormalities constitutes metabolic syndrome.

From Cook S, Weizman M, Auinger P, et al: Prevalence of a metabolic syndrome phenotype in adolescents: Findings from the third National Health and Nutrition Examination Survey, 1988–1994. Arch Pediatr Adolsc Med 157:821–827, 2003.

circumference than counterparts of other ethnicity. Children with waist circumference in the 75th and 90th percentile need to be identified because they are at an increased risk for cardiovascular and metabolic disorders (with significantly higher levels of total cholesterol, blood pressure, and triglycerides and lower levels of HDL cholesterol). Note that the 75th percentile of waist circumference of African American and Mexican American girls 16 and 17 years old exceeds the waist circumference value of 88 cm identified as the cutoff point for increased risk of obesity-related comorbidities in adult women. BMI percentile curves are presented as Figures C–1 and C–2, Appendix C.

The American Diabetic Association and the European Association for the Study of Diabetes issued a joint statement in September 2005 distancing their organizations from the concept of metabolic syndrome. They cautioned that there is as yet no strong evidence that treatment targeting insulin resistance, the putative root cause of the syndrome, produces any outcome benefit superior to treatment targeting the individual component disorders of the syndrome. Aside from the controversy surrounding the terminology of metabolic syndrome, the concept of the metabolic syndrome is useful for practicing physicians because its components are all important risk factors for CVD and type 2 diabetes. It reminds practitioners that the patients at highest risk for CVD have not just one or two but multiple risk factors and that more aggressive management should be applied to these patients.

The most important aspect of the syndrome is its prevention. The mainstay of the treatment of metabolic syndrome for both adults and children with the syndrome is weight control through dietary intervention and promotion of an active lifestyle to achieve and maintain optimum weight, normal blood pressure, and normal lipid profile for age (Grundy et al, 2004; Singh, 2006). Pharmacologic intervention is usually not required in children, but drugs may be used in selected high-risk patients. Each component of the syndrome present should be treated aggressively because children with the metabolic syndrome are at a higher risk for the development of CVDs and diabetes.

1. The principles of managing overweight are presented in the section of obesity to follow in this chapter.

2. Treatments of dyslipidemia are also presented in some detail in the section to follow.

3. Metformin therapy may be effective in preventing or delaying the development of diabetes.

4. For the prothrombotic state, aspirin therapy may be used in adults.

5. In patients with elevated C-reactive protein, more intense lifestyle therapies should be applied, including aspirin and control of dyslipidemia.

6. The basic principles of managing other risk factors, such as physical inactivity and smoking, are also presented in later sections of this chapter.

There appears to be a difference in susceptibility to different risk factors for different populations when they gain weight (Grundy, 2002). For example:

1. The white population of European origin appears to be more predisposed to atherogenic dyslipidemia than other populations when they gain weight.

2. Blacks of African origin are susceptible to hypertension when they gain weight; they also appear to be susceptible to type 2 diabetes. On the other hand, they develop less atherogenic dyslipidemia than whites with the same degree of weight gain.

3. Native Americans and Hispanics are especially susceptible to type 2 diabetes but less likely to develop hypertension than blacks.

4. People of South and Southeast Asia also have a high frequency of insulin resistance and type 2 diabetes. They appear more susceptible to CAD than East Asians.

Dyslipidemia

The pathogenesis of atherosclerosis and death from coronary atherosclerosis are importantly related to high levels of total cholesterol and LDL cholesterol and low levels of HDL cholesterol. Multiple trials in adults have demonstrated that cholesterol reduction results in reduced angiographic progression of CAD and even modest regression in some cases. A link has been established between increased levels of triglycerides and coronary heart disease. This association appears to be stronger among women than men. The NCEP Expert Panel on Blood Cholesterol Levels in Children and Adolescents (1991) recommended strategies for the prevention and detection of hyperlipidemia in children in the hope of preventing or retarding the progress of atherosclerosis.

LIPIDS AND LIPOPROTEINS

Lipids represent an essential constituent of our daily diet. Four major lipids of plasma are cholesterol, triglycerides, phospholipids, and free fatty acids. Triglycerides form an important energy source for cellular metabolism. Phospholipids are, because of their amphiphilic behavior, excellent emulsifiers of fats and constitute the predominant element of all biologic membranes. Cholesterol has an ambivalent nature: on the one hand, it is necessary for the stabilization of biologic membrane structure and an essential precursor of hormones and bile acids in hepatic metabolism; on the other hand, a surplus of cholesterol is generally considered to trigger atherosclerosis.

Plasma lipids that are hydrophobic do not circulate freely but rather circulate in the form of lipid-protein macromolecular complexes known as *lipoproteins*. Free fatty acids are bound to albumin. The nonpolar lipids (cholesterol esters and triglycerides) are present in the lipoprotein core surrounded by a monolayer composed of specific proteins (apoproteins) and the polar lipids (unesterified or free cholesterol and phospholipids). This monolayer allows the lipoprotein to remain miscible in plasma. Lipoproteins function as transport vehicles for water-insoluble lipid fractions and lead them to their sites of metabolism or deposition, or both.

The plasma lipoproteins have been classified into four major groups based on their density: chylomicrons, very low-density lipoprotein (VLDL), LDL, and HDL. Electrophoretic techniques permit the separation of the serum lipoproteins based on differences in electrostatic charges: chylomicrons (which remain at the origin), β-lipoproteins (LDL), pre-β-lipoprotein (VLDL), and α-lipoproteins (HDL).

The principal lipid of chylomicrons and VLDL is triglyceride. LDL is mostly cholesterol and phospholipids, and HDL is mostly protein with cholesterol and phospholipid as its major lipids. The proteins contained in lipoproteins (*apoproteins*) serve as enzymatic cofactors and recognition elements in binding to specific receptors.

LIPID AND LIPOPROTEIN METABOLISM

A review of simplified lipid and lipoprotein metabolism is presented in Figure 33–1 for readers who wish a quick refresher on the metabolism of lipids and lipoproteins before reading clinical aspects of dyslipidemia.

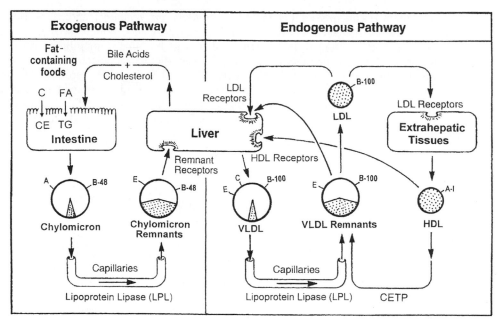

Figure 33–1. *Endogenous and exogenous pathways of plasma lipid and lipoprotein metabolism. Free fatty acid (FA) and cholesterol (C) are esterified in the intestinal mucosa to form triglyceride (TG) and cholesteryl ester (CE), respectively. They combine with apoA and apoB-48 to form chylomicron and are secreted into the circulation. The clear portion in the circles represents TG and the shaded portion represents CE. Chylomicron undergoes lipolysis in the capillary endothelium near adipose tissue and muscle tissue, losing TG through lipoprotein lipase (LPL). The resulting chylomicron remnants are taken up by hepatic apoE receptors for degradation by lysosomes. In the liver, TG and CE are combined with apoB-100, apoC, and apoE and then secreted as very low-density lipoprotein (VLDL). VLDL undergoes lipolysis in the capillary endothelium near adipose tissue and muscle tissue, losing TG through LPL, similar to what happens with chylomicron remnants. The resulting VLDL remnants (or intermediate-density lipoprotein, IDL) are either converted to low-density lipoprotein (LDL) for transport to peripheral cells by LDL receptor-mediated uptake or taken up by hepatic receptors. The other major class of lipoprotein, high-density lipoprotein (HDL), participates in the conversion of free cholesterol from peripheral tissues to cholesteryl ester by the action of lecithin-cholesterol acyltransferase (LCAT). Cholesteryl esters are then directly taken up by the HDL receptors in the liver or transferred to VLDL remnants and LDL by cholesteryl ester transfer protein (CETP), to be ultimately taken up by the liver. This process is known as reverse cholesterol transport. (Modified from Goldstein JL, Kita T, Brown MS: Defective lipoprotein receptors and atherosclerosis: Lessons from an animal counterpart of familial hypercholesterolemia. N Engl J Med 309:288–295, 1983.)*

Exogenous Pathway

Following ingestion of fat-containing foods, triglycerides and cholesterol are absorbed into intestinal cells as fatty acids and free cholesterol. Within the intestinal wall, free fatty acids and cholesterol are reesterified to form triglycerides and cholesteryl ester, respectively. These lipids are then combined with phospholipids and apoproteins (apos) A-I, A-IV, and B-48 to form triglyceride-rich *chylomicron* particles. ApoB-48 is an obligatory protein.

Chylomicrons rapidly enter plasma through the thoracic duct. In the circulation, chylomicrons acquire additional apoproteins (mainly ApoE and several forms of ApoC). Triglyceride-rich chylomicrons are hydrolyzed by the enzyme lipoprotein lipase (LPL) at the capillary endothelium, leaving a smaller and denser, remnant particle because they have lost much of their triglycerides. (The free fatty acid products of this hydrolysis are transferred primarily to adipose tissues for storage as triglycerides and to muscle for β-oxidation.) This particle is called a *chylomicron remnant*, and it is rich in cholesterol and has gained apoE from HDL (losing apoA and apoC to HDL).

These remnants are bound and internalized in part by hepatic membrane receptors specific for ApoE on the particle. By this mechanism, dietary cholesterol is delivered to the liver, where it plays a role in the regulation of hepatic cholesterol metabolism. In normal persons, chylomicrons and chylomicron remnants are very short-lived in the circulation and none of them exist in the plasma following a 12-hour fast. Chylomicrons and chylomicron remnants may be atherogenic. Delayed clearance of chylomicron occurs in inherited deficiency of LPL or its activator, apoC-II (type I hypertriglyceridemia).

Endogenous Pathway

Triglycerides synthesized in the liver are packaged with cholesteryl esters and apos B-100, C, and E and then secreted as VLDL. The synthesis of VLDL by the liver is increased by excess carbohydrate, alcohol, or caloric intake and is decreased in the fasting state.

In the capillary beds, triglyceride in the core of the VLDL is hydrolyzed by LPL, with a cofactor apoC-II, to produce a smaller denser particle called *VLDL remnant* or *intermediate-density lipoprotein* (IDL), which is analogous to chylomicron remnant. (The surface components, except for apos B-100 and E, are transferred to HDL.) Free fatty acids generated by hydrolysis of triglyceride are delivered to adipose tissue and muscle. Compared with VLDL, VLDL remnants have more cholesterol ester and less triglyceride.

Some of these remnant particles (IDLs) are taken up by the hepatic receptors specific for ApoE, whereas some undergo conversion to LDL by hepatic triglyceride lipase. Elevation of VLDL remnants may predispose the patient to premature CAD and peripheral artery disease (characteristically seen in Fredrickson's type III hyperlipoproteinemia).

LDL is usually formed by means of enhanced conversion of VLDL remnants (see Fig. 33–1) or by direct hepatic production of apoB-containing lipoproteins. LDLs are almost entirely made up of cholesteryl esters and apoB-100.

The content of cholesterol ester in the LDL particle may vary as much as 40%. LDL particles that contain lower amounts of cholesterol ester are known as *small, dense LDL particles*. Patients with increased amounts of small, dense LDL particles are at increased risk for CAD. Small, dense LDL is commonly associated with male gender, diabetes, low HDL cholesterol levels, high triglyceride levels, and familial combined hyperlipidemia (FCH).

LDLs are transported to peripheral cells or liver cells. ApoB-100, the only protein found in LDL, is recognized by a high-affinity LDL receptor on the surfaces of hepatic and certain nonhepatic cells where LDLs are internalized into the cells. By this mechanism, LDL particles can deliver cholesterol to extrahepatic tissues for use in membrane or steroid hormone synthesis. LDL receptor expression by the liver is a major regulator of plasma LDL cholesterol levels. LDL particles have a half-life of 3 to 4 days.

The liver and small intestine secrete HDL as nascent discoid particles composed primarily of phospholipids and apolipoproteins (nascent HDL). (Nascent HDL particles secreted by the intestine are rich in apoA-I and apoA-IV, whereas those secreted by the liver contain predominantly apoA-I and apoA-II.) Nascent lipid-poor apoA-I accepts free (unesterified) cholesterol from tissues, and the free cholesterol transferred to the surface of HDL is esterified by the action of enzyme lecithin-cholesterol acyltransferase (LCAT).

HDL cholesteryl esters may be directly transferred to and selectively taken up by the liver through a hepatic HDL receptor called scavenger receptor class BI (SR-BI). Alternatively, HDL cholesteryl esters may be transferred from HDL to VLDL and LDL by the cholesteryl ester transfer protein (CETP), after which they may be taken up by the liver or redistributed to peripheral tissues. Thus, HDLs have two pathways by which they return tissue-derived cholesterol to the liver. The removal of cholesterol from cells by HDL for ultimate disposal in the liver has been termed *reverse cholesterol transport*. These reactions may explain how HDL and apoA-I can protect against the development of atherosclerosis.

Among the several subtypes of HDL particles, HDL_2 and HDL_3 are clinically important. HDL_2 is closely associated with statistical protection against premature atherosclerosis. Alcohol consumption predominantly increases the HDL_3 subfraction. Lower levels of both subfractions are associated with male gender, hypertriglyceridemia, diabetes mellitus, obesity, uremia, smoking, and the use of androgens and progesterones. Estrogen raises HDL levels.

Cholesterol returning to the liver is converted into bile acids by the enzymatic hydroxylation of cholesterol, or cholesterol and phospholipids are excreted directly into the bile. A large portion of secreted bile acid is reabsorbed in the enterohepatic circulation and recycled. Bile acid sequestrants reduce the reabsorption of secreted bile acids, eventually reducing serum cholesterol levels by increasing the conversion of hepatic cholesterol to bile acids, thus reducing the cholesterol content of the hepatocytes. The reduced hepatic cholesterol stimulates the production of surface receptors for LDL cholesterol, clearing more LDL from the serum.

The hepatic and extrahepatic cells can control their own cholesterol content through a feedback control system. In conditions of cellular cholesterol excess, the cell can (1) suppress endogenous cholesterol production by inhibiting the activity of 3-hydroxy-3-methylglutaryl coenzyme A (HMG-CoA) reductase, the rate-limiting enzyme in cholesterol synthesis, (2) decrease its input of cholesterol by suppressing the production of LDL surface receptors through a feedback mechanism, and (3) promote the removal of cholesterol by increasing its movement to the plasma membrane for efflux.

MEASUREMENT OF CHOLESTEROL AND LIPOPROTEINS

Cholesterol levels are reasonably consistent after 2 years of age (with some small increment during adolescence). Cholesterol and LDL levels are not measured before the age of 2 years, and no treatment is recommended for this age group.

1. For the measurement of total cholesterol, the child does not have to be fasting for the test.

2. A lipoprotein analysis is obtained by measuring total cholesterol, HDL, and triglyceride levels after an overnight fast of 12 hours. The LDL level is usually estimated by the Friedewald formula:

$$LDL = \text{total cholesterol} - HDL - (\text{triglyceride}/5)$$

This formula is not accurate if the child is not fasting, if the triglyceride level is greater than 400 mg/dL, or if chylomicrons or dysbetalipoproteinemia (type III hyperlipoproteinemia) is present. Methods are currently available to measure LDL cholesterol directly, which allow LDL cholesterol determination on specimens with triglyceride level greater than 400 mg/dL. Direct LDL cholesterol measurement does not require a fasting specimen.

Normal Levels of Lipids and Lipoproteins. The cross-sectional age and gender-specific distribution of plasma lipids and lipoprotein were reported for American children by NCEP in 1991. Table C–4, Appendix C, provides age-specific percentile values for total cholesterol, LDL cholesterol, HDL cholesterol, and triglycerides. Children and adolescents with total cholesterol greater than 200 mg/dL, LDL cholesterol greater than 130 mg/dL, HDL cholesterol less than 40 mg/dL, or triglycerides greater than 200 mg/dL need to be evaluated for possible dyslipidemia. (For adults, the desirable level of triglycerides is less than 150 mg/dL.)

The following derivatives of lipid profile are useful in the assessment of risks for CVD.

1. TC to HDL-C ratio: The total cholesterol to HDL cholesterol ratio is a useful parameter for assessing risk for CVD. The usual TC/HDL-C ratio in children is approximately 3 (based on TC of 150 mg/dL and an HDL-C of 50 mg/dL). According to the Framingham study, the ratio for average risk was 5.0 for men and 4.2 for women. The higher the ratio, the higher is the risk of developing CVD. The ratio of 3.4 halves the risk of developing CVD for both men and women.

2. Non-HDL cholesterol: Serum non-HDL cholesterol (total cholesterol minus HDL cholesterol) is considered a better screening tool than LDL cholesterol for the assessment of CAD risk in adults because it includes all classes of atherogenic (apoB-containing) lipoproteins. It includes VLDL cholesterol, intermediate-density lipoproteins, LDL, and lipoprotein(a) or Lp(a). An additional advantage of non-HDL-C is that its measurement does not require overnight fasting.

According to the report of the Bogalusa Heart Study (Srinivasan et al, 2002), there is no important racial difference, although girls had higher levels than boys. Non-HDL-C was higher than LDL-C by 13.2 to 17.3 mg/dL (with the equation non-HDL cholesterol = 7.56 + 1.05 × LDL cholesterol). Serum non-HDL-C values equivalent to NHCEP's LDL cholesterol cut points of 110, 130, 170, and 200 are 123, 144, 186, and 218, respectively.

SELECTED PRIMARY LIPOPROTEIN DISORDERS

Primary lipoprotein disorders may manifest with increased levels of cholesterol or triglycerides, or both, or a decreased level of HDL cholesterol.

1. Primary hypercholesterolemia manifests as familial hypercholesterolemia (FH) and familial combined hyperlipidemia (FCH), which are the two most common familial lipoprotein disorders with elevated LDL cholesterol levels. One should, however, rule out secondary causes of hypercholesterolemia (see later). Screening of all family members is recommended to determine whether the disorder is familial. Family screening is important not only to detect hypercholesterolemia in other members of the family but also to emphasize the need for all family members to change their eating patterns. Young patients with elevated LDL levels are more likely to have a familial disorder of LDL metabolism.

2. Primary lipoprotein disorders that arise with an increased level of triglycerides are FCH, familial hypertriglyceridemia, and familial dysbetalipoproteinemia (type III hyperlipoproteinemia). Some hypertriglyceridemias are also secondary to other disease state (see later).

3. Familial hypoalphalipoproteinemia (low HDL syndrome).

The clinical features of hyperlipoproteinemias are summarized in Table 33–1 according to the Fredrickson and Lees phenotype.

Familial Hypercholesterolemia. FH is due to a lack of or a reduction in LDL receptors. Heterozygotes have about a 50% reduction in LDL receptors, whereas homozygotes have little or no receptor activity.

FH heterozygous disorder is fairly common, occurring in 1 of every 500 people. It is inherited in an autosomal dominant mode. An evaluation of family members is important in the diagnosis of this condition. In this condition, one parent and one out of two siblings have elevated total and LDL cholesterol levels, but unaffected first-degree relatives have completely normal levels. In heterozygotes, total cholesterol and LDL levels are two to three times higher than normal. Their total cholesterol levels are most often greater than 240 mg/dL, with an average of 300 mg/dL, and their LDL levels are above 160 mg/dL, with an average of 240 mg/dL. Triglyceride levels are usually normal. The presence of xanthomas of the extensor tendon in the parents of such children almost confirms the diagnosis. A heterozygous child or adolescent has normal physical findings. Tendon xanthomas are rarely found before the age of 10 years; they develop in the second decade, primarily in the Achilles tendons and extensor tendons of the hands, in only 10% to 15% of patients. These patients are likely to develop premature CVD; rarely, angina pectoris develops in the late teenage years.

Treatment of heterozygotes includes a diet low in cholesterol and saturated fat and high in water-soluble fibers. Bile acid sequestrants are safe and moderately effective but difficult to tolerate over the long term because of gritty texture and gastrointestinal complaints (see Table 33–3 for the dosage). Recent reports show that statins are safe, effective, and well tolerated (see later section). The addition to the statin of bile acid sequestrant or a cholesterol absorption inhibitor is often necessary to achieve LDL cholesterol goals. Niacin is generally not used to treat FH heterozygous children.

Table 33–1. **Clinical Summary of Hyperlipoproteinemia**

Fredrickson Phenotype	Elevated Lipids or Lipoproteins	Prevalence in Childhood	Etiology	Symptoms and Signs	Treatment
Type I	Triglyceride (usually >1000 mg/dL) Chylomicrons identified	Rare	LPL deficiency (familial hyperchylomicronemia), apoC-II deficiency Systemic lupus erythematosus	Childhood onset (70%) Abdominal pain due to pancreatitis Eruptive xanthomas Lack of coronary heart disease during childhood	Very low-fat diet (10%–15% calories), supplemented with medium-chain triglycerides
Type IIa	LDL-C (≥130 mg/dL)	Common	FH, FCH, Polygenic hyper-cholesterolemia Hypothyroidism Renal disease* Biliary tract disease Diabetes mellitus	Childhood or adulthood onset Xanthomas of eyelids and palms Tendinitis of Achilles tendon Arcus corneae Coronary heart disease (common in homozygotes)	Low-cholesterol, high-unsaturated-fat diet Weight loss if obese Statins, if condition does not respond to diet alone. Bile acid sequestrant, occasionally
Type IIb	LDL-C (≥130 mg/dL and triglycerides (≥125 mg/dL)	Uncommon	Similar to type IIa	Late childhood onset Lack of symptoms and signs (often)	Low-cholesterol, low-fat diet Weight loss if obese Statins, if condition does not respond to diet alone Fibric acid and niacin, occasionally
Type III	Triglycerides and LDL-C (approximately equal values); chylomicron remnant and IDL elevated	Very rare	Dysbetalipoproteinemia ApoE-2 homozygosity (E-2/E-2) plus obesity Diabetes mellitus Renal disease* Hypothyroidism Liver disease	Palmar and tuberosum xanthomas Coronary heart disease (±)	Low-fat, low-cholesterol diet Weight control Statins are effective
Type IV	Triglycerides (≥125 mg/dL) VLDL elevated	Relatively uncommon	FCH FH Familial hypertrigly-ceridemia Metabolic or endocrine disease[†] Renal disease Liver disease Ethanol use/abuse Pregnancy Drug use[‡]	Obesity Eruptive xanthomas Abdominal pain	Low-fat, low-cholesterol diet Weight control Statins, if condition does not respond to diet alone Fibric acid and niacin, occasionally
Type V	Triglycerides (>1000 mg/dL); chylomicron and elevated VLDL	Very rare	Usually results from a combination of any two conditions that cause type IV	Obesity Eruptive xanthomas Coronary heart disease (infrequent)	Low-fat diet Weight control

*Renal disease (e.g., nephrosis).
[†]Metabolic/endocrine disease (e.g., obesity, diabetes, hypothyroidism, Cushing's disease, acromegaly).
[‡]Drug use (e.g., glucocorticoids, growth hormone, androgens, thiazides, β-blockers, estrogen).
IDL, intermediate-density lipoprotein; LDL-C, low-density lipoprotein cholesterol; VLDL, very low-density lipoprotein.
Adapted from the following articles:
Winter W, Schartz D: Pediatric lipid disorders in clinical practice. eMedicine, last updated January 19, 2005.
Trxoler RG, Park MK: Hyperlipidemia in childhood. In Pediatric Cardiology for Practitioners, 4th ed. St. Louis, Mosby, 2002.
Holmes KW, Kwiterovich PO Jr: Treatment of dyslipidemia in children and adolescents. Curr Cardiol Rep 7:445–456, 2005.

Homozygosity occurs in children who have inherited two mutant FH genes; it is rare (one in a million). The total cholesterol and LDL cholesterol levels in these children are five to six times greater than normal. Such children have cholesterol levels that average 700 mg/dL but may reach higher than 1000 mg/dL. Clinical signs such as planar xanthomas, which are flat, orange-colored skin lesions, may be present by the age of 5 years in the webbing of the hands and over the elbows and buttocks. Tendon xanthomas, arcus corneae, and clinically significant coronary heart disease are often present by the age of 10 years. The generalized atherosclerosis often affects the aortic valve, with resulting aortic stenosis.

FH homozygous children respond somewhat to high doses of potent statins and to niacin. Cholesterol absorption inhibitor also lowers LDL in FH homozygotes, especially in combination with a more potent statin. However, most FH homozygotes invariably require LDL apheresis (with extracorporeal affinity LDL absorption column and plasma reinfusion) every 2 weeks to lower LDL to a range that is less atherogenic. The Liposorber system is an example, which selectively binds apoB-containing lipoproteins—LDL, Lp(a),* and VLDL.

Familial Combined Hyperlipidemia. FCH is more common than FH, occurring in 1 of every 200 to 300 people. It occurs in families of survivors of myocardial infarction as an autosomal dominant with variable phenotypic expression: elevated LDL level alone (type IIa), elevated LDL with hypertriglyceridemia (type IIb), or normal LDL with hypertriglyceridemia (type IV). Clinically, it may be difficult to separate this entity from FH. The diagnosis of FCH is suspected when a first-degree family member (often a parent or sibling) has a different lipoprotein phenotype than the proband. Levels of total and LDL cholesterol are somewhat lower than in patients with FH, and LDL levels fluctuate from time to time, with triglyceride levels fluctuating in the opposite direction. These children usually have plasma total cholesterol levels between 190 and 220 mg/dL. The LDL cholesterol level is usually normal or only mildly elevated. In FCH, most patients lack tendon xanthomas, and extreme hyperlipidemia is absent in childhood.

The phenotypes often have other characteristics such as hyperinsulinemia, glucose intolerance, hypertension, and visceral obesity. The combined expression of three or more of these traits constitutes the metabolic syndrome (see earlier section).

Treatment of FCH includes a low-fat diet, reduction to ideal body weight, and regular aerobic exercise. The statins are the most effective in lowering LDL cholesterol and the total number of atherogenic small dense LDL particles. Fibric acid and niacin, which are effective in adults, are not ordinarily used in pediatric patients. Metformin has been used to treat obese hyperinsulinemic adolescents with the metabolic syndrome. Metformin may enhance insulin sensitivity and reduce fasting blood glucose, insulin levels, plasma lipids, free fatty acids, and leptin.

Familial Hypertriglyceridemia. In the pediatric age group, this disorder is caused by LPL deficiency, resulting in hepatic overproduction of VLDL cholesterol. When hypertriglycerides exceed 1000 mg/dL, pancreatitis is a major concern. Eruptive xanthomas and lipemia retinalis (a creamy appearance of the retinal veins and arteries related to a high concentration of lipids in the blood) can also be found. In this situation, the treatment should reflect the risk of pancreatitis. When the level of triglycerides is between 200 and 500 mg/dL, the goal of the treatment is to reduce CAD. When hypertriglyceridemia occurs as part of primary hypercholesterolemia, the levels of triglycerides are much lower than in familial hypertriglyceridemia. Metabolic consequences of hypertriglyceridemia include (1) a lowering of HDL cholesterol, (2) the production of smaller, denser LDL particles with more atherogenicity, and (3) a hypercoagulable state.

Treatment is based first on lifestyle modification, including withdrawal of hormones (estrogen, progesterone), limiting alcohol intake, reducing caloric intake, and increasing exercise.

---

*Lp(a) is an apoB-100 (and another antigenically unique apoprotein)-containing lipoprotein that is normally a minor plasma constituent. In some individuals, it is markedly elevated. It appears to be an autosomal dominant inheritance. Elevated levels of Lp(a) have been correlated with increased risk of heart disease.

Dysbetalipoproteinemia (Type III Hyperlipoproteinemia). This familial disorder is a rare genetic disorder caused by a defect in apoE, which results in increased accumulation of chylomicron remnants and VLDL remnants. Patients with this disorder have increased cardiovascular risk. Clinical manifestation may include palmar xanthoma. Cholesterol and triglyceride levels are equally elevated to greater than 300 mg/dL, but this disorder is not usually seen in childhood. A low-fat diet, correction of metabolic syndrome, and drug treatment (fibric acid or statin) are very effective.

Familial Hypoalphalipoproteinemia (Low HDL Syndrome). In this condition, apoA-I and apoA-II concentrations are decreased and apoC-III is absent. In *Tangier disease*, HDL cholesterol is nearly absent (with markedly enlarged yellow tonsils). The LDL levels are low, which appears to have a protective effect. This condition is not included in the Fredrickson classification. A low-fat diet is also indicated in children with inherited disorders of HDL metabolism. Exercise and weight loss are also helpful. Drugs are rarely used.

SECONDARY DYSLIPOPROTEINEMIA

Secondary dyslipoproteinemias result from other underlying disorders, but they may mimic primary forms of hyperlipidemia and can have similar consequences. They may result in increased predisposition to premature CAD, or when associated with marked hypertriglyceridemia, they may lead to the development of pancreatitis and other features of hyperchylomicronemia.

Common causes in children include obesity, oral contraceptive use, and isotretinoin (Accutane) use or anabolic steroid therapy. Medications such as diuretics, β-blockers, and estrogens; medical conditions including hypothyroidism, renal failure, and nephrotic syndrome; and alcohol usage are less common causes of secondary dyslipoproteinemia. Box 33–4 lists causes of secondary dyslipoproteinemia.

All children with LDL levels >130 mg/dL or triglycerides >150 mg/dL need to be evaluated for possible secondary dyslipoproteinemia. In addition to a careful history and physical examination, determination of blood glucose levels and appropriate tests of liver, kidney, and thyroid function may be indicated.

Treatment of the underlying condition, when possible, or discontinuation of the offending drugs usually leads to an improvement in the hyperlipidemia. Specific lipid-lowering therapy may be required in certain circumstances.

CHOLESTEROL-LOWERING STRATEGIES

The NCEP Expert Panel has recommended two complementary approaches to lowering blood cholesterol levels for children and adolescents: a population approach and an individualized approach.

Population Approach

The population approach encourages changes in nutrient intake and eating patterns for the entire population of the United States. For children older than 2 years, the following are recommended:

1. Nutritional adequacy should be achieved by eating a wide variety of foods.
2. Adequate calories should be provided for normal growth and development.
3. The following pattern of nutrient intake is recommended:
   a. Saturated fatty acids less than 10% of total calories.
   b. Total fat ≤30% of total calories.
   c. Dietary cholesterol less than 300 mg/day.

These recommendations are the same as a step-one diet (Table 33–2). Children younger than 2 years may require a higher percentage of calories from fat.

Individualized Approach

The individualized approach identifies and treats children and adolescents at risk of having high cholesterol levels. See Table C–4, Appendix C, for normal levels of total cholesterol, LDL, HDL, and serum triglycerides in American children and adolescents.

BOX 33–4	CAUSES OF SECONDARY DYSLIPOPROTEINEMIA

METABOLIC
Metabolic syndrome
Diabetes
Lipodystrophies
Glycogen storage disorders

CHRONIC RENAL DISEASE
Chronic renal failure
Nephrotic syndrome
Glomerulonephritis

HEPATIC
Biliary atresia
Cirrhosis

HORMONAL
Estrogen
Progesterone
Growth hormone
Hypothyroidism
Corticosteroids

LIFESTYLE
Obesity
Physical inactivity
Diets rich in fat and saturated fat
Alcohol intake

MEDICATIONS
Isotretinoin (Accutane)
Certain oral contraceptives
Anabolic steroids
Thiazide diuretics
β-Adrenergic blockers
Anticonvulsants
Glucocorticoids
Estrogen
Testosterone
Immunosuppressive agents (cyclosporine)
Antiviral agents (human immunodeficiency virus protease inhibitor)

The NCEP Expert Panel recommends *selective* screening of children and adolescents with family histories of premature CVD or at least one parent with high serum cholesterol levels because there is strong evidence demonstrating a familial aggregation of coronary heart disease, high serum cholesterol levels, and other risk factors. Patients who meet the following specific criteria should be screened:

1. Children and adolescents whose parents or grandparents, at 55 years of age or younger for men and 65 years of age or younger for women, had coronary atherosclerosis after angiography or underwent balloon angioplasty or coronary artery bypass surgery.

2. Children and adolescents whose parents or grandparents, at 55 years of age or younger for men and 65 years of age or younger for women, had documented myocardial infarction, angina pectoris, peripheral vascular disease, cerebrovascular disease, or sudden cardiac death.

3. The offspring of a parent who had high total cholesterol levels (≥240 mg/dL).

4. Children and adolescents whose parental or grandparental history is unobtainable, particularly those with other risk factors.

Table 33–2. **Nutrient Composition of Step-One and Step-Two Diets**

Nutrient	Step-One Diet	Step-Two Diet
Total fat (% total calories)	<30%	<30%
Saturated fatty acids	<10%	<7%
Polyunsaturated fatty acids	Up to 10%	Up to 10%
Monounsaturated fatty acids	10%–15%	10%–15%
Carbohydrates (% total calories)	50%–60%	50%–60%
Protein (% total calories)	10%–20%	10%–20%
Cholesterol (per day)	<300 mg	<200 mg
Total calories	To achieve and maintain desirable weight	To achieve and maintain desirable weight

The recommendations for selective screening are somewhat controversial. Several studies published in the pediatric literature have indicated that about 50% of children with high LDL levels will be missed if a positive family history of premature coronary heart disease is used as the sole screening criterion. The results of the Bogalusa Heart Study, in particular, show that 60% of white and 80% of African American children with high LDL cholesterol levels (≥95th percentile) did not have positive family histories of CAD (Dennison et al, 1989). Universal screening should theoretically detect all children with high LDL levels, and some authorities recommend general screening of preschool children. Although the NCEP Expert Panel believed that, given the current state of knowledge, universal screening should not be recommended, optional cholesterol testing by the practicing physician may be appropriate in children judged to be at higher risk for coronary heart disease (such as those who smoke, have high blood pressure, are obese, or have excessive fat intake).

The panel's recommendations are summarized in Figure 33–2. The screening protocol varies according to the reasons for testing.

1. For young people being tested because they have at least one parent with high blood cholesterol levels, the initial step is measurement of total cholesterol.

2. For children who have family histories of premature CVD, a lipoprotein analysis is recommended because a high proportion of these children have some lipoprotein abnormality.

Depending on total cholesterol and LDL levels, patients' conditions are categorized as acceptable, borderline, or high.

1. For those who had total cholesterol levels measured (see Fig. 33–2), the patient's condition is categorized as *acceptable* (<170 mg/dL), *borderline* (170–199 mg/dL), or *high* (≥200 mg/dL).

   a. If total cholesterol levels are acceptable (<170 mg/dL), cholesterol measurement is repeated within 5 years.

   b. If total cholesterol levels are borderline (170 to 199 mg/dL), a second measurement is taken.

   c. If the average is borderline or high (>200 mg/dL), a lipoprotein analysis is recommended.

2. For those who had lipoprotein analysis done (Fig. 33–3), regardless of indications, a lipoprotein analysis should be repeated and the average LDL levels determined. The patient's condition is then categorized as *acceptable* (LDL cholesterol <110 mg/dL), *borderline* (110 to 129 mg/dL), or *high* (≥130 mg/dL).

   a. If LDL levels are acceptable (<110 mg/dL), education about the eating pattern recommended for all children and adolescents and about coronary heart disease risk factors is provided (see Box 33–1). Lipoprotein analysis is repeated in 5 years.

   b. If LDL levels are in the borderline range (110 to 129 mg/dL), advice about risk factors is provided, the step-one diet is initiated (Table 33–3), and the patient's status is evaluated in 1 year.

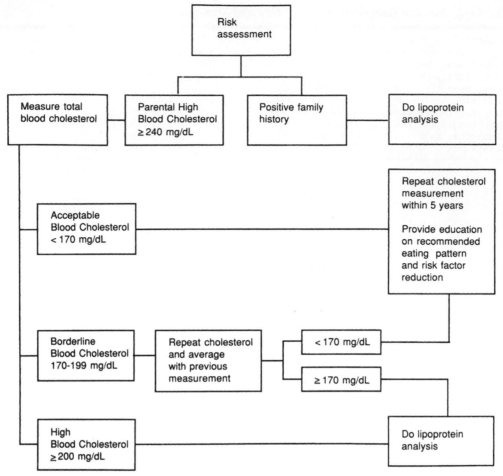

Figure 33–2. Risk assessment for cardiovascular disease or CVD. (From Expert Panel on Blood Cholesterol Levels in Children and Adolescents: National Cholesterol Education Program. NIH Publication No. 91-2732, September 1991.)

      c. If LDL levels are high (≥130 mg/dL), the patient is evaluated for secondary causes and familial disorders; all family members are screened; and the step-one diet is initiated, followed, if necessary, by the step-two diet (see Table 33–3) and, in extreme cases, by drug therapy (see later section).

MANAGEMENT

Diet Therapy

Diet therapy is prescribed in two steps that progressively reduce the intake of saturated fatty acids and cholesterol. The step-one diet calls for the same nutrient intake recommended in the population approach to lowering cholesterol levels (see Table 33–2): less than 10% of total calories from saturated fatty acids, no more than 30% of calories from total fat, less than 300 mg of cholesterol a day, and adequate calories to support growth and development and to reach or maintain a desirable body weight. Involvement of a registered dietitian or other qualified health professional is recommended.

If the step-one diet fails to achieve the minimal goals of therapy in 3 months, the step-two diet is prescribed (see Table 33–2). This diet further reduces the saturated fatty acid intake to less than 7% of calories and the cholesterol intake to less than 200 mg a day. Adequate amounts of nutrients, vitamins, and minerals should be provided. A registered dietitian or other qualified nutrition professional should be consulted. See Appendix C, Table C–5, for detailed information on specific food choices.

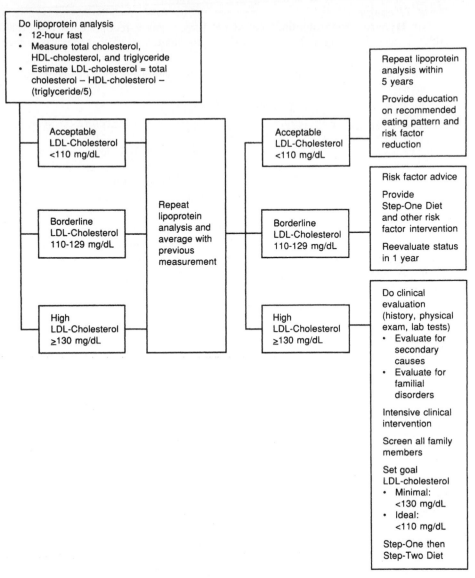

Figure 33–3. *Classification, education, and follow-up based on low-density lipoprotein (LDL) levels. HDL, high-density lipoprotein. (From Expert Panel on Blood Cholesterol Levels in Children and Adolescents: National Cholesterol Education Program. NIH Publication No. 91-2732, September 1991.)*

Table 33–3. **Suggested Initial Dosage of a Bile Acid Sequestrant for Treatment of Familial Hypercholesterolemia in Children and Adolescents**

	TC and LDL Levels after Diet (mg/100 dL)	
Daily Doses[*]	*TC*	*LDL*
1	<245	<195
2	245–300	195–235
3	301–345	236–280
4	345	

[*]One dose is the equivalent of a 9-g packet of cholestyramine (containing 4 g of cholestyramine and 5 g of filler), one bar of cholestyramine, or 5 g of colestipol.
LDL, low-density lipoprotein; TC, total cholesterol.

Drug Therapy

For Hypercholesterolemia.

The NCEP Expert Panel recommends drug therapy in children aged 10 years and older if, after an adequate trial of diet therapy (6 months to 1 year):

1. The LDL level remains at or above 190 mg/dL, with a negative or unobtainable family history of premature coronary CVD.

2. The LDL level remains at or above 160 mg/dL *plus*:
   a. There is a positive family history of premature CVD (before 55 years of age in men and before 65 years in women).
   b. Two or more other CVD risk factors (e.g., low HDL levels, cigarette smoking, high blood pressure, obesity, diabetes) (see Box 33–1) or metabolic syndrome is present (see Box 33–3 for the definition of the metabolic syndrome in children).

For children and adolescents with hypercholesterolemia, two classes of pharmaceutical agents are currently used in children older than 10 years with sufficiently elevated LDL cholesterol levels. They are bile acid sequestrants (cholestyramine, colestipol) and HMG-CoA reductase inhibitors (statins). Ezetimibe, a cholesterol absorption inhibitor, is also effective but is not yet approved by the Food and Drug Administration (FDA) for use in children, except the rare children with homozygous FH. Nicotinic acid and fibrates are not routinely used in pediatrics.

Bile acid sequestrants were the only agents recommended by NCEP in 1991 for pharmacologic lipid-lowering therapy. These agents suffer from a low compliance rate (secondary to gritty texture and gastrointestinal complaints) and provide only a modest LDL cholesterol reduction. The dosage of bile acid sequestrant is determined by the levels of total cholesterol and LDL cholesterol, not by the patient's weight (see Table 33–3).

Statins are widely used to lower total cholesterol and LDL cholesterol in adults. Numerous studies have demonstrated the safety and efficacy of the statins in male and female adolescents with FH (Holmes and Kwiterovich, 2005). Four statins, atorvastatin, lovastatin, pravastatin, and simvastatin, are currently approved by the FDA for use in adolescents. A double-blind, placebo-controlled trial with 2 years of pravastatin treatment has shown not only significant reduction of LDL cholesterol but also regression of carotid atherosclerosis in children and adolescents with FH (Wiegman et al, 2004).

Increases in liver enzymes up to three times the upper limits of normal have been reported in several cases treated with high doses of simvastatin (40 mg/day) and atorvastatin (20 mg/day). Instances of asymptomatic increases in creatine phosphokinase (CPK), although unusual, have been reported. Muscle pain or weakness, myositis, and rhabdomyolysis with renal failure have been reported in adults. Therefore, periodic measurements of alanine aminotransferase (ALT), aspartate aminotransferase (AST, preferred because it is also found in muscles), and CPK should be done for possible adverse effects of the statins (when lipid levels are measured). The mechanisms of action, side effects, and ranges of adult dosages of lipid-lowering agents are presented in Table 33–4.

Based on published clinical trials in children and adolescents, the following may be reasonable pediatric dosages of the four statins that are approved for pediatric use (Holmes and Kwiterovich, 2005).

The maintenance dosage of the drug is decided by periodic determinations of cholesterol levels.

1. Atorvastatin: Starting dose of 10 mg is increased to 20 mg at 4 to 6 weeks and further to a dose of 40 mg/day (maximum adult dose is 80 mg/day).

2. Lovastatin: Starting dose 10 mg/day for 6 to 8 weeks, with a 10-mg increase every 6 to 8 weeks, to a maximum 40 mg/day.

3. Pravastatin: Starting dose of 10 mg/day is increased to 20 or 40 mg/day.

4. Simvastatin: Starting dose 10 mg, increment of 10 mg every 6 to 8 weeks to maximum 40 mg/day.

In pediatric trials, starting doses were usually half of the adult lower range dose, depending on the age of the child, increased by 10 mg every 4 to 8 weeks to the half or full dose of the upper range dosage with periodic measurements of cholesterols.

Table 33–4. **Summary of Lipid-Lowering Drugs**

Agent	Mechanism of Action	Side Effects	Daily Dosage Range
Bile acid sequestrants: Cholestyramine (Questran) Colestipol (Colestid) Colesevelam (WelChol)	Increases excretion of bile acids in stool; increases LDL receptor activity	Constipation, nausea, bloating, flatulence, transient increase in transaminase and alkaline phosphatase levels, increased triglyceride levels (±), possible prevention of absorption of fat-soluble vitamins	Related to levels of cholesterol, not body weight; for specific dosage, see Table 33–3 for pediatric dosages
HMG-CoA reductase inhibitors ("statins"): Atorvastatin (Lipitor), Fluvastatin (Lescol), Lovastatin (Mevacor), Pravastatin (Pravachol), Rosuvastatin (Crestor), Simvastatin (Zocor)	Inhibits HMG-CoA reductase, with resulting decrease in cholesterol synthesis; increases LDL receptor activity; and reduces LDL and VLDL secretion by the liver	Mild gastrointestinal symptoms, myositis syndrome, elevated hepatic transaminase levels, increased CPK levels (Contraindicated during pregnancy because of potential risk to a developing fetus)	*Children*: See text for suggested pediatric dosages Adult dose ranges (of statins approved for pediatric use): Atrovastatin: 10–80 mg Lovastatin: 20–80 mg Pravastatin: 10–40 mg Simvastatin: 10–80 mg
Cholesterol absorption inhibitors: Ezetimibe (Zetia; Ezetrol)	Selective inhibition of intestinal sterol absorption	Abdominal pain, rhabdomyolysis (±)	*Adult*: 10 mg/day.
Nicotinic acid (niacin, vitamin B₃)	Decreases plasma levels of free fatty acid; possibly inhibits cholesterol synthesis; decreases hepatic VLDL synthesis	Cutaneous flushing, pruritus, gastrointestinal upset, liver function abnormalities, increased uric acid levels, increased glucose intolerance	*Children*: only short-term efficacy reported for homozygous FH; not recommended for routine use *Adults*: 1–3 g
Fibric acid derivatives: Gemfibrozil (Lopid), Clofibrate	Decrease hepatic VLDL synthesis; increase LPL activity	Increased incidence of gallstones and perhaps gastrointestinal cancer, myositis, diarrhea, nausea, rash, altered liver function, increased CPK levels, potentiation of warfarin	*Children*: not recommended *Adults*: gemfibrozil, 600–1200 mg; clofibrate, 1–2 g

CPK, creatine phosphokinase; FH, familial hypercholesterolemia; HDL, high-density lipoprotein; HMG-CoA, 3-hydroxy-3-methylglutaryl coenzyme A; LDL, low-density lipoprotein; LPL, lipoprotein lipase; VLDL, very low-density lipoprotein.

For High Levels of Triglycerides. Treatment of this condition includes a very low fat diet (10% to 15% of calories) that can be supplemented by medium-chain triglycerides (see Table 33–1). Portagen, a soybean-based formula enriched in medium-chain triglycerides, is available for infants with LPL deficiency. Lipid-lowering drugs are ineffective in LPL deficiency.

In adult patients, the primary aim of therapy is to reach the LDL goal by the use of statins, intense weight management, and increasing physical activity. If triglycerides are ≥200 mg/dL when the LDL goal is reached, nicotinic acid or fibrate alone, or better in combination with a statin, may be used to reduce the non-HDL cholesterol level to the level of 30 mg/dL plus the LDL goal. A prescription omega-3 fatty acid product (e.g., Omacor) at 4 and 8 g/day reduced triglyceride levels by 30% and 43%, respectively, from baseline values. (Most fish oil capsules have an omega-3 fatty acid content only one third of that in Omacor.) Omega-3 fatty acid plus a statin may be an effective alternative to a fibrate or niacin plus a statin.

For Low Levels of HDL Cholesterol. A low HDL level is defined as less than 40 mg/dL in men and less than 50 mg/dL in women. HDL cholesterol is inversely related to fatal myocardial infarction. A rise of 1 mg/dL in HDL cholesterol lowers the risk of fatal myocardial infarction by about 3%. Statins that are effective in lowering LDL cholesterol are not very effective in raising HDL cholesterol. The following has been suggested for adults to raise the low levels of HDL cholesterol (Ashen et al, 2005).

1. Regular exercise—30 minutes of brisk aerobic exercise every day or every other day.

2. Quitting smoking—provides an average 4 mg/dL rise.

3. Weight control—every 3 kg weight loss results in 1 mg/dL rise.

4. Mild to moderate consumption of alcohol (one to two drinks a day)—rise of 4 mg/dL (not for those with liver or addiction problems).

5. Diet low in saturated fat and rich in the polyunsaturated fatty acids. Examples are oils (olive, canola, soy, flaxseed), nuts (almonds, peanuts, walnuts, pecans), cold-water fish (salmon, mackerel), and shellfish.

6. Restrict consumption of carbohydrate (especially high glycemic products), which lowers HDL.

7. Drug.
   a. Niacin is the most effective therapy for raising HDL-C (20% to 35% rise).
   b. Fibrate raises 10% to 25%.
   c. Statins are the least effective.

Other Risk Factors

There are other cardiovascular risk factors beside dyslipidemia that need attention in order to prevent CVD and diabetes. In this section, a brief discussion is presented on the topics of obesity and smoking. Another risk factor, hypertension, has been presented in Chapter 28.

OBESITY

Information provided in this section is only to assist health care providers in making a diagnosis of overweight and obesity, recognizing the complications of obesity, providing the basic knowledge needed in counseling patients, and helping patients with appropriate time for referral to a weight management specialist. This section is not meant to describe in detail treatment of obesity; successful treatment of obesity requires special skills and facilities with availability of a multidisciplinary team consisting of registered dietitians, specialized nurses, psychologists, and exercise specialists. Such specialized programs are costly and, unfortunately, are insufficient in number.

Prevalence. Obesity continues to be a leading public health concern in the United States. Between 1980 and 2002, obesity prevalence doubled in adults and overweight prevalence tripled in children and adolescents aged 6 to 19 years (Hedley et al, 2004). Between 1999 and 2004, the prevalence of overweight among children and adolescents and obesity among men increased significantly during the 6-year period, although the prevalence among women appeared to be leveling off. According to the latest statistics (as of 2004), 17.1% of children and adolescents are overweight and 32.2% of adults are obese (Ogden et al, 2006). There was an increasing trend in the prevalence of overweight in children and adolescents from 1999–2000 to 2003–2004. For females, the rate increased from 13.9% to 16.0% and for males it increased from 14.0% to 18.2%. Among men, the prevalence of obesity increased significantly between 1999–2000 (27.5%) and 2003–2004 (31.1%). Among women, no significant increase in obesity was observed in the same period of time.

As discussed earlier in this chapter, obesity is an independent risk factor for CVD and is a component of the metabolic syndrome. An increase in the prevalence of obesity is of particular concern because it may increase the prevalence of atherosclerotic heart disease and diabetes.

Physiology. Some interesting physiologic facts are as follows:

1. Changes in BMI occur with normal growth. There is a rapid increase in BMI (and total fat) during the first year of life. After 9 to 12 months of age, BMI declines and reaches a minimum at around 5 to 6 years of age before beginning a gradual increase through adolescence and most of adulthood. The point of maximal leanness or minimal BMI has been called the *adiposity rebound*. Studies have shown that an early adiposity rebound (younger age at the point of adiposity rebound) is associated with higher BMI in adolescence and in adults.

2. Fully differentiated adipocytes appear in the human fetus at around 15 weeks of gestation. A rapid increase in total fat occurs during the third trimester (with percent body fat reaching 15%). There is a rapid increase in percent body fat during the first year after birth, which is mostly due to enlargement of existing adipocytes (hypertrophy) rather than an increase in number (hyperplasia). Between 2 and 14 years of age, no significant change in fat cell volumes is seen in nonobese children (with a slight increase in cell number); in obese children, there is continual enlargement of adipocytes without hyperplasia.

3. There is evidence that energy expenditure changes to oppose alterations in body weight (either gain or loss), which may in part explain difficulties in maintaining new weight status in dieting adults. Decreases in body weight of both obese and nonobese adults are resisted by equivalent declines in energy expenditure. A formerly obese individual requires 10% to 15% fewer calories to maintain a normal body weight than a never-obese individual of the same body composition. The decline in energy expenditure in this case reflects a decrease primarily in energy expenditure during physical activity and possibly an additional decrease in resting energy expenditure. For previously nonobese individuals, maintenance of an increased body weight is also resisted with equal metabolic force. Thus, a lean or obese individual who has gained weight to 10% above usual body weight required about 15% more calories to maintain an elevated body weight.

Pathogenesis. The pathogenesis of obesity may be, in part, inherited, but genetics alone cannot account for the rapid increases in overweight in the U.S. population. Environmental factors appear importantly related to the rise in the prevalence of obesity in this country. The concept of energy balance applies to the pathogenesis of obesity (Fig. 33–4). When energy intake exceeds energy expenditure on a chronic basis, obesity results. When energy intake is less than energy expenditure, weight loss may result. An increase in caloric intake (overnutrition) and a decline in leisure and work-related physical activity have been associated with the increase in the prevalence of obesity. Increased consumption of calorie-dense foods and a decrease in physical activity or increased time spent on television and video games may be causally related to the increasing prevalence of obesity seen in children and adolescents (Gortmaker et al, 1996; Gutin and Manos, 1993).

Practically all energy intake comes from ingestion of macronutrients. The caloric value of fat is 9 kcal/g, and that of protein and carbohydrate is 4 kcal/g; an important reason for recommending reduced fat intake to control weight. A large portion of energy expenditure is the resting metabolic rate (RMR), accounting for 60% to 75% of energy expenditure. Approximately 10% of energy expenditure is dissipated through the thermic effect of food (TEF), which is mainly the result of the energy cost of nutrient absorption, processing, and storage. The TEF has two components: obligatory and facultative. The latter can be blocked by β-adrenergic blockade, suggesting that the sympathetic nervous system is important. Energy expenditure resulting from physical activity varies greatly from individual to individual, with a large portion of energy expenditure seen in physically active persons and a small amount of expenditure seen in sedentary individuals. Energy expenditure from RMR and TEF, and possibly that from physical activity, may be importantly determined by genetic factors.

Health Consequences of Obesity. A number of disease states are associated with obesity in adults, which are not only risk factors for heart disease and diabetes but also

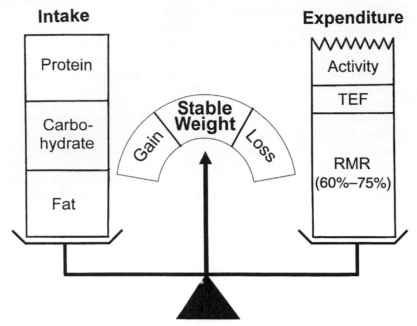

Figure 33–4. *Energy balance. In order to maintain a stable weight, energy intake (protein, carbohydrate, and fat) of a person should be equal to energy expenditure, which is composed of resting metabolic rate (RMR), thermic effect of food (TEF), and expenditure associated with physical activities. When intake is greater than expenditure, weight gain results; when expenditure of energy is greater than the intake, weight loss may result.*

responsible for significant health care costs: approximately 5% of total health care costs (over $100 billion) can be attributed to overweight. Common conditions associated with adult obesity include hyperlipidemia, heart disease, hypertension, type 2 diabetes, stroke, and osteoarthritis. Obesity also increases the prevalence of some cancers, gallbladder disease, sleep disorders, gout, and mood disorders.

Health consequences of obesity in children are somewhat different from those seen in obese adults (Dietz, 1998).

1. Psychosocial consequences.
   a. Early discrimination (in childhood).
   b. Inappropriate expectation to be more mature because of their large size. This may lead to frustration, a sense of failure, and social isolation.
   c. Negative self-esteem (in adolescence).
   d. Learning difficulties.
   e. Eating disorders (in white girls).
   f. Obese men tend to attain lower socioeconomic status and social achievement. Obese women tend to have lower educational level, family income, and rates of marriage and higher rates of living in poverty.

2. Common medical consequences of obesity.
   a. Early maturation with advanced bone age (and early onset of menarche).
   b. Cardiovascular risk factors (data from Becque, 1988; Srinivasan et al, 1999).
      1). Hypercholesterolemia—31%
      2). Hypertriglyceridemia—64%
      3). Low HDL cholesterol—64%
   c. Glucose intolerance, which is linked to the increase in the prevalence of type 2 diabetes.

   d. Hypertension is present in 10% to 30% of overweight children.

   e. Acanthosis nigricans (~25%), an indication of hyperinsulinemia.

   f. Hepatic steatosis (fatty degeneration) with elevated liver enzymes (seen in >10% of overweight children), cholelithiasis (due to increased cholesterol synthesis), and cholecystitis (occurring more often with weight reduction).

3. Less common medical consequences of obesity.

   a. Pseudotumor cerebri (with manifestations of headache, visual impairment or blindness, papilledema, occurring before adolescence) requires aggressive treatment. About 50% of children with the condition are obese.

   b. Sleep apnea occurs in less than 7% of obese children. This requires aggressive treatment including tonsillectomy and adenoidectomy or weight reduction.

   c. Orthopedic complications: Blount's disease (bowing of the tibia and femur with resulting overgrowth of the medial aspect of the proximal tibial metaphysis) or slipped capital femoral epiphysis.

   d. Polycystic ovary disease: Menstrual abnormalities and hirsutism in association with obesity, acanthosis, hyperinsulinemia, and hyperandrogenemia suggest this condition.

Diagnosis

1. The BMI (weight in kg divided by square of the height in meters, kg/m^2) is a simple, valid measure of relative weight and is recommended in clinical diagnosis of overweight states. Although parents tend to better understand the term relative weight (the child's weight divided by the ideal weight of the child for his or her height), physicians should use BMI percentile in following up overweight children. Age- and gender-specific BMI standards for the U.S. pediatric population have been published as percentile curves by the Centers for Disease Control and Prevention (see Appendix C, Figs. C–1 and C–2).

2. *Classification*: In adults, obesity is present when BMI is greater than 30 and overweight is present when BMI is between 25.0 and 29.9. For children, a statistical definition of overweight is used. Children whose BMI is at the 85th to 95th percentile are mildly to moderately overweight (children "at risk of overweight," adult equivalent of overweight) and children whose BMI is at or greater than the 95th percentile are more significantly overweight (overweight children; adult equivalent of obesity).

3. Percent body fat may be more accurate in determining obesity than BMI, although the method of determining body fat is cumbersome and costly. A large BMI does not necessarily indicate an increase in body fat: lean, muscular individuals may have a large BMI. There is no accurate and reliable conversion equation between BMI and percent body fat. Although highly significant relationships exist between BMI and percent fat, for a given value of BMI, an adolescent's percentage fat can change by as much as −3% to +7% (Hannan et al, 1995).

   The percent body fat is 12% to 20% in normal adult men and 20% to 30% in normal adult women. The amount of body fat in well-trained athletes is less than 10%, and it is nearly 50% in obese patients. Obesity is present when percent body fat is over 25% in men and over 33% in women. When percent body fat is between the range of normal and obesity, it is called borderline obesity. Percent body fat of 25% for male adolescents and 30% for female adolescents may be an indication of obesity.

4. Physicians should consider identifiable underlying causes of obesity, such as genetic or endocrine disorders.

   a. Genetic causes: Prader-Willi, Bardet-Biedl, and Alström syndromes all have early onset of severe obesity, out of proportion to the family history, often with dysmorphic features.

   b. Endocrine abnormalities, such as hypothyroidism, Cushing's syndrome, and generalized hypothalamic dysfunction, should be considered. Children with hypothyroidism and cortisol excess have short stature and delayed puberty rather than the tall stature and early puberty seen in most obese children. When questions arise, determination of free thyroxine and thyroid-stimulating hormone and 24-hour urinary free cortisol or diurnal salivary cortisol levels should clarify the questions.

5. Check for the presence of other risk factors for CVD or diabetes (metabolic syndrome; see Box 33–2).
   a. Blood pressure measurement.
   b. Lipoprotein analysis, fasting insulin, and blood glucose.
   c. Glycosylated hemoglobin (HbA_{1c}) may also be useful.

6. Search for possible obesity-related complications by history and physical examination, such as the following.
   a. Acanthosis nigricans is associated with hyperinsulinemia and a higher risk of developing type 2 diabetes.
   b. Thyroid enlargement may be associated with hypothyroidism.
   c. History of nighttime snoring, breathing difficulties, or daytime somnolence may indicate obstructive sleep apnea or obesity hypoventilation syndrome.
   d. Hip or knee pain may be a manifestation of slipped capital femoral epiphysis.
   e. Abdominal pain or tenderness may be associated with gallbladder disease.
   f. Headaches and blurred optic disk margins may indicate pseudotumor cerebri.
   g. Hepatomegaly may be associated with hepatic steatosis.
   h. Oligomenorrhea, amenorrhea, striae, or hirsutism may indicate polycystic ovary disease or Cushing's syndrome.
   i. Signs of depression, bulimia nervosa, binge eating disorder, or other serious psychological disorders would require further evaluation and treatment by a child psychiatrist or psychologist.

Management. All successful pediatric weight management programs include four components: (1) dietary component, (2) exercise, (3) behavior modification, and (4) family component. Among these, dietary intervention and regular exercise combined are the cornerstones of weight management. Only through behavior modification can long-term healthy eating and activity patterns be established; attempts at employing diet and exercise for quick weight loss usually fail. Without involvement of the parents and family, behavior modifications in children and adolescents are difficult to achieve. Currently, there are no pharmacologic agents available for weight management in children and adolescents that have been shown to be safe and effective. A physician or other health care professional alone is usually inadequate in managing weight problems because of lack of training and limited time in weight management; thus, consultations with registered dietitians, psychologists, or exercise specialists may be sought or a referral to a multidisciplinary weight management program may become necessary.

Physicians should first assess usual diet and activity patterns of overweight children and adolescents and counsel them and their parents about the risk of childhood obesity and the need to adopt a healthy lifestyle. Physicians' counseling should include at least the following points.

1. The diet of choice is a diet low in saturated fat and cholesterol that includes 5 or more daily servings of vegetables and fruits and 6 to 11 servings of whole grain and other complex carbohydrate foods.

2. A "healthy plate" should be introduced, of which half is filled with salad and vegetables, one fourth with starch (e.g., potatoes, rice), and one fourth with a protein source (e.g., meat, poultry, fish, soy).

3. Children should participate in at least 30 minutes of moderate physical activity at least 4 or more days of the week, and preferably every day.

4. Parents should be encouraged to help their children reduce excessive time spent on sedentary behaviors such as watching television and videotapes, playing on a computer, listening to music, and talking on the telephone. The television set should be removed from the child's bedroom.

5. More physical activity should be part of the lifestyle, such as walking or biking to school instead of driving, skating, stairs instead of elevators, and helping with active chores inside and outside the house.

Further discussion of important components of successful pediatric obesity treatment follows.

1. Early intervention (beginning at or before adolescence) is important for the following reasons.
   a. Many lifestyle habits (eating and exercise habits) are established early in childhood. Parents have much control of their children's behaviors in early school years.
   b. There is a tracking of cardiovascular risk factors from childhood to adulthood. About 80% of obese adolescents became obese adults. Once established, obesity is difficult to cure. Only palliation is possible, with an enormous cost.
   c. Successful treatment of obesity has been shown to improve dyslipidemia and glucose intolerance and thus eventually will result in the prevention of CVD.

2. Dietary modification is an integral part of the treatment. Assessment of eating habits and parent education and consultation with dietitians are needed.
   a. Assessment of eating habits.
      1). Ask about consumption of high-calorie drinks (soda pops, fruit juices).
      2). Number and types of fast foods per week.
   b. Physicians may use the following as handout materials for counseling.
      1). Box 33–5 (dietary strategies) and Box 33–6 (tips for parents).
      2). Tables C–5 and C–6 in Appendix C specify foods to choose and to decrease and the serving sizes of each food group, respectively.
      3). Serving size of various food groups according to age and gender (Table C–6).
   c. Physicians may recommend that parents read about the new food guide pyramid recommended by the U.S. Department of Agriculture (*http://www.mypyramid.gov*).

3. Exercise is also an integral part of the management. Without regular exercise, dietary modification alone is insufficient for successful weight management. Physicians should first assess the level of physical activity of overweight children and utilize their influential position to counsel children and their family to adopt a healthy lifestyle.
   a. The following questions are useful in assessing physical activity in children.
      1). Amount of time regularly spent walking, bicycling, swimming, and in backyard play.

BOX 33–5	AMERICAN HEART ASSOCIATION'S PEDIATRIC DIETARY STRATEGIES FOR INDIVIDUALS OLDER THAN 2 YEARS: RECOMMENDATIONS TO ALL PATIENTS AND FAMILIES

- Balance dietary calories with physical activity to maintain normal growth.
- 60 minutes of moderate to vigorous play or physical activity daily.
- Eat vegetables and fruits daily, limit juice intake.
- Use vegetable oil and soft margarines low in saturated fat and trans fatty acids instead of butter or most other animal fats in the diet.
- Eat whole grain breads and cereals rather than refined grain products.
- Reduce the intake of sugar-sweetened beverages and foods.
- Use nonfat (skim) or low-fat milk and dairy products daily.
- Eat more fish, especially oily fish, broiled or baked.
- Reduce salt intake, including salt from processed foods.

From Gidding SS, Dennison BA, Birch LL, et al, American Heart Association; American Academy of Pediatrics: Dietary recommendations for children and adolescents: A guide for practitioners. Pediatrics 117:544–559, 2006.

BOX 33–6	TIPS FOR PARENTS TO IMPLEMENT AMERICAN HEART ASSOCIATION PEDIATRIC DIETARY GUIDELINES

- Reduce added sugars, including sugar-sweetened drinks and juices.

- Use canola, soybean, corn oil, safflower oil, or other unsaturated oils in place of solid fats during food preparation.

- Use recommended portion size on food labels when preparing and serving food.

- Use fresh, frozen, and canned vegetables and fruits and serve at every meal; be careful with added sauces and sugar.

- Introduce and regularly serve fish as an entrée.

- Remove the skin from poultry before eating.

- Use only lean cuts of meat and reduced-fat meat products.

- Limit high-calorie sauces such as Alfredo, cream sauces, cheese sauces, and hollandaise sauce.

- Eat whole grain breads and cereals rather than refined products; read labels and ensure that "whole grain" is the first ingredient on the food label of these products.

- Eat more legumes (beans) and tofu in place of meat for some entrées.

- Breads, breakfast cereals, and prepared foods, including soups, may be high in salt and/or sugar; read food labels for content and choose high-fiber, low-salt/low-sugar alternatives.

From Gidding SS, Dennison BA, Birch LL, et al, American Heart Association; American Academy of Pediatrics: Dietary recommendations for children and adolescents: A guide for practitioners. Pediatrics 117:544–559, 2006.

2). Use of stairs, playgrounds, and gymnasiums and interactive physical play with other children.
3). Number of hours per day spent watching television or videotapes and playing video or computer games.
4). Time spent participating in organized sports, lessons, clubs, or league games.
5). Time spent in school physical education that includes a minimum of 30 minutes of coordinated large-muscle exercise.
6). Participation in household chores.
7). Positive role modeling for a physically active lifestyle by parents and other caretakers.
b. Physician's counseling and education should include the following areas.
1). Formally address the subject of exercise, emphasizing the benefits of regular physical activity. The health benefits associated with increased physical activity include:
      Helps weight control by lowering level of weight gain
      Metabolic benefits include improved glucose tolerance and insulin sensitivity (even in the absence of weight loss)
      Reduction in VLDL and rise in HDL cholesterol levels
      Lowers blood pressure
      Improves psychological well-being
      Predisposition to increased physical activity in adulthood
2). Advise parents to establish limits for sedentary activities of their children and encourage a daily time for physical activity. The American Academy of Pediatrics has recommended that television viewing or games be limited to 1 to 2 hours a day and that television sets be removed from children's bedrooms. A 30-minute regular exercise daily or nearly daily is encouraged.

       3). Encourage children to participate in sports that can be enjoyed throughout life, summer camp, and school physical education programs.

       4). Teach parents the importance of being role models for an active lifestyle and providing children with opportunities for increased physical activity.

4. Behavior modification is essential for permanent changes in dietary and exercise habits.

  a. Promotion of long-term permanent changes in behavior patterns, rather than short-term diet or exercise program for rapid weight loss, should be the goal of the treatment.

  b. Emphasis should be on small and gradual behavior changes.

5. Family involvement is very important in pediatric weight management programs.

  a. Willingness on the part of both child and family to participate and involvement of the entire family and other caregivers are important.

  b. Education of families about the medical complications of obesity should be included (as discussed earlier in this chapter).

  c. Parents need to learn certain skills and commit themselves to the program, such as:

       1). Parent role modeling of healthful dietary and activity habits

       2). Understanding the new food guide pyramid

       3). Ability to learn how to read food labels

       4). Appropriate ways of praising and rewarding good progress

       5). Changes in family environment, such as removing high-calorie foods, reducing the number of meals eaten outside the home, serving portion-controlled meals to the child, and promoting active lifestyles and discouraging sedentary lifestyles

       6). Inclusion of activities to help families monitor their eating and physical activity behaviors and establishing formal routine exercise program at a scheduled time each day or evening

Primary emphasis should be the lifestyle change; the weight change itself is of secondary importance. An active lifestyle improves risk factors even when weight loss is minimal. When a weight loss goal is set, it should be realistic and should not attempt to normalize weight fully. In children without many complications of obesity, maintenance of the current weight or modest weight loss, while children continue to grow in height, reduces their degree of overweight. Children with complications of obesity (e.g., hypertension, hyperlipidemias, insulin resistance, hepatic steatosis) should attempt to lose weight to correct those complications. Even a modest weight loss of 5 to 10 pounds may result in substantial reductions in CVD risks.

CIGARETTE SMOKING

Cigarette smoking has been called the chief single avoidable cause of death in our society and the most important public health issue of our time, costing over $167 billion a year. Cigarette smoking is a powerful independent risk factor for myocardial infarction, sudden death, and peripheral vascular disease. Even passive exposure to smoke causes alterations in the risk factors in children.

Prevalence. The prevalence of cigarette smoking nationwide among high school students (grades 9 to 12) increased during the 1990s, peaking during 1996 to 1997, and then declined slightly, but a significant number of children and adolescents continue to be smokers. An estimated 6.4 million children younger than 18 years who are living today will die prematurely as adults because they began to smoke cigarettes during adolescence.

Some important statistics on the prevalence of smoking among youth are presented here, based on the most recent report from Centers for Disease Control and Prevention (Marshall et al, 2006) and other recent reports.

1. Current use of any tobacco product (cigarettes, cigar, pipes, and smokeless tobacco) ranges from 13% among middle school students to 28% among high school students. Among college students, 33% are current users of tobacco products and nearly 50% used a tobacco product in the past year (Rigotti et al, 2000).

Tobacco use was significantly higher among white students than black students. Cigarette smoking was the most prevalent and cigar smoking was the second most prevalent form of tobacco use.

2. Approximately 80% of tobacco users initiate use before age 18 years.

3. There were smokers in the households of 72% of middle school student smokers and 58% of high school student smokers.

4. Nearly 50% of middle school student smokers and 62% of high school student smokers reported a desire to stop smoking cigarettes, and most of them have made at least one cessation attempt during the last 12 months. On the other hand, among students who have never smoked cigarettes, 21% of middle school students and 23% of high school students were susceptible to initiating cigarette smoking in the next year. These data show the urgency of providing means to prevent smoking in children and the need to help them stop smoking.

Pathophysiologic Effects of Smoking. The following are some pathophysiologic effects of smoking on the cardiovascular system (Lu and Creager, 2004), all of which appear likely to be involved in accelerating atherosclerosis in the coronary artery and peripheral arteries or increasing the probability of thrombosis (with potential for stroke). Physicians could use this information in counseling sessions with smokers.

1. Smoking causes atherogenic dyslipidemia.
   a. It increases levels of LDL and VLDL cholesterols and triglycerides.
   b. It lowers HDL cholesterol levels.

   These effects are greater in children and adolescents than in adults. Even passive smoking lowers HDL cholesterol.

2. Smoking contributes to a prothrombotic predisposition.
   a. It increases levels of fibrinogen, factor VII, and other factors involved in the fibrin clotting cascade and decreases the concentration of plasminogen.
   b. It activates platelets, increasing their ability to adhere to the vessel wall.

3. Smoking increases blood viscosity by increasing hemoglobin levels (through carbon monoxide–induced increase in carboxyhemoglobin) and by an elevation of plasma fibrinogen levels.

4. Smoking accelerates the atherosclerotic process by:
   a. Increasing monocyte adhesion to endothelial cells (the initial step in atherogenesis)
   b. Decreasing nitric oxide synthesis (with resulting endothelial dysfunction)
   c. Decreasing synthesis of prostacyclin

5. Smoking causes peripheral arterial disease through endothelial dysfunction.

6. Smoking raises blood pressure transiently, raises heart rate, and increases myocardial contractility and myocardial oxygen consumption (by stimulation of sympathetic nervous system).

Psychosociology of Smoking. Physicians should be aware of the psychosociology of initiating smoking in order to help prevent smoking in children.

1. *Age*: Most smoking starts during adolescence. The high-risk period is the transition from elementary school to middle school and first and second years of middle school. This should be the target age group to counsel individually or through school systems.

2. Known predictors of smoking include peer influence (the most important), family members who smoke (siblings and parents), less educated parents, being a more independent and rebellious child, and having less academic success.

3. Cited reasons for starting to smoke include wanting to fit into a group, to lose weight, and to appear more mature.

Management. Physicians and health care professionals should assess the status of smoking, provide smoking prevention messages, help counsel parents and children about smoking cessation, and encourage school and community antismoking efforts.

1. Physicians should assess the status of smoking during office visits.
   a. Smoking history should be obtained for all children older than 8 years during routine health assessments and updated. History regarding any siblings and friends who smoke should also be obtained.
   b. For current smokers, onset of smoking; number and type of cigarettes smoked per day, week, or month; and whether they want to quit smoking and need help to quit the habit.
   c. Smoking history should also be obtained for parents and be updated.

2. Parents who smoke should be encouraged to quit. Physicians should emphasize adverse effects of passive smoking on their children and the need to be a role model for their children. Physicians should refer parent smokers to community smoking cessation programs.

3. Physicians' offices should be nonsmoking environments (without ashtrays), and anti-smoking posters, pamphlets, and videos in the waiting room may be productive.

4. Counseling techniques may vary with the age of the child.
   a. For elementary school children, an antismoking message at each well-child assessment may counterbalance any negative pro-smoking influences exerted by friends or family. Emphasize the harmful physical consequences of smoking and the addictive nature of cigarettes. Parental assistance in child's cessation of smoking should also be sought.
   b. For adolescents, emphasis should be on current negative physiologic and social effects of smoking rather than long-term health consequences. Adolescents understand the health consequences of smoking but see them as remote and irrelevant. More immediate negative effects include bad breath, smelling like smoke, yellow-stained fingers, smell in clothing and hair, increasing heart rate and blood pressure, lack of stamina for sports, and shortness of breath.

Some adolescents quit smoking on the advice of their physician, and a cessation message as brief as 3 minutes may be effective. Many adolescents require repeated efforts to quit smoking. Physicians should also encourage activities that tend to preclude cigarette smoking, such as regular physical activity and a variety of school and after-school activities.

Pharmacologic Approach. For established adult smokers, if counseling is ineffective, physicians may try nicotine replacement and bupropion to help them quit smoking.

1. Nicotine replacement (by nicotine polacrilex gum or transdermal patch) delivers less nicotine than cigarette smoking, which delivers a bolus of nicotine. It also eliminates carbon monoxide inhalation.

2. Bupropion, an antidepressant, stimulates dopamine release and curbs the severe withdrawal symptoms of smoking cessation.

Practice of Preventive Cardiology

The primary mission of pediatrics has been prevention of disease and ensuring normal growth and development. It is natural for pediatricians to pay attention to early detection of children at risk for developing CVD (and type 2 diabetes) and provide counseling, intervention, or treatment whenever possible.

Atherosclerotic CVD, the leading cause of both death and disability in this country, has an early onset, and its presence and extent correlate positively and significantly with established cardiovascular risk factors, namely LDL cholesterol, triglycerides, blood pressure, BMI, and presence of cigarette smoking (see Box 33–1). There is a disturbing increase in the prevalence of obesity during childhood and it is closely related to the development of other risk factors for CAD and diabetes, which is known as the metabolic syndrome (see Box 33–3).

Acquisition of behaviors associated with risk factors occurs in childhood, such as dietary habits, physical activity behaviors, and the use of tobacco. Intervention to reduce the risk factors in childhood has been successful with low-calorie diets, smoking prevention,

Table 33–5. **Summary Guidelines for Preventive Pediatric Cardiology**

Risk Identification	Treatment Goals	Recommendations
Blood Cholesterol		
Total cholesterol: >170 mg/dL is borderline >200 mg/dL is elevated LDL-C: >110 mg/dL is borderline >130 mg/dL is elevated.	Goals: LDL-C <160 mg/dL (<130 mg/dL is even better) For patients with diabetes, LDL-C <100 mg/dL	If LDL-C is above goals, initiate additional therapeutic lifestyle changes, including diet (<7% of calories from saturated fat; <200 mg cholesterol per day), in conjunction with a trained dietitian. Consider LDL-lowering dietary options (increase soluble fiber by using age [in years] plus 5 to 10 g up to age 15, when the total remains at 25 g per day) in conjunction with a trained dietitian. Emphasize weight management and increased physical activity. If LDL-C is persistently above goals, evaluate for secondary causes (thyroid-stimulating hormone, liver function tests, renal function tests, urinalysis). Consider pharmacologic therapy for individuals with LDL >190 mg/dL with no other risk factors for CVD or >160 mg/dL with other risk factors present (blood pressure elevation, diabetes, obesity, strong family history of premature CVD). Pharmacologic intervention for dyslipidemia should be accomplished in collaboration with a physician experienced in treatment of disorders of cholesterol in pediatric patients.
Other Lipids and Lipoprotein		
Triglycerides: >150 mg/dL HDL-C <40 mg/dL	Goals: Fasting TG <150 mg/dL HDL-C >40 mg/dL	Elevated fasting TG and reduced HDL-C are often seen in the context of overweight with insulin resistance. Therapeutic lifestyle change should include weight management with appropriate energy intake and expenditure. Decrease intake of simple sugars. If fasting TGs are persistently elevated, evaluate for secondary causes such as diabetes, thyroid disease, renal disease, and alcohol abuse. No pharmacologic interventions are recommended in children for isolated elevation of fasting TG unless this is very marked (treatment may be initiated at TG >400 mg/dL to protect against postprandial TG of 1000 mg/dL or greater, which may be associated with an increased risk of pancreatitis).
Blood Pressure		
Systolic and diastolic pressure >95th percentile for age, sex and height percentile.	Goal: Systolic and diastolic blood pressure <95th percentile for age, sex, and height	Promote achievement of appropriate weight. Reduce sodium in the diet. Emphasize increased consumption of fruits and vegetables. If BP is persistently above the 95th percentile, consider possible secondary causes (e.g., renal disease, coarctation of the aorta). Consider pharmacologic therapy for individuals above the 95th percentile if lifestyle modification brings no improvement and there is evidence of target organ changes (left ventricular hypertrophy, microalbuminuria, retinal vascular abnormalities). Start blood pressure medication individualized to other requirements and characteristics of the patient (i.e., age, race, need for drugs with specific benefits). Pharmacologic management of hypertension should be accomplished in collaboration with a physician experienced in pediatric hypertension.
Weight		
BMI: >85th percentile is at risk of overweight >90th percentile is overweight	Goal: Achieve and maintain BMI <95th percentile for age and sex	For children who are at risk of overweight (>85th percentile) or obesity (>95th percentile), a weight management program should be initiated with appropriate energy balance achieved through changes in diet and physical activity. For children of normal height, a secondary cause of obesity is unlikely. Weight management should be directed at all family members who are overweight, using a family-centered, behavioral management approach. Weight management should be done in collaboration with a trained dietitian.

Table 33–5. **Summary Guidelines for Preventive Pediatric Cardiology** *(Continued)*

Risk Identification	Treatment Goals	Recommendations
Diabetes		
	Near-normal fasting plasma glucose (<120 mg/dL) Near-normal HbA$_{1c}$ (<7%) (goals for fasting glucose and HbA$_{1c}$ should take into consideration age and risk of hypoglycemia)	Management of type 1 and type 2 diabetes in children and adolescents should be accomplished in collaboration with a pediatric endocrinologist. For type 2 diabetes, the first step is weight management with improved diet and exercise. Because of risk for accelerated vascular disease, other risk factors (e.g., blood pressure, lipid abnormalities) should be treated more aggressively in patients with diabetes.
Cigarette Smoking		
	Complete cessation of smoking for children and parents who smoke	Advise every tobacco user (parents and children) to quit and be prepared to provide assistance with this (counseling/referral to develop a plan for quitting using available community resources to help with smoking cessation).

BP, blood pressure; CVD, cardiovascular disease; HbA$_{1c}$, hemoglobin A$_{1c}$; HDL-C, high-density lipoprotein cholesterol; LDL-C, low-density lipoprotein cholesterol; TG, triglyceride.
Modified from Kavey RW, Daniels SR, Lauer RM, et al: American Heart Association guidelines for primary prevention of atherosclerotic cardiovascular disease beginning in childhood. Circulation 107:1562–1566, 2003.

increasing physical activities, and family-based weight control programs. This is due to the fact that some risk factors are detectable, modifiable, or treatable.

1. Family history of CVD is very important in assessing a child's risk for developing CAD later in life. Although it is not modifiable, its presence is a marker for a high risk of heart disease. A history of premature CAD in first- or second-degree relatives (parents, siblings, grandparents, or blood-related aunts and uncles) before age 55 for males and before age 60 for females should prompt physicians to check on other risk factors.

2. Hypercholesterolemia is one of the major risk factors that are identifiable and treatable. A detailed discussion of this topic has been presented earlier in this chapter.

3. Hypertension is also an identifiable and treatable risk factor (see Chapter 28).

4. Other risk factors, such as smoking, consumption of atherogenic diets, and physical inactivity, are all modifiable by behavior changes.

5. Obesity is easily detectable. Although treatment of obesity can be frustrating to both patients and physicians, patients' education and behavior modification can be productive.

6. Inclusion of HbA$_{1c}$ should be considered in the screening protocol to detect a diabetic or prediabetic state.

The American Heart Association has updated a guideline for the prevention of CVD. Table 33–5 is a summary that presents goals and recommendations to achieve the goals of reducing risks in children and adolescents identified as at high risk for future CVD.

Chapter 34

Athletes with Cardiac Problems

Competitive athletes are those who participate in an organized team or individual sport that requires regular competition against others. This definition is most easily applied to high school, college, and professional sports. Athletic competitions substantially increase the sympathetic drive, and the resulting increase in catecholamine levels increases blood pressure, heart rate, and myocardial contractility, thereby increasing myocardial oxygen demand. The increase in sympathetic tone can cause arrhythmias and may worsen existing myocardial ischemia. An athlete with a cardiac problem is at an increased risk for developing serious morbidity and even sudden death during athletic competition in comparison with nonathletes with a similar cardiac problem. Undiagnosed heart conditions or cardiac arrhythmias can cause problems during athletic competitions.

Many physicians are involved in medical clearance for participation in school sports activities. In order to help reduce or prevent sudden death or other serious events occurring during athletic competitions, physicians should be aware of cardiac conditions that may cause problems. In addition, physicians should have general understanding of the eligibility guidelines and have access to the participation eligibility for patients with specific cardiovascular conditions.

This chapter discusses the knowledge base required to accomplish physicians' roles in school sports clearance. The following major areas are discussed: sudden unexpected death, preparticipation screening of athletes, classification of sports, participation eligibility for athletes with congenital and acquired heart disease, athletes with cardiac arrhythmias, and athletes with hypertension. The recommendations are mostly from the 36th Bethesda Conference (36th Bethesda Conference, 2005).

Sudden Unexpected Death in Young Athletes

Sudden unexpected death in young athletes is estimated to occur in about 1 per 200,000 high school participants per academic year. Although it is rare, when a sudden unexpected death of an athlete related to a cardiac condition occurs, the public becomes disbelieving, suspicious, and even angry. Sometimes, these feelings have been directed at the physicians involved. It is, therefore, important for primary care physicians to have a good understanding of cardiac conditions that could result in sudden death in order to reduce that possibility.

Among a variety of congenital or acquired heat diseases that can cause sudden death during athletic competition, hypertrophic cardiomyopathy and coronary artery anomalies or diseases are the two most important groups. The previously implicated diseases for sudden cardiac death are shown in Box 34–1.

BOX 34–1	CARDIOVASCULAR ANOMALIES IN 134 YOUNG COMPETITIVE ATHLETES WITH SUDDEN DEATH	
Primary Cardiovascular Lesions		**Percent**
Hypertrophic cardiomyopathy		36.0
Unexplained increase in cardiac mass (possible hypertrophic cardiomyopathy)		10.0
Aberrant coronary arteries		13.0
Other coronary anomalies		6.0
Ruptured aortic aneurysm		5.0
Tunneled left anterior descending coronary artery (myocardial "bridges")		5.0
Aortic valve stenosis		4.0
Myocarditis		3.0
Idiopathic myocardial scarring		3.0
Idiopathic dilated cardiomyopathy		3.0
Arrhythmogenic right ventricular dysplasia		3.0
Mitral valve prolapse		2.0
Atherosclerotic coronary artery disease		2.0
Other congenital heart disease		1.5
Long QT syndrome		0.5
Sarcoidosis		0.5
Sickle cell trait		0.5
Normal heart		2.0

From Maron BJ, Shirani J, Poline LC, et al: Sudden death in young competitive athletes: Clinical, demographic and pathological profiles. JAMA 276:199–208, 1996.

1. Hypertrophic cardiomyopathy (HCM). The single most common cardiovascular abnormality among the causes of sudden death in young athletes is HCM (up to 40%) and its variants (10%), accounting for nearly half of the cases (see Box 34–1).

2. Congenital anomalies and acquired diseases of the coronary arteries are the next important group of causes of sudden death, accounting for about 30%.
   a. Aberrant origin of the left coronary artery at an acute angle from the right sinus of Valsalva or the right coronary artery from the left sinus of Valsalva.
   b. Acquired coronary artery diseases such as atherosclerotic coronary artery disease or coronary artery stenosis as the result of Kawasaki disease.

3. Myocarditis. Sudden cardiac death has been reported at rest and during exercise with both acute and chronic myocarditis (up to 17% of sudden death) by way of ventricular arrhythmias. Rarely, myocardial fibrosis can be a cause of sudden death.

4. Cardiac arrhythmias (from long QT syndrome, Wolff-Parkinson-White [WPW] syndrome, sinus node dysfunction, and arrhythmogenic right ventricular dysplasia [ARVD]) are rare causes of sudden death.

5. Other rare causes of sudden death in athletes include:
   a. Severe obstructive lesions (such as aortic stenosis or pulmonary stenosis)
   b. Marfan syndrome (from ruptured aortic aneurysm)
   c. Mitral valve prolapse
   d. Dilated cardiomyopathy
   e. Primary pulmonary hypertension
   f. Unexpected blow to the chest (by such objects as a baseball or hockey puck)
   g. Sarcoidosis
   h. Sickle cell trait

Most patients die while they are sedentary or during mild exertion, but many collapse during or just after vigorous physical activity. On occasion, athletes may die suddenly without evidence of structural heart disease on autopsy. In such instances, the death may be due to a noncardiac cause such as drug abuse.

Preparticipation Screening

The objective of preparticipation screening is the recognition of "silent" cardiovascular disease that can progress to or cause sudden cardiac death. There are, however, no cost-effective practical guidelines for the screening that have been proved to be effective in identifying the potential candidates for sudden death at this time. Prospective cardiovascular screening of a large athletic population is impractical because only 0.3% of the general athletic population have congenital malformations relevant to athletic screening. The total number of competitive athletes in the United States may be in the range of 8 million to 10 million. Even with the use of specialized tools available to cardiologists, complete prevention of such death is nearly impossible, given the rarity of some of the causes of sudden expected death. Consequently, medical clearance for sports does not necessarily imply the absence of cardiovascular disease or complete protection from sudden death.

Customary screening for U.S. high school and college athletes is confined to history taking and physical examination, which are known to be limited in their power to identify consistently important cardiovascular abnormalities. The American Heart Association's recommendations for preparticipation screening are shown in Box 34–2. This screening method has the capability of raising clinical suspicion of several cardiovascular abnormalities by virtue of the history and physical examination.

History and Physical Examination. Although screening history and physical examination are important, they do not have sufficient power to guarantee detection of many critical cardiovascular abnormalities. Despite these major limitations, simple history and physical examination can raise the suspicion of cardiovascular disease in some at-risk athletes.

1. History of syncope, chest pain, dyspnea, and fatigue, particularly when associated with exertion, is important.

2. Family history of premature cardiac death, sudden unexpected death, and heritable diseases should be noted.

BOX 34–2	AMERICAN HEART ASSOCIATION CONSENSUS PANEL RECOMMENDATIONS FOR PREPARTICIPATION ATHLETE SCREENING

Family History

 1. Premature sudden cardiac death

 2. Heart disease in surviving relative younger than 50 years

Personal History

 3. Heart murmur

 4. Systemic hypertension

 5. Fatigue

 6. Syncope/near syncope

 7. Excessive/unexplained exertional dyspnea

 8. Exertional chest pain

Physical Examination

 9. Heart murmur (supine/standing*)

10. Femoral arterial pulses (to exclude coarctation of the aorta)

11. Stigmata of Marfan syndrome

12. Brachial blood pressure measurement (sitting)

*In particular, to identify heart murmur consistent with dynamic obstruction to the LV outflow tract.
From Maron BJ, Thompson PD, Puffer JC, et al: Cardiovascular preparticipation screening of competitive athletes. Circulation 94:850–856, 1996.

3. Significant aortic or pulmonary stenosis or coarctation of the aorta may be one of a few lesions most likely to be detected by physical examination alone.

4. Identification of HCM by the standard history and physical examination is unreliable because (a) most patients with HCM have the nonobstructive form of the disease (and, thus, no audible heart murmur) and (b) most athletes with HCM do not experience exertional syncope or have a family history of the disease or premature sudden death.

If cardiovascular abnormalities are suspected from the preceding screening questionnaire, ECG and echo studies are carried out.

Electrocardiography. The 12-lead ECG is a practical and cost-effective strategic alternative to routine echocardiography.

1. The ECG is abnormal in up to 75% to 95% of patients with HCM.

2. It is expected to be abnormal in those with coronary artery abnormalities.

3. It also identifies other abnormalities such as the long QT syndrome, Brugada syndrome (right bundle branch block [RBBB] with ST-segment elevation), and other inherited syndromes associated with ventricular arrhythmias.

4. It may also raise suspicion of myocarditis (premature ventricular contractions [PVCs], ST-T changes) or arrhythmogenic right ventricular cardiomyopathy (by T-wave inversion in leads V1 through V3).

5. However, abnormal ECGs are seen in about 40% of trained athletes and may be a source of confusion. ECG abnormalities seen in trained athletes include increased R- or S-wave voltages, Q-wave and repolarization abnormalities, and frequent and/or complex ventricular tachyarrhythmias on Holter ECG monitors.

Echocardiography. Echo study is the principal diagnostic imaging modality for clinical identification of HCM and other cardiac abnormalities.

1. HCM can be reliably diagnosed by two-dimensional echo. A diastolic left ventricular (LV) wall thickness 15 mm or greater (or, on occasion, 13 or 14 mm), usually with LV dimension less than 45 mm, is accepted for the clinical diagnosis of HCM in adults. For children, a z-score of 2 or more relative to body surface area is theoretically compatible with the diagnosis.

The heart of some highly trained athletes may show hypertrophy of the LV wall, making the differentiation between physiologic hypertrophy and HCM difficult. An LV wall thickness of 13 mm and greater is very uncommon in highly trained athletes and is always associated with an enlarged LV cavity (with LV diastolic dimension greater than 54 mm, with range 55 to 63 mm). Therefore, athletes with LV wall thickness greater than 16 mm and a nondilated LV cavity are likely to have HCM (Pelliccia et al, 1991).

2. Echo is also expected to detect other congenital structural abnormalities, such as valvular heart disease (aortic stenosis, pulmonary stenosis), Marfan syndrome (aortic root dilatation, mitral valve prolapse), myocarditis, or dilated cardiomyopathy (LV dysfunction and/or enlargement).

3. Definitive diagnosis of congenital coronary artery anomalies may not be accomplished by echo studies; it may require other tests such as coronary angiography.

When a potentially serious condition is found by screening or following cardiology consultation, the physician should make recommendations to the athlete and to the team but should not be put in the position of being solely responsible for whether or not an athlete is permitted to participate. In many situations, physicians have been wrongly put into a situation in which they have to make a recommendation whether to allow or disallow the participation of an athlete. The physician's recommendation may be against the wishes of the team, school, or even the community. Therefore, the final decision should be made jointly by the physician, player, player's parents, the team, and the sponsoring organization. Financial considerations and the importance of the player to the team should be secondary factors to be weighed by the other participants in the decision-making process.

Classification of Sports

Sports can be classified according to the type and intensity of exercise performed and also with regard to the danger of bodily injury from collision as well as the consequences of syncope. Exercise can be divided into two broad types: dynamic and static.

Dynamic (isotonic) exercise involves changes in muscle length and joint movement with rhythmic contractions that develop relatively small intramuscular force; static (isometric) exercise involves development of relatively large intramuscular force with little or no change in muscle length or joint movement. Most sports activities are combinations of static and dynamic exercises. The terms *dynamic* and *static* exercise characterize activity on the basis of the mechanical action of the muscles involved and are different from the terms *aerobic* and *anaerobic* exercise. The latter characterize activity on the basis of the type of muscle metabolism.

Dynamic exercise causes a marked increase in oxygen consumption with a substantial increase in cardiac output, heart rate, stroke volume, and systolic blood pressure (BP) and a decrease in diastolic pressure and systemic vascular resistance. Static exercise, in contrast, causes a small increase in oxygen consumption, cardiac output, and heart rate and no change in stroke volume. There is a marked increase in systolic, diastolic, and mean arterial pressures and no appreciable change in total peripheral resistance. Thus, dynamic exercise primarily causes a volume load on the left ventricle, whereas static exercise causes a pressure load.

For the purpose of making recommendations on athletes' participation eligibility, Task Force 8 of the 36th Bethesda Conference (Mitchel et al, 2005) presented the following classification of sports (Fig. 34–1). In this classification, sports are classified into dynamic

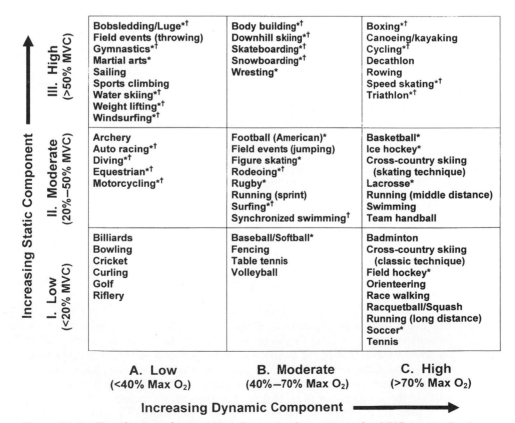

Figure 34–1. *Classification of sports. Max O₂, maximal oxygen uptake; MVC, maximal voluntary contraction; *danger of bodily collision, †increased risk if syncope occurs. (Modified from Mitchel JH, Haskel W, Snell P, Van Camp SP: Task Force 8: Classification of sports. J Am Coll Cardiol 45:1364–1367, 2005.)*

and static exercises and each sport is categorized by the level of intensity (low, medium, high). It should not be regarded as a rigid classification but rather a spectrum in which some athletes in the same sport could possibly deserve placement in different categories.

Eligibility Determination for Athletes with Cardiovascular Diseases

For the purpose of eligibility recommendations for athletes with cardiovascular abnormalities, recommendations for specific conditions are presented according to the following types of cardiac conditions: acyanotic congenital heart diseases, cyanotic congenital heart defects, coronary artery anomalies (including Kawasaki disease), valvular heart diseases, and myocardial and pericardial diseases. Most of the recommendations are excerpts from the 36th Bethesda Conference (Maron et al, 2005). These recommendations apply to athletes in high school and college. For middle school and elementary school children, less strict restriction may apply because of less strenuous training and sports activities. However, these guidelines will still be useful in making final recommendations for this group of athletes.

It should be noted that β-blockers that are used to treat certain heart conditions and arrhythmias are expressly banned in sports such as riflery (class IA) and archery (class IIA) in which the athlete would benefit from a slow heart rate. In these sports, β-blockers are banned substances, and prescribing β-blockers for athletes would risk them having a positive drug test.

ACYANOTIC CONGENITAL HEART DEFECTS

Participation eligibility of athletes with acyanotic heart diseases (which include left-to-right shunt lesions and obstructive lesions) is importantly determined by the level of pulmonary artery (PA) systolic pressure and the status of LV systolic function. Note that the following PA pressure levels are those obtained in the cardiac catheterization laboratory, and Doppler-derived pressure gradients are higher than these (see Chapter 29).

1. PA systolic pressure:
   a. When PA systolic pressure is ≤30 mm Hg (or Doppler-estimated PA systolic pressure <36 to 40 mm Hg), full participation in all competitive sports is allowed.
   b. When PA systolic pressure is greater than 30 mm Hg (or Doppler-estimated PA systolic pressure >36 to 40 mm Hg), a full evaluation determines limitations in participation eligibility.
   c. With mild pulmonary hypertension, low-intensity sports (IA) are permitted. With pulmonary vascular obstructive disease, no competitive sports are allowed.

2. LV systolic function:
   a. When LV systolic function is normal (with ejection fraction [EF] ≥50%), full participation is allowed.
   b. With mild LV dysfunction (EF 40% to 50%), low-intensity static sports (class IA, IB, and IC) are allowed.
   c. With moderate to severe LV dysfunction (EF <40%), no competitive sports are allowed.

Detailed participation recommendations for specific left-to-right shunt lesion and obstructive lesion are presented in Table 34–1.

CYANOTIC CONGENITAL HEART DEFECTS

In patients with arterial oxygen desaturation from cyanotic congenital heart disease, moderate to severe restriction in sport participation is recommended.

1. Patients with cyanotic congenital heart defects that are unoperated or for which palliative procedures have been done can participate only in low-intensity competitive sports, such as class IA sports.

2. Most patients with cyanotic heart defects for which surgical repair has been done can participate only in low-intensity sports.

Table 34–1. **Participation Recommendations for Acyanotic Congenital Heart Defects**

Heart Defects	Clinical Status	Can Participate in:
ASD, untreated	Small ASD with normal PA pressure	All competitive sports
	Moderate to large ASD with mild PH	Class IA sports
	Large ASD with severe PH (cyanosis)	No competitive sports
ASD, closed by surgery or device	Postclosure ASD in the absence of PH, symptomatic arrhythmias, or second- or third-degree AV block	All sports (3–6 mo after closure)
	Athletes with PH, arrhythmias, or AV block	Determined by level of PH and Table 34–6 recommendations
VSD, untreated	VSD with normal PA pressure	All competitive sports
	Large VSD (without marked PH) requires surgery	All competitive sports, 3–6 mo after surgical repair
VSD, closed	Asymptomatic, no or small residual defect, and no PH	All sports (3–6 mo after closure)
	Symptomatic arrhythmias, or second- or third-degree AV block	See Table 34–6 recommendations
	Persistent severe PH	No competitive sports
PDA	Small PDA	All competitive sports
	Moderate to large PDA requires surgery.	All competitive sports, 3–6 mo after surgical repair
	Moderate or large PDA with severe PH and cyanosis	No competitive sports
PDA, closed	Asymptomatic, with no PH and no LV enlargement	All sports (after 3 mo)
	Residual PH	Class IA or no competitive sports
PS, untreated	Mild PS (peak Doppler gradient <40 mm Hg) and normal RV function	All competitive sports (annual reevaluation needed)
	Moderate PS (peak Doppler gradient 40–60 mm Hg) and severe PS (peak gradient >60 mm Hg)	Classes IA and IB until balloon valvuloplasty is performed
PS, treated	No or mild residual PS and normal ventricular function	All competitive sports (2–4 wk after balloon or 3 mo after surgery)
	Residual Doppler gradient >40 mm Hg	Classes IA and IB
	Severe PR with marked RV enlargement	Classes IA and IB
AS, untreated	Mild AS (peak Doppler gradient <40 mm Hg), with normal ECG, normal EST, no symptoms, and no symptomatic arrhythmias	All competitive sports
	Moderate AS (peak Doppler gradient 40–70 mm Hg), asymptomatic, with mild or no LVH (echo); no strain pattern on ECG; normal EST	Classes IA, IB, and IIA
	Moderate AS with SVT or multiple or complex ventricular arrhythmias at rest or with exercise	Classes IA and IB
	Severe AS (peak Doppler gradient >70 mm Hg)	No competitive sports
AS, treated by surgery or balloon	Residual mild, moderate or severe AS	Same as untreated AS
	Moderate to severe AR following procedure	See Table 34–4 recommendations
COA, untreated	Mild COA (no aortic root dilatation, normal EST, arm to leg SP gradient at rest <20 mm Hg, and arm SP <230 mm Hg with exercise)	All competitive sports
	Arm to leg SP gradient >20 mm Hg, or exercise-induced hypertension with arm SP >230 mm Hg	Only class IA until treated
COA, treated by surgery or balloon	Arm to leg SP gradient <20 mm Hg at rest and normal arm SP during rest and exercise	All competitive sports 3 mo after repair
	Significant aortic dilatation, wall thinning, or aneurysm formation	Classes IA and IB

AR, aortic regurgitation; AS, aortic (valve) stenosis; ASD, atrial septal defect; AV, atrioventricular; COA, coarctation of the aorta; EST, exercise stress test; LV, left ventricle; MR, mitral regurgitation; PA, pulmonary artery; PDA, patent ductus arteriosus; PH, pulmonary hypertension; PR, pulmonary regurgitation; PS, pulmonary (valve) stenosis; RV, right ventricle; SP, systolic pressure; SVT, supraventricular arrhythmia; VSD, ventricular septal defect.

Adapted from Graham TP, Driscoll DJ, Gerosny WM, et al: 36th Bethesda Conference: Eligibility recommendations for competitive athletes with cardiovascular abnormalities. Task Force 2: Congenital heart disease. J Am Coll Cardiol 45:1326–1333, 2005.

3. Patients who have received an excellent result from the surgical repair of tetralogy of Fallot or arterial switch operation for transposition of the great arteries may participate in all competitive sports.

Detailed recommendations are provided for specific cyanotic heart defects in Table 34–2.

Table 34–2. **Participation Recommendations for Cyanotic Congenital Heart Defects**

Heart Defects	Clinical Status	Can Participate in:
Cyanotic CHD, unoperated	Untreated cyanotic CHDs, in general	Class IA sport
Cyanotic CHDs, palliated	Palliated patients with the following criteria: Arterial O_2 saturation >80%, No history of syncope or presyncope from tachyarrhythmias, and Absence of moderate or severe ventricular dysfunction (EF < 40%)	Class IA sports
TOF, postoperative	Excellent repair with the following findings: Normal or near-normal RV pressure No or only mild RV volume overload No significant residual shunt No atrial or ventricular tachyarrhythmias on ambulatory ECG or exercise testing	All competitive sports
	Residual problems with the following findings. Marked PR and RV volume overload, Residual RV hypertension (RV SP ≥ 50% systemic pressure), or Atrial or ventricular tachyarrhythmias	Class IA sports
TGA, post–atrial repair surgery (Senning)	Athletes with the following findings: Mild or no cardiac chamber enlargement on CXR No history of atrial flutter, SVT, or ventricular tachyarrhythmias Normal EST (normal duration, workload, heart rate, ECG, and BP response)	Classes IA and IIA sports
	Athletes not in the above category	Individualized exercise prescription
TGA, post–arterial switch operation	Athletes with normal ventricular function, normal EST, no atrial or ventricular tachyarrhythmias	All competitive sports
	Athletes with more than mild hemodynamic abnormalities or ventricular dysfunction, but with normal EST	Classes IA, IB, IC, and IIA sports
Congenitally corrected TGA	Asymptomatic patients without other cardiac abnormalities with the following findings. No systemic ventricular enlargement, No atrial or ventricular tachyarrhythmias on ambulatory ECG or exercise testing, or Normal EST	Classes IA and IIA sports
	Periodic reevaluation is required to detect arrhythmias or systemic ventricular dysfunction and systemic AV valve regurgitation	Not allowed in classes IIIA, IIIB, and IIIC, or power weightlifting
Fontan operation, postoperative	Post-Fontan patients	Class IA sports
	Post-Fontan patients with normal ventricular function and O_2 saturation	Class IB sports
Ebstein's anomaly	Mild Ebstein's anomaly (with no cyanosis, normal RV size, no atrial or ventricular arrhythmias)	All competitive sports
	Moderate TR, but no arrhythmia on Holter ECG other than isolated premature contractions	Class IA sports
	Severe Ebstein's anomaly	No competitive sports
Ebstein's postoperative	Mild or no TR, with No cardiac chamber enlargement No symptomatic atrial or ventricular arrhythmias	Class I sports
	Excellent hemodynamics after repair	May be permitted additional participation

AV, atrioventricular; BP, blood pressure; CHD, congenital heart defects; CXR, chest x-ray; ECG, electrocardiogram; EF, ejection fraction; EST, exercise stress test; LV, left ventricle; PR, pulmonary regurgitation; RV, right ventricle; SP, systolic pressure; SVT, supraventricular tachycardia; TGA, transposition of the great arteries; TR, tricuspid regurgitation; TOF, tetralogy of Fallot; VSD, ventricular septal defect.

Adapted from Graham TP, Driscoll DJ, Gerosny WM, et al: 36th Bethesda Conference: Eligibility recommendations for competitive athletes with cardiovascular abnormalities. Task Force 2: Congenital heart disease. J Am Coll Cardiol 45:1326–1333, 2005.

CORONARY ARTERY ABNORMALITIES

For most patients with congenital abnormalities of the coronary arteries or following Kawasaki disease, moderate to severe restriction in sports participation is recommended. Children who had no coronary artery involvement during the acute phase of Kawasaki disease may participate in all sports 6 to 8 weeks after the illness. Stress testing is often required before prescribing participation eligibility. Detailed participation recommendations for specific conditions with coronary artery abnormalities are presented in Table 34–3.

VALVULAR HEART DISEASES

The severity of the valvular lesion determines eligibility for participation in competitive sports.

1. With mild valvular lesions (such as mitral stenosis, mitral regurgitation, aortic stenosis, and aortic regurgitation), participation in all competitive sports is allowed.
2. With moderate valvular lesions, participation is limited to low- to moderate-intensity sports.
3. With severe obstructive lesions such as aortic stenosis, participation in competitive sports is not permitted.
4. With valvular lesions that produce significant pulmonary hypertension, no participation in competitive sports is permitted.
5. For patients with prosthetic valves and taking warfarin, no sport involving the risk of bodily contact is allowed.

Detailed participation recommendations for specific valvular heart diseases are presented in Table 34–4.

Table 34–3. **Participation Recommendations for Coronary Anomalies**

Heart Condition	Clinical Status	Can Participate in:
Congenital CA anomalies	Presurgery: CA arising from wrong sinus, passing between great arteries	Exclusion from all competitive sports
	Postsurgery: without ischemia, ventricular dysfunction, or arrhythmias during maximal EST	All competitive sports, 3 mo after successful surgery
Kawasaki disease	No CA abnormalities or transient CA ectasia resolving during the convalescent phase	All competitive sports (after 6–8 wk)
	Regressed aneurysm, with no evidence of exercise-induced ischemia by EST with myocardial perfusion scan	All competitive sports
	Isolated small to medium-sized aneurysm in one or more CAs (but with normal LV function, no exercise-induced ischemia or arrhythmia)	Classes IA, IB, IIA, and IIB sports (EST every 1–2 yr)
	One or more large CA aneurysms or multiple or complex aneurysm, with or without obstruction to coronary blood flow, with normal LV function, and no exercise-induced arrhythmias	Classes IA and IIA sports
	Recent MI or revascularization.	No competitive sports for 6–8 wk
	1. Those with normal LV function and EST, no reversible ischemia on myocardial perfusion scan, no exercise-induced arrhythmia	1. Classes IA and IB sports
	2. Those with LV EF < 40%, exercise intolerance, or exercise-induced ventricular arrhythmia	2. No competitive sports
	Patients with CA lesions and taking warfarin and/or aspirin	No competitive sports

CA, coronary artery; EF, ejection fraction; EST, exercise stress test; LV, left ventricle; MI, myocardial infarction.
Adapted from Graham TP, Driscoll DJ, Gerosny WM, et al: 36th Bethesda Conference: Eligibility recommendations for competitive athletes with cardiovascular abnormalities. Task Force 2: Congenital heart disease. J Am Coll Cardiol 45:1326–1333, 2005.

CARDIOMYOPATHY, PERICARDITIS, AND OTHER MYOCARDIAL DISEASES

Detailed participation recommendations for specific disorders of the myocardium and pericardium and other related cardiovascular diseases are presented in Table 34–5.

1. Athletes who have either a confirmed or probable diagnosis of HCM or ARVD are excluded from most competitive sports, with the possible exception of class IA sports.

2. Athletes with myocarditis or pericarditis of any etiology should be excluded from all competitive sports during the acute phase. After complete recovery from these illnesses, they may gradually participate in sports.

3. Athletes with Marfan syndrome can participate only in class IA or IB sports.

*Table 34–4. **Participation Recommendations for Valvular Heart Disease***

Heart Condition	Clinical Status	Can Participate in:
Mitral stenosis (MS)	Mild MS (valve area >1.5 cm^2; rest PA SP ≤20 mm Hg)	All competitive sports
	Moderate MS (valve area 1.0–1.5 cm^2; rest PA SP ≤50 mm Hg)	Classes IA, IB, IIA, and IIB sports
	Severe MS (valve area <1.0 cm^2; rest PA SP >50 mm Hg)	No participation in any competitive sports
	MS of any severity with AF or history of AF (with anticoagulation)	No participation in any competitive sports
Mitral regurgitation (MR)	Mild to moderate MR with sinus rhythm, normal LV size and function, and normal PA pressure	All competitive sports
	Mild to moderate MR with sinus rhythm, normal LV systolic function, and mild LV enlargement (<60 mm)	Classes IA, IB, IC, IIA, IIB, and IIC sports
	Severe MR + definite LV enlargement (≥60 mm), PH, or any degree of LV systolic dysfunction at rest	No participation in any competitive sports
	Patients in AF or history of AF, receiving anticoagulation	No participation in any competitive sports
Aortic stenosis (AS)	Mild AS (mean gradient <25 mm Hg)	All competitive sports
	Moderate AS (mean gradient 25–40 mm Hg) with abnormalities in any of the above categories	Class IA sports
	Moderate AS with EST performed to the level comparable to a competitive sport with no symptoms, ST depression or ventricular arrhythmias, and normal BP response	Classes IA, IB, and IIA sports
	Severe AS (mean gradient >40 mm Hg) or symptomatic patients	No participation in any competitive sports
Aortic regurgitation (AR)	Mild or moderate AR (with slight or no LVE)	All competitive sports
	Mild to moderate AR (with moderate LVE) but with good EST to the level of that sport with no symptom or ventricular arrhythmia	Classes IA, IB, IC, IIA, IIB, and IIC sports
	Mild to moderate AR with asymptomatic nonsustained ventricular tachycardia	Class IA sports
	Severe AR and LVE (>65 mm) or those with mild to moderate AR and symptoms	No participation in any competitive sports
	AR and significant dilatation of the proximal ascending aorta (>45 mm) who are not Marfan patients	Only in class IA sports
Bicuspid aortic valve (BAV)	No aortic root dilatation and no significant AS or AR	All competitive sports
	BAV with dilated aortic root (40–45 mm)	Classes IA, IB, IIA, and IIB sports
	BAV with dilated aortic root (>45 mm)	Class IA sports only
Prosthetic heart valves	Bioprosthetic *mitral* valve, not taking warfarin, and with normal valve function and normal or near-normal LV function	Classes IA, IB, IIA, and IIB sports
	Mechanical or bioprosthetic *aortic* valve, with normal valve function and normal LV function	Classes IA, IB, and IIA sports
	Those with prosthetic aortic or mitral valve taking warfarin	No sports involving the risk of bodily contact.

AF, atrial fibrillation; AS, aortic stenosis; AR, aortic regurgitation; BAV, bicuspid aortic valve; LV, left ventricle or ventricular; LVE, left ventricular enlargement; MR, mitral regurgitation; MS, mitral stenosis; PA, pulmonary artery; PH, pulmonary hypertension; SP, systolic pressure.

Bonow RO, Cheitlin MD: Bethesda Conference Report. Task Force 3: Valvular heart disease. J Am Coll Cardiol 45: 1334–1340.

Table 34–5. **Participation Recommendations for Cardiomyopathy, Pericarditis, and Other Select Cardiovascular Diseases**

Heart Condition	Clinical Status	Can Participate in:
Hypertrophic cardiomyopathy (HCM)	Probable or definite diagnosis of HCM (regardless of age, gender, symptoms, LVOT obstruction, prior drug treatment or ICD)	No participation in most competitive sports, with the possible exception of class IA sports
Arrhythmogenic RV dysplasia	Diagnosis of arrhythmogenic RV dysplasia	No competitive sports, with possible exception of class IA sports
Myocarditis	Probable or definite myocarditis	No participation in competitive sports
	When the following occurs: Normal LV function No arrhythmias on ambulatory ECG No serum markers of inflammation and heart failure Normal 12-lead ECG	May return to training or competition
Pericarditis	Pericarditis, regardless of etiology	No competitive sports during the acute phase
Mitral valve prolapse (MVP)	Athletes with MVP without any of the following features: Prior syncope, judged to be due to arrhythmia Sustained or nonsustained SVT and/or complex VT on ambulatory ECG Severe MR LV systolic dysfunction (EF < 50%) Prior embolic event FH of MVP-related sudden death	All competitive sports
	Athletes with MVP with any of the aforementioned features	Class IA sports only
Marfan syndrome	If patients with Marfan syndrome do not have the following: Aortic root dilatation (≥2 SD from mean in children; ≥40 mm in adults) Moderate to severe MR FH of dissection or sudden death	Classes IA and IIA sports. (Repeat echo every 6 mo to measure aortic root dimension)
	Athletes with aortic root dilatation (≥ 40 mm), prior aortic root reconstruction, moderate to severe MR, FH of dissection or sudden death	Class IA sports only
Ehlers-Danlos syndrome	Diagnosis of Ehlers-Danlos syndrome	No competitive sports
Myocardial bridging	Myocardial bridging without evidence of myocardial ischemia at rest or during exercise	All competitive sports
	Myocardial bridging with objective evidence of myocardial ischemia or prior MI.	Class IA sports only
	Asymptomatic athletes who had surgical resection or stenting for myocardial bridging and normal EST 6 mo after the procedure.	All competitive sports

EF, ejection fraction; EST, exercise stress testing; FH, family history; HCM, hypertrophic cardiomyopathy; ICD, implantable cardioverter-defibrillator; LV, left ventricle; LVOT, left ventricular outflow tract; MI, myocardial infarction; MR, mitral regurgitation; MVP, mitral valve prolapse; RV, right ventricle; SD, standard deviation; SVT, supraventricular tachycardia; VT, ventricular tachycardia.
Adapted from Maron BJ, Ackerman MJ, Towbin JA: Bethesda Conference Report. Task Force 4: HCM and other cardiomyopathies, mitral valve prolapse, myocarditis, and Marfan syndrome. J Am Coll Cardiol 45:1340–1345, 2005.

4. Athletes with mitral valve prolapse who have any symptoms or abnormalities in ECG, LV function, or arrhythmias are permitted to participate only in low-intensity sports.

5. Athletes with myocardial bridging without ischemia at rest and during exercise may participate in all sports.

Cardiac Arrhythmias and Sports

Although sudden unexpected death in the young athlete is rare, a significant portion of these deaths occur in relation to exercise and are probably related to cardiac arrhythmias.

Cardiac arrhythmias occurring while playing sports, however, manifest more often with syncope or near syncope than sudden death. A cardiac arrhythmia should be considered a possible cause of syncope, particularly when it occurs during or immediately after exercise, and a thorough evaluation is required. Although syncope may signal the presence of a serious cardiac problem, it may also be due to a benign mechanism such as vasovagal syncope, which is a common finding in highly trained athletes. However, the diagnosis of such a benign mechanism should not be made without first excluding underlying structural disease or electrical disorders (see Chapter 31).

Arrhythmias may be associated with a variety of structural heart diseases. In the absence of identifiable structural abnormalities of the heart, they may be due to primary electrical disorders, such as a supraventricular tachycardia (SVT) associated with WPW preexcitation or ventricular tachycardia secondary to long QT syndrome. A number of stimulant-containing drinks that are popular among young athletes can trigger certain arrhythmias. Abuse with drugs such as cocaine or ephedra can precipitate life-threatening arrhythmias.

Young athletes with an arrhythmia who are permitted to engage in athletics should be reevaluated at 6- to 12-month intervals to determine whether the training process affected the arrhythmia. Follow-up evaluation should be done to check on compliance with antiarrhythmic drugs. Use of certain drugs, such as β-adrenergic blocking agents, is banned in some competitive sports, such as archery and riflery, in which athletes benefit from slow heart rates.

DIAGNOSTIC WORK-UP

In general, all athletes with possible cardiac arrhythmias being considered for athletic activity should have a careful history and cardiac examination, a 12-lead ECG, and an echocardiogram. In most cases, a 24-hour Holter ambulatory ECG recording and exercise stress testing are also indicated.

History. The screening questionnaires recommended by the American Heart Association (see Box 34–2) are useful starting points in eligibility evaluation. However, review of an athlete's medical history and careful cardiac examination are often negative. The following are some important aspects of the history that should prompt one to consider the possibility of arrhythmia in an athlete.

History of syncope, near syncope, dizziness or lightheadedness, seizures, palpitation, chest pain, or pallor

History of known heart disease (congenital or acquired) and medications or surgery for it

Family history of arrhythmias or sudden death

Certain medications or drugs of abuse (e.g., tricyclic antidepressant, inhalants, or cocaine)

Physical Examination. Physical examination may reveal irregularity of heart rate, but a regular heart rate on examination does not rule our arrhythmias.

Recording of Electrocardiogram. All athletes with history suggestive of significant cardiac arrhythmias should have a 12-lead ECG, echocardiogram, exercise stress test, and a 24-hour Holter ambulatory ECG recording, if possible during the specific type of exercise being considered. A normal ambulatory ECG monitor does not provide absolute safety or absence of arrhythmias because arrhythmias are commonly evanescent, often disappearing unpredictably for long periods of time in some cases, and the athlete may not develop the arrhythmia during each sporting event.

Although most high school and college athletes are not fully trained athletes, it is important to understand the range of normal heart rate and rhythm for the trained athlete recorded on 24-hour Holter ECG recordings.

1. Heart rates of 25 beats/minute and sinus pauses greater than 2 seconds may be found.

2. Mobitz type I second-degree atrioventricular (AV) block and single uniform PVCs may each occur in about 40% of trained athletes.

3. Complex ventricular arrhythmias (multiform PVCs, couplets, nonsustained ventricular tachycardia) are rare.

Detailed participation recommendations are provided in Table 34–6 for arrhythmias and in Table 34–7 for AV and intraventricular blocks, based on the 36th Bethesda Conference (Zipes et al, 2005). The following are general statements regarding participation eligibility for athletes with cardiac arrhythmias and conduction disturbances.

1. The presence of a symptomatic cardiac arrhythmia requires exclusion from physical activity until this problem can be adequately evaluated and controlled by a cardiologist.

Table 34–6. **Eligibility Recommendations for Athletes with Cardiac Arrhythmias**

Arrhythmias	Clinical Situation	Can Participate in:
Sinus node dysfunction	Bradycardia, structurally normal heart, and appropriate increase in HR by physical activity	All competitive sports
	Bradycardia, structural HD, and appropriate increase in HR by physical activity	Limitation determined by the nature of the structural HD
	Symptomatic bradycardia (syncope or near syncope)	No sports until the cause has been determined and treated, and asymptomatic
	Tachycardia/bradycardia syndrome, with no structural HD—should be treated	All competitive sports (when asymptomatic for 2–3 mo after successful treatment)
	Athlete with pacemaker	No sports with danger of bodily collision. Protective padding for soccer, basketball, baseball, softball, etc
Premature atrial contraction (PAC)	Asymptomatic PACs, structurally normal heart	All competitive sports
Atrial flutter	Atrial flutter, normal heart, appropriate ventricular rate response during exercise (receiving no therapy or AV nodal blocking agents)	Class IA sports only Full participation allowed only when no recurrence after 2–3 mo of treatment. (note that β-blockers are prohibited in some sports)
	Atrial flutter, structural HD, no recurrence for 2–4 wk	Class IA sports
	Atrial flutter, normal heart, postablation with no recurrence for 2–4 wk	All competitive sports
	Atrial flutter, on anticoagulation	No sports with danger of bodily collision
Atrial fibrillation (AF)	Asymptomatic AF, normal heart, appropriate ventricular rate response during exercise (receiving no therapy or AV nodal blocking agents)	All competitive sports (note that β-blockers are prohibited in some sports)
	AF, structural HD (receiving no therapy or AV nodal blocking agents)	Sports consistent with the limitation of the structural heart disease
	AF in normal heart, postablation with no recurrence for 4–6 wk (or EPS confirmed success)	All competitive sports
	AF on anticoagulation	No sports with danger of bodily collision
AV junctional escape beats/ rhythm	Usually associated with sinus node dysfunction	The same as those for sinus node dysfunction
Premature AV junctional complexes	Structurally normal heart, normal HR response without sustained tachycardia	All competitive sports
AV junctional tachycardia (AVJT)	Asymptomatic AVJT, normal heart, appropriate ventricular rate response during activity (with or without therapy)	All competitive sports
	Asymptomatic AVJT, structural HD or incompletely controlled ventricular rate	Class IA sports
	Inappropriately rapid ventricular rate, successful treatment to control ventricular rate, with or without HD	With normal heart—class IA sports Structural HD—limitation consistent with the structural heart disease

Table 34–6. **Eligibility Recommendations for Athletes with Cardiac Arrhythmias** *(Continued)*

Arrhythmias	Clinical Situation	Can Participate in:
Supraventricular tachycardia (SVT)	Asymptomatic patients with normal hearts, whose reproducible exercise-induced SVT has been successfully treated and verified by appropriate testing	All competitive sports
	Patients with sporadic recurrences of SVT (but without exercise-induced SVT), after successful treatment to prevent recurrence	All competitive sports
	Asymptomatic, episodes of SVT lasting <5–15 sec, no worsening with exercise	All competitive sports
	Syncope, near syncope, or significant symptoms, structural HD	Class IA sports, only after adequate treatment for 2–4 wk
	Normal heart, successful catheter or surgical ablation, with no recurrence for 2–4 wk (or EPS confirmed success)	All competitive sports
WPW syndrome	Young adults (20–25 year old), normal heart, no history of palpitation or tachycardia	All competitive sports
	Younger patients, normal heart, no history of palpitation or tachycardia	In-depth evaluation before allowing competitive sports
	Episodes of reciprocating SVT with the shortest cycle length <250 ms—should undergo ablation	All competitive sports after successful ablation
	Episodes of AF/flutter (with rate >240 bpm), syncope or near syncope—should receive catheter ablation	All competitive sports after successful ablation
	Normal heart, successful catheter or surgical ablation, asymptomatic	All competitive sports (in several days if normal EPS study or in 2–4 wk without recurrence of SVT)
Premature ventricular complexes (PVCs)	Normal heart, asymptomatic PVCs at rest and during exercise, normal exercise test	All competitive sports
	Normal heart, PVCs increasing in frequency or becoming symptomatic during exercise (near syncope, significant fatigue or dyspnea)	Class IA sports only
	Structural HD, PVCs (with or without treatment)	Class IA sports only
Ventricular tachycardia (VT)	Normal heart, monomorphic nonsustained or sustained VT with a specific site of origin should receive catheter ablation	All competitive sports after successful ablation
	Normal heart, monomorphic VT, treated with drugs, VT not inducible by exercise, EST or EPS	All competitive sports
	VT with structural HD, regardless of whether VT is suppressed or ablated	Class IA sports only
	Normal heart, asymptomatic, brief episodes of VT (<8–10 consecutive monomorphic VT) with VT rate <150 bpm, suppression or no worsening of VT during EST compared with the baseline	All competitive sports
	ICD implantation (Athlete's desire to continue sports is not an indication for ICD implantation)	Class IA sports only
Ventricular flutter and VT	Generally requires ICD implantation	Class IA sports, only after no episodes for more than 6 mo
Long QT syndrome (LQTS)	Patients with history of cardiac arrest or LQTS-precipitated syncopal episode, regardless of QTc or genotype	Class IA sports only
	Asymptomatic patients with baseline QTc ≥470 ms in males, ≥480 ms in females	Class IA sports only
	Patients with ICD/pacemaker	Class IA sports only

AF, atrial fibrillation; AVJT, atrioventricular junctional tachycardia; bpm; beats/min; EPS, electrophysiologic study; EST, exercise stress test; HD, heart disease; HR, heart rate; ICD, implantable cardioverter-defibrillator; LQTS, long QT syndrome; VT, ventricular tachycardia; WPW, Wolff-Parkinson-White.

Adapted from Zipes DP, Ackerman MJ, Estes MAM, et al: Task Force 7: Arrhythmias, 36th Bethesda Conference: Eligibility recommendations for competitive athletes with cardiovascular abnormalities. J Am Coll Cardiol 45:1354–1363, 2005.

2. Sinus arrhythmias and premature atrial contractions are benign if the heart is structurally normal; participation in all competitive sports is allowed.

3. Asymptomatic athletes with atrial flutter or fibrillation and a structurally normal heart may participate in competitive sports when the arrhythmias are fully under control by either medication or ablation.

*Table 34–7. **Eligibility Recommendations for Athletes with Atrioventricular or Intraventricular Block***

Type of AV Block	Clinical Situation	Can Participate in:
First-degree AV block	Normal heart, first-degree AV block that does not worsen with exercise	All competitive sports
Second-degree AV block, Mobitz type I (Wenckebach)	Normal heart, type 1 AV block that does not worsen with exercise	All competitive sports
	Structural HD, type 1 AV block that does not worsen with exercise	As determined by the limitation of the cardiac abnormality
	Structural HD, type 1 AV block that worsens during or after exercise	Further evaluation (may require pacemaker)
	Athletes with pacemaker	No sports with danger of bodily collision
Second-degree AV block, Mobitz type II	The same as in acquired complete heart block—should receive pacemaker	Permanent pacing before any athletic activity
Congenital complete heart block	Normal heart, normal ventricular function, no syncope or near syncope; narrow QRS complex; ventricular rate > 40–50 bpm; HR increasing appropriately with exercise	All competitive sports
	Ventricular arrhythmia, symptoms of fatigue, syncope or near syncope: should receive pacemaker	No sports with danger of bodily collision
		Sports category to be determined after EST
	Structural HD (such as shunt lesions) should receive pacemaker	No sports with danger of bodily collision
		Sports category to be determined after EST
Acquired complete heart block	Should receive pacemaker	No sports with danger of bodily collision
Complete RBBB	Asymptomatic, no ventricular arrhythmias, who do not develop AV block with exercise	All competitive sports
Complete LBBB	Adult athletes with acquired LBBB follow the same recommendations as RBBB	
	Normal HV interval and normal AV conduction response to pacing	All competitive sports categories consistent with their cardiac status
	Abnormal AV conduction with HV interval >90 ms or His-Purkinje block should have pacemaker	No sports with danger of bodily collision
		Sports category consistent with their cardiac status

AF, atrial fibrillation; AV, atrioventricular; bpm; beats/min; EPS, electrophysiologic study; HD, heart disease; HR, heart rate; LBBB, left bundle branch block; PVC, premature ventricular contraction; RBBB, right bundle branch block; VT, ventricular tachycardia; WPW, Wolff-Parkinson-White.

Adapted from Zipes DP, Ackerman MJ, Estes MAM, et al: Task Force 7: Arrhythmias, 36th Bethesda Conference: Eligibility recommendations for competitive athletes with cardiovascular abnormalities. J Am Coll Cardiol 45:1354–1363, 2005.

4. Athletes with SVT and a structurally normal heart may participate in all competitive sports when the SVT is in full control with medication or following successful ablation.

5. For athletes with a structurally normal heart who have PVCs or more complex arrhythmias, an exercise stress test is a useful technique. If the PVCs disappear when the heart rate reaches 140 to 150 beats/minute, the PVCs are benign and full participation may be permitted.

6. Athletes with ventricular tachycardia (VT) who had successful treatment to prevent recurrence of the arrhythmias may participate in sports provided that VT is not inducible by exercise stress test or electrophysiologic study.

7. Asymptomatic adult athletes with WPW preexcitation with no history of SVT may participate in all competitive sports, but children with the same diagnosis require in-depth evaluation.

8. Athletes with long QT syndrome can participate only in class IA sports.

9. Athletes who had a successful ablation for any of the arrhythmias may participate in all competitive sports after verification of the success by appropriate tests.

10. Athletes with structural heart disease and an arrhythmia can participate in sports within the limits determined by the structural defect, usually class IA sports.

11. Athletes who have a pacemaker implanted and those who are receiving antico-agulation (usually for atrial flutter or fibrillation) should not be permitted to engage in activities with danger of bodily collision. Participation in class IA sports is usually permitted.

12. Athletes with first-degree AV block or Mobitz type I second-degree AV block can participate in all sports provided the block does not worsen with exercise.

13. Athletes with Mobitz type II second-degree AV block or complete heart block usually require pacemaker implantation before being permitted to participate in any sports (with participation permitted only in sports without danger of bodily collision).

14. Asymptomatic athletes with RBBB or LBBB who do not have ventricular arrhyth-mias or develop AV block during exercise can participate in all sports. However, patients with LBBB who have an abnormal prolongation of the HV interval on electrophysiologic study should receive a pacemaker.

Athletes with Systemic Hypertension

Reports of cerebrovascular accident during maximal exercise have raised concerns that the rise in BP accompanying strenuous activity may cause harm. However, changes in BP depend on the type of exercise the athlete is engaged in. For example:

1. Dynamic exercise causes a substantial increase in cardiac output, heart rate, stroke volume, and systolic pressure. A moderate increase in mean arterial pressure and a decrease in diastolic pressure occur, with a marked decrease in total peripheral resistance.

2. Static exercise, in contrast, causes a small increase in cardiac output and heart rate and no change in stroke volume. There is a marked increase in systolic, diastolic, and mean arterial pressures and no appreciable change in total peripheral resistance.

Hypertension is classified as the following (as discussed in Chapter 28):

1. Prehypertension is classified as BP levels 120–139/80–89 mm Hg in adults and BP values between the 90th and 95th percentiles for children.

2. Stage 1 hypertension is classified as BP levels 140–159/90–99 mm Hg in adults and BP values between the 95th and 99th percentiles for children.

3. Stage 2 hypertension is classified as BP levels above 160/100 mm Hg in adults and BP values ≥5 mm Hg above the 99th percentile values for children. In athletes older than 18 years, the adult definition of hypertension can be used.

On each occasion, two or more BP readings should be taken, and when the readings vary by more than 5 mm Hg, additional readings should be taken until two consecutive readings are close. Initially high BP (>140/90 mm Hg) should have out-of-office measurement obtained to exclude "white-coat" hyper-tension. When categorizing BP elevation, if systolic and diastolic pressures fall into different categories, the higher category should be selected to classify the patient's BP status. The diagnosis of hypertension should be made only after several elevated BP values are obtained on separate occasions. When the diagnosis of hypertension is confirmed, an evaluation including a history, thorough physical examination, and appropriate laboratory testing should be performed (see Chapter 28).

Task Force 5: Systemic hypertension of the 36th Bethesda Conference has recommended the following (Kaplan et al, 2005).

1. Athletes with prehypertension:
   a. May participate in physical activity but should be encouraged to modify lifestyle.
   b. If prehypertension persists, echo studies are done to see if there is left ventricular hypertrophy (LVH) (beyond that seen with "athletes' heart").
   c. If LVH is present, athletic participation is limited until BP is normalized by appropriate drug therapy.

2. Athletes with stage 1 hypertension:
   a. May participate in any competitive sports, in the absence of target organ damage, including LVH or concomitant heart disease. However, hypertension should be checked every 2 to 4 months (or more frequently) to monitor the impact of exercise.
   b. If LVH is present, athletic participation is limited until BP is normalized by appropriate drug therapy.

3. Athletes with stage 2 (severe) hypertension: Even in the absence of target organ damage (such as LVH), athletic participation should be restricted, particularly from high static sports (class IIIA, IIIB, and IIIC), until the hypertension is controlled by either lifestyle modification or drug therapy.

All drugs being taken must be registered with appropriate governing bodies to obtain a therapeutic exemption. When hypertension coexists with another cardiovascular disease, eligibility for participation in competitive sports is usually based on the type and severity of the associated condition.

With respect to the treatment of hypertension, β-blockers are not banned for most sports, including football and basketball, whereas β-blockers are banned for riflery or archery. However, athletes with essential hypertension do not tolerate the drugs well because they reduce their maximum performance. One should, therefore, avoid treating hypertensive athletes with β-blockers. Instead, angiotensin-converting enzyme (ACE) inhibitors are preferred. However, one should be aware of potential teratogenic effects of ACE inhibitors if taken during pregnancy. Calcium channel blockers may also be used instead of β-blockers in treating hypertension.

Chapter 35

Cardiac Transplantation

Lower and Shumway at Stanford University performed the first successful orthotopic heart transplantation in a dog in 1960. Barnard in South Africa unexpectedly performed the first successful human heart transplantation in 1966. This was followed by an explosive interest in heart transplantation but almost uniformly poor results because of organ rejection. Introduction of cyclosporine in 1980 markedly improved the results of adult heart transplantation. This success has extended to pediatric patients, and the first infant cardiac transplantation was carried out by Bailey at Loma Linda University in 1985. Cardiac transplantation is considered standard therapy for children with selected complex congenital heart defects in some centers and those with certain end-stage heart diseases in many cardiac centers. Although many ethical and medical issues exist, cardiac transplantation will find steady applications and contribute substantially to the treatment of children with some heart diseases.

Pediatricians will have an increasing chance to participate in the care of cardiac transplant recipients. Therefore, practitioners should have some basic knowledge on the topic, and that is the aim of this chapter. Although rapid advances are being made in this field, especially with immunosuppression, it is not the aim of this chapter to review the advances. This chapter describes the steps involved in donor and recipient selection, postoperative management, immunosuppressive therapy, long-term complications, and prognosis. Cardiac transplantation should be done only by transplantation centers with a multidisciplinary team of professionals and supporting staff including social workers.

Indications

The majority of pediatric transplant patients are those with pre- and postoperative complex congenital heart defects and those with cardiomyopathies. In infants younger than 12 months, which accounts for about 23% of pediatric cardiac transplantation, hypoplastic left heart syndrome (HLHS) is the most common indication, followed by dilated cardiomyopathy. In children, cardiomyopathies (dilated and restrictive) account for about 60% of the cases. Most of the other indications for the transplant were patients who had surgical repairs for complex congenital heart defects (such as single ventricle, atrioventricular canal defect, truncus arteriosus, L-TGA). Rarely, patients with unresectable cardiac tumor are candidates for the transplantation.

Selection of the Recipient

Careful selection of appropriate recipients remains the most important determinant of a favorable outcome. Multidisciplinary evaluation of the recipient includes assessment of cardiopulmonary, renal, hepatic, neurologic, and infectious disease status and socioeconomic assessment. Cardiopulmonary evaluation includes physical examination, ECG, Holter monitoring, echocardiography, and usually cardiac catheterization (with exception of infants with HLHS). In general, the recipient should satisfy the following selection criteria:

1. Terminal heart disease with death expected within 6 to 12 months.

2. The presence of adequate dimension of hilar pulmonary arteries (if the pulmonary vascular resistance [PVR] is high or if severe hypoplasia or stenosis of the pulmonary arteries is present, the patient may be a candidate for heart and lung transplantation).

3. Other general requirements:
   a. Normal function or reversible dysfunction of the kidneys and liver.
   b. Lack of systemic infection.
   c. Malignancy under complete remission for longer than 1 year.
   d. Lack of systemic disease (such as diabetes and degenerative neuromuscular disease) that would limit recovery or survival.
   e. Lack of drug addiction.
   f. Lack of mental deficiency.

4. Equally important for successful pediatric heart transplantation are a family history of stability, past history of compliance, and evidence of strong motivation for the transplant as assessed by physicians and social workers. The child and parents should demonstrate sufficient responsibility, resources, and psychological strength to cope with multiple outpatient clinic visits, routine endomyocardial biopsy, and a lifetime of vigilance in the immunosuppressed state. Unique to pediatric transplantation is the requirement of a reliable caregiver for the recipient child. The caregiver identified need not be a parent but must have legal responsibility for total care and be prepared to deal with the strict medical regimen required.

Cardiac transplantation is contraindicated:

1. If PVR ≥ 6 Wood units/m^2 and/or

2. Transpulmonary gradient (TPG = PA pressure − PA wedge pressure) is ≥ 15 mm Hg, which does not respond to vasodilators.

Following the decision for heart transplantation and complete multidisciplinary evaluation, the patient is placed on the cardiac transplantation waiting list (to the United Network of Organ Sharing [UNOS] and the Regional Organ Bank). Each listing is specific for ABO blood type and the recipient's weight.

Evaluation and Management of the Cardiac Donor

1. The cardiac donor must meet the legal definition of *brain death*. Most neonatal donors were victims of sudden infant death syndrome or birth asphyxia. Most older children donors were victims of car accident or violence.

2. The screening of the donor is accomplished in three phases:
   a. *Primary screening is* done by organ procurement specialists to obtain information on body size, ABO blood type, serologic data on hepatitis B and human immunodeficiency virus (HIV), cause of death, clinical course, and routine laboratory data.
   b. *Secondary screening is* performed by cardiac surgeons or cardiologists, who pay attention to the extent of other (especially thoracic) injuries, the extent of treatment required to sustain acceptable hemodynamic status, ECG, chest x-ray films, arterial blood gas analysis, and echocardiogram.
   c. *Tertiary screening is* inspection of the heart by a "harvesting" surgeon to ensure that there is no evidence of a palpable thrill over the heart and great arteries, obvious arteriosclerotic heart disease, or myocardial contusion.

3. The donor heart should have:
   a. No evidence of cardiac abnormalities by echo, ECG, or myocardial enzyme tests.
   b. Left ventricular fractional shortening greater than 28%, regardless of inotropic support.

4. Specific compatibility should exist between the donor and recipient in three aspects:
   a. ABO blood group compatibility. (Unlike renal transplantation, histocompatibility typing and matching do not predict success in heart transplantation.)
   b. The donor's body weight should be within 20% of the recipient's weight; a larger donor heart is better tolerated than a smaller one. A donor-recipient weight ratio of up to 3.0 is acceptable.
   c. The donor should be within close geographic range so that the donor heart can be harvested, transported, and implanted within 4 hours. For infant transplantation, a longer duration is acceptable (up to 9 hours).

5. Medical management of the donor heart before transplantation. The donor should be managed in the intensive care unit with routine monitoring. The systolic blood pressure should be maintained in the normal range (>100 mg Hg for adults). Fluid resuscitation may be necessary initially if fluids were restricted (to prevent brain edema, for example). Hypotension despite adequate filling pressure is treated with dopamine. Normal serum electrolyte levels, acid-base balance, and oxygenation should be maintained. The hematocrit should be above 30%.

Informed Consent from the Family and Recipient

The public often misunderstands what transplantation can accomplish. The recipient and parents must fully understand the short- and long-term implications of transplantation by knowing the following facts, which are not well publicized:

1. Unlike most cardiac surgeries, cardiac transplantation is not a cure for the condition for which it is being considered. It can be viewed as another medical problem that will require *lifelong* medical attention, including frequent hospital visits or admissions for noninvasive and invasive procedures, frequent adjustments of immunosuppressive and antibiotic medications, varying degrees of limitations in activity, and adjustments in lifestyle.

2. There is always a threat of rejection and infection throughout the patient's life. Even with full compliance, rejection can occur, resulting in death or a need for retransplantation.

3. The heart received will not last for an indefinite period; it will eventually develop allograft coronary artery disease, requiring consideration of retransplantation (see later section "Allograft Coronary Artery Disease").

4. Immunosuppressive therapy may cause malignancies (especially lymphoma in children) and an increased risk of infection (see later section for further discussion).

5. Lifelong medical attention will place a tremendous financial, emotional, and social burden on the family. A dysfunctional family could result.

Operative Technique

There are currently two surgical techniques used in cardiac transplantation: the "right atrial" technique and the "bicaval" technique. The latter is a more recent technique and has become more popular than the former.

In right atrial cardiac transplantation, when the native heart is explanted, the posterior walls of both atria of the recipient heart are left in place and are anastomosed to the donor heart. End-to-end anastomoses are also made between the donor and recipient aortas and pulmonary arteries (Fig. 35–1). This technique is similar to those described by Lower and Shumway in 1960. The hospital mortality rate is 10% to 15%.

A modification of that technique, called bicaval cardiac transplantation, has become popular in some institutions (Fig. 35–2). In this technique, the right atrium is also explanted from the recipient, leaving only the posterior wall of the left atrium with four pulmonary veins attached. Anastomoses are made between the venae cavae, the aorta, the pulmonary artery, and the left atrium.

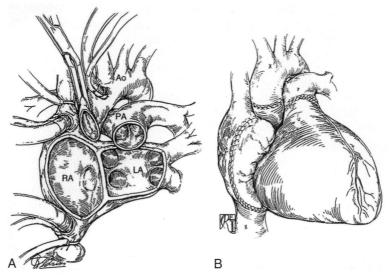

Figure 35–1. *Right atrial technique of cardiac transplantation.* ***A,*** *The recipient cardiectomy has been completed, leaving the anastomosis to be performed in the following sequence: (1) left atrial (LA), (2) aortic (AO), (3) right atrial (RA), and (4) pulmonary artery (PA).* ***B,*** *The completed transplant.* (From Backer CL, Mavroudis C: Pediatric transplantation, Part A: Heart transplantation. In Stuart FP, Abecassis MM, Kaufman DB [eds]: *Organ Transplantation,* Georgetown, Tex, Landes Bioscience, 2000.)

For most babies with HLHS, the donor cardiectomy is modified in that the entire aortic arch is harvested well beyond the insertion of the ligamentum arteriosus to augment the ascending aorta and aortic arch, such as those shown in Figure 35–3.

Early Postoperative Management

Early postoperative management is directed toward the detection and treatment of acute rejection and infection, two most common complications. Each institution has a detailed

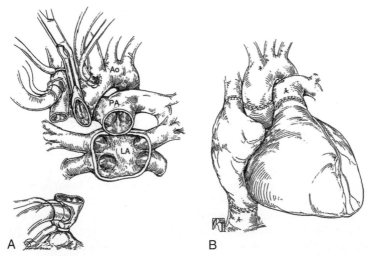

Figure 35–2. *Bicaval technique of cardiac transplantation.* ***A,*** *The recipient cardiectomy has been completed. Note that the entire right atrium has been removed. The sequence of the anastomosis is (1) left atrial (LA), (2) aortic (AO), (3) inferior vena cava, (4) pulmonary artery (PA), and (5) superior vena cava.* ***B,*** *The completed transplant.* (From Backer CL, Mavroudis C: Pediatric transplantation, Part A: Heart transplantation. In Stuart FP, Abecassis MM, Kaufman DB [eds]: *Organ Transplantation,* Georgetown, Tex, Landes Bioscience, 2000.)

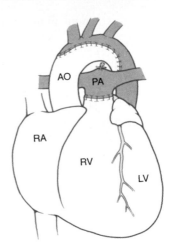

Figure 35–3. *Modification of heart transplantation surgery for hypoplastic left heart syndrome. AO, aorta; LV, left ventricle; PA, pulmonary artery; RA, right atrium; RV, right ventricle.*

management plan established by the transplantation team, which may be somewhat different from the following description.

Postoperative care is similar to that for most patients who have had cardiac surgery; the exception is immunosuppression. Inotropic support with isoproterenol, dobutamine, or amrinone for 2 or 3 days is usually needed. Antibiotics (usually vancomycin and ceftazidime) are administered intravenously during the first 48 hours after transplantation.

IMMUNOSUPPRESSIVE THERAPY

Successful immunosuppression depends on a delicate balance between suppression of the host mechanisms that would reject the foreign graft and preservation of the mechanisms of the immune response that protect against bacterial, fungal, and viral invasion. Immunosuppressive therapy is begun 4 to 12 hours before surgery and continued throughout the patient's life. The so-called triple-drug therapy consists of three classes of medications (Table 35–1).

1. Calcineurin inhibitors, such as cyclosporine (Neoral) or tacrolimus (Prograf, FK506), block T-cell cytokine gene expression.

2. Corticosteroids (methylprednisolone or prednisone).

3. Antiproliferative agents (or cell toxins), such as azathioprine (Imuran) or mycophenolate mofetil (CellCept), prevent rejection by interfering with purine synthesis, resulting in antiproliferative effects on T and B cells.

Table 35–1. **Dosages of Immunosuppressive Agents**

Drug	Preoperative	Early Postoperative	Late Postoperative
Cyclosporine*	10 mg/kg IV	0.5–1 mg/kg/day IV	3–6 mg/kg/day PO*
Methylprednisolone	10 mg/kg IV	2 mg/kg IV q8h × 3	
Prednisone		1 mg/kg/day PO	Taper to 0.2 mg/kg/day PO by 3 mo; stop by 6 mo
Azathioprine		1–2 mg/kg PO or IV	1–2 mg/kg/day (adjust according to white blood cell count)

*Adjust cyclosporine dosage by PO bid dosing (or q8h dosing for infants younger than 6 mo) to maintain target trough level as follows:

0–3 mo postoperatively	300 ng/mL
3–12 mo postoperatively	200–250 ng/mL
>12 mo postoperatively	150–200 ng/mL

Adapted from Canter CE: Pediatric cardiac transplantation. In Moller JH, Hoffman JIE (eds): Pediatric Cardiovascular Medicine. New York, Churchill Livingstone, 2000, pp 942–952.

Newer immunosuppressive agents, such as sirolimus (Rapamycin), basiliximab (Simulect), and daclizumab (Zenapax), are gaining clinical experience.

Cyclosporine. Cyclosporine is the most commonly used agent of maintenance therapy. It is a fungal metabolite that inhibits the production and release of the lymphokines interleukin-1 from the activated macrophage and interleukin-2 (T-cell growth factor) from the activated T helper cells, thus preventing the formation of cytotoxic T cells without affecting suppressor T cells. The first dose of cyclosporine (10 mg/kg) is administered before surgery because it may be most effective when given before the antigenic challenge. After surgery, the dosage is 0.5 to 1 mg/kg per day given intravenously in two or three doses. This dose is soon switched to 3 to 6 mg/kg per day in two to three doses by mouth to produce the desired therapeutic whole blood trough levels of 200 to 300 ng/mL (see Table 35–1). Cyclosporine is continued as long as the patient lives.

The drug's primary toxic effects are hypertension and associated renal insufficiency. Other side effects of the drug include hyperlipidemia, hirsutism, gingival hyperplasia, and facial dysmorphism (with widening of the nose, thickening of the nares and lips, and prominence of the supraorbital ridge and eyebrows).

Blood levels of cyclosporine decrease when used with phenobarbital, phenytoin, or carbamazepine, requiring higher doses of the drug (because these drugs increase cyclosporine metabolism in the liver, the major organ of elimination). Macrolides (erythromycin, clarithromycin [Biaxin], or azithromycin) increase blood levels and should be avoided because they potentially cause renal failure. When renal function is impaired, this dose is reduced to as low as 1 mg/kg per day.

Tacrolimus (Prograf), a newer agent in the same class as cyclosporine, is being used increasingly by some centers as a primary calcineurin agent. It is associated with remarkably lower rates of hypertension and hyperlipidemia and does not cause hirsutism, gingival hyperplasia, or the facial dysmorphism associated with cyclosporine.

Corticosteroids. Methylprednisolone (10 mg/kg for children) is administered intravenously as the sternotomy is made. After cardiopulmonary bypass has been discontinued, a 2 mg/kg intravenous dose is given every 8 hours, totaling three doses. After 24 hours, prednisone is administered in high doses (1 mg/kg per day by mouth). After about 3 weeks, the dose is tapered to 0.2 mg/kg per day by 3 months after surgery (see Table 35–1). Further tapering or discontinuation depends on the institution's protocol and the presence or absence of rejection. Some centers discontinue it after 6 months, particularly in neonates and infants, but in many centers this regimen continues as long as the patient lives.

Azathioprine. Azathioprine (Imuran) is added as an immunosuppressive agent in most protocols. Azathioprine is a purine analogue antimetabolite with some selective anti-T-cell activity. It is given immediately after the transplantation surgery. The starting dose is 1 to 2 mg/kg per day to produce a peripheral white blood cell count around 5000/mm^3. If the count falls below 4000/mm^3, the drug is reduced, or it is stopped if the reduction is severe (see Table 35–1). The major toxicity of azathioprine is bone marrow depression and less frequently hepatotoxicity. The drug is generally continued indefinitely.

Mycophenolate mofetil (CellCept) is a new agent in the antiproliferative agent group. A clinical study has demonstrated a lower rate of rejection than with azathioprine when it is used with cyclosporin and corticosteroids. This resulted in replacing azathioprine with mycophenolate mofetil by some centers. This agent also allowed reduction of the dosage of cyclosporin and tacrolimus, which may potentially reduce side effects of these drugs. The dose is 600 mg/m^2/dose by mouth twice a day. Its side effects include gastrointestinal symptoms (in 30%), bone marrow suppression (anemia), hypertension, headache, fever, and increased risk of developing lymphomas or other malignancies. The target level of the drug appears to be approximately 5 to 7 ng/mL.

ACUTE REJECTION

Identification. Endomyocardial biopsy remains the most important method for identifying acute rejection and is performed once a week for the first 4 to 6 weeks after surgery in older children and adults. Thereafter, biopsies are performed every 3 to

Table 35–2. **Standardized Endomyocardial Biopsy Grading: International Society of Heart and Lung Transplantation Scale**

Grade	"New" Nomenclature	"Old" Nomenclature
0	No rejection	No rejection
1A	Focal (perivascular or interstitial) infiltrate without necrosis	Mild rejection
1B	Diffuse but sparse infiltrate without necrosis	
2	One focus only, with aggressive infiltration and/or focal myocyte damage	"Focal" moderate rejection
3A	Multifocal aggressive infiltrates and/or myocyte damage	"Low" moderate rejection
3B	Diffuse inflammatory process with necrosis	"Borderline/severe" rejection
4	Diffuse aggressive polymorphous infiltrate ± edema, ± hemorrhage, ± vasculitis, with necrosis	"Severe acute" rejection

Adapted from Billingham ME, Cary NR, Hammond ME, et al: A working formulation for the standardization of nomenclature in the diagnosis of heart and lung rejection: Heart Rejection Study Group. J Heart Transplant 9:587–593, 1990.

4 months. For newborns and small infants, a routine endomyocardial biopsy is not performed; these patients are followed primarily by echo and other noninvasive means.

1. Subtle symptoms may be the only indication of the beginning of a rejection episode. These symptoms include unexplained fever, tachycardia, fatigue, shortness of breath, joint pain, and personality changes.

2. Echo techniques rely on a physiologic abnormality of the rejecting heart (myocardial edema or decreased left ventricular contractility) (see "Monitoring for and Treatment of Rejection" later).

3. The endomyocardial biopsy is graded according to the International Society of Heart and Lung Transplantation scale (1990) (Table 35–2).

Treatment. Rejection treatment is dependent on the grade of rejection. Generally, mild rejection (grade 1) does not warrant acute treatment, although about 25% of patients may progress to a higher grade of rejection. With moderate or severe rejection (grade 3 or 4), specific antirejection therapy is initiated.

1. Methylprednisolone (1000 mg for adults; 15 mg/kg for children weighing <50 kg) given intravenously or prednisone (100 mg for adults) given orally for 3 days is followed by tapering to the baseline dose over the next 2 weeks.

2. If rejection does not respond to steroids or if hemodynamic compromise occurs, antithymocyte sera such as antithymocyte globulin (ATG) or the monoclonal antibody to T3 lymphocytes (OKT3) are used for 5 or 10 days, respectively.

3. If all measures prove ineffective, retransplantation is considered.

INFECTION

Immunosuppressive medications used to prevent allograft rejection increase the risk of infection. Although cyclosporine has reduced the severity and frequency of rejection, infection remains a leading cause of death after heart transplantation. There are two peak incidences for infection after transplantation.

1. The "early" infection, occurring within the first month of transplantation, is dominated by nosocomial, often catheter-related, infection caused by *Staphylococcus* species and gram-negative organisms.

2. The "late" infection, occurring within 2 to 5 months, is caused by opportunistic infections from organisms such as cytomegalovirus (CMV), *Pneumocystis*, and fungal pathogens (see later section). The lung is the most common site of infection in heart transplant recipients, followed by the blood, urine, gastrointestinal tract, and sternal wound.

Late Post-Transplantation Follow-up

In following up post-transplantation patients, physicians should first be aware of the unique physiology of the transplanted heart, which responds differently to exercise and to certain medications.

The transplanted heart remains largely, but not entirely, denervated throughout the life of the recipient.

1. The response of the transplanted heart to exercise or stress is less than normal but adequate for most activities. With exercise, the heart rate accelerates slowly, and it parallels the rise in circulating catecholamine levels.

2. Most patients with denervated hearts experience no chest pain, even with significant coronary artery disease.

3. Transplant recipients are supersensitive to catecholamines, in part because of the upregulation of β-adrenergic receptors and in part because of a loss of norepinephrine uptake in sympathetic neurons.

4. Coronary vasodilator response may be abnormal if coronary artery disease has developed.

Follow-up examinations are intended to detect rejection, infection, and the side effects of immunosuppression. Infection and rejection remain the most common causes of death after heart transplantation. Graft failure, lymphoma, and coronary artery disease are responsible for the remaining deaths.

MONITORING FOR SIDE EFFECTS OF IMMUNOSUPPRESSION

1. Hypertension and renal toxicity are common side effects and malignancies are rare side effects of cyclosporine therapy. Less severe adverse side effects of the drug include reversible hepatotoxicity, fluid retention, hirsutism, gum hypertrophy, and gastrointestinal symptoms.
   a. The mechanism of cyclosporine-associated nephrotoxicity is probably related to the vasoconstrictor effect of the drug and decreased renal blood flow.
   b. Hypertension occurs in 50% to 90% of heart transplant recipients who take cyclosporine. The mechanisms of cyclosporine-associated hypertension include nephrotoxicity, increased sympathetic tone, volume expansion, increased endothelin levels, and stimulation of the renin-angiotensin system. Calcium channel blockers, angiotensin-converting enzyme inhibitors, and β- and α-blockers have been used with varying degrees of success.
   c. Rarely (10% of patients), lymphoma develops with a larger dose of the drug.
2. Growth retardation may occur with large doses of steroids. The dosage of steroids is kept at a minimum, or steroids are not given at all.

3. Azathioprine may produce bone marrow depression (e.g., thrombocytopenia, leukocytopenia, anemia), alopecia, and gastrointestinal symptoms.

MONITORING FOR AND TREATMENT OF REJECTION

The risk of rejection is greatest in the first 3 months after transplantation, occurring in approximately 70% of patients. However, the rate of lethal rejection is low in infants (6%). A high index of suspicion is necessary to detect rejection, particularly in the early months after transplantation, because many rejections occur without symptoms. Therefore, endomyocardial biopsy at a regular interval is required to detect rejection.

1. Clinically evident cardiac dysfunction or congestive heart failure (CHF) is usually absent. Nonspecific clinical signs and symptoms (e.g., fever, tachycardia, malaise, personality changes, gallop rhythm, arrhythmias, hypotension) may be the only indications of rejection. These symptoms are often due to infection rather than rejection. Decreased ECG voltages and decreased ventricular function (by echo) are late signs of acute rejection.

2. Some centers have used serial echocardiography to assess rejection, but this method has not been universally accepted. The endomyocardial biopsy provides the

earliest detectable indication of rejection. Cardiac rejection is characterized by cellular infiltration of the myocardium, particularly around blood vessels, with or without damage to or destruction of the myocytes. In so-called *chronic rejection*, endothelial cells are also damaged or destroyed. This is believed to be the basis for accelerated coronary artery disease (see later section).

3. Patients with no or mild rejection (grade 0 or 1) on the biopsy receive no change in drug dosage. Moderate rejection (grade 3) is treated with higher doses of steroids, whereas severe rejection (grade 4) is treated with higher doses of steroids and/or antithymocyte sera, with hospitalization and hemodynamic monitoring (see previous section).

MONITORING FOR INFECTION

Infection after the immediate post-transplantation period is caused by opportunistic infective agents such as CMV, *Pneumocystis* organisms, and fungus. Infection is a common cause of death and is probably related to the immunosuppressive therapy. The average mortality rate from infection is about 12%; that of fungal infection is about 36%. The lung is the most commonly infected organ; the mortality rate of patients with infected lungs is 22%. CMV remains the most common single infection, but the specific antiviral agent for CMV, ganciclovir, does not appear to reduce the incidence of primary CMV infection. Pediatric patients have a higher incidence of otitis media and sinusitis as well as the gastrointestinal manifestations of many childhood illnesses. The efficacy of pyrimethamine and trimethoprim-sulfamethoxazole has been proved for the prophylaxis of toxoplasmosis and *Pneumocystis* infection, respectively. The risk-benefit ratio of using influenza vaccines after transplantation remains controversial.

Most researchers agree that children receiving immunosuppressive therapy, as well as their siblings, should not receive all live vaccines, including varicella, measles, mumps, rubella, and oral polio. Because of their immunosuppressed status, there is an increased risk for these patients developing active disease from the vaccine strains.

ALLOGRAFT CORONARY ARTERY DISEASE

An unusual, accelerated form of coronary artery disease, probably an immune-mediated disease, is the third most common cause of death, following infection and rejection. Coronary artery disease is the major determinant of long-term survival. Virtually all patients have some histopathologic evidence of coronary artery disease by 1 year after transplantation. It may occur in up to 40% of transplanted hearts in 3 years and in more than 50% in 5 years. This disease also occurs in pediatric patients, perhaps to a lesser degree, but 28% of pediatric patients surviving 6 months to 6 years after transplantation develop coronary artery disease.

Coronary angiography is necessary to diagnose the disease. The unique angiographic hallmark of this disease is diffuse, concentric, longitudinal, and rapid pruning and obliteration of distal branch vessels. Many centers recommend performing the first coronary angiography within 2 to 4 weeks of transplantation to obtain a baseline; some centers also recommend performing an exercise stress test, if appropriate for the patient's age, and coronary angiography 1 year after transplantation to evaluate graft function and to detect premature and aggressive coronary atherosclerosis.

Most patients with transplanted, denervated hearts fail to experience typical chest pain. Life-threatening ventricular arrhythmias, CHF, silent myocardial infarction, and sudden death may result. The only effective treatment of allograft coronary artery disease is retransplantation.

MALIGNANCY

Another side effect of chronic immunosuppressive treatment is the development of a malignant neoplasm, occurring in 1% to 2% of patients each year, or 12.5% during a mean follow-up period of 50 months. A unique form of lymphoma, *post-transplantation lymphoproliferative disease*, is the most common tumor reported (80%) with cyclosporine-based immunosuppression; it occurs more frequently in young patients. Most of these tumors are thought to be the result of Epstein-Barr virus infection. The use of OKT3 and ATG, as well as higher initial doses of cyclosporine and prednisone, appears to increase the risk of post-transplantation lymphoproliferative disease. There is a rapid proliferation of lymph cells that can occur throughout the body. Common sites are the tonsils and adenoids, cervical lymph nodes, lungs, and abdomen. Symptoms may include fever, malaise, sore throat, tonsillitis, abdominal pain, or palpable mass. About 40% of patients respond to a reduction in immunotherapy, but chemotherapy and radiation therapy may be needed. Reported mortality rates vary widely (ranging from 20% to over 8%).

Cutaneous malignancy (squamous cell and basal cell carcinoma) is the most common tumor associated with the use of azathioprine, perhaps related to the drug's enhanced photosensitivity. The mortality rate from post-transplantation tumors is high (38%).

OTHER MEDICATIONS USED BY TRANSPLANT PATIENTS

In addition to the triple-drug regimen, the heart transplant patient is taking several other medications to treat side effects of immunosuppressive agents.

1. Antihypertensive medications—calcium channel blockers and/or ACE inhibitors.
2. Cholesterol-lowering medications (such as pravastatin and other statins). Hypercholesterolemia occurs in 35% to 50% of transplant patients taking immunosuppressive drugs. Pravastatin has been shown to be effective in reducing total cholesterol and LDL cholesterol levels in post-transplantation patients (Seipelt et al, 2004). Serial CPK and liver enzyme determination are recommended.
3. Supplemental calcium and magnesium (for side effects of cyclosporine).
4. Iron supplementation.
5. Prophylactic antibiotics for fungal and pneumocystis pneumonia.

Prognosis

The pediatric survival rate is 70% to 80% at 1 year, 65% to 75% at 3 years, and 60% to 70% at 5 years. Newborns and infants appear to have better survival rates after transplantation; the 5-year actuarial survival rate is 80%. The survival rate among newborn recipients at 5 years is 84%, with no subsequent deaths occurring in a 5-year follow-up.

Appendices

Appendix A: Miscellaneous

Table A–1. **Recurrence Risks Given One Sibling Who Has a Cardiovascular Anomaly**

Anomaly	Suggested Risk (%)
Ventricular septal defect	3.0
Patent ductus arteriosus	3.0
Atrial septal defect	2.5
Tetralogy of Fallot	2.5
Pulmonary stenosis	2.0
Coarctation of the aorta	2.0
Aortic stenosis	2.0
Transposition of the great arteries	1.5
Atrioventricular canal (complete endocardial cushion defect)	2.0
Endocardial fibroelastosis	4.0
Tricuspid atresia	1.0
Ebstein's anomaly	1.0
Persistent truncus arteriosus	1.0
Pulmonary atresia	1.0
Hypoplastic left heart syndrome	2.0

Modified from Nora JJ, Nora AH: The evaluation of specific genetic and environmental counseling in congenital heart diseases. Circulation 57:205–213, 1978.

Table A–2. **Affected Offspring Given One Parent with a Congenital Heart Defect**

Defect	Mother Affected (%)	Father Affected (%)
Aortic stenosis	13.0–18.0	3.0
Atrial septal defect	4.0–4.5	1.5
Atrioventricular canal (complete endocardial cushion defect)	14.0	1.0
Coarctation of the aorta	4.0	2.0
Patent ductus arteriosus	3.5–4.0	2.5
Pulmonary stenosis	4.0–6.5	2.0
Tetralogy of Fallot	6.0–10.0	1.5
Ventricular septal defect	6.0	2.0

From Nora JJ, Nora AH: Maternal transmission of congenital heart disease: New recurrence risk figures and the questions of cytoplasmic inheritance and vulnerability to teratogens. Am J Cardiol 59:459–463, 1987.

Table A–3. **Classification of Antiarrhythmic Drugs According to Their Mechanism of Action**

Class	Action	Drugs
I	Sodium channel blockade	
A	Moderate phase 0 depression and slow conduction (2+)*; prolonged repolarization	Quinidine, procainamide, disopyramide
B	Minimal phase 0 depression and slow conduction (0 to 1+); shortened repolarization	Lidocaine, phenytoin, tocainide, mexiletine
C	Marked phase 0 depression and slow conduction (4+); little effect on repolarization	Encainide, lorcainide, flecainide
II	β-Adrenergic blockade	Propranolol, others
III	Prolong repolarization	Amiodarone, bretylium
IV	Calcium channel blockade	Diltiazem, verapamil

*Relative magnitude of effect on conduction velocity is indicated on a scale of 1+ to 4+.
Adapted from Gilman AG, Goodman LS, Rall TW, Murad F (eds): Goodman and Gilman's The Pharmacological Basis of Therapeutics, 7th ed. New York, Macmillan, 1985.

Table A–4. **New York Heart Association Functional Classification**

Class	Impairment
I	The patient has the disease, but the condition is asymptomatic.
II	The patient experiences symptoms with moderate activity.
III	The patient has symptoms with mild activity.
IV	The patient's condition is symptomatic at rest.

This is a classification of functional impairment in exercise capacity based on symptoms of dyspnea and fatigue. It is simple and useful in the evaluation of cardiac patients.

Table A–5. *Oxygen Consumption per Body Surface Area**

Age (yr)	Heart Rate (beats/min)												
	50	*60*	*70*	*80*	*90*	*100*	*110*	*120*	*130*	*140*	*150*	*160*	*170*
Male Patients													
3				155	159	163	167	171	175	178	182	186	190
4			149	152	156	160	163	168	171	175	179	182	186
6		141	144	148	151	155	159	162	167	171	174	178	181
8		136	141	145	148	152	156	159	163	167	171	175	178
10	130	134	139	142	146	149	153	157	160	165	169	172	176
12	128	132	136	140	144	147	151	155	158	162	167	170	174
14	127	130	134	137	142	146	149	153	157	160	165	169	172
16	125	129	132	136	141	144	148	152	155	159	162	167	
18	124	127	131	135	139	143	147	150	154	157	161	166	
20	123	126	130	134	137	142	145	149	153	156	160	165	
25	120	124	127	131	135	139	143	147	150	154	157		
30	118	122	125	129	133	136	141	145	148	152	155		
35	116	120	124	127	131	135	139	143	147	150			
40	115	119	122	126	130	133	137	141	145	149			
Female Patients													
3				150	153	157	161	165	169	172	176	180	183
4			141	145	149	152	156	159	163	168	171	175	179
6		130	134	137	142	146	149	153	156	160	165	168	172
8		125	129	133	136	141	144	148	152	155	159	163	167
10	118	122	125	129	133	136	141	144	148	152	155	159	163
12	115	119	122	126	130	133	137	141	145	149	152	156	160
14	112	116	120	123	127	131	134	133	143	146	150	153	157
16	109	114	118	121	125	128	132	136	140	144	148	151	
18	107	111	116	119	123	127	130	134	137	142	146	149	
20	106	109	114	118	121	125	128	132	136	140	144	148	
25	102	106	109	114	118	121	125	128	132	136	140		
30	99	103	106	110	115	118	122	125	129	133	136		
35	97	100	104	107	111	116	119	123	127	130			
50	94	98	102	105	109	112	117	121	124	128			

*In mL/min/m^2. From LaFarge CG, Miettinen OS: The estimation of oxygen consumption. Cardiovasc Res 4:23, 1970.

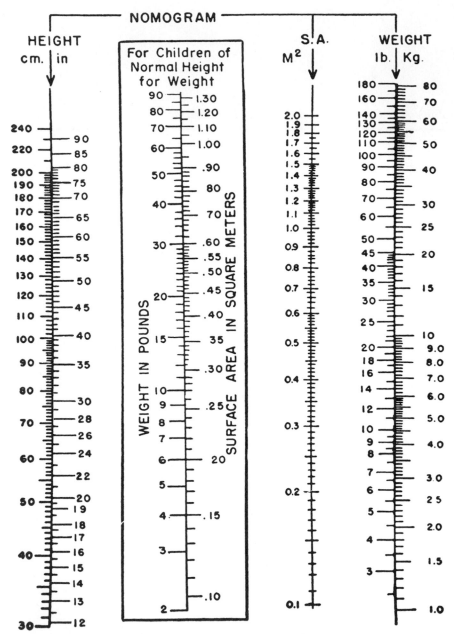

Figure A–1. *Body surface area nomogram.*

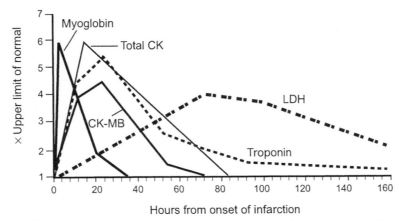

Figure A–2. *Time course of elevation of selected serum markers after acute myocardial infarction in an adult. This figure summarizes the relative timing, rate of rise, peak values, and duration of elevation above the upper limit of normal for the serum markers. Myoglobin rises quickly soon after the onset of infarction, but it is not specific for cardiac muscle; it may also come from skeletal muscles. Total creatine kinase (CK) rises within 4 to 8 hours, reaches a peak at 24 hours, and declines to normal levels within 2 to 3 days. There are three isoenzymes (BB, MM, and MB) of CK identified by electrophoresis. The CK-MB isoenzyme occurs primarily in cardiac muscles, the BB enzyme occurs primarily in the brain and kidneys, and the MM isoenzyme occurs in cardiac and skeletal muscles. Lactate dehydrogenase (LDH) elevation occurs several days after the onset of myocardial infarction. False elevation of LDH occurs in patients with hemolysis, leukemia, liver disease or congestion, renal disease, pulmonary embolism, skeletal muscle disease, shock, and myocarditis. Cardiac-specific troponin I may be useful for the diagnosis of infarction even 3 to 4 days after the event. In children, the normal value of cardiac troponin I has been reported to be 2 ng/mL or less, and it is frequently below the level of detection for the assay. (From Antman EM: General hospital management. In Julian DG, Braunwald E [eds]: Management of Acute Myocardial Infarction. London, WB Saunders, 1994, p 63.)*

Appendix B: Blood Pressure Values

Table B–1. *BP Levels for Boys by Age and Height Percentile (NHBPEP*)*

Age	BP Percentile	Systolic BP (mm Hg) Percentile of Height							Diastolic BP (mm Hg) Percentile of Height						
		5th	10th	25th	50th	75th	90th	95th	5th	10th	25th	50th	75th	90th	95th
1	50th	80	81	83	85	87	88	89	34	35	36	37	38	39	39
	90th	94	95	97	99	100	102	103	49	50	51	52	53	53	54
	95th	98	99	101	103	104	106	106	54	54	55	56	57	58	58
	99th	105	106	108	110	112	113	114	61	62	63	64	65	66	66
2	50th	84	85	87	88	90	92	92	39	40	41	42	43	44	44
	90th	97	99	100	102	104	105	106	54	55	56	57	58	58	59
	95th	101	102	104	106	108	109	110	59	59	60	61	62	63	63
	99th	109	110	111	113	115	117	117	66	67	68	69	70	71	71
3	50th	86	87	89	91	93	94	95	44	44	45	46	47	48	48
	90th	100	101	103	105	107	108	109	59	59	60	61	62	63	63
	95th	104	105	107	109	110	112	113	63	63	64	65	66	67	67
	99th	111	112	114	116	118	119	120	71	71	72	73	74	75	75
4	50th	88	89	91	93	95	96	97	47	48	49	50	51	51	52
	90th	102	103	105	107	109	110	111	62	63	64	65	66	66	67
	95th	106	107	109	111	112	114	115	66	67	68	69	70	71	71
	99th	113	114	116	118	120	121	122	74	75	76	77	78	78	79
5	50th	90	91	93	95	96	98	98	50	51	52	53	54	55	55
	90th	104	105	106	108	110	111	112	65	66	67	68	69	69	70
	95th	108	109	110	112	114	115	116	69	70	71	72	73	74	74
	99th	115	116	118	120	121	123	123	77	78	79	80	81	81	82
6	50th	91	92	94	96	98	99	100	53	53	54	55	56	57	57
	90th	105	106	108	110	111	113	113	68	68	69	70	71	72	72
	95th	109	110	112	114	115	117	117	72	72	73	74	75	76	76
	99th	116	117	119	121	123	124	125	80	80	81	82	83	84	84
7	50th	92	94	95	97	99	100	101	55	55	56	57	58	59	59
	90th	106	107	109	111	113	114	115	70	70	71	72	73	74	74
	95th	110	111	113	115	117	118	119	74	74	75	76	77	78	78
	99th	117	118	120	122	124	125	126	82	82	83	84	85	86	86
8	50th	94	95	97	99	100	102	102	56	57	58	59	60	60	61
	90th	107	109	110	112	114	115	116	71	72	72	73	74	75	76
	95th	111	112	114	116	118	119	120	75	76	77	78	79	79	80
	99th	119	120	122	123	125	127	127	83	84	85	86	87	87	88
9	50th	95	96	98	100	102	103	104	57	58	59	60	61	61	62
	90th	109	110	112	114	115	117	118	72	73	74	75	76	76	77
	95th	113	114	116	118	119	121	121	76	77	78	79	80	81	81
	99th	120	121	123	125	127	128	129	84	85	86	87	88	88	89
10	50th	97	98	100	102	103	105	106	58	59	60	61	61	62	63
	90th	111	112	114	115	117	119	119	73	73	74	75	76	77	78

Table continued on the following page

585

Table B–1. **BP Levels for Boys by Age and Height Percentile (NHBPEP*)** *(Continued)*

		Systolic BP (mm Hg) Percentile of Height							Diastolic BP (mm Hg) Percentile of Height						
Age	BP Percentile	5th	10th	25th	50th	75th	90th	95th	5th	10th	25th	50th	75th	90th	95th
	95th	115	116	117	119	121	122	123	77	78	79	80	81	81	82
	99th	122	123	125	127	128	130	130	85	86	86	88	88	89	90
11	50th	99	100	102	104	105	107	107	59	59	60	61	62	63	63
	90th	113	114	115	117	119	120	121	74	74	75	76	77	78	78
	95th	117	118	119	121	123	124	125	78	78	79	80	81	82	82
	99th	124	125	127	129	130	132	132	86	86	87	88	89	90	90
12	50th	101	102	104	106	108	109	110	59	60	61	62	63	63	64
	90th	115	116	118	120	121	123	123	74	75	75	76	77	78	79
	95th	119	120	122	123	125	127	127	78	79	80	81	82	82	83
	99th	126	127	129	131	133	134	135	86	87	88	89	90	90	91
13	50th	104	105	106	108	110	111	112	60	60	61	62	63	64	64
	90th	117	118	120	122	124	125	126	75	75	76	77	78	79	79
	95th	121	122	124	126	128	129	130	79	79	80	81	82	83	83
	99th	128	130	131	133	135	136	137	87	87	88	89	90	91	91
14	50th	106	107	109	111	113	114	115	60	61	62	63	64	65	65
	90th	120	121	123	125	126	128	128	75	76	77	78	79	79	80
	95th	124	125	127	128	130	132	132	80	80	81	82	83	84	84
	99th	131	132	134	136	138	139	140	87	88	89	90	91	92	92
15	50th	109	110	112	113	115	117	117	61	62	63	64	65	66	66
	90th	122	124	125	127	129	130	131	76	77	78	79	80	80	81
	95th	126	127	129	131	133	134	135	81	81	82	83	84	85	85
	99th	134	135	136	138	140	142	142	88	89	90	91	92	93	93
16	50th	111	112	114	116	118	119	120	63	63	64	65	66	67	67
	90th	125	126	128	130	131	133	134	78	78	79	80	81	82	82
	95th	129	130	132	134	135	137	137	82	83	83	84	85	86	87
	99th	136	137	139	141	143	144	145	90	90	91	92	93	94	94
17	50th	114	115	116	118	120	121	122	65	66	66	67	68	69	70
	90th	127	128	130	132	134	135	136	80	80	81	82	83	84	84
	95th	131	132	134	136	138	139	140	84	85	86	87	87	88	89
	99th	139	140	141	143	145	146	147	92	93	93	94	95	96	97

*National High Blood Pressure Education Program.
From The Fourth Report on the Diagnosis, Evaluation, and Treatment of High Blood Pressure in Children and
   Adolescents. National High Blood Pressure Education Program Working Group on High Blood Pressure in Children
   and Adolescents. Pediatrics 114:555–576, 2004.

Table B–2. **BP Levels for Girls by Age and Height Percentile (NHBPEP*)**

		Systolic BP (mm Hg) Percentile of Height							Diastolic BP (mm Hg) Percentile of Height						
Age	BP Percentile	5th	10th	25th	50th	75th	90th	95th	5th	10th	25th	50th	75th	90th	95th
1	50th	83	84	85	86	88	89	90	38	39	39	40	41	41	42
	90th	97	97	98	100	101	102	103	52	53	53	54	55	55	56
	95th	100	101	102	104	105	106	107	56	57	57	58	59	59	60
	99th	108	108	109	111	112	113	114	64	64	65	65	66	67	67
2	50th	85	85	87	88	89	91	91	43	44	44	45	46	46	47
	90th	98	99	100	101	103	104	105	57	58	58	59	60	61	61
	95th	102	103	104	105	107	108	109	61	62	62	63	64	65	65
	99th	109	110	111	112	114	115	116	69	69	70	70	71	72	72
3	50th	86	87	88	89	91	92	93	47	48	48	49	50	50	51
	90th	100	100	102	103	104	106	106	61	62	62	63	64	64	65
	95th	104	104	105	107	108	109	110	65	66	66	67	68	68	69
	99th	111	111	113	114	115	116	117	73	73	74	74	75	76	76

Table B–2. **BP Levels for Girls by Age and Height Percentile (NHBPEP*)** *(Continued)*

Age	BP Percentile	Systolic BP (mm Hg) Percentile of Height							Diastolic BP (mm Hg) Percentile of Height						
		5th	10th	25th	50th	75th	90th	95th	5th	10th	25th	50th	75th	90th	95th
4	50th	88	88	90	91	92	94	94	50	50	51	52	52	53	54
	90th	101	102	103	104	106	107	108	64	64	65	66	67	67	68
	95th	105	106	107	108	110	111	112	68	68	69	70	71	71	72
	99th	112	113	114	115	117	118	119	76	76	76	77	78	79	79
5	50th	89	90	91	93	94	95	96	52	53	53	54	55	55	56
	90th	103	103	105	106	107	109	109	66	67	67	68	69	69	70
	95th	107	107	108	110	111	112	113	70	71	71	72	73	73	74
	99th	114	114	116	117	118	120	120	78	78	79	79	80	81	81
6	50th	91	92	93	94	96	97	98	54	54	55	56	56	57	58
	90th	104	105	106	108	109	110	111	68	68	69	70	70	71	72
	95th	108	109	110	111	113	114	115	72	72	73	74	74	75	76
	99th	115	116	117	119	120	121	122	80	80	80	81	82	83	83
7	50th	93	93	95	96	97	99	99	55	56	56	57	58	58	59
	90th	106	107	108	109	111	112	113	69	70	70	71	72	72	73
	95th	110	111	112	113	115	116	116	73	74	74	75	76	76	77
	99th	117	118	119	120	122	123	124	81	81	82	82	83	84	84
8	50th	95	95	96	98	99	100	101	57	57	57	58	59	60	60
	90th	108	109	110	111	113	114	114	71	71	71	72	73	74	74
	95th	112	112	114	115	116	118	118	75	75	75	76	77	78	78
	99th	119	120	121	122	123	125	125	82	82	83	83	84	85	86
9	50th	96	97	98	100	101	102	103	58	58	58	59	60	61	61
	90th	110	110	112	113	114	116	116	72	72	72	73	74	75	75
	95th	114	114	115	117	118	119	120	76	76	76	77	78	79	79
	99th	121	121	123	124	125	127	127	83	83	84	84	85	86	87
10	50th	98	99	100	102	103	104	105	59	59	59	60	61	62	62
	90th	112	112	114	115	116	118	118	73	73	73	74	75	76	76
	95th	116	116	117	119	120	121	122	77	77	77	78	79	80	80
	99th	123	123	125	126	127	129	129	84	84	85	86	86	87	88
11	50th	100	101	102	103	105	106	107	60	60	60	61.	62	63	63
	90th	114	114	116	117	118	119	120	74	74	74	75	76	77	77
	95th	118	118	119	121	122	123	124	78	78	78	79	80	81	81
	99th	125	125	126	128	129	130	131	85	85	86	87	87	88	89
12	50th	102	103	104	105	107	108	109	61	61	61	62	63	64	64
	90th	116	116	117	119	120	121	122	75	75	75	76	77	78	78
	95th	119	120	121	123	124	125	126	79	79	79	80	81	82	82
	99th	127	127	128	130	131	132	133	86	86	87	88	88	89	90
13	50th	104	105	106	107	109	110	110	62	62	62	63	64	65	65
	90th	117	118	119	121	122	123	124	76	76	76	77	78	79	79
	95th	121	122	123	124	126	127	128	80	80	80	81	82	83	83
	99th	128	129	130	132	133	134	135	87	87	88	89	89	90	91
14	50th	106	106	107	109	110	111	112	63	63	63	64	65	66	66
	90th	119	120	121	122	124	125	125	77	77	77	78	79	80	80
	95th	123	123	125	126	127	129	129	81	81	81	82	83	84	84
	99th	130	131	132	133	135	136	136	88	88	89	90	90	91	92
15	50th	107	108	109	110	111	113	113	64	64	64	65	66	67	67
	90th	120	121	122	123	125	126	127	78	78	78	79	80	81	81
	95th	124	125	126	127	129	130	131	82	82	82	83	84	85	85
	99th	131	132	133	134	136	137	138	89	89	90	91	91	92	93
16	50th	108	108	110	111	112	114	114	64	64	65	66	66	67	68
	90th	121	122	123	124	126	127	128	78	78	79	80	81	81	82
	95th	125	126	127	128	130	131	132	82	82	83	84	85	85	86
	99th	132	133	134	135	137	138	139	90	90	90	91	92	93	93
17	50th	108	109	110	111	113	114	115	64	65	65	66	67	67	68
	90th	122	122	123	125	126	127	128	78	79	79	80	81	81.	82
	95th	125	126	127	129	130	131	132	82	83	83	84	85	85	86
	99th	133	133	134	136	137	138	139	90	90	91	91	92	93	93

*National High Blood Pressure Education Program.
From The Fourth Report on the Diagnosis, Evaluation, and Treatment of High Blood Pressure in Children and Adolescents. National High Blood Pressure Education Program Working Group on High Blood Pressure in Children and Adolescents. Pediatrics 114:555–576, 2004.

Table B–3. **Auscultatory Blood Pressure Values for Boys 5 to 17 Years Old**
(San Antonio Children's Blood Pressure Study)

Age (yr)				Percentiles				
	5th	*10th*	*25th*	*Mean*	*75th*	*90th*	*95th*	*99th**
Systolic Pressure								
5	78	81	87	92	98	103	106	112
6	81	84	89	95	100	105	108	114
7	82	85	90	96	102	107	110	116
8	83	86	92	97	103	108	111	117
9	85	88	93	99	104	109	113	118
10	86	89	95	100	106	111	114	120
11	88	91	97	102	108	113	116	122
12	91	94	99	105	111	116	119	125
13	94	97	102	108	113	118	122	127
14	96	99	105	110	116	121	122	130
15	99	102	107	113	118	124	127	132
16	100	103	108	114	120	125	128	134
17	100	103	109	114	120	125	128	134
Diastolic Pressure (K5)								
5	34	37	43	49	55	60	63	70
6	38	41	47	53	59	64	67	73
7	40	44	49	55	61	66	70	76
8	42	45	50	56	62	68	71	77
9	42	45	51	57	63	68	71	77
10	42	45	51	57	63	68	71	77
11	42	45	51	57	63	68	71	77
12	42	45	50	56	62	68	71	77
13	42	45	51	56	62	68	71	77
14	42	45	51	57	63	68	71	77
15	43	46	51	57	63	69	72	78
16	45	48	53	59	65	71	74	80
17	47	51	56	62	68	73	77	83

*The 99th percentile values were computed after publication of the source paper (Park et al, 2001).
K5 = Korotkoff phase 5.
Data presented in graphic form in Park MK, Menard SW, Yuan C: Comparison of blood pressure in children
  from three ethnic groups. Am J Cardiol 87:1305–1308, 2001.

Table B–4. **Auscultatory Blood Pressure Values for Girls 5 to 17 Years Old**
(San Antonio Children's Blood Pressure Study)

	Percentiles							
Age (yr)	*5th*	*10th*	*25th*	*Mean*	*75th*	*90th*	*95th*	*99th**
Systolic Pressure								
5	79	82	87	92	97	102	105	110
6	80	83	88	93	98	103	106	111
7	81	84	89	94	99	104	107	112
8	83	86	91	96	101	106	109	114
9	85	88	93	98	103	108	111	116
10	87	90	95	100	105	110	113	118
11	89	92	97	102	107	112	115	120
12	91	94	98	104	109	113	116	122
13	92	95	100	105	110	115	118	123
14	93	96	101	106	111	116	119	124
15	94	97	101	107	112	117	119	125
16	94	97	102	107	112	117	120	125
17	95	98	103	108	113	118	121	126
Diastolic Pressure (K5)								
5	35	38	44	49	55	60	63	69
6	38	41	47	52	58	63	66	72
7	40	41	49	54	60	65	68	74
8	42	45	50	56	61	67	70	75
9	43	46	51	56	62	67	70	76
10	43	46	51	57	63	68	71	77
11	43	46	51	57	63	68	71	77
12	43	46	52	57	63	68	71	77
13	43	47	52	57	63	68	71	77
14	44	47	52	58	63	68	72	77
15	44	47	52	58	64	69	72	78
16	45	48	53	59	64	69	73	78
17	46	49	54	59	65	70	73	79

*The 99th percentile values were computed after publication of the source paper (Park et al, 2001).
K5 = Korotkoff phase 5.
Data presented in graphic form in Park MK, Menard SW, Yuan C: Comparison of blood pressure in children
    from three ethnic groups. Am J Cardiol 87:1305–1308, 2001.

Table B–5. **Dinamap (Model 1846) BP Percentiles for Neonates to 5-Year-Old Children**

Age	Percentiles						
	5th	*10th*	*25th*	*Mean*	*75th*	*90th*	*95th*
Systolic Pressure							
1–3 days	52	56	58	65	71	74	77
2–3 wk	62	66	71	78	84	89	92
1–5 mo	76	79	88	94	102	106	111
6–11 mo	79	84	88	94	99	104	109
1 yr	80	84	89	94	99	104	108
2 yr	82	85	91	95	101	106	109
3 yr	84	87	92	98	103	108	112
4 yr	86	90	95	100	105	110	114
5 yr	89	93	96	102	107	113	116
Diastolic Pressure							
1–3 days	31	33	37	41	45	50	52
2–3 wk	31	37	42	47	63	58	61
1–5 mo	45	48	53	59	64	71	75
6–11 mo	41	44	52	57	63	67	69
1 yr	44	48	52	57	73	67	69
2 yr	45	47	52	56	61	65	68
3 yr	44	47	52	56	61	65	69
4 yr	44	48	52	56	61	65	68
5 yr	44	48	53	57	62	66	68

Data presented in graphic form in Park MK, Menard SM: Normative oscillometric BP values in the first 5 years in an office setting. Arch J Dis Child 143:860–864, 1989.

Table B–6. **Dinamap (Model 8100) Blood Pressure Values for Boys 5 to 17 Years Old (San Antonio Children's Blood Pressure Study)**

Age (yr)	Percentiles							
	5th	*10th*	*25th*	*Mean*	*75th*	*90th*	*95th*	*99th**
Systolic Pressure								
5	90	93	98	104	110	115	118	124
6	92	95	100	106	112	117	120	126
7	93	96	102	107	113	118	121	127
8	94	97	103	108	114	119	123	128
9	95	99	104	110	115	121	124	130
10	97	100	105	110	117	122	125	131
11	99	102	107	113	119	124	127	133
12	101	104	109	115	121	126	129	135
13	104	107	112	118	123	129	132	138
14	106	109	114	120	126	131	134	140
15	108	111	116	122	128	133	136	141
16	109	112	117	123	128	134	137	143
17	109	112	117	123	129	134	137	143
Diastolic Pressure								
5	46	49	53	58	63	68	71	76
6	47	49	54	59	64	68	71	76
7	47	50	54	59	64	69	72	77
8	48	51	55	60	65	70	72	78
9	49	51	56	61	66	70	73	78
10	49	52	56	61	66	71	74	79
11	49	52	57	62	67	71	74	79
12	50	52	57	62	67	71	74	79
13	50	52	57	62	67	71	74	79
14	50	52	57	62	67	72	74	79
15	50	52	57	62	67	72	74	79
16	50	53	57	62	67	72	74	80
17	50	53	57	62	67	72	75	80

*The 99th percentile values were computed after publication of the source paper (Park et al, 2005).
From Park MK, Menard SW, Schoolfield J: Oscillometric blood pressure standards for children. Pediatr Cardiol 26:601–607, 2005.

Table B–7. **Dinamap (Model 8100) Blood Pressure Values for Girls 5 to 17 Years Old (San Antonio Children's Blood Pressure Study)**

Age (yr)	\ 5th	\ 10th	Percentiles\ 25th	\ Mean	\ 75th	\ 90th	\ 95th	\ 99th*
Systolic Pressure								
5	90	93	98	103	109	114	117	122
6	91	94	99	1043	110	115	118	123
7	92	95	100	106	111	116	119	125
8	94	97	102	107	113	118	121	126
9	95	98	103	109	114	119	122	128
10	97	100	105	110	116	121	124	129
11	98	101	106	112	117	122	125	131
12	100	103	107	113	118	123	126	132
13	101	104	109	114	120	125	128	133
14	102	104	109	115	120	125	128	134
15	102	105	110	115	121	126	129	134
16	102	105	110	115	121	126	129	134
17	102	105	110	115	121	126	129	134
Diastolic Pressure								
5	46	48	53	59	64	68	71	76
6	47	49	54	59	64	68	71	76
7	47	50	54	60	65	69	72	77
8	48	50	55	60	65	70	73	78
9	49	51	55	61	66	70	73	78
10	49	51	56	61	66	71	74	79
11	49	52	56	62	67	71	74	79
12	50	52	57	62	67	71	74	79
13	50	53	57	62	67	71	74	79
14	50	53	58	62	67	72	74	79
15	50	54	58	62	67	72	74	79
16	50	54	58	62	67	72	74	80
17	50	54	58	62	67	72	75	80

*The 99th percentile values were computed after publication of the source paper (Park et al, 2001).
From Park MK, Menard SW, Schoolfield J: Oscillometric blood pressure standards for children. Pediatr Cardiol 26:601–607, 2005.

Appendix C: Cardiovascular Risk Factors

Table C–1. *Estimated Value for Percentile Regression of Waist Circumference (in cm) for European-American Children and Adolescents According to Sex*[*]

Age (yr)	Percentile for Boys					Percentile for Girls				
	10th	25th	50th	75th	90th	10th	25th	50th	75th	90th
2	42.9	46.9	47.1	48.6	50.6	43.1	45.1	47.4	49.6	52.5
3	44.7	48.8	49.2	51.2	54.0	44.7	46.8	49.3	51.9	55.4
4	46.5	50.6	51.3	53.8	57.4	46.3	48.5	51.2	54.2	58.2
5	48.3	52.5	53.3	56.5	60.8	47.9	50.2	53.1	56.5	61.1
6	50.1	54.3	55.4	59.1	64.2	49.5	51.8	55.0	58.8	64.0
7	46.5	50.6	51.3	53.8	57.4	46.3	48.5	51.2	54.2	58.2
8	48.3	52.5	53.3	56.5	60.8	47.9	50.2	53.1	56.5	61.1
9	50.1	54.3	55.4	59.1	64.2	49.5	51.8	55.0	58.8	64.0
10	46.5	50.6	51.3	53.8	57.4	46.3	48.5	51.2	54.2	58.2
11	59.1	63.6	65.8	72.2	81.1	57.5	60.2	64.4	70.3	78.3
12	60.9	65.5	67.9	74.9	84.5	59.1	61.9	66.3	72.6	81.2
13	62.7	67.4	70.0	77.5	87.9	60.7	63.6	68.2	74.9	84.1
14	64.5	69.2	72.1	80.1	91.3	62.3	65.3	70.1	77.2	86.9
15	66.3	71.1	74.1	82.8	94.7	63.9	67.0	72.0	79.5	89.8
16	68.1	72.9	76.2	85.4	98.1	65.5	68.6	73.9	81.8	92.7
17	69.9	74.8	78.3	88.0	101.5	67.1	70.3	75.8	84.1	95.5
18	71.7	76.7	80.4	90.6	104.9	68.7	72.0	77.7	86.4	98.4

[*]Waist circumference was measured with a tape at just above the uppermost lateral border of the right ileum at the end of normal expiration.

From Fernandez JR, Redden DT, Pietrobelli A, Allison DB: Waist circumference percentiles in nationally representative samples of African-American, European-American, and Mexican-American children and adolescents. J Pediatr 145:439–444, 2004.

Table C–2. **Estimated Value for Percentile Regression of Waist Circumference (in cm) for African-American Children and Adolescents According to Sex**[*]

Age (yr)	Percentile for Boys					Percentile for Girls				
	10th	*25th*	*50th*	*75th*	*90th*	*10th*	*25th*	*50th*	*75th*	*90th*
2	43.2	44.6	46.4	48.5	50.0	43.0	44.6	46.0	47.7	50.1
3	44.8	46.3	48.3	50.7	53.2	44.6	46.3	48.1	50.6	53.8
4	46.3	48.0	50.1	52.9	56.4	46.1	48.0	50.2	53.4	57.5
5	47.9	49.7	52.0	55.1	59.6	47.7	49.7	52.3	56.2	61.1
6	49.4	51.4	53.9	57.3	62.8	49.2	51.4	54.5	59.0	64.8
7	51.0	53.1	55.7	59.5	66.1	50.8	53.2	56.6	61.8	68.5
8	52.5	54.8	57.6	61.7	69.3	52.4	54.9	58.7	64.7	72.2
9	54.1	56.4	59.4	63.9	72.5	53.9	56.6	60.9	67.5	75.8
10	55.6	58.1	61.3	66.1	75.7	55.5	58.3	63.0	70.3	79.5
11	57.2	59.8	63.2	68.3	78.9	57.0	60.0	65.1	73.1	83.2
12	58.7	61.5	65.0	70.5	82.1	58.6	61.7	67.3	75.9	86.9
13	60.3	63.2	66.9	72.7	85.3	60.2	63.4	69.4	78.8	90.5
14	61.8	64.9	68.7	74.9	88.5	61.7	65.1	71.5	81.6	94.2
15	63.4	66.6	70.6	77.1	91.7	63.3	66.8	73.6	84.4	97.9
16	64.9	68.3	72.5	79.3	94.9	64.8	68.5	75.8	87.2	101.6
17	66.5	70.0	74.3	81.5	98.2	66.4	70.3	77.9	90.0	105.2
18	68.0	71.7	76.2	83.7	101.4	68.0	72.0	80.0	92.9	108.9

[*]Waist circumference was measured with a tape at just above the uppermost lateral border of the right ileum at the end of normal expiration.

From Fernandez JR, Redden DT, Pietrobelli A, Allison DB: Waist circumference percentiles in nationally representative samples of African-American, European-American, and Mexican-American children and adolescents. J Pediatr 145:439–444, 2004.

Table C–3. **Estimated Value for Percentile Regression of Waist Circumference (in cm) for Mexican-American Children and Adolescents According to Sex**[*]

Age (yr)	Percentile for Boys					Percentile for Girls				
	10th	*25th*	*50th*	*75th*	*90th*	*10th*	*25th*	*50th*	*75th*	*90th*
2	44.4	45.6	47.6	49.8	53.2	44.5	45.7	48.0	50.0	53.5
3	46.1	47.5	49.8	52.5	56.7	46.0	47.4	50.1	52.6	56.7
4	47.8	49.4	52.0	55.3	60.2	47.5	49.2	52.2	55.2	59.9
5	49.5	51.3	54.2	58.0	63.6	49.0	51.0	54.2	57.8	63.0
6	51.2	53.2	56.3	60.7	67.1	50.5	52.7	56.3	60.4	66.2
7	52.9	55.1	58.5	63.4	70.6	52.0	54.5	58.4	63.0	69.4
8	54.6	57.0	60.7	66.2	74.1	53.5	56.3	60.4	65.6	72.6
9	56.3	58.9	62.9	68.9	77.6	55.0	58.0	62.5	68.2	75.8
10	58.0	60.8	65.1	71.6	81.0	56.5	59.8	64.6	70.8	78.9
11	59.7	62.7	67.2	74.4	84.5	58.1	61.6	66.6	73.4	82.1
12	61.4	64.6	69.4	77.1	88.0	59.6	63.4	68.7	76.0	85.3
13	63.1	66.5	71.6	79.8	91.5	61.1	65.1	70.8	78.6	88.5
14	64.8	68.4	73.8	82.6	95.0	62.6	66.9	72.9	81.2	91.7
15	66.5	70.3	76.0	85.3	98.4	64.1	68.7	74.9	83.8	94.8
16	68.2	72.2	78.1	88.0	101.9	65.6	70.4	77.0	86.4	98.0
17	69.9	74.1	80.3	90.7	105.4	67.1	72.2	79.1	89.0	101.2
18	71.6	76.0	82.5	93.5	108.9	68.6	74.0	81.1	91.6	104.4

[*]Waist circumference was measured with a tape at just above the uppermost lateral border of the right ileum at the end of normal expiration.

From Fernandez JR, Redden DT, Pietrobelli A, Allison DB: Waist circumference percentiles in nationally representative samples of African-American, European-American, and Mexican-American children and adolescents. J Pediatr 145:439–444, 2004.

Table C–4. Serum Lipid and Lipoprotein Levels in U.S. Children and Adolescents (mg/dL)

	Sex	Age (yr)	Percentile Values					
			5th	25th	50th	75th	90th	95th
Total cholesterol	Boys	0–4	117	141	156	176	192	209
		5–9	125	147	164	180	197	209
		10–14	123	144	160	178	196	208
		15–19	116	136	150	170	188	203
	Girls	0–4	115	143	161	177	195	206
		5–9	130	150	168	184	201	211
		10–14	128	148	163	179	196	207
		15–19	124	144	160	177	197	209
LDL cholesterol	Boys	5–9	65	82	93	106	121	133
		10–14	66	83	97	112	126	136
		15–19	64	82	96	112	127	134
	Girls	5–9	70	91	101	118	129	144
		10–14	70	83	97	113	130	140
		15–19	61	80	96	114	133	141
HDL cholesterol	Boys	5–9	39	50	56	65	72	76
		10–14	38	47	57	63	73	76
		15–19	31	40	47	54	61	65
	Girls	5–9	37	48	54	63	69	75
		10–14	38	46	54	60	66	72
		15–19	36	44	53	63	70	76
Triglycerides	Boys	0–4	30	46	53	69	87	102
		5–9	31	45	53	67	88	104
		10–14	33	56	61	80	105	129
		15–19	38	55	71	94	124	152
	Girls	0–4	35	46	61	79	99	115
		5–9	33	45	57	73	93	108
		10–14	38	56	72	93	117	135
		15–19	40	55	70	90	117	136

HDL, high-density lipoprotein; LDL, low-density lipoprotein.
From Report of the Expert Panel on Blood Cholesterol Levels in Children and Adolescents. National Cholesterol
  Education Program, U. S. Department of Health and Human Services, National Institutes of Health. NIH Publication
  91-2732, September 1991.

Table C–5. Foods to Choose and Decrease for the Step-One* and Step-Two Diets

Foods to Choose	Food to Decrease
Meat, Poultry, and Fish	
Beef, pork, lamb—lean cuts well trimmed before cooking	Beef, pork, lamb—regular ground beef, fatty cuts, spare ribs, organ meats, sausage, regular luncheon meats, wieners, bacon
Poultry without skin	Poultry with skin, fried chicken
Fish, shellfish	Fried fish, fried shellfish
Processed meat—prepared from lean meat (e.g., turkey, ham, tuna wieners)	Regular luncheon meats (e.g., bologna, salami, sausage, wieners)
Eggs	
Egg whites (two whites equal one whole egg in recipes), cholesterol-free egg substitute	Egg yolk (if more than four per week on step one or if more than two per week on step two); includes eggs used in cooking
Dairy Products	
Milk—skim or 1% fat (fluid, powdered, evaporated), buttermilk	Whole milk (fluid, evaporated, condensed), 2% low-fat milk, imitation milk
Yogurt—nonfat or low-fat yogurt or yogurt beverages	Whole-milk yogurt, whole-milk yogurt beverages
Cheese—low-fat natural or processed cheese (part skim mozzarella, ricotta) with no more than 6 g of fat per ounce on step one or 2 g of fat per ounce on step two	Regular cheese (American, blue, Brie, cheddar, Colby, Edam, Monterey jack, whole-milk mozzarella, Parmesan, Swiss), cream cheese, Neufchatel cheese

Table continued on the following page

Table C–5. **Foods to Choose and Decrease for the Step-One* and Step-Two Diets** *(Continued)*

Foods to Choose	Food to Decrease
Cottage cheese—low fat, nonfat, or dry curd (0% to 2% fat)	Cottage cheese (4% fat)
Frozen dairy dessert—ice milk, frozen yogurt (low fat or nonfat)	Ice cream
	Cream, half-and-half, whipping cream, nondairy creamer, whipped topping, sour cream
Fats and Oils	
Unsaturated oils—safflower, sunflower, corn, soybean, cottonseed, canola, olive, peanut	Coconut oil, palm kernel oil, palm oil
Margarine—made from unsaturated oils previously listed, light or diet margarine	Butter, lard, shortening, bacon fat
Salad dressings—made with unsaturated oils previously listed, low fat or oil free	Dressing made with egg yolk, cheese, sour cream, whole milk
Seeds and nuts—peanut butter, other nut butters	Coconut
Cocoa powder	Chocolate
Breads and Cereals	
Breads—whole grain bread, hamburger and hot dog buns, corn tortilla	Bread in which eggs are a major ingredient, croissants
Cereals—oat, wheat, corn, multigrain	Granola made with coconut
Pasta	Egg noodles and pasta containing egg yolk
Rice	
Dry beans and peas	
Crackers—low-fat animal-type, graham, saltine	High-fat crackers
Homemade baked goods using unsaturated oil, skim or 1% milk, and egg substitute—quick breads, biscuits, cornbread muffins, bran muffins, pancakes, waffles	Commercially baked pastries, muffins, biscuits
Soup—chicken or beef noodle, minestrone, tomato, vegetarian, potato	Soup containing whole milk, cream, meat fat, poultry fat, or poultry skin
Vegetables	
Fresh, frozen, or canned vegetables	Vegetables prepared with butter, cheese, or cream sauce
Fruits	
Fruit—fresh, frozen, canned, or dried	Fried fruit or fruit served with butter or cream sauce
Fruit juice—fresh, frozen, or canned	
Sweets and Modified Fat Desserts	
Beverages—fruit-flavored drinks, lemonade, fruit punch	
Sweets—sugar, syrup, honey, jam, preserves, candy made without fat (candy corn, gumdrops, hard candy), fruit-flavored gelatin	Candy made with chocolate, coconut oil, palm kernel oil, palm oil
Frozen desserts—sherbet, sorbet, fruit ice, popsicles	Ice cream and frozen treats made with ice cream
Cookies, cakes, pies, puddings—prepared with egg whites, egg substitute, skim milk or 1% milk, and unsaturated oil or margarine; gingersnaps; fig bar cookies; angel food cake	Commercially baked pies, cakes, doughnuts, high-fat cookies, cream pies

*The step-one diet has the same nutrient recommendations as the eating pattern recommended for the general population.
From National Cholesterol Education Program: Report of the Expert Panel on Blood Cholesterol Levels in Children and Adolescents. NIH Publication No. 91-2732, September 1991.

Table C–6. **Serving Size of Various Food Groups According to Age and Gender**[*]

	Grains[†]	Vegetables	Fruits	Dairy	Meat and Beans[‡]	Fats, Oils, and Sweets
2–3 yr	3 oz	1 cup	1 cup	2 cup	2 oz	Use sparingly.
4–8 yr	4–5 oz	1½ cups	1½ cups	2 cups	3–4 oz	Sugars are quickly absorbed into
9–13 yr girls	5 oz	2 cups	1½ cups	3 cups	5 oz	bloodstream and unused sugars
9–13 yr boys	6 oz	2½ cups	1½ cups	3 cups	5 oz	are stored as fat.
14–18 yr girls	6 oz	2½ cups	1½ cups	3 cups	5 oz	
14–18 yr boys	7 oz	3 cups	2 cups	3 cups	6 oz	

[*]These guidelines are for children who get about 30 minutes of exercise per day.
[†]An ounce equals 1 slice of bread, 1/2 cup of cooked rice or pasta, or 1/2 cup of oatmeal.
[‡]An ounce equals 1/2 cup cooked dry beans, 1/2 cup of tofu, 1 egg, 1 tablespoon of peanut butter, 1/2 cup of nuts or seeds, or 1 ounce of meat, poultry, or fish.
Adapted from The Food Guide Pyramid, http://www.kidshealth.org/parent/food/general/pyramid.html.

CDC Growth Charts: United States

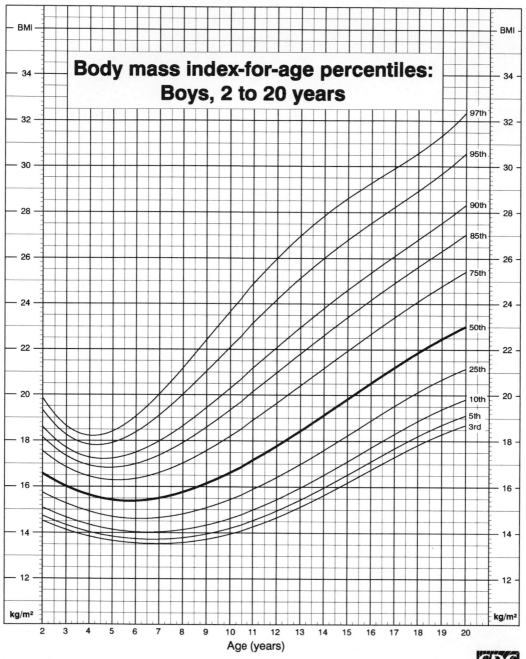

Body mass index-for-age percentiles: Boys, 2 to 20 years

Published May 30, 2000.
SOURCE: Developed by the National Center for Health Statistics in collaboration with
the National Center for Chronic Disease Prevention and Health Promotion (2000).

SAFER · HEALTHIER · PEOPLE™

Figure C–1. *Body mass index percentile curves for boys 2 to 20 years old.*

CDC Growth Charts: United States

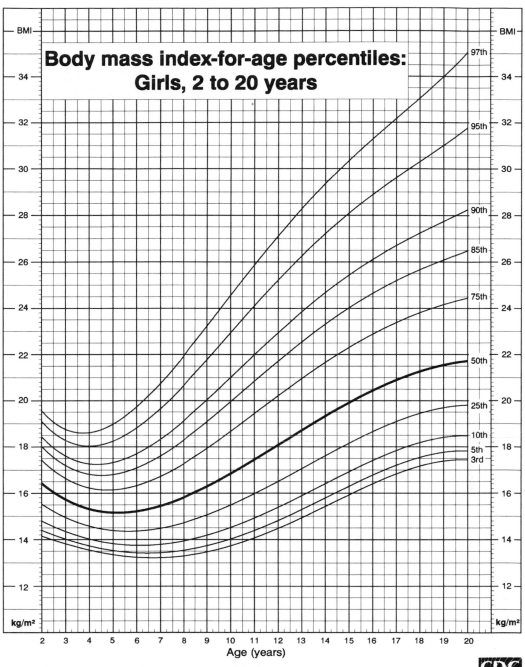

Body mass index-for-age percentiles:
Girls, 2 to 20 years

Published May 30, 2000.
SOURCE: Developed by the National Center for Health Statistics in collaboration with
the National Center for Chronic Disease Prevention and Health Promotion (2000).

Figure C–2. *Body mass index percentile curves for girls 2 to 20 years old.*

Appendix D: Normal Echocardiographic Values and Images

Table D–1. Stand-alone M-Mode Echo Measurements: LA, RV, and LV Size and Thickness of LV Wall by Body Surface Area: Mean (90% Tolerance Limits) (in mm)

BSA (m²) BW in (kg)*	0.25 3	0.3 4	0.4 7	0.5 10	0.6 13	0.7 16	0.8 19	0.9 23	1.0 28	1.2 37	1.4 46	1.6 55	1.8 70	2.0 80
AO dimension (diastolic)	11 (7–15)	12 (7.5–16)	13 (9–17.5)	14 (9.5–19)	15 (10.5–21)	16 (11.5–22)	17 (12.5–24)	18 (13–24.5)	19 (13.5–25)	21 (14.5–27)	22 (15.5–29)	23 (16–30.5)	24 (16–32)	24 (16–33)
LA dimension (systolic)	15 (7–22)	16 (8–23)	18 (9–25)	19 (11–27)	20 (12–29)	22 (13–31)	23 (14–33)	24 (15–34)	26 (16–35)	27 (17–38)	28 (17–40)	29 (18–42)	29 (18–43)	30 (18–44)
RV dimension (diastolic)	8 (0–16)	9.5 (0–17)	10 (0–17)	10 (2.5–18)	11 (3–19)	12 (3.5–21)	13 (4–22)	14 (4.5–23)	14 (5–24)	16 (6–26)	18 (6.5–29)	20 (7–32)	22 (7.5–35)	23 (8–42)
LV diastolic dimension	20 (11–29)	22 (13–30)	25 (16–33)	27 (18–37)	30 (21–40)	33 (23–43)	35 (25–45)	37 (27–47)	39 (28–50)	42 (30–53)	43 (31–56)	45 (32–58)	45 (32–61)	46 (32–62)
LV systolic dimension	12 (7–17)	13 (8–19)	15 (9–21)	17 (11–23)	19 (12–25)	20 (14–27)	22 (15–28)	23 (16–30)	24 (17–31)	26 (18–34)	27 (19–36)	28 (19–37)	28 (19–38)	28 (19–39)
IVS thickness (diastolic)	3.5 (1.5–5.5)	3.5 (1.5–5.5)	4 (1.5–6)	4 (2–6.5)	4.5 (2–7)	5 (2–7)	5 (2.5–7.5)	5.5 (2.5–8)	5.5 (3–8.5)	6 (3–9)	7 (3.5–10)	7.5 (4–11)	8 (4–12)	8.5 (4.5–13)
LVPW thickness (diastolic)	3.5 (1.5–5.5)	3.5 (1.5–5.5)	4 (2–6)	4 (2–6.5)	4.5 (2–7)	5 (2.5–7.5)	5 (2.5–7.5)	5 (3–8)	5.5 (3–8.5)	6 (3–9.5)	7 (3.5–10)	7.5 (4–11)	8 (4–12)	8.5 (4.5–13)

*Approximate weight for average sized individual.
Values rounded off to the nearest 0.5 mm for measurements <10 mm and to the nearest 1 mm for measurements ≥10 mm.
AO, aorta; BSA, body surface area; BW, body weight; IVS, interventricular septum; LA, left atrium; LV, left ventricle; LVPW, LV posterior wall; RV, right ventricle.
Values have been derived from graphic data of Roge CL, Silverman NH, Hart PA, Ray RM: Cardiac structure growth pattern determined by echocardiography. Circulation 57:285–290, 1978.

Table D–2. Two-Dimensional Echo–Derived M-Mode Measurements: Aortic Annulus, LA, and LV Dimensions by Age (Mean and 95% Confidence Limit) (in mm)

Age (yr)	1	2	3	4	5	6	7	8	9	10	11	12	13	14	15	16	17	18
Aortic annulus (PL)	10 (7–13)	11 (8.5–4)	12 (9.5–15)	13 (10–16)	14 (11–17)	15 (12–18)	15 (13–19)	16 (14–19)	17 (14–20)	17 (15–20)	18 (15–21)	18 (16–21)	19 (16–21)	19 (16–22)	19 (16–22)	19 (17–22)	19 (17–22)	19 (17–22)
LA diameter (PL)	17 (12–22)	18 (13–23)	20 (15–25)	21 (16–26)	22 (17–27)	23 (18–28)	24 (19–29)	25 (20–30)	26 (21–31)	27 (22–32)	27 (22–32)	28 (23–33)	28 (23–33)	29 (23–34)	29 (24–34)	29 (24–34)	29 (24–34)	29 (24–34)
LV diameter (PL)	24 (17–32)	27 (19–33)	28 (22–36)	31 (24–38)	33 (26–39)	34 (28–41)	36 (29–43)	37 (31–44)	38 (32–45)	40 (33–47)	41 (34–48)	42 (35–49)	43 (36–50)	43 (37–51)	43 (37–51)	44 (38–52)	44 (38–52)	45 (38–52)

Values have been derived from graphic data of Nidorf SM, Picard MH, Triulzi MO, et al: New perspectives in the assessment of cardiac chamber dimensions during development and adulthood. J Am Coll Cardiol 19:983–988, 1992.

Values rounded off to the nearest 0.5 mm for measurements <10 mm and to the nearest 1 mm for measurements ≥10 mm.

LA, left atrium; LV, left ventricle; PL, parasternal long-axis view.

Table D–3. M-mode Echo Measurements: LA and LV Dimensions by Height (in mm) (Mean and 95% Confidence Limit)

Height (cm)	40	50	60	70	80	90	100	110	120	130	140	150	160	170	180	190	200
LA diameter (PL)	12	14	15	17	18	19	20	22	23	24	26	27	28	30	31	32	33
	(7–18)	(8.5–19)	(10–20)	(11–22)	(13–23)	(14–24)	(15–26)	(17–27)	(18–28)	(19–30)	(21–31)	(22–32)	(23–33)	(24–35)	(26–36)	(27–38)	(28–39)
LV diameter (PL)	17	19	22	24	26	28	30	32	35	37	39	42	44	46	48	50	52
	(10–24)	(13–26)	(14–28)	(17–31)	(19–33)	(21–35)	(23–37)	(25–40)	(27–42)	(30–45)	(32–47)	(34–49)	(37–51)	(39–53)	(41–55)	(43–57)	(45–59)

Values have been derived from graphic data of Nidorf SM, Picard MH, Triulzi MO, et al: New perspectives in the assessment of cardiac chamber dimensions during development and adulthood. J Am Coll Cardiol 19:983–988, 1992.

Values rounded off to the nearest 0.5 mm for measurements <10 mm and to the nearest 1 mm for measurements ≥10 mm.

LA, left atrium; LV, left ventricle; PL, parasternal long-axis view.

Table D–4. Dimensions of Aorta and Pulmonary Arteries by Two-Dimensional Echo[*][†]

Echo Views	BSA (m²)	0.25	0.3	0.4	0.5	0.6	0.7	0.8	1.0	1.2	1.4	1.6	1.8	2.0
	Approx. BW (kg)	3	4	7	10	13	16	19	28	37	46	55	70	80
	AA	10 (7–13)†	11 (7.5–15)	13 (9–16)	14 (10–18)	15 (11–19)	16 (12–20)	17 (12–21)	18 (14–23)	20 (15–25)	22 (16–27)	23 (18–29)	25 (19–31)	26 (20–32)
	MPA	9 (5–12)	10 (6–13)	11 (7–14)	12 (8–16)	13 (9–17)	14 (9–18)	15 (11–19)	16 (12–21)	17 (13–23)	19 (14–24)	21 (14–26)	22 (14–28)	23 (15–29)
	RPA	5.5 (3.5–8)	6 (4–8.5)	6.5 (4.5–9)	7.5 (5–10)	8 (5.5–10)	8.5 (6–11)	9 (7–11)	10 (7–12)	10 (8–14)	11 (8–15)	12 (8.5–16)	13 (9–16)	13 (9–17)
	AA	7.5 (4–10)	8 (4.5–11)	9 (6–12)	10 (6.5–13)	11 (7.5–14)	12 (8.5–15)	12 (9–16)	14 (11–18)	15 (12–19)	17 (14–21)	18 (13–23)	19 (14–24)	20 (15–25)
	TA	6 (4–8.5)	7 (4.5–9)	8 (5.5–11)	9 (6.5–11)	10 (7.5–12)	11 (8–13)	11 (8.5–14)	13 (10–16)	14 (11–17)	15 (12–18)	17 (13–19)	18 (14–21)	19 (15–22)
	RPA	6 (4–8)	6.5 (4.5–9)	7.5 (5–10)	8.5 (6–11)	9 (6.5–11)	9.5 (7–12)	10 (8–13)	12 (9–15)	13 (10–16)	14 (11–17)	15 (11–18)	16 (12–19)	16 (13–20)
	TA	9 (6–11)	10 (7–12.5)	11 (8–14)	12 (9.5–15)	13 (10.5–16)	14 (11–17)	15 (13–18)	17 (14–20)	19 (15–22)	20 (17–24)	22 (18–27)	24 (19–28)	25 (20–30)
	RPA	6 (4–8)	6.5 (4.5–9)	7 (5–10)	8 (6–10)	9 (6.5–11)	9.5 (7.5–11)	10 (8–12)	11 (9–14)	12 (10–15)	13 (11–16)	15 (12–18)	16 (12–19)	16 (13–20)

*Values are rounded off to the nearest 0.5 mm for measurements <10 mm and to the nearest 1 mm for measurements ≥10 mm. Measurements are made at the end of diastole (the Q wave), using a leading-edge technique.

†Figures in parentheses are the tolerance limits weighted for body surface area for prediction of normal values for 80% of the future population with 50% confidence.

AA, ascending aorta; AO, aorta; BSA, body surface area; BW, body weight; LA, left atrium; MPA, main pulmonary artery; RA, right atrium; RPA, right pulmonary artery; RV, right ventricle; SVC, superior vena cava; TA, transverse aorta.

Values have been derived from graphic data of Snider AR, Enderlein MA, Teitel DJ, Juster RP: Two-dimensional echocardiographic determination of aortic and pulmonary artery sizes from infancy to adulthood in normal subjects. Am J Cardiol 53:218–224, 1984.

Table D–5. Aortic Root Dimension by Two-Dimensional Echo: Mean (95% Confidence Limit)

Height (cm)	50	60	70	80	90	100	110	120	130	140	150	160	170	180	190
Aortic annulus	7 (4–10)	8 (5.5–11.5)	9.5 (6.5–13)	10.5 (7–13.5)	12 (8.5–14.5)	13 (9.5–16)	14 (11–17)	15 (12–18)	16.5 (13.5–19)	17 (14–20)	18.5 (15.5–21.5)	19 (16.5–23)	20.5 (17.5–24)	21.5 (18.5–24.5)	23 (19.5–25.5)
Sinus of Valsalva	9 (5–13.5)	11 (7–15)	13 (8–17)	14 (10–18.5)	15.5 (12–20)	17.5 (13.5–22)	19 (15–23.5)	20.5 (16.5–25)	22.5 (18–26.5)	24 (20–27.5)	26 (21.5–29.5)	27.5 (23–31.5)	29 (25–33)	30 (26–34.5)	32 (28–36)
Supra-aortic ridge	7 (4–10)	8.5 (5.5–11.5)	10 (7–13)	11.5 (8–14)	12.5 (9–15.5)	14 (10.5–17)	15 (12–18.5)	16.5 (13.5–19.5)	18 (14.5–20.5)	19 (16–22)	20 (17.5–23.5)	21.5 (18.5–25)	23 (20–26)	24 (21.5–27.5)	25.5 (22.5–28.5)
Ascending aorta	7.5 (3–11.5)	9 (5–12.5)	10.5 (6.5–14)	12 (8–15.5)	13.5 (9.5–17)	15 (11–18.5)	16.5 (12.5–20)	18 (14–21.5)	19 (15–22.5)	20.5 (17–24)	21.5 (18–25.5)	23 (19.5–27)	24 (21–28)	26 (22–30)	27.5 (23.5–32)

SOV/annulus   1.37 (95% CL, 1.18–1.56)
SAR/annulus   1.11 (95% CL, 0.95–1.28)
AAO/annulus   1.16 (95% CL, 0.97–1.35)

*Measurements were obtained in the parasternal long-axis view, perpendicular to the long axis, using a leading edge technique, during systole. Values are rounded off to the nearest 0.5 mm.
AAO, ascending aorta; SAR, supra-aortic ridge; SOV, sinus of Valsalva.
Values are derived from graphic data of Sheil ML, Jenkins O, Sholler GF: Echocardiographic assessment of aortic root dimensions in normal children based on measurement of a new ratio of aortic size independent of growth. Am J Cardiol 75:711–715, 1995.

Table D–6. Mitral and Tricuspid Valve Annulus Diameter by Two-Dimensional Echo: Mean (95% Confidence Interval)

BSA (m²) BW (kg)*	0.2 2	0.25 3	0.3 4	0.4 7	0.5 10	0.6 13	0.7 16	0.8 19	0.9 23	1.0 28	1.2 37	1.4 46
Mitral valve (PL)	10 (7–13)	12 (9–15)	13 (10–16)	16 (13–19)	18 (15–21)	19 (16–23)	21 (18–24)	22 (18–26)	23 (19–26)	24 (20–27)	25 (22–28)	26 (23–30)
Mitral valve (A4C, S4C)†	12 (7–17)	15 (10–20)	17 (12–22)	20 (16–25)	23 (18–28)	25 (20–31)	27 (22–32)	29 (23–35)	31 (25–36)	32 (26–37)	35 (28–40)	36 (31–42)
Tricuspid valve (A4C, S4C)†	12 (8–17)	15 (10–19)	17 (12–22)	21 (16–26)	23 (18–29)	26 (20–31)	27 (22–33)	29 (33–36)	31 (24–37)	32 (25–38)	34 (25–42)	36 (28–44)

Measurements made at onset of R waves on ECG, using inner edge–to–inner edge method.

* Approximate weight for average-sized individuals.

† Measurements greater of two projections A4C and S4C.

A4C, apical four-chamber view; PL, parasternal long-axis view; S4C, subcostal four-chamber view.

Adapted from data presented in graphic form by King DH, Smith EO, Huhta LC, Gutgessel HP: Mitral and tricuspid valve annular diameter in normal children determined by two-dimensional echocardiography. Am J Cardiol 55:787–789, 1985.

Table D-7. Selected Two-Dimensional Echo Measurements of Valve Annuli in Neonates: 95% Prediction Interval (mm)*

Body Weight (kg)	0.5	1.0	1.5	2.0	2.5	3.0	3.5	4.0	4.5	5.0
Aortic valve annulus (PL)	4–5.5	4.5–6	4.5–6.5	5–7	5.5–7.5	6–8	6.5–8.5	7–9	7.5–9	8–9.5
Pulmonary valve annulus (PL)	4–7.5	4.5–8	5.5–9	6–9.5	6.5–10	7.5–11	8–11.5	8.5–12	9.5–13	10–13.5
Mitral valve annulus (PL)	5.5–9.5	6–10	6.5–11	7–11.5	8–12	8.5–13	9–13.5	9.5–14	10–14.5	11–15.5
Mitral valve annulus (apical view)	6–9.5	6.5–10	7.5–11	8–11.5	8.5–12	9–12.5	9.5–13	10.5–14	11–14.5	11.5–15
Tricuspid valve annulus (apical view)	6.5–9.5	7–10.5	8–11	8.5–12	9.5–12.5	10–13.5	11–14	11.5–15	12–15.5	13–16

*Values rounded off to the nearest 0.5 mm.

PL, parasternal long-axis view.

Data are derived from graphic presentation by Tacy TA, Vermillion RP, Ludomirsky A: Range of normal valve annulus size in neonates. Am J Cardiol 75:541–543, 1995.

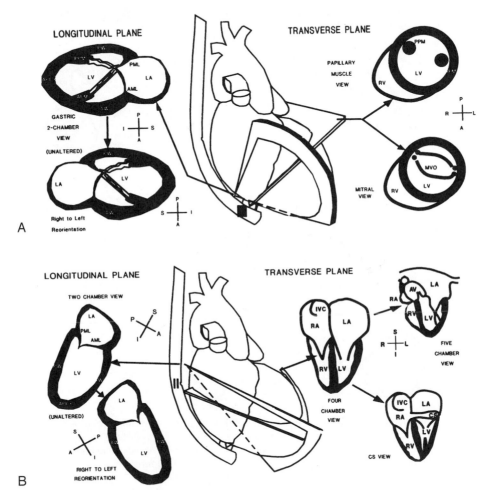

Figure D–1. A, *Biplane transesophageal echocardiographic views from transgastric position III.* ***B,*** *Biplane transesophageal echocardiographic views at midesophageal position II.*

Figure continued on the following page

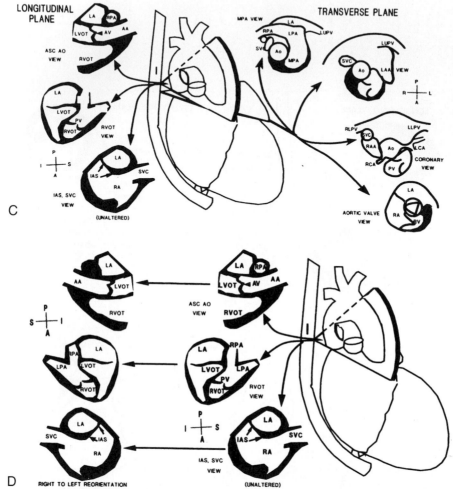

Figure D–1. Continued. ***C,*** *Biplane transesophageal echocardiography views from the base of the heart at position I.* ***D,*** *Basal views of the heart and great vessels with use of the longitudinal plane probe at position I. A, anterior; AA, ascending aorta; AML, anterior mitral leaflet; AO, aorta; ASC, ascending; AV, aortic valve; CS, coronary sinus; I, inferior; IAS, interatrial septum; IVC, inferior vena cava; L, left; LA, left atrium; LAA, left atrial appendage; LCA, left coronary artery; LPA, left pulmonary artery; LUPV, left upper pulmonary vein; LV, left ventricle; LVOT, left ventricular outflow tract; MPA, main pulmonary artery; MVO, mitral valve orifice; P, posterior; PML, posterior mitral leaflet; PPM, posterior papillary muscle; PV, pulmonary valve; R, right; RA, right atrium; RAA, right atrial appendage; RCA, right coronary artery; RLPV, right lower pulmonary vein; RPA, right pulmonary artery; RV, right ventricle; RVOT, right ventricular outflow tract; S, superior; SVC, superior vena cava. (From Bansal RC, Shakudo M, Shah PM, Shah PM: Biplane transesophageal echocardiography: Technique, image orientation, and preliminary experience in 131 patients. J Am Soc Echocardiogr 3:348–366, 1990.)*

Appendix E: Drugs Used in Pediatric Cardiology

Table E–1. **Drug Index (for Drugs Used in Pediatric Cardiology)**

Trade Name	Generic Name	Class
Abbokinase	Urokinase	Thrombolytic agent
Actiq	Fentanyl	Narcotic analgesic
Adalat	Nifedipine	Calcium channel blocker
Adalat CC	Nifedipine, sustained release	Calcium channel blocker
Adenocard	Adenosine	Antiarrhythmic
Adrenaline	Epinephrine HCl	Nonselective adrenergic stimulator
Aldactone	Spironolactone	Aldosterone antagonist
Aldomet	Methyldopa	Antihypertensive
Alprostadil	Prostaglandin E_1	Vasodilator
Anacin	Aspirin	Antiplatelet agent, analgesic
Apresoline	Hydralazine HCl	Peripheral vasodilator
Aquachloral Supprettes	Chloral hydrate	Sedative and hypnotic
Aramine	Metaraminol	α- and β-Adrenoceptor stimulant
Atarax	Hydroxyzine	Sedative
Atromid-S	Clofibrate	Antilipidemic, triglyceride-lowering agent
Bretylol	Bretylium tosylate	Class III antiarrhythmic
Brevibloc	Esmolol	β_1-Selective adrenergic blocking agent, antihypertensive
Bumex	Bumetanide	Loop diuretic
Calan	Verapamil	Class IV antiarrhythmic agent
Capoten	Captopril	ACE inhibitor
Cardioquin	Quinidine	Class IA antiarrhythmic agent
Cardizem	Diltiazem	Calcium channel blocker
Carnitor	Carnitine	L-Carnitine
Colestid	Colestipol	Lipid-lowering agent
Cordarone	Amiodarone	Class III antiarrhythmic
Coreg	Carvedilol	Nonselective β-adrenergic blocker
Coreg Tiltab	Carvedilol	Nonselective β-adrenergic blocker
Coumadin	Warfarin	Anticoagulant
Cozaar	Losartan	Angiotensin-receptor blocker
Demerol	Meperidine	Narcotic analgesic
Digibind	Digoxin immune Fab (ovine)	Antidigoxin antibody
Dilacor XR	Diltiazem	Calcium channel blocker
Dilantin	Phenytoin	Class IB antiarrhythmic
Diulo	Metolazone	Thiazide-like diuretic
Diurigen	Chlorothiazide	Thiazide diuretic
Diuril	Chlorothiazide	Diuretic
Dobutrex	Dobutamine	β_1-Adrenergic stimulator
Dopastat	Dopamine	Sympathomimetic agent
Duragesic	Fentanyl	Narcotic analgesic
DynaCirc	Isradipine	Calcium channel blocker
Dyrenium	Triamterene	Potassium-conserving diuretic
Edecrin	Ethacrynic acid	Loop diuretic
Esidrix	Hydrochlorothiazide Hydro-Par, Oretic	Thiazide diuretic

Table continued on the following page

Table E–1. **Drug Index (for Drugs Used in Pediatric Cardiology)** *(Continued)*

Trade Name	Generic Name	Class
Florinef	Fludrocortisone acetate	Corticosteroids
Fluohydrisone	Fludrocortisone acetate	Corticosteroids
Furomide	Furosemide	Loop diuretic
Hyperstat	Diazoxide	Peripheral vasodilator
HydroDIURIL	Hydrochlorothiazide	Diuretic
Hydro-Par	Hydrochlorothiazide	Thiazide diuretic
Imuran	Azathioprine	Immunosuppressive
Inderal	Propranolol	β-Adrenoceptor blocker, class II antiarrhythmic agent
Indocin	Indomethacin	Nonsteroidal anti-inflammatory agent
Inocor	Amrinone lactate	Noncatecholamine inotropic agent with vasodilating effects
Intropin	Dopamine	Natural catecholamine inotropic agent
Isoptin	Verapamil	Class IV antiarrhythmic agent
Isuprel	Isoproterenol	β_1- and β_2-Adrenergic stimulator
Kabikinase	Streptokinase	Thrombolytic agent
Kayexalate	Sodium polystyrene sulfonate	Potassium-lowering agent
Ketalar	Ketamine	Dissociate anesthetic
Kionex	Sodium polystyrene sulfonate	Potassium-lowering agent
Lanoxin	Digoxin	Cardiac glycoside
Lasix	Furosemide	Loop diuretic
Levocarnitine	Carnitine	L-Carnitine
Levophed	Norepinephrine bitartrate	α- and β-Adrenergic stimulator
Lipitor	Atorvastatin	Lipid-lowering agent, "statin"
Loniten	Minoxidil	Peripheral vasodilator
Lopressor	Metoprolol	β-Adrenoceptor blocker
Lovenox	Enoxaparin	Low-molecular weight heparin (anticoagulant)
Mevacor	Lovastatin	HMG-CoA reductase inhibitor, lipid-lowering agent
Mexitil	Mexiletine	Class IB antiarrhythmic
Minipress	Prazosin HCl	Postsynaptic α-adrenergic blocker, antihypertensive
Mykrox	Metolazone	Thiazide-like diuretic
Narcan	Naloxone	Narcotic antagonist
Neo-Calglucon	Calcium glubionate	Calcium supplement
Neo-Synephrine	Phenylephrine HCl	α-Adrenoceptor stimulant
Neoral	Cyclosporin microemulsion	Immunosuppressive agent
Nipride	Nitroprusside	Peripheral vasodilator
Nitro-bid	Nitroglycerin	Peripheral vasodilator
Nitrostat	Nitroglycerin	Peripheral vasodilator
Noctec	Chloral hydrate	Sedative, hypnotic
Normodyne	Labetalol	α- and β-Adrenergic antagonist
Norpace	Disopyramide phosphate	Class IA antiarrhythmic agent
Norvasc	Amlodipine	Calcium channel blocker
Oretic	Hydrochlorothiazide	Thiazide diuretic
Phenergan	Promethazine	Sedative, antiemetic
Pravachol	Pravastatin	Lipid-lowering agent, HMG-CoA reductase inhibitor
Prevalite	Cholestyramine	Cholesterol-lowering agent
Primacor	Milrinone	Phosphodiesterase inhibitor, noncatecholamine inotropic, vasodilator
Prinivil	Lisinopril	ACE inhibitor
Priscoline	Tolazoline	α-Adrenoceptor blocker
Procan SR	Procainamide	Class IA antiarrhythmic
Procardia	Nifedipine	Calcium-channel blocker
Procardia XL	Nifedipine, sustained release	Calcium-channel blocker
Proglycem	Diazoxide	Antihypertensive agent
Prograf	Tacrolimus	Immunosuppressive agent
Pronestyl	Procainamide	Class IA antiarrhythmic
Prostin VR	Prostaglandin E_1	Vasodilator
Questran	Cholestyramine	Cholesterol-lowering agent
Questran Light	Cholestyramine	Lipid-lowering agent
Quinidex	Quinidine sulfate	Class IA antiarrhythmic

Table E–1. **Drug Index (for Drugs Used in Pediatric Cardiology) (Continued)**

Trade Name	Generic Name	Class
Quinaglute	Quinidine gluconate	Class IA antiarrhythmic
Regitine	Phentolamine mesylate	α-Adrenoceptor blocker
Rogaine	Minoxidil	Peripheral vasodilator
Sandimmune	Cyclosporine	Immunosuppressive
Sofarin	Warfarin	Anticoagulating agent
Streptase	Streptokinase	Thrombolytic agent
Sublimaze	Fentanyl	Narcotic analgesic
Tambocor	Flecainide acetate	Class IC antiarrhythmic
Tenormin	Atenolol	β1-Adrenoceptor blocker
Thorazine	Chlorpromazine	Sedative, antiemetic
Tiazac	Diltiazem	Calcium channel blocker
Tonocard	Tocainide	Class IB antiarrhythmic agent
Trandate	Labetalol	α- and β-Adrenergic antagonist
Tridil	Nitroglycerin	Peripheral vasodilator
Valium	Diazepam	Sedative, antianxiety, antiseizure agent
Vasotec	Enalapril maleate	ACE inhibitor, vasodilator
Vistaril	Hydroxyzine	Sedative
VitaCarn	Carnitine	L-Carnitine
Xylocaine	Lidocaine	Class IB antiarrhythmic
Zestril	Lisinopril	ACE inhibitor
Zocor	Simvastatin	Lipid-lowering agent, HMG-CoA reductase inhibitor
Zaroxolyn	Metolazone	Thiazide-like diuretic

Table E–2. **Dosages of Drugs Used in Pediatric Cardiology**

Drug	Route and Dosage	Toxicities or Side Effects	How Supplied
Adenosine (Adenocard) (antiarrhythmic)	*For supraventricular tachycardia:* *Children and adults:* IV: 50 µg/kg Repeat q1–2 min, with increment of 50 µg/kg, to maximum of 250 µg/kg	Transient bradycardia and tachycardia Transient AV block in atrial flutter/fibrillation (±)	Inj: 3 mg/mL (2 mL)
Amiodarone (Cordarone) (class III antiarrhythmic)	*Children:* IV (in emergency situation): *Loading:* 1 mg/kg, given over a 5–10 min period, 5 doses May be repeated 30 min later Alternatively, IV infusion at a dose of 10–15 mg/ kg/24 hr PO: 5–10 mg/kg/24 hr in 2 doses for 10 days If responsive, 3–5 mg/kg once a day May be reduced to 2.5 mg/kg for 5–7 days thereafter (Therapeutic level: 0.5–2.5 mg/L) *Adults:* PO: *Loading:* 800–1600 mg/ day for 1–3 wk, then reduce to 600–800 mg/ day for 1 mo *Maintenance:* 400 mg/day	Progressive dyspnea and cough (pulmonary fibrosis), worsening of arrhythmias, hepatotoxicity, nausea and vomiting, corneal microdeposits, hypotension and heart block, ataxia, alteration of thyroid function (hypo- or hyperthyroidism), photosensitivity Contraindications: AV block, sinus node dysfunction, sinus bradycardia.	Tab: 200 mg Inj: 50 mg/mL Suspension: 5 mg/mL

Table continued on the following page

Table E–2. **Dosages of Drugs Used in Pediatric Cardiology** *(Continued)*

Drug	Route and Dosage	Toxicities or Side Effects	How Supplied
Amlodipine (Norvasc) (calcium channel blocker, antihypertensive)	*For hypertension:* *Children:* PO: Initial 0.1 mg/kg/dose QD-BID May be increased gradually to a maximum of 0.6 mg/kg/24 hr. *Adults:* PO: 5–10 mg/dose QD (max. 10 mg/24 hr)	Edema, dizziness, flushing, and palpitation. Other side effects include headache, fatigue, nausea, abdominal pain, somnolence	Tab: 2.5, 5, 10 mg Suspension: 1 mg/mL
Amrinone (Inocor) (noncatecholamine inotropic agent with vasodilator effects)	*Children:* IV: *Loading:* 0.5 mg/kg over 2–3 min in ½NS (not D5W) *Maintenance:* 5–20 µg/kg/min *Adults:* IV: *Loading:* 0.75 mg/kg over 2–3 min *Maintenance:* 5–10 µg/ kg/min	Thrombocytopenia, hypotension, tachyarrhythmias, hepatotoxicity, nausea and vomiting, fever	Inj: 5 mg/mL (20 mL)
Acetylsalicylic acid (aspirin)	*Antiplatelet therapy:* *Children:* PO: 3–5 mg/kg every day *Antipyretic/analgesic:* PO: 10–15 mg/kg/dose, q4–6hr (Max. 4 g/24 hr) *Anti-inflammatory:* *Children:* PO: 80–100 mg/kg/24 hr in 4 doses	Rash, nausea, hepatotoxicity, GI bleeding, bronchospasm, GI distress, tinnitus Contraindications: hepatic failure, blooding disorder, hypersensitivity, children <16 yr old with chickenpox or flu symptoms (due to the association with Reye's syndrome)	Tab: 325, 500 mg Tab, enteric-coated: 81,165, 325, 500, 650 mg Tab, chewable: 81 mg Suppository: 60, 120, 125, 130, 195, 200, 300, 325, 600, 650 mg, and 1.2 g.
Atenolol (Tenormin) (β_1-adrenoceptor blocker, antihypertensive, antiarrhythmic)	*Children:* PO: 1–2 mg/kg/24 hr *Adults:* PO: 50 mg once a day for 1–2 wk (alone or with diuretic for hypertension) May increase to 100 mg once a day	CNS symptoms (dizziness, tiredness, depression), bradycardia, postural hypotension, nausea and vomiting, rash, blood dyscrasias (agranulocytosis, purpura)	Tab: 25, 50, 100 mg Suspension: 2 mg/mL Inj: 0.5 mg/mL
Atorvastatin (Lipitor) (lipid-lowering agent, ("statin"), HMG-CoA reductase inhibitor)	*Children:* PO: Starting dose 10 mg QD, for 4–6 wk Increase to 20 mg and 40 mg as needed. (Adult max. dose 80 mg/day)	Headache, constipation, diarrhea, elevated liver enzymes, rhabdomyolysis, myopathy	Tab: 10, 20, 40, 80 mg
Azathioprine (Imuran) (immunosuppressive)	*Children:* PO: *Starting dose*: 1–2 mg/kg/day (to produce WBC count around 5000/mm³); may be reduced if WBC count falls below 4000/mm³	Bone marrow suppression (leukopenia, thrombocytopenia), GI symptoms (nausea and vomiting), hyperlipidemia.	Tab: 50 mg Suspension: 50 mg/mL Inj: 5 mg/mL
Bosentan (nonselective endothelin receptor blocker)	*For pulmonary hypertension (experimental):* *Children:* PO: *<20 kg*: 31.25 mg BID *20–40 kg*: 62.5 mg BID *>40 kg*: 125 mg BID *Adults:* PO: 125 mg BID	Liver dysfunction, decrease in hemoglobin, fluid retention, heart failure, headache	Tab: 62.5, 125 mg

Table E–2. **Dosages of Drugs Used in Pediatric Cardiology** *(Continued)*

Drug	Route and Dosage	Toxicities or Side Effects	How Supplied
Bretylium tosylate (Bretylol) (class III antiarrhythmic)	***For ventricular fibrillation or tachycardia:*** *Children:* IV: 5 mg/kg/dose over 8 min, then 10 mg/kg/dose q15–30 min (maximum 30 mg/kg) *Adults:* IV: 5–10 mg/kg bolus over 8 min q6hr or 1–2 mg/min IV infusion	Hypotension, worsening of arrhythmias, aggravation of digitoxicity, nausea and vomiting	Inj: 50 mg/mL (10-mL ampule)
Bumetanide (Bumex) (loop diuretic)	*Children:* PO, IM, IV: >6 mo: 0.015–0.1 mg/kg/dose, QD-QOD (max. dose: 10 mg/24 hr) *Adults:* PO: 0.5–2 mg/dose, QD-BID MI, IV: 0.5–1 mg over 1–2 min, q2–3hr prn.	Hypotension, cramps, dizziness, headache, electrolyte losses (hypokalemia, hypocalcemia, hyponatremia, hypochloremia), metabolic alkalosis	Tab: 0.5, 1, 2 mg Inj: 0.25 mg/mL
Calcium glubionate (Neo-Calglucon 6.4% elemental calcium) (calcium supplement)	***For neonatal hypocalcemia:*** PO: 1200 mg/kg/24 hr, q4–6hr Maintenance *Infant and child:* PO: 600–2000 mg/kg/day, in 4 doses *Adults:* PO: 6–18 g/day, QID	GI irritation, diarrhea, dizziness, headache. Best absorbed when given before meals.	Syrup: 1.8 g/5 mL (480 mL) (1.2 mEq Ca/mL)
Captopril (Capoten) (angiotensin-converting enzyme inhibitor, antihypertensive, vasodilator)	*Children:* PO: *Newborn:* 0.1–0.4 mg/kg/24 hr, in QD-QID; *Infant:* Initially 0.15–0.3 mg/kg/dose. Titrate upward if needed. Max. dose 6 mg/kg/24 hr, QD-QID. *Child:* Initially 0.3–0.5 mg/kg/dose q8hr. Titrate upward if needed. Max. 6 mg/kg/24 hr, BID-QID. *Adolescent and adult:* Initially 12.5–25 mg/dose, BID-TID. Increase weekly if needed by 25 mg/dose to max. dose 450 mg/24 hr. Smaller dose in renal impairment	Neutropenia/agranulocytosis, proteinuria, hypotension and tachycardia, rash, taste impairment, small increase in serum potassium levels ($\pm$) Evidence of fetal risk if given during second and third trimesters (same with all other ACE inhibitors)	Tab: 12.5, 25, 50, 100 mg Suspension: 0.75, 1 mg/mL
Carnitine (Carnitor)	*Children:* PO: 50–100 mg/kg/24 hr, q8-12hr Increase slowly as needed (max. 3 g/day) *Adults:* PO: 330 mg–1 g/dose, BID-TID	Nausea/vomiting, abdominal cramp, diarrhea	Tab: 330 mg Caps: 250 mg Solution: 100 mg/mL (118 mL) Inj: 200 mg/mL (5 mL)
Carvedilol (Coreg, Coreg Tiltabs) (nonselective β-adrenergic blocker)	*Children:* PO: Initial 0.09 mg/kg/dose, q12hr Increase gradually to 0.36 and 0.75 mg/kg as tolerated to adult max. dose of 50 mg/24 hr.	Dizziness, hypotension, headache, diarrhea, rarely AV block.	Tabs, scored:. 125 mg, 6.125, 12.5, 25 mg

Table continued on the following page

Table E–2. **Dosages of Drugs Used in Pediatric Cardiology** *(Continued)*

Drug	Route and Dosage	Toxicities or Side Effects	How Supplied
	Adults: PO: 3.125 mg, BID for 2 wk; increase slowly to a max. dose of 25 mg BID as needed (for heart failure) (Max. 25 mg BID for <85 kg; 50 mg BID for >85 kg)		
Chloral hydrate (Noctec) (sedative, hypnotic)	*As sedative:* *Children:* PO, PR: 25 mg/kg/dose q8hr *Adults:* PO, PR: 250 mg/dose q8hr *As hypnotic:* *Children:* PO, PR: 50–75 mg/kg/dose *Adults:* PO, PR: 500-2000 mg/dose	Mucous membrane irritation (laryngospasm if aspirated), GI irritation, excitement/delirium (contraindicated in hepatic and renal impairment)	Caps: 500 mg Syrup: 250, 500 mg/ 5 mL Suppository: 324, 500, 648 mg
Chlorothiazide (Diuril) (diuretic)	*Children:* PO: 20–40 mg/kg/24 hr, BID *Adults:* PO: 250–500 mg/dose once a day or intermittently	May increase serum calcium, ↑bilirubin, glucose, and uric acid. Hypochloremic alkalosis, hypokalemia, hyponatremia, prerenal azotemia, rarely pancreatitis, blood dyscrasias, allergic reactions	Tab: 250, 500 mg Suspension: 250 mg/ 5 mL (237 mL) Inj: 500 mg (vial, for reconstruction with 18 mL sterile water)
Chlorpromazine (Thorazine) (sedative, antiemetic)	*For sedation or nausea:* *Children >6 mo:* IM: 0.5 mg/kg/dose q6-8hr prn PO: 0.5 mg/kg/dose q4-6hr prn PR: 1–2 mg/kg/dose q6-8hr prn *Adults:* IM: 25-mg test dose, then 25–50 mg q3-4hr PO: 10–25 mg q4-6hr PR: 100 mg q6-8hr	Hypotension, arrhythmias, first- degree AV block, ST-T changes, hepatotoxicity, leukopenia or agranulocytosis	Syrup: 10 mg/5 mL (120 mL) Tab: 10, 25, 50, 100, 200 mg Supp: 25, 100 mg Oral concentrate: 30 mg/mL, 100 mg/mL. Inj: 25 mg/mL
Cholestyramine (Questran, Prevalite) (cholesterol-lowering agent)	*Children:* PO: 250–1500 mg/kg/24 hr in 2–4 doses *Adults:* PO: *Starting:* 1 packet (or scoopful) of Questran powder or Questran Light 1–2 times/day *Maintenance:* 2–4 packets or scoopfuls/day in 2 doses (or 1–6 doses) *Maximum:* 6 packets/day	Constipation and other GI symptoms, hyperchloremic acidosis, bleeding	Packet of 9-g Questran powder or 5-g Questran Light, each packet containing 4 g anhydrous cholestyramine resin
Clofibrate (Atromid-S) (antilipidemic, triglyceride-lowering agent)	*Children:* PO: 0.5–1.5 mg/day in 2–3 doses *Adults:* PO: *Initial and* *maintenance:* 2 g/day in 2–3 doses	Nausea and other GI symptoms (vomiting, diarrhea, flatulence), headache, dizziness, fatigue, rash, blood dyscrasias, myalgia, arthralgia, hepatic dysfunction	Caps: 500 mg
Clopidogrel (Plavix) (antiplatelet agent)	*Children:* PO: 1 mg/kg/day to max. (adult dose) of 75 mg/day	Bleeding, especially when used with aspirin, neutropenia or agranulocytosis, abdominal pain,	Tab: 75 mg

Table E–2. **Dosages of Drugs Used in Pediatric Cardiology** (*Continued*)

Drug	Route and Dosage	Toxicities or Side Effects	How Supplied
Colestipol (Colestid) (lipid-lowering agent)	*Adults:* PO: 75 mg once a day *Children:* PO: 300–1500 mg/24 hr in 2–4 doses *Adults:* PO: *Starting dose:* 5 g 1–2 times/day, increment of 5 g q1–2mo *Maintenance:* 5–30 g/day in 2–4 doses (mix with 3–6 oz water or another fluid)	constipation, rash, syncope, palpitation Constipation and other GI symptoms (abdominal distention, flatulence, nausea and vomiting, diarrhea), rarely rash, muscle and joint pain, headache, dizziness	Packet: 5 g
Cyclosporine, Cyclosporin microemulsion (Sandimmune, Gengraf, Neonal) (immunosuppressive)	*Children:* PO: 15 mg/kg as a single dose given 4–12 hr pretransplantation; give same daily dose for 1–2 wk post-transplantation, then reduce by 5% per wk to 5–10 mg/kg/24 hr in QD-BID Blood trough level 200–300 ng/mL IV. 5–6 mg/kg as a single dose given 4–12 hr pretransplantation; administer over 2–6 hr; give same dose post-transplantation until patient able to tolerate oral form.	Nephrotoxicity, tremor, hypertension, less commonly hepatotoxicity, hyperlipidemia, hirsutism, gum hypertrophy, rarely lymphoma, hypomagnesemia Reduced blood levels by phenobarbital, phenytoin, or carbamazepine. Increased level by macrolides (erythromycin, azithromycin)	Oral sol: 100 mg/ mL (50 mL) Neoral solution: 100 mg/mL (50 mL) Caps: 25, 50, 100 mg Neonal caps: 25, 100 mg Inj: 50 mg/mL
Diazepam (Valium) (sedative, antianxiety, antiseizure agent)	*For sedation:* *Children >6 mo:* IM, IV: 0.1–0.3 mg/kg/dose q2–4hr (maximum 0.6 mg/kg in 8 hr) PO: 0.2–0.8 mg/kg/24 hr in 3–4 doses, or 1–2.5 mg 3–4 times/day initially and increase prn *Adults:* IM, IV: 2–10 mg/dose q3–4hr prn PO: 2–10 mg/dose q6–8hr prn	Apnea, drowsiness, ataxia, rash, hypotension, bradycardia, hyperexcited state	Tab: 2, 5, 10 mg Oral solution: 1 mg/mL, 5 mg/mL Inj: 5 mg/mL
Diazoxide (Hyperstat, Proglycem) (peripheral vasodilator)	*For hypertensive crisis:* *Children and adults:* IV: 1–3 mg/kg (maximum 150-mg single dose), repeat q5–15 min, titrate to desired effect	Hypotension, transient hyperglycemia, nausea and vomiting, sodium retention (CHF±)	Inj: 15 mg/mL
Digoxin (Lanoxin) (cardiac glycoside)	*Children:* *TDD:* PO: Premature infant: 20 μg/kg; Full-term newborn: 30 μg/kg; Child 1 mo–2 yr: 40-50 μg/kg; Child >2 yr: 30–40 μg/kg IV: 75%–80% of PO dose *Maintenance:* PO: 25%–30% of TDD/day in 2 doses *Adults:* PO: *Loading:* 8–12 μg/kg *Maintenance:* 0.10–0.25 mg/day	AV conduction disturbances, arrhythmias, nausea and vomiting (see Box 30–1 for ECG changes)	Elixir: 50 μg/mL (60 mL) Tab: 125, 250, 500 μg Caps: 50, 100, 200 μg. Inj: 100, 250 μg/mL

Table continued on the following page

Table E–2. **Dosages of Drugs Used in Pediatric Cardiology** *(Continued)*

Drug	Route and Dosage	Toxicities or Side Effects	How Supplied
Digoxin immune Fab (Digibind) (digoxin antidote)	*Infants and children:* IV: 1 vial (40 mg) dissolved in 4 mL H$_2$O, over 30 min *Adults:* IV: 4 vials (240 mg)	Allergic reaction (rare), hypokalemia, rapid AV conduction in atrial flutter	Vial (38 mg)
Diltiazem (Cardizem, Cardizem SR, Cardizem CD, Dilacor XR, Tiazac) (calcium channel blocker, antihypertensive)	*Children:* PO: 1.5–2 mg/kg/24 hr TID-QID Max. dose: 3.5 mg/kg/24 hr *Adolescents:* Immediate release: PO: 30–120 mg/dose, TID-QID; Usual range 180–360 mg/24 hr Extended release: PO: 120–300 mg/24 hr QD-BID (BID dosing with Cardizem SR; QD dosing with Cardizem CD, Dilacor XR, Tiazac)	Dizziness, headache, edema, nausea, vomiting, heart block, and arrhythmias Contraindicated in second- and third-degree AV block, sinus node dysfunction, acute MI with pulmonary congestion. Maximum antihypertensive effect seen within 2 weeks	Tab: 30, 60, 90, 120 mg Extended-release tab: 120, 180, 240 mg Extended-release caps: *Cardizem SR:* 60, 90, 120 mg; *Cardizem CD:* 120, 180, 240, 300, 360 mg *Dilacor XR:* 120, 180, 240 mg *Tiazac:* 120, 180, 240, 300, 360, 420 mg Inj: 5 mg/mL
Dipyridamole (Persantine) (antiplatelet agent)	*Children:* PO: 2–6 mg/kg/day in 3 doses *Adults:* PO: 75–100 mg QID (As an adjunct to warfarin therapy. Not to use with aspirin)	Rare. Dizziness, angina	Tab: 25, 50, 75 mg
Disopyramide (Norpace) (class IA antiarrhythmic)	*Children:* PO: <1 yr: 10–30 mg/kg/24 hr q6hr; 1–4 yr: 10–20 mg/kg/24 hr q6hr; 4–12 yr: 10–15 mg/kg/24 hr q6hr; 12–18 yr: 6–15 mg/kg/24 hr q6hr (q4hr dosing when using regular caps) *Adults:* PO: 150 mg/dose q6hr or 300 mg (extended release) q12hr Max. dose 1.6 g/24 hr	Heart failure or hypotension, anticholinergic effects (urinary retention, dry mouth, constipation), nausea and vomiting, hypoglycemia	Caps: 100, 150 mg CR caps: 100, 150 mg Suspension: 1 mg/mL, 10 mg/mL
Dobutamine (Dobutrex) (β$_1$-adrenergic stimulator)	*Children:* IV: 2–15 μg/kg/min in D5W or NS (incompatible with alkali solution) *Adults:* IV: 2.5–10 μg/kg/min (maximum 40 μg/kg/min)	Tachyarrhythmias, hypertension, nausea and vomiting, headache (contraindicated in IHSS and atrial flutter/fibrillation)	Inj: 12.5 mg/mL (20-mL vial)
Dopamine (Intropin, Dopastat) (natural catecholamine inotropic agent)	*Children:* IV: Effects are dose dependent: 2–5 μg/kg/min—increases RBF and urine output 5–15 μg/kg/min—increases heart rate, cardiac contractility and cardiac output. >20 μg/kg/min— α-adrenergic effects with	Tachyarrhythmias, nausea and vomiting, hypotension or hypertension, extravasation (tissue necrosis [treat with local infiltration of phentolamine])	Inj: 40 mg/mL (5 mL), 80 mg/mL (5 mL), 160 mg/mL (5 mL)

Table E–2. **Dosages of Drugs Used in Pediatric Cardiology** *(Continued)*

Drug	Route and Dosage	Toxicities or Side Effects	How Supplied
	decreased RBF (±) (Incompatible with alkali solution)		

Enalapril, Enalaprilat
(Vasotec)
(ACE inhibitor,
vasodilator)
	Children:
	PO: 0.1 mg/kg/dose QD or
	    BID (maximum 0.5 mg/
	    kg/day)
	Adults:
	For CHF:
	PO: Start with 2.5 mg once
	    or twice daily (usual
	    range 5–20 mg/day)
	For hypertension:
	PO: Start with 5 mg once
	    a day (usual dose
	    10–40 mg/day)
		Hypotension, dizziness, fatigue,
		  headache, rash, diminishing taste,
		  neutropenia, hyperkalemia,
		  chronic cough
		Evidence of fetal risk if given
		  during second and third trimesters
		  (same with all other ACE
		  inhibitors)
			Tab: 2.5, 5, 10,
			  20 mg
			Oral suspension:
			  1 mg/dL
			Inj: 1.25 mg/mL

Enoxaparin
(Lovenox)
(low-molecular-
weight heparin)
(anticoagulant)
	For DVT treatment:
	Infants <2 mo:
	SC: 1.5 mg/kg/dose, q12hr
	Infants ≥2 mo to adults:
	SC: 1 mg/kg/dose, q12hr
	    [Adjust dose to achieve
	    target anti-factor Xa levels
	    of 0.5–1 units/mL]
	For DVT prophylaxis:
	Infants <2 mo:
	SC: 1 mg/kg/dose, q12hr
	Infants ≥2 mo up to 18 yr:
	SC: 0.5 mg/kg/dose, q12hr,
	Adults:
	SC: 30 mg, BID for 7–10 days
		Bleeding	Inj (ampule): 30 mg/
			  0.3 mL

Epinephrine (Adrenalin)
(α-, β$_1$-, and β$_2$-
adrenergic stimulator)
	Children:
	IV: 1:10,000 sol—begin with
	    0.1 μg/kg/min; increase
	    to 1 μg/kg/min to achieve
	    desired effect
		Tachyarrhythmias, hypertension,
		  nausea and vomiting, headache,
		  tissue necrosis (±)
			Inj: 0.01 mg/mL
			  (1:100,000 sol,
			  5 mL)
			0.1 mg/mL
			  (1:10,000 sol,
			  10 mL)
			1 mg/mL (1:1000
			  sol, 1 mL)

Esmolol (Brevibloc)
(β$_1$-selective
adrenergic
blocking agent,
antihypertensive.
class II antiarrhythmic)
	Children:
	IV infusion:
	    Loading dose: 100–
	    500 μg/kg over 1 min.
	    Maintenance: 25–100 μg/
	    kg/min as infusion,
	    increase by 50 μg/kg to
	    a maximum of 300 μg/
	    kg/min
	    (Usual maintenance dose
	    50–500 μg/kg/min)
		Bronchospasm, CHF, hypotension,
		  nausea/vomiting
			Inj: 10, 250 mg/mL

Ethacrynic acid
(Edecrin)
(loop diuretic)
	Children:
	PO: 25 mg/dose once a day
	    (maximum 2–3 mg/
	    kg/ 24 hr)
	IV: 1 mg/kg/dose
	Adults:
	PO: 50–100 mg once a day
	    (maximum 400 mg)
	IV: 0.5–1 mg/kg/dose or
	    50 mg/dose
		Dehydration, hypokalemia, prerenal
		  azotemia, hyperuricemia, eighth
		  cranial nerve damage (deafness),
		  abnormal LFT, agranulocytosis or
		  thrombocytopenia, GI irritation,
		  rash
			Tab: 25, 50 mg
			Inj: (50 mg vial for
			  reconstitution with
			  50 mL D5W)

Fentanyl (Sublimaze,
Duragesic, Fentanyl
Oralet) (narcotic
analgesic)
	For sedation:
	Children:
	IV: 1–3 yr: 2–3 μg/kg/dose;
	    3–12 yr: 1–2 μg/kg/dose;
		Respiratory depression, apnea,
		  rigidity, bradycardia
			Inj: 50 μg/mL
			Fentanyl Oralet:
			  100, 200, 300,
			  400 μg.

Table continued on the following page

Table E–2. **Dosages of Drugs Used in Pediatric Cardiology** (*Continued*)

Drug	Route and Dosage	Toxicities or Side Effects	How Supplied
	>12 yr: 0.5–1 µg/kg/dose; may repeat q30–60 min PO (Fentanyl Oralet) for sedation: 10–15 µg/kg/dose. (Max. 400 µg/dose) *Adults:* IV: 50–100 µg/dose		
Flecainide (Tambocor) (Class IC antiarrhythmic)	*For sustained ventricular tachycardia:* *Children:* PO: Initial 1–3 mg/kg/day, q8hr. Usual range: 3–6 mg/kg/day, q8hr Monitor serum level to adjust dose if needed. [Therapeutic trough level after 2–3 days of continuous dosing: 0.2–1 mg/L] *Adults:* PO: 100 mg, q12hr. May increase by 50 mg q12hr every 4 days to max. dose of 600 mg/24 hr	Worsening of HF, bradycardia, AV block, dizziness, blurred vision, dyspnea, nausea, headache, increased PR and QRS duration Reserve for life-threatening cases.	Tab: 50, 100, 150 mg Suspension: 5, 20 mg/mL
Fludrocortisone acetate (Florinef, Fluohydrisone) (corticosteroids)	*For syncopal episodes:* *Children:* PO: 0.1 mg/dose, once or 2 times a day *Adults:* PO: 0.2 mg/dose, once or 2 times	Hypertension, hypokalemia, acne, rash, bruising, headache, GI ulcers, and growth suppression. Weight gain (1–2 kg in 2–3 wk)	Tab: 0.1 mg
Furosemide (Lasix, Furomide) (loop diuretic)	*Children:* IV: 0.5–2 mg/kg/dose 2–4 times/day PO: 1–2 mg/kg/dose 1–3 times/day prn (maximum 6 mg/kg/dose) *Adults:* IV: 20–40 mg/dose 2–4 times/day PO: 20–80 mg/dose 1–4 times/day prn	Hypokalemia, hyperuricemia, prerenal azotemia, ototoxicity, rarely bloody dyscrasias, rash	Oral liquid: 10 mg/mL 40 mg/5 mL Tab: 20, 40, 80 mg Inj: 10 mg/mL
Heparin (anticoagulant)	*Infants and children:* IV: Initial: 50 U/kg IV bolus Maintenance: 10–25 U/kg/hr as IV infusion, or 50–100 U/kg q4hr IV [Adjust dose to give PTT 1.5–2.5 times control, 6–8 hr after IV infusion (or 3.5–4 hr after injection)] *Adults:* IV: *Initial:* 10,000 U IV inj *Maintenance:* 5000–10,000 U q4-6hr IV drip: *Initial dose:* 5000 U followed by 20,000–40,000 U/24 hr	Bleeding Antidote: protamine sulfate (1 mg per 100 U heparin in previous 4 hr)	Inj: 1000, 2500, 5000, 7500, 10,000 U/mL

Table E–2. **Dosages of Drugs Used in Pediatric Cardiology** *(Continued)*

Drug	Route and Dosage	Toxicities or Side Effects	How Supplied
Hydralazine (Apresoline) (peripheral vasodilator, antihypertensive)	*Children:* IM, IV: 0.15–0.2 mg/kg/dose (for emergency); may be repeated q4–6hr PO: 0.75–3 mg/kg/day in 2–4 doses *Adults:* IM, IV: 20–40 mg/dose (for emergency); repeat prn PO: Start with 10 mg 4 times/day for 3–4 days, increase to 25 mg 4 times/day for 3–4 days, then up to 50 mg 4 times/day	Hypotension, tachycardia and palpitation, lupus-like syndrome with prolonged use (fever, arthralgia, splenomegaly and positive LE-cell preparation), blood dyscrasias	Tab: 10, 25, 50, 100 mg Oral liquid: 1.25, 2, 4 mg/mL Inj: 20 mg/mL
Hydrochlorothiazide (HydroDIURIL, Esidrix, Hydro-Par, Oretic) (thiazide diuretic)	*Children:* PO: 2–4 mg/kg/24 hr in 2 doses *Adults:* PO: 25–100 mg/24 hr, single or divided doses May be given intermittently	Same as for chlorothiazide	Tab: 25, 50, 100 mg Caps: 12.5 mg Solution: 10 mg/mL
Hydroxyzine (Vistaril, Atarax) (sedative)	*Children:* IM: 1 mg/kg/dose q4–6hr prn PO: <6 yr: 50 mg/day in 4 doses; >6 yr: 50–100 mg/day in 4 doses *Adults:* IM: 25–100 mg q4–6 hr (maximum 600 mg/24 hr) PO: 50–100 mg/dose q6hr	CNS symptoms (drowsiness, tremor, convulsion), anticholinergic effects (dry mouth, blurred vision, palpitations, hypotension, urinary frequency)	Suspension; 25 mg/ 5 mL Syrup: 10 mg/5 mL Tab: 10, 25, 50, 100 mg Caps: 25, 50, 100 mg Inj: 25, 50 mg/mL
Indomethacin (Indocin) (nonsteroidal anti-inflammatory, antipyretic agent, PG synthesis inhibitor)	***For PDA closure in premature infants:*** IV: *<48 hr:* 0.2, 01, and 0.1 mg/kg/dose, q12–24 hr. *2–7 days:* 0.2, 0.2, and 0.2 mg/kg/dose, q12–24 hr >7 days: 0.2, 0.25, and 0.25 mg/kg/dose, q12–24 hr	GI or other bleeding, GI disturbances, renal impairment, electrolyte disturbances (decreased sodium and increased potassium levels)	Vial: 1 mg
Isoproterenol (Isuprel) (β_1- and β_2-adrenergic stimulator)	*Children:* IV: 0.1–0.5 µg/kg/min, titrated to desired effect *Adults:* IV: 2–20 µg/min, titrated to desired effect (incompatible with alkali solution)	Similar to epinephrine	Inj: 0.2 mg/mL (1:5000 solution: 1.5 mL)
Isradipine (DynaCirc) (calcium channel blocker, dihydropyridine agent)	***For hypertension*** *Children:* PO: 0.15–0.2 mg/kg/24 hr TID-QID (max, 0.8 mg/kg/24 hr up to 20 mg/24 hr) *Adults:* PO: Initial 2.5 mg BID Max. 20 mg daily	Pedal edema, headache, dizziness, flushing, lightheadedness, asthenia	Caps: 2.5, 5 mg
Ketamine (Ketalar) (dissociate anesthetic)	*Children:* IM: 8–12 mg/kg Repeat smaller doses q30min prn	Hypertension/tachycardia, respiratory depression or apnea, CNS symptoms (dream-like state, confusion, agitation)	Inj: 10, 50, 100 mg/mL

Table continued on the following page

Table E–2. **Dosages of Drugs Used in Pediatric Cardiology** *(Continued)*

Drug	Route and Dosage	Toxicities or Side Effects	How Supplied

Labetalol (Normodyne, Trandate) (α- and β-adrenergic antagonist)	IV: 2–3 mg/kg/dose
	  Repeat smaller doses
	  q30min prn
	Children:
	PO: Initial 4 mg/kg/24 hr,
	  BID
	  Max. 40 mg/kg/24 hr.
	IV: (for hypertensive
	  emergency)
	Initial 0.1–1 mg/kg/dose
	  q10min, prn
	  (Max. 20 mg/dose)
		Orthostatic hypotension, edema, CHF, bradycardia.
		Contraindicated in asthma.
			Tab: 100, 200, 300 mg
			Inj: 5 mg/mL
			Suspension: 10 mg/mL

Lidocaine (Xylocaine) (class IB antiarrhythmic)	*Children:*
	IV: Loading: 1 mg/kg/dose
	  q5–10min prn
	  Maintenance: 30 µg/
	  kg/min IV drip (range
	  20–50 µg/kg/min)
	Adults:
	IV: *Loading:* 1 mg/kg/dose
	  q5min
	  Maintenance: 1–4 mg/min
	  IV drip
		Seizure, respiratory depression, CNS symptoms (anxiety, euphoria or drowsiness), arrhythmias, hypotension or shock	Inj: 10 mg/mL (5-mL ampule), 20 mg/mL (5-, 10- mL ampule)

Lisinopril (Zestril, Prinivil) (ACE inhibitor, antihypertensive)	**For hypertension**
	Children:
	PO: Initial 0.07 mg/kg/day,
	  May increase up to 5 mg/day
	  (max, 0.6 mg/kg/day or
	  40 mg/day)
	Adults:
	PO: Initial 10 mg QD
	  May increase upward as
	  needed to max. 80 mg/day
		Dry nonproductive cough, rash, hypotension, hyperkalemia, angioedema, rarely marrow depression
		Evidence of fetal risk if given during second and third trimesters (same with all other ACE inhibitors)
			Tab: 2.5, 5, 10, 20, 30, 40 mg

Losartan (Cozaar) (angiotensin receptor blocker)	**For hypertension**
	Children:
	PO: 0.7 mg/kg/24 hr,
	  QD-BID, up to 50 mg/24 hr
	Adults:
	PO: Initial dose 50 mg, QD
	  with maximum dose of
	  100 mg QD
		Hypotension, dizziness, nasal congestion, muscle cramps.	Tab: 25, 50, 100 mg

Lovastatin (Mevacor) (HMG-CoA reductase inhibitor, lipid-lowering agent)	*Adolescents (10–17 yr):*
	PO: starting dose 10 mg/day, QD
	  for 6–8 wk; increase to
	  20 mg/day for 8 wk and
	  then increase to 40 mg/day
	  for 8 wk
	Adults:
	PO: starting dose 20 mg/day
	  (range 40–80 mg/day)
		Mild GI symptoms, myositis syndrome, elevated transaminase levels, increased CK levels	Tab: 10, 20, 40 mg

Meperidine (Demerol) (narcotic analgesic)	*Children:*
	IM, IV, PO: 1–1.5 mg/kg/dose
	  q3–4hr prn
	Adults:
	IM, IV, PO: 50–100 mg/dose
	  q3–4hr prn
		Respiratory depression, hypotension, bradycardia, nausea and vomiting	Inj: 25, 50, 75, 100 mg/mL
			Tab: 50, 100 mg
			Syrup: 50 mg/5 mL

Metaraminol (Aramine) (α- and β-adrenoceptor stimulant)	*Children:*
	IV: 0.01 mg/kg/dose IV
	  bolus
	  5 µg/kg/min IV infusion
	  initially, titrated to
	  achieve desired effect
	Adults:
	IV: 0.5–5 mg IV bolus
	  q5–10min prn 1–4 µg/
	  kg/min IV infusion
		Similar to norepinephrine	Inj: 10 mg/mL

Table E–2. **Dosages of Drugs Used in Pediatric Cardiology** *(Continued)*

Drug	Route and Dosage	Toxicities or Side Effects	How Supplied
Methyldopa (Aldomet) (antihypertensive)	*Children:* IV: 5–10 mg/kg/dose over 30–60 min; then 20–40 mg/kg/day in 4 doses (maximum 65 mg/kg/24 hr or 3 g/24 hr) PO: 10 mg/kg/day in 2–4 doses May be increased or decreased (maximum 65 mg/kg/24 hr or 3 g/24 hr) *Adults:* IV: 250–500 mg q6hr (maximum 1 g q6hr) PO: 250 mg 2–3 times/day for 2 days May be increased or decreased q2 days (Usual dose: 0.5–2 g/day in 2–4 doses; maximum 3 g/day)	Sedation, orthostatic hypotension and bradycardia, lupus-like syndrome, Coombs (+) hemolytic anemia and leukopenia, hepatitis or cirrhosis, colitis, impotence	Inj: 50 mg/mL Suspension: 250 mg/mL (16 oz) Tab: 125, 250, 500 mg
Metoprolol (Lopressor) (β_1-adrenoceptor blocker)	*Children >2 yr:* PO: Initial 0.1–0.2 mg/kg/dose BID Gradually increase to 1–3 mg/kg/24 hr. *Adults:* PO: 100 mg/day in 1–3 doses initially May increase to 450 mg/24 hr in 2–3 doses (Usual dose 100–450 mg/24 hr) (Usually used with hydrochlorothiazide 25–100 mg/day)	CNS symptoms (dizziness, tiredness, depression), bronchospasm, bradycardia, diarrhea, nausea and vomiting, abdominal pain	Tab: 50, 100 mg
Metolazone (Zaroxolyn, Diulo, Mykrox) (thiazide-like diuretic)	*Children:* PO: 0.2–0.4 mg/kg/24 hr QD-BID *Adults:* PO: For hypertension: 2.5–5 mg QD For edema: 5–20 mg, QD	Electrolyte imbalance, GI disturbance, hyperglycemia, bone marrow depression, chills, hyperuricemia, hepatitis, rash. May be more effective than thiazide diuretics in impaired renal function	Tab: 0.5 (Mykrox), 2.5, 5, 10 mg Suspension: 1 mg/mL
Mexiletine (Mexitil) (class 1B antiarrhythmic)	*Children:* PO: 6–8 mg/kg/day BID-TID for 2–3 days, then 2–5 mg/kg/dose q6–8hr. Increase 1–2 mg/kg/dose q2–3 days until desired effect achieved (with food or antacid) *Adults:* PO: 200 mg q8hr for 2–3 days Increase to 300–400 mg q8hr (Usual dose 200–300 mg q8hr) Therapeutic level: 0.75–2 µg/mL	Nausea and vomiting, CNS symptoms (headache, dizziness, tremor, paresthesia, mood changes), rash, hepatic dysfunction (±)	Caps: 150, 200, 250 mg
Milrinone (Primacor) (phosphodiesterase inhibitor, noncatecholamine inotropic, vasodilator)	*Children:* IV: *Loading:* 10–50 µg/kg over 10 min, then 0.1–1 µg/kg/min IV drip	Arrhythmias, hypotension, hypokalemia, thrombocytopenia	Inj: 1 mg/mL

Table continued on the following page

Table E–2. **Dosages of Drugs Used in Pediatric Cardiology** *(Continued)*

Drug	Route and Dosage	Toxicities or Side Effects	How Supplied

	Adults:
	IV: *Loading:* 50 µg/kg over
	    10 min
	    0.5 µg/kg/min IV drip
	    (range 0.375–0.75 µg/
	    kg/min)		

Minoxidil
  (Loniten, Rogaine)
  (peripheral
  vasodilator)
	Children <12 yr:
	PO: 0.2 mg/kg/day in
	    1–2 doses initially
	    Increase 0.1–0.2 mg/kg/day
	    q3days until desired
	    effect achieved
	    (Usual dose 0.25–1 mg/kg/
	    day in 1–2 doses;
	    maximum 50 mg/day)
	Children >12 yr and adults:
	PO: 5 mg once a day initially
	    May be increased to 10, 20,
	    40 mg in single or divided
	    doses
	    (Usual dose 10–40 mg/day
	    in 1–2 doses; maximum
	    100 mg/day)
		Reflex tachycardia and fluid
		  retention (used with a beta blocker
		  and diuretic), pericardial effusion,
		  hypertrichosis, rarely blood
		  dyscrasias (leukopenia,
		  thrombocytopenia)
			Tab: 2.5, 10 mg

Morphine sulfate
  (narcotic analgesic)
	Children:
	  SC, IM, IV: 0.1–0.2 mg/kg/
	    dose q2–4hr (maximum
	    15 mg/dose)
	Adults:
	  SC, IM, IV: 2.5–20 mg/dose
	    q2–6hr prn
		CNS depression, respiratory
		  depression, nausea and vomiting,
		  hypotension, bradycardia
			Inj: 8, 10, 15 mg/mL

Mycophenolate mofetil
  (CellCept)
  (immunosuppressant
  agent)
	Children:
	PO: 600 mg/m²/dose, BID
	    Maximum 2000 mg/24 hr.
	    Target drug level: 5–7 ng/mL
	Adults:
	PO/IV: 2000–3000 g/24hr BID
		Headache, GI symptoms,
		  hypertension, bone marrow
		  suppression (anemia), fever,
		  increased risk of developing
		  lymphomas or other malignancies
			Tab: 500 mg
			Caps: 250 mg
			Oral suspension:
			  200 mg/mL
			Inj: 500 mg

Naloxone (Narcan)
  (narcotic antagonist)
	Children:
	IM, IV: 5–10 µg/kg/dose
	    q2–3min for 1–3 doses
	    prn (may need 5–10 doses)
	Adults:
	IM, IV: 0.4–2 mg/dose
	    q2–3min for 1–3 doses prn
		Ventricular arrhythmia, pulmonary
		  edema (±), nausea and vomiting,
		  seizure
			Inj: 0.4, 10 mg/mL
			Neonatal inj:
			  0.02 mg/mL

Nifedipine
  (Procardia, Adalat)
  (calcium channel
  blocker)
	***For hypertrophic
	  cardiomyopathy:***
	Children:
	PO: 0.6–0.9 mg/kg/24 hr
	    in 3–4 doses
	For hypertension:
	Children:
	PO: 0.25-0.5 mg/kg/24 hr
	    in 1–2 doses
	    (max. 3 mg/kg/24 hr up to
	    120 mg/24 hr)
	Adults:
	PO: Initially 10 mg
	    3 times/day
	    Titrate up to 20 or 30 mg
	    3–4 times/day over
	    7–14 days
	    (Usual dose 10–20 mg
	    3 times/day; maximum
	    180 mg/day)
		Hypotension, peripheral edema,
		  CNS symptoms (headache,
		  dizziness, weakness), nausea
			Caps (Adalat,
			  Procardia): 10,
			  20 mg
			Sustained release
			  tabs (Adalat CC,
			  Procardia XL): 30,
			  60, 90 mg:

Table E–2. **Dosages of Drugs Used in Pediatric Cardiology** *(Continued)*

Drug	Route and Dosage	Toxicities or Side Effects	How Supplied

Nitroglycerine (Nitrobid, Tridil, Nitrostat) (peripheral vasodilator)	*Children:*
	IV: 0.5–1 µg/kg/min
	    Increase 1 µg/kg/min
	       q20min to titrate to effect
	       (maximum 6 µg/kg/min)
	       (Dilute in D5W or NS
	         with final concentration
	         <400 µg/mL; light
	         sensitive)
	Adults:
	IV: Initial dose: 5 µg/min
	      through infusion pump
	    Increase 5 µg/min q3–5min
	      until desired effect
	      achieved
		Hypotension, tachycardia, headache, nausea and vomiting	Inj: 5 mg/mL

Nitroprusside (Nipride) (peripheral vasodilator)	*Children:*
	IV: 0.5–8 µg/kg/min,
	      with BP monitoring
	    (Usual dose 2–3 µg/kg/min)
	    (Dilute stock solution
	      [50 mg] in 250–2000 mL
	      D5W; light sensitive)
		Hypotension, sweating and palpitation, nausea and vomiting, cyanide toxicity (metabolic acidosis earliest and most reliable evidence; monitor thiocyanate level when used >48 hr and in renal failure)	Inj: 50 mg (vial for reconstitution with 2–3 mL D5W)

Norepinephrine (Levophed, levarterenol) (α- and β-adrenoceptor stimulant)	*Children:*
	IV: 0.1 µg/kg/min initially;
	      increase dose to attain
	      desired effect
	Adults:
	IV: Add 4 mL levarterenol
	      to 1000 mL D5W, start
	      at 2–3 mL/min (8–12
	      µg/min) and adjust rate
		Hypertension, bradycardia (reflex), arrhythmias, tissue necrosis (treat with phentolamine infiltration)	Inj: 1 mg/mL

Phentolamine (Regitine) (α-adrenoceptor blocker)	***For pheochromocytoma:***
	Children:
	IM, IV: 0.05–0.1 mg/kg/dose
	    Repeat q5min until
	      hypertension is controlled,
	      then q2–4hr prn
	Adults:
	IM, IV: 2.5–5 mg/dose
	    Repeat q5min until
	      hypertension is controlled,
	      then q2–4hr prn
	For treatment of extravasated
	α-adrenergic drugs:
	SC: 0.1–0.2 mg/kg locally
	    within 12 hr (maximum
	    10 mg)
		Hypotension, tachycardia or arrhythmias, nausea and vomiting	Inj: 5 mg/mL

Phenylephrine (Neo-Synephrine) (α-adrenoceptor stimulant)	***For hypotension:***
	Children:
	IM, SC: 0.1 mg/kg/dose
	    q1–2hr prn
	IV: 5–10 µg/kg/dose IV
	    bolus q10–15min or
	    0.1–0.5 µg/kg/ min
	    IV infusion
	Adults:
	IM, SC: 2–5 mg/dose
	    q1–2hr prn
	IV: 0.1–0.5 mg/dose IV
	    bolus q10–15min prn
		Arrhythmias, hypertension, angina	Inj: 10 mg/mL

Table continued on the following page

Table E–2. **Dosages of Drugs Used in Pediatric Cardiology** *(Continued)*

Drug	Route and Dosage	Toxicities or Side Effects	How Supplied
	Start IV infusion at 100–180 μg/min; maintain at 40–60 μg/min		
Phenytoin (Dilantin) class IB antiarrhythmic)	*Children:* IV: 2–4 mg/kg/dose over 5–10 min followed by: PO: 2–5 mg/kg/day in 2–3 doses (Therapeutic level: 5–18 μg/mL for arrhythmias, 10–20 μg/mL for seizures) *Adults:* IV: 100 mg q5min (total 500 mg) PO: 250 mg 4 times for 1 day, 250 mg twice for 2 days, and 300–400 mg/day in 1–4 doses	Rash, Stevens-Johnson syndrome, CNS symptoms (ataxia, dysarthria), lupus-like syndrome, blood dyscrasias, peripheral neuropathy, gingival hypertrophy	Inj: 50 mg/mL Suspension: 125 mg/5 mL (240 mL) Chewable tabs: 50 mg (Infatab) Caps: 100 mg
Potassium chloride	***Supplement in diuretic therapy:*** *Children:* PO: 1–2 mEq/kg/day in 3–4 doses (0.8–1.5 mL 10% potassium chloride/kg/day, or 0.4–0.7 mL 20% potassium chloride/kg/day in 3–4 doses)	GI disturbances, ulcerations, hyperkalemia	10% sol: 1.3 mEq/mL 20% sol: 2.7 mEq/mL Sustained release caps: 8, 10 mEq Sustained release tab: 6, 7, 8, 10, 20 mEq
Potassium gluconate	***Supplement in diuretic therapy:*** *Children:* PO: 1–2 mEq/kg/day in 3–4 doses or 0.8–1.5 mL/kg/day in 3–4 doses	Same as for potassium chloride	Elixir: 1.3 mEq/mL
Pravastatin (Pravachol) (lipid-lowering agent, HMG-CoA reductase inhibitor)	*Children:* PO: Starting dose 10 mg, QD for 4–6 wk Increase to 20 or 40 mg as needed. (Adult max. dose 80 mg/day)	Headache, constipation, diarrhea, elevated liver enzymes, rhabdomyolysis, myopathy	Tab: 10, 20, 40, 80 mg
Prazosin (Minipress) (postsynaptic α-adrenergic blocker; antihypertensive)	*Children:* PO: 5 μg/kg as a test dose, then 25–150 μg/kg/day in 4 doses *Adults:* PO: 1 mg 2–3 times/day initially Increase to 20 mg/day in 2–4 doses (Usual dose 6–15 mg/day)	CNS symptoms (dizziness, headache, drowsiness), palpitation, nausea	Caps: 1, 2, 5 mg
Procainamide (Pronestyl) (class IA antiarrhythmic)	*Children:* IV: *Loading:* 3–6 mg/kg/dose over 5 min repeated q10–30min (maximum 100 mg) *Maintenance:* 20–80 μg/kg/min by IV infusion (maximum 2 g/24 hr) PO: 15–50 mg/kg/day q3–6hr (maximum 4 g/24 hr) *Adults:* IV: *Loading:* 50–100 mg/dose q5min prn *Maintenance:* 1–6 mg/min by IV infusion	Nausea and vomiting, blood dyscrasias, rash, lupus-like syndrome, hypotension, confusion or disorientation	Tab: 250, 375, 500 mg Tab, sustained release: 250, 500, 750, 1000 mg Caps: 250, 375, 500 mg Suspension: 6, 50, 100 mg/mL Inj: 100, 500 mg/mL

Table E–2. **Dosages of Drugs Used in Pediatric Cardiology** *(Continued)*

Drug	Route and Dosage	Toxicities or Side Effects	How Supplied
	PO: 250–500 mg/dose q3-6hr (usual dose 2–4 g/day). Therapeutic level: 4–10 µg/mL		
Promethazine (Phenergan) (sedative, antiemetic)	*For nausea and vomiting:* *Children:* IM, PR: 0.25–0.5 mg/kg q4–6hr prn *Adults:* IM, PR: 12.5–25 mg q6hr prn *For sedation before surgery:* *Children:* IM, PO, PR: 0.5–1 mg/kg/dose q6hr prn *Adults:* IM, PO, PR: 25–50 mg q4-6hr prn	CNS stimulation, anticholinergic effects	Tab: 12.5, 25, 50 mg Syrup: 6.25 mg/5 mL, 25 mg/5 mL Supp: 12.5, 25, 50 mg Inj: 25, 50 mg/mL
Propranolol (Inderal) (β-adrenoceptor blocker, class II antiarrhythmic)	*For hypertension:* *Children:* PO: 2–4 mg/kg/24 hr in 2–4 doses (maximum 16 mg/kg/24 hr) *For arrhythmias:* *Children:* IV: 0.01–0.15 mg/kg/dose over 10 min (maximum 1 mg/dose) PO: 2–4 mg/kg/24 hr in 3–4 doses (maximum 16 mg/kg/24 hr) *Adults:* IV: 1 mg/dose q5min (maximum 5 mg) PO: 40–320 mg/24 hr in 3–4 doses	Hypotension, syncope, bronchospasm, nausea and vomiting, hypoglycemia, lethargy or depression, heart block	Tab: 10, 20, 40, 60, 80, 90 mg Extended-release caps: 60, 80, 120, 160 mg Oral solution: 20, 40 mg/5 mL Concentrated solution: 80 mg/mL Inj: 1 mg/mL
Prostaglandin E$_1$ or alprostadil (Prostin VR) (vasodilator)	*For patency of ductus arteriosus:* IV: Begin infusion at 0.05–0.1 µg/kg/min When desired effect achieved, reduce to 0.05, 0.025, and 0.01 µg/kg/min If unresponsive, dose may be increased to 0.4 µg/kg/min	Apnea, flushing, bradycardia, hypotension, fever	Ampule: 500 µg/mL
Protamine sulfate (heparin antidote)	*Antidote to heparin overdose:* IV: Each 1-mg protamine neutralizes approx 100 U heparin given in preceding 3–4 hr Slow IV infusion at rate not exceeding 20 mg/min or 50 mg/10 min Check APTT	Hypotension, bradycardia, dyspnea, flushing, coagulation problem	Inj: 10 mg/mL
Quinidine (Cardioquin, Quinidex, Quinaglute) (class IA antiarrhythmic)	*Children:* Test dose for idiosyncrasy: 2 mg/kg once (PO as sulfate; IM/IV as gluconate) Therapeutic dose: IV (as gluconate): 2–10 mg/kg/dose, q3–6hr, prn PO (as sulfate): 15–60 mg/kg/24 hr q6hr)	Nausea and vomiting, ventricular arrhythmias, prolonged QRS complex, depressed myocardial contractility, blood dyscrasias, symptoms of cinchonism	*Gluconate* (62% quinidine): Slow-release tab: 330 mg Inj: 80 mg/mL *Sulfate* (83% quinidine): Tab: 200, 300 mg

Table continued on the following page

Table E–2. **Dosages of Drugs Used in Pediatric Cardiology** *(Continued)*

Drug	Route and Dosage	Toxicities or Side Effects	How Supplied

	Adults:
	Test dose: 200 mg once
	  PO/IM
	Therapeutic dose:
	PO (as sulfate) immediate
	  release:
	  100–600 mg/dose q4–6hr.
	  Begin at 200 mg/dose
	  and titrate to desired
	  effect, or
	PO (sulfate, sustained release):
	  300–600 mg/
	  dose q8–12hr
	IM (as gluconate): 400 mg/dose
	  q4–6hr
	IV (as gluconate): 200–400 mg/
	  dose, infused at a rate of
	  ≤10 mg/min
	PO (as gluconate):
	  324–972 mg q8–12hr
			Slow-release tabs:
			  300 mg
			Suspension:
			  10 mg/mL

Simvastatin
  (Zocor)
  (lipid-lowering agent,
  HMG-CoA reductase
  inhibitor)
	Children:
	PO: Starting dose 10 mg, QD
	  Increment of 10 mg
	  q6–8wk to max. dose of
	  40 mg/day as needed.
	  (Adult max. dose 80 mg/day)
		Headache, constipation, diarrhea,
		  elevated liver enzymes,
		  rhabdomyolysis, myopathy
			Tab: 5, 10, 20, 40,
			  80 mg

Sodium polystyrene
  sulfonate
  (Kayexalate, Kionex)
  (potassium-lowering
  agent)
	For hyperkalemia (slowly
	  effective, taking hours to days):
	Children:
	PO, NG: 1 g/kg/dose q6hr
	PR: 1 g/kg/dose q2–6hr
	Adults:
	PO, NG, PR: 15 g (4 level
	  tsp) 1–4 times/day
		(Cation exchange resin with
		  practical exchange rates of 1 mEq
		  potassium per 1 g resin)
		(Note: Delivers 1 mEq sodium for
		  each mEq of potassium removed)
		Nausea and vomiting, constipation,
		  severe hypokalemia (muscle
		  weakness, confusion [monitor
		  serum potassium levels, ECG]),
		  hypocalcemia or hypernatremia
		  (edema)
			Powder: 454,
			  480 g/lb
			Suspension:
			  15 g/60 mL

Spironolactone
  (Aldactone)
  (aldosterone
  antagonist)
	Children:
	PO: 3 mg/kg/day in 1–2 doses
	Adults:
	PO: 50–100 mg/day in
	  3–4 doses (maximum
	  200 mg/day)
		Hyperkalemia (when given with
		  potassium supplements), GI
		  distress, rash, gynecomastia,
		  agranulocytosis
		Contraindicated in renal failure.
			Tab: 25, 50, 100 mg
			Suspension: 1, 2, 5,
			  25 mg/mL

Streptokinase
  (Streptase, Kabikinase)
  (thrombolytic agent)
	For thrombolysis:
	Children:
	IV: 3500–4000 U/kg over
	  30 min, followed by
	  1000–1500 U/kg/hr, or
	  2000 U/kg load over
	  30 min followed by
	  2000 U/kg/hr,
	  [Duration of infusion based
	  on response but generally
	  does not exceed 3 days]
	Obtain tests at baseline and
	  q4hr: APTT, TT, fibrinogen,
	  PT, hematocrit, platelet
	  count
	APTT and TT should be
	  <2 times control
		Potential for allergic reaction with
		  repeated use; premedicate with
		  acetaminophen and antihistamine,
		  and repeat q4-6hr
			Inj:
			  250,000, 600,000,
			  750,000, 1,500,000
			  U/6.5-mL vial

Tocainide
  (Tonocard)
  (class IB
  antiarrhythmic)
	Children:
	PO: 20–40 mg/kg/day in
	  3 doses
		Dizziness and vertigo, nausea and
		  vomiting, blood dyscrasias (±)
			Tab: 400, 600 mg

Table E–2. **Dosages of Drugs Used in Pediatric Cardiology** *(Continued)*

Drug	Route and Dosage	Toxicities or Side Effects	How Supplied
	Adults: PO: 400 mg q8hr May increase to 600 mg q8hr (Usual dose 400–600 mg q8hr)		
Tolazoline (Priscoline) (α-adrenoceptor blocker)	*For neonatal pulmonary* *hypertension:* IV: *Loading:* 1–2 mg/kg over 10 min *Maintenance:* 1–2 mg/kg/hr IV infusion	Hypotension and tachycardia, pulmonary hemorrhage, GI bleeding, arrhythmias, thrombocytopenia, leukopenia	Inj: 25 mg/mL
Triamterene (Dyrenium) (potassium- sparing diuretic)	*Children:* PO: 2–4 mg/kg/24 hr in 1–2 doses. May increase up to max. 6 mg/kg/24 hr or 300 mg/24 hr *Adults:* PO: 50–100 mg/24 hr in 1–2 doses (maximum 300 mg/24 hr)	Nausea and vomiting, leg cramps, dizziness, hyperuricemia, rash, prerenal azotemia	Caps: 50, 100 mg
Urokinase (Abbokinase) (thrombolytic agent)	*Children:* *For clot lysis:* IV: *Loading:* 4400 U/kg over 10 min *Maintenance:* 4400 U/kg/H for 6–12 hr. Some patients may require 12–72 hr of therapy. Monitor same laboratory tests as for streptokinase *For catheter clearance:* IV: Infuse 1 mL (containing 5000 U/mL) into catheter, aspirate with 5-mL syringe q5min 6 times; may repeat urokinase infusion prn *Adults:* *For pulmonary embolism:* IV: Priming dose: 4400 U/kg IV infusion 4400 U/kg/H for 12 hr by infusion pump	Bleeding, allergic reactions, rash, fever and chills, bronchospasm	Inj: 5000 U/mL
Verapamil (Isoptin, Calan) (calcium channel blocker, class IV antiarrhythmic agent)	*For dysrhythmia (SVT):* *Children:* IV: 1-15 yr 0.1–0.3 mg/kg over 2 min May repeat same dose in 15 min. Max. dose 5 mg first dose; 10 mg second dose *Adults:* IV: 5–10 mg, 10 mg second dose *For hypertension:* *Children:* PO: 4–8 mg/kg/24 hr in 3 doses *Adults:* PO: 240–480 mg/24 hr in 3–4 doses	Hypotension, bradycardia, cardiac depression	Tab: 40, 80, 120 mg Extended-release tab: 120, 180, 240 mg Extended-release caps: 100, 120, 180, 200, 240, 300, 360 mg Suspension: 50 mg/mL Inj: 2.5 mg/mL
Vitamin K$_1$	*Antidote to dicumarol or* *warfarin:* PO/IM/SC/IV: 2.5–10 mg/dose in 1 dose for correction of excessive PT from		Tab: 5 mg Inj: 2, 10 mg/mL

Table continued on the following page

Table E–2. **Dosages of Drugs Used in Pediatric Cardiology** *(Continued)*

Drug	Route and Dosage	Toxicities or Side Effects	How Supplied
	dicumarol or warfarin overdose		
Warfarin (Coumadin, Sofarin) (anticoagulant)	*Children:* PO: *Initial:* 0.1–0.2 mg/kg/dose QD for 2 days in evening (Max. dose 10 mg/dose) [Liver dysfunction, 0.1 mg/kg/ day, max. 5 mg/dose] *Maintenance:* 0.1 mg/kg/ 24 hr QD. Monitor INR after 5–7 days of new dosage. Keep INR at 2.5–3.5 for mechanical prosthetic valve; 2–3 for prophylaxis of DVT, pulmonary emboli. Heparin preferred initially for rapid anticoagulation; warfarin may be started concomitantly with heparin or may be delayed 3–6 days *Adults:* PO: *Initial:* 5–15 mg/day for 2–5 days *Maintenance:* 2–10 mg/day. Adjust dosage based on INR	Bleeding (antidote: vitamin K or fresh-frozen plasma) *Increased PT response:* salicylates, acetaminophen, alcohol, lipid- lowering agents, phenytoin, ibuprofen, some antibiotics *Decreased PT response:* antihistamines, barbiturates, oral contraceptives, vitamin C, diet high in vitamin K Onset of action: 36–72 hr. and full effects in 45 days. Mode of action: inhibits hepatic synthesis of vitamin-K dependent factors (I, VII, IX, X).	Tab: 1, 2, 2.5, 3, 4, 5, 6, 7.5, 10 mg Inj: 5 mg

ACE, angiotensin-converting enzyme; APTT, activated partial thromboplastin time; AV, atrioventricular; BP, blood pressure; caps, capsule; CHF, congestive heart failure; CK, creatine kinase; CNS, central nervous system; CR, controlled release; D5W, 5% dextrose in water; DVT, deep vein thrombosis; ECG, electrocardiogram; GI, gastrointestinal; HMG-CoA, 3-hydroxy-3-methylglutaryl coenzyme A; IHSS, idiopathic hypertrophic subaortic stenosis; IM, intramuscular; inj, injection; INR, international normalized ratio; IV, intravenous; LFT, liver function test; NE, norepinephrine; NG, nasogastric; NS, normal saline; PDA, patent ductus arteriosus; PG, prostaglandin; PO, by mouth; PR, per rectum; prn, as necessary; PT, prothrombin time; q, every; RBF, renal blood flow; SC, subcutaneous; sol, solution; supp, suppository; susp, suspension; tab, tablet; TDD, total digitalizing dose; TT, thrombin time; WBC, white blood cell; (±), may occur.

Suggested Readings

GENERAL REFERENCES

Allen HD, Gutgesell HP, Clark EB, Driscoll DJ: Moss and Adams' Heart Disease in Infants, Children, and Adolescents, Including the Fetus and Young Adult, 6th ed. Philadelphia, Lippincott Williams & Wilkins, 2001.

Gillette PC, Garson A Jr: Clinical Pediatric Arrhythmias, 2nd ed. Philadelphia, WB Saunders, 1999.

Jonas RA: Comprehensive Surgical Management of Congenital Heart Disease. London, Arnold, 2004.

Mavroudis C, Backer CL: Pediatric Cardiac Surgery, 3rd ed. Philadelphia, Mosby, 2003.

Moller JH, Hoffman JIE: Pediatric Cardiovascular Medicine. New York, Churchill Livingstone, 2000.

Park MK, Guntheroth WG: How to Read Pediatric ECGs, 4th ed. Philadelphia, Mosby, 2006.

Snider AR, Serwer GA, Ritter SB: Echocardiography in Pediatric Heart Disease, 2nd ed. St. Louis, Mosby, 1997.

Walsh EP, Saul JP, Triedman JK: Cardiac Arrhythmias in Children and Young Adults With Congenital Heart Disease. Philadelphia, Lippincott Williams & Wilkins, 2001.

CHAPTER 1. HISTORY TAKING

Copel JA, Kleinman CS: Congenital heart disease and extracardiac anomalies: Association and indications for fetal echocardiography. Am J Obstet Gynecol 154:1121–1132, 1986.

Greenwood RD, Rosenthal A, Nadas AS: Cardiovascular malformations associated with congenital diaphragmatic hernia. Pediatrics 57:92–97, 1976.

Nora JJ: Etiologic aspects of heart disease. In Adams FH, Emmanouilides GC, Riemenschneider TA (eds): Moss' Heart Disease in Infants, Children, and Adolescents, 4th ed. Baltimore, Williams & Wilkins, 1989.

Schafer AI: The hypercoagulable states. Ann Intern Med 102:814–828, 1985.

CHAPTER 2. PHYSICAL EXAMINATION

Braunwald E, Perloff JK: Physical examination of the heart and circulation. In Braunwald E, Zipes DP, Libby P (eds): Heart Disease, 6th ed. Philadelphia, WB Saunders, 2001, pp 45–81.

Chobanian AV, Bakris GL, Black HR, et al: The Seventh Report of the Joint National Committee on Prevention, Detection, Evaluation, and Treatment of High Blood Pressure: The JNC 7 report. JAMA 289:2560–2572, 2003.

Fourth Report on the Diagnosis, Evaluation, and Treatment of High Blood Pressure in Children and Adolescents. National High Blood Pressure Education Program Working Group on High Blood Pressure in Children and Adolescents. Pediatrics 111:555–576, 2004.

Frolich ED, Labarth DR, Maxwell MH, et al: Recommendations for human blood pressure determination by sphygmomanometers: Report of a special task force appointed by the Steering Committee, American Heart Association. Circulation 77:501A–514A, 1988.

Leatham A: Auscultation of the heart. Lancet 2:757–766, 1958.

National High Blood Pressure Education Program Working Group on Hypertension Control in Children and Adolescents: Update on the 1987 Task Force on high blood pressure in children: a working group report from the National High Blood Pressure Education Program. Pediatrics 98:649–658, 1996.

O'Rourke MF, Blazek JV, Morreels CL Jr, Krovetz LJ: Pressure wave transmission along the human aorta: Changes with age and in arterial degenerative disease. Circ Res 23:567–579, 1968.

Park MK: Blood Pressure Tables [letter]. Pediatrics 115:826–827, 2005.

Park MK, Guntheroth WG: Accurate blood pressure measurement in children: A review. Am J Noninvas Cardiol 3:297–309, 1989.

Park MK, Lee D-H: Normative blood pressure values in the arm and calf in the newborn. Pediatrics 83:240–243, 1989.

Park MK, Lee D-H, Johnson GA: Oscillometric blood pressure in the arm, thigh and calf in healthy children and those with aortic coarctation. Pediatrics 91:761–765, 1993.

Park MK, Menard SW: Accuracy of blood pressure measurement by the Dinamap Monitor in infants and children. Pediatrics 79:907–914, 1987.

Park MK, Menard SW, Schoolfield J: Oscillometric blood pressure standards for children. Pediatr Cardiol 26:601–607, 2005.

Park MK, Menard SW, Yuan C: Comparison of auscultatory and oscillometric blood pressure. Arch Pediatr Adolesc Med 155:50–53, 2001.

Park MK, Menard SW, Yuan C: Comparison of blood pressure in children from three ethnic groups. Am J Cardiol 87:1305–1308, 2001.

Pelech AN: Evaluation of the pediatric patient with a cardiac murmur. Pediatr Clin North Am 46: 167–188, 1999.

Perloff JK: Physical Examination of the Heart and Circulation, 3rd ed. Philadelphia, WB Saunders, 2000.

Report of the Second Task Force on Blood Pressure Control in Children. Pediatrics 79:1–25, 1987.

Rosenthal A: How to distinguish between innocent and pathologic murmurs in childhood. Pediatr Clin North Am 31:1229–1240, 1984.

Rudolph AM: Congenital Diseases of the Heart: Clinical-Physiologic Considerations in Diagnosis and Management. St. Louis, Mosby, 1974.

CHAPTER 3. ELECTROCARDIOGRAPHY

Park MK, Guntheroth WG: How to Read Pediatric ECGs, 3rd ed. St. Louis, Mosby, 1992.

Towbin JA, Bricker JT, Garson A: Electrocardiographic criteria for diagnosis of acute myocardial infarction in childhood. Am J Cardiol 69:1545–1548, 1992.

CHAPTER 4. CHEST ROENTGENOGRAPHY

Amplatz K: Plain film diagnosis of congenital heart disease. In Moller JH, Hoffman JIE (eds): Pediatric Cardiovascular Medicine. New York, Churchill Livingstone, 2000, pp 143–155.

CHAPTER 5. FLOW DIAGRAMS

Kawabori I: Cyanotic congenital heart defects with decreased pulmonary blood flow. Pediatr Clin North Am 25:759–776, 1978.

Kawabori I: Cyanotic congenital heart defects with increased pulmonary blood flow. Pediatr Clin North Am 25:777–795, 1978.

Stevenson JG: Acyanotic lesions with normal pulmonary blood flow. Pediatr Clin North Am 25:725–742, 1978.

Stevenson JG: Acyanotic lesions with increased pulmonary blood flow. Pediatr Clin North Am 25: 743–758, 1978.

CHAPTER 6. NONINVASIVE TECHNIQUES

Ahmad F, Kavey R-E, Kveselis DA, Gaum WE: Response of non-obese white children to treadmill exercise. J Pediatr 139:284–290, 2001.

Chatrath R, Shenoy R, Serratto M, Thoele DG: Physical fitness of urban American children. Pediatr Cardiol 23:608–612, 2002.

Cumming GR, Everatt D, Hartman L: Bruce treadmill test in children: Normal values in a clinic population. Am J Cardiol 41:69–75, 1978.

Gibbons RJ, Balady GJ, Bricker JT, et al: ACC/AHA 2002 Guideline Update for Exercise Testing. J Am Coll Cardiol 40:1531–1540, 2005.

Huhta JC, Gutgesell HP, Murphy DJ Jr, et al: Segmental analysis of congenital heart disease. Dynamic Cardiovasc Imaging 1:117–125, 1987.

Nishimura RA, Abel MD, Hatle LK, et al: Assessment of diastolic function of the heart: Background and current applications of Doppler echocardiography. II. Clinical studies. Mayo Clin Proc 64:181–204, 1989.

Paridon SM, Alpert BS, Boas SR, Cabrera ME, et al: Clinical stress testing in the pediatric age group. A statement from the American Heart Association Council on Cardiovascular Disease in the Young, Committee on Atherosclerosis, Hypertension, and Obesity in Youth. Circulation 113:1905–1920, 2006.

Rowell LB, Brengelmann GL, Blackmon JR, et al: Disparities between aortic and peripheral pulse pressure induced by upright exercise and vasomotor changes in man. Circulation 37:954–964, 1968.

Soergel M, Kirschstein M, Busch C, et al: Oscillometric twenty-four-hour ambulatory blood pressure values in healthy children and adolescents: A multicenter trial including 1141 subjects. J Pediatr 130:178–184, 1997.

Sorof J, Portman RJ: Ambulatory blood pressure monitoring in pediatric patients. J Pediatr 165: 578–586, 2000.

Southall DP, Johnson AM, Shinebourne EA, et al: Frequency and outcome of disorder of cardiac rhythm and conduction in a population of newborn infants. Pediatrics 68:58–66, 1981.

Southall DP, Richards J, Mitchell P, et al: Study of cardiac rhythm in healthy newborn infants. Br Heart J 43:14–20,1980.

CHAPTER 7. INVASIVE PROCEDURES

Cassidy SC, Schmidt KG, Van Hare GF, et al: Complications of pediatric cardiac catheterization: A 3-year study. J Am Coll Cardiol 19:1285–1293, 1992.

Lock JE, Keane JF, Mandell VS, et al: Cardiac catheterization. In Fyler DC (ed): Nadas' Pediatric Cardiology. St. Louis, Mosby, 1992.

Mullins CE, Nihil MR: Cardiac catheterization hemodynamics and intervention. In Moller JH, Hoffman HE (eds): Pediatric Cardiovascular Medicine. New York, Churchill Livingstone, 2000, pp 203–215.

CHAPTER 8. FETAL AND PERINATAL CIRCULATION

Guntheroth WG, Kawabori I, Stevenson JG: Physiology of the circulation: Fetus, neonate, and child. In Kelly VC (ed): Practice of Pediatrics, vol 8. Philadelphia, Harper & Row, 1982–1983.

Rudolph AM: Congenital Diseases of the Heart: Clinical-Physiologic Considerations in Diagnosis and Management. Chicago, Mosby, 1974.

CHAPTERS 9, 10, AND 11. PATHOPHYSIOLOGY OF LEFT-TO-RIGHT SHUNT LESIONS, PATHOPHYSIOLOGY OF OBSTRUCTIVE AND VALVULAR REGURGITANT LESIONS, AND PATHOPHYSIOLOGY OF CYANOTIC CONGENITAL HEART DEFECTS

Duc G: Assessment of hypoxia in the newborn: Suggestions for a practical approach. Pediatrics 48: 469–481, 1971.

Guntheroth WG, Morgan BC, Mullins GL, Baum D: Venous return with knee-chest position and squatting in tetralogy of Fallot. Am Heart J 75:313–318, 1968.

Guntheroth WG, Morgan BC, Mullins GL: Physiologic studies of paroxysmal hyperpnea in cyanotic congenital heart disease. Circulation 31:66–76, 1965.

Heath D, Edwards JE: The pathology of hypertensive pulmonary vascular disease. Circulation 18:533–547, 1958.

King SB, Franch RH: Production of increased right-to-left shunting by rapid heart rates in patients with tetralogy of Fallot. Circulation 44:265–271, 1971.

Moller JH, Amplatz K, Edwards JE: Congenital Heart Disease. Kalamazoo, Mich, Upjohn, 1971.

Rudolph AM: Congenital Diseases of the Heart. Chicago, Mosby, 1974.

CHAPTER 12. LEFT-TO-RIGHT SHUNT LESIONS

Atrial Septal Defect

Laussen PC, Bichell DP, McGowan FX, et al: Postoperative recovery in children after minimum versus full length sternotomy. Ann Thorac Surg 69:591–596, 2000.

Radzik D, Davignon A, van Doesburg N, et al: Predictive factors for spontaneous closure of atrial septal defect diagnosed in the first 3 months of life. J Am Coll Cardiol 22:851–853, 1993.

Rao V, Freedom RM, Black MD: Minimally invasive surgery with cardioscopy for congenital heart defects. Ann Thorac Surg 68:1742–1745, 2000.

Shivaprakahas K, Murthy KS, Coelho R, et al: Role of limited posterior thoracotomy for open-heart surgery in the current era. Ann Thorac Surg 68:2310–2313, 1999.

Wax DF: Therapeutic cardiac catheterization in children. The Children's Doctor. Journal of Children's Memorial Hospital, Chicago. http://www.childsdoc.org/Fall99/catheterization.asp.

Ventricular Septal Defect

Fyler DC: Ventricular septal defect. In Fyler DC (ed): Nadas' Pediatric Cardiology. Philadelphia, Hanley & Belfus, 1992.

Graham TP Jr, Bender HW, Spach MS: Ventricular septal defect. In Adams FH, Emmanouilides GC, Riemenschneider TA (eds): Moss' Heart Disease in Infants, Children and Adolescents, 4th ed. Baltimore, Williams & Wilkins, 1989.

Hoffman JI: Natural history of congenital heart disease. Problems in its assessment with special reference to ventricular septal defects. Circulation 37:97–125, 1968.

Soto B, Becker AE, Moulaezt AH, et al: Classification of ventricular septal defects. Br Heart J 43:332–363, 1980.

Patent Ductus Arteriosus

Desfrere L, Zohar S, Morville P, et al: Dose-finding study of ibuprofen in patent ductus arteriosus using the continual reassessment method. J Clin Pharm Ther 30:121–132, 2005.

Musewe NN, Poppe D, Smallhorn JF, et al: Doppler echocardiographic measurement of pulmonary artery pressure from ductal Doppler velocities in the newborn. J Am Coll Cardiol 15:446–456, 1990.

Musewe NN, Smallhorn JF Benson LN, et al: Validation of Doppler-derived pulmonary arterial pressure in patients with ductus arteriosus under different hemodynamic states. Circulation 76:1081–1091, 1987.

Rao PS, Sideris EB, Haddad J, et al: Transcatheter occlusion of patent ductus arteriosus with adjustable buttoned device: Initial clinical experience. Circulation 88:1119–1126, 1993.

Van Overmeire B, Smets K, Lecoutere D, et al: A comparison of ibuprofen and indomethacin for closure of patent ductus arteriosus. N Engl J Med 343:674–681, 2000.

Varvarigou A, Bardin CL, Beharry K, et al: Early ibuprofen administration to prevent patent ductus arteriosus in premature newborn infants. JAMA 275:539–544, 1996.

Endocardial Cushion Defect

Anderson RH, Macartney FJ, Shineboume EA, et al: Atrioventricular septal defects. In Anderson RH, Macartney FJ, Shinebourne EA, et al (eds): Pediatric Cardiology. New York, Churchill Livingstone, 1987.

Piccoli GP, Gerlis LM, Wilkinson JL, et al: Morphology and classification of atrioventricular defects. Br Heart J 42:621–632, 1979.

Rastelli GC, Kirklin JW, Titus JL: Anatomic observation on complete form of persistent common atrioventricular canal with special reference to atrioventricular valves. Mayo Clin Proc 41: 296–308, 1966.

Partial Anomalous Pulmonary Venous Return

Ward KE, Mullins CE: Anomalous pulmonary venous connections; pulmonary vein stenosis; atresia of the common pulmonary vein. In Garson A Jr, Bricker JT, McNamara DG (eds): The Science and Practice of Pediatric Cardiology. Philadelphia, Lea & Febiger, 1990.

CHAPTER 13. OBSTRUCTIVE LESIONS

Pulmonary Stenosis

Cournay V, Peiechaud JF, Delogu A, et al: Balloon valvotomy for critical stenosis or atresia or pulmonary valve in newborns. J Am Coll Cardiol 26:1725–1731, 1995.

Nugent EW, Freedom RM, Nora JJ, et al: Clinical course in pulmonic stenosis. Circulation 56:15–28, 1977.

Stanger P, Cassidy SC, Dried DA, et al: Balloon pulmonary valvuloplasty: Results of the valvuloplasty and angioplasty of congenital anomalies registry. Am J Cardiol 65:775–783, 1990.

Aortic Stenosis

ACC/AHA 2006 guidelines for the management of patients with valvular heart disease. Circulation 114:e84–e231, 2006 or J Am Coll Cardiol 48:e1–e148, 2006.

Farivar RS, Cohn LH: Hypercholesterolemia is a risk factor for bioprosthetic valve calcification and explantation. J Thorac Cardiovasc Surg 126:969–975, 2003.

Kouchoukos NT, Davila-Roman VG, Spray TL, et al: Replacement of the aortic root with a pulmonary autograft in children and young adults with aortic valve disease. N Engl J Med 330:1–6, 1994.

Lupinetti FM, Pridjian AK, Callow LB, et al: Optimum treatment of discrete subaortic stenosis. Ann Thorac Surg 54:467–471, 1992.

Van Son JAM, Schaff HV, Danielson GK, et al: Surgical treatment of discrete and tunnel subaortic stenosis. II. Late survival and risk of reoperation. Circulation 88:159–169, 1993.

Wilson WR, Greer GE, Durzinsky DS, Curtis JJ: Ross procedure for complex left ventricular outflow tract obstruction, J Cardiovasc Surg 41:387–392, 2000.

Coarctation of the Aorta

Cowley CG, Orsmond GS, Feola P, et al: Long-term, randomized comparison of balloon angioplasty and surgery for native coarctation of the aorta in childhood. Circulation 111:3453–3456, 2005.

Hellenbrand WE, Allen HD, Golinko RJ, et al: Balloon angioplasty for aortic recoarctation: Results of valvuloplasty and angioplasty of congenital anomalies registry. Am J Cardiol 65:793–797, 1990.

Hornberger LK, Weintraub RG, Pesonen E, et al: Echocardiographic study of the morphology and growth of the aortic arch in the human fetus. Observations related to the prenatal diagnosis of coarctation. Circulation 86:741–747, 1992.

Peuster M, Wohlsein P, Brugman M, et al: A novel approach to temporary stenting: Degradable cardiovascular stents produced from corrodible metal-results 6-18 months after implantation into New Zealand white rabbits. Heart 86:563–569, 2001.

Tynan M, Finley JP, Fontes V, et al: Balloon angioplasty for the treatment of native coarctation: Results of valvuloplasty and angioplasty of congenital anomalies registry. Am J Cardiol 65:790–793, 1990.

CHAPTER 14. CYANOTIC CONGENITAL HEART DEFECTS

Complete Transposition of the Great Arteries

Blume ED, Altman K, Mayer JE, et al: Evolution of risk factors influencing early mortality of the arterial switch operation. J Am Coll Cardiol 33:1702–1709, 1999.

Jex RK, Puga FJ, Julsrud PR, et al: Repair of transposition of the great arteries with intact ventricular septum and left ventricular outflow tract obstruction. J Thorac Cardiovasc Surg 100:682–686, 1990.

Lupinetti FM, Bove EL, Minich LL, et al: Intermediate-term survival and functional results after arterial repair for transposition of the great arteries. J Thorac Cardiovasc Surg 103:421–427, 1992.

Morell VO, Jacobs JP, Quintessenza JA: Aortic translocation in the management of transposition of the great arteries with ventricular septal defect and pulmonary stenosis: Results and follow-up. Ann Thorac Surg 79:2089–2093, 2005.

Waldeman JD, Lamberti JJ, George L, et al: Experience with Damus procedure. Circulation 78(suppl III): III-32–III-39, 1988.

Yacoub M, Bernhard A, Lange P, et al: Clinical and hemodynamic results of the two-stage anatomic correction of simple transposition of the great arteries. Circulation 62(suppl I):I-190–I-196, 1980.

Congenitally Corrected Transposition of the Great Arteries

Dabizzi RP, Barletta GA, Caprioli G, et al: Coronary artery anatomy in corrected transposition of the great arteries. J Am Coll Cardiol 12:486–491, 1988.

Graham TP, Bernard YD, Mellen BG, et al: Long-term outcome in congenitally corrected transposition of the great arteries. J Am Coll Cardiol 36:255–261, 2000.

Lundstrom U, Bull C, Wyse RKH, et al: The natural and "unnatural" history of congenitally corrected transposition. Am J Cardiol 65:1222–1229, 1990.

Tetralogy of Fallot

Bonhoeffer P, Boudjemline Y, Saliba Z, et al: Percutaneous replacement of pulmonary valve in a right-ventricle to pulmonary-artery prosthetic conduit with valve dysfunction. Lancet 356:1403–1405, 2000.

Gupta A, Odim J, Levi D, et al: Staged repair of pulmonary atresia with ventricular septal defect and major aortopulmonary collateral arteries: Experience with 104 patients. J Thorac Cardiovasc Surg 126:1746–1752, 2003.

Khambadkone S, Coats L, Taylor A, et al: Percutaneous pulmonary valve implantation in humans: Results in 59 consecutive patients. Circulation 112:1189–1197, 2005.

Kirklin JW, Blackstone EH, Jonas RA, et al: Morphologic and surgical determinant of outcome events after repair of tetralogy of Fallot and pulmonary stenosis: A two-institution study. J Thorac Cardiovasc Surg 103:706–723, 1992.

Lakier JB, Stanger P, Heymann MA, et al: Tetralogy of Fallot with absent pulmonary valve: Natural history and hemodynamic considerations. Circulation 50:167–175, 1974.

Need LR, Powell AJ, del Nide P, et al: Coronary echocardiography in tetralogy of Fallot: Diagnostic accuracy, resource utilization and surgical implications over 13 years. J Am Coll Cardiol 36:1371–1377, 2000.

Puga FJ, Leoni FE, Julsrud PR, et al: Complete repair of pulmonary atresia, ventricular septal defect, and severe peripheral arborization abnormalities of the central pulmonary arteries. J Thorac Cardiovasc Surg 98:1018–1029, 1989.

Reddy VM, Liddicoat JR, Hanley FL: Midline one-stage complete unifocalization and repair of pulmonary atresia with ventricular septal defect and major aortopulmonary collaterals. J Thorac Cardiovasc Surg 109:832–844, 1995.

Sawatari K, Imai Y, Kurosawa H, et al: Staged operation for pulmonary atresia and ventricular septal defect with major aortopulmonary collateral arteries. J Thorac Cardiovasc Surg 98:738–750, 1989.

Watterson KG, Wilkinson JL, Karly TR, Mee RBB: Very small pulmonary arteries: Central end-to-side shunt. Ann Thorac Surg 52:1131–1137, 1991.

Total Anomalous Pulmonary Venous Return

Lupinetti FM, Kulik TJ, Beekman RH, et al: Correction of total anomalous pulmonary venous connection in infancy. J Thorac Cardiovasc Surg 106:880–885, 1993.

Van der Velde ME, Parness IA, Colan SD, et al: Two-dimensional echocardiography in pre- and postoperative management of totally anomalous pulmonary venous connection. J Am Coll Cardiol 18:1746–1751, 1991.

Tricuspid Atresia

Bjork VO, Olin CL, Bjarke BB, et al: Right atrial-right ventricular anastomosis for correction of tricuspid atresia. J Thorac Cardiovasc Surg 77:452–458, 1979.

Bridges ND, Mayer JE, Lock JE, et al: Effects of baffle fenestration on outcome of the modified Fontan operation. Circulation 86:1762–1769, 1992.

Castaneda AR: From Glenn to Fontan: A continuing evolution. Circulation 86(suppl II):II-80–II-84, 1992.

Chang RK, Alejos JC, Atkinson D, et al: Bubble contrast echocardiography in detecting pulmonary arteriovenous shunting in children with univentricular heart after cavopulmonary anastomosis. J Am Coll Cardiol 33:2052–2058, 1999.

Fontan F, Baudet E: Surgical repair of tricuspid atresia. Thorax, 26:240–248, 1971.

Gentles TL, Mayer JE Jr, Gauvreau K, et al: Fontan operation in five hundred consecutive patients: Factors influencing early and late outcome. J Thorac Cardiovasc Surg 114:376–391, 1997.

Giannico S, Como A, Marino B, et al: Total extracardiac right heart bypass. Circulation 86(suppl II):II-110–II-117, 1992.

Hsu DT, Wuaegebeur JM, Ing FF, et al: Outcome after the single-stage, nonfenestrated Fontan procedure. Circulation 96:11-335–11-340, 1997.

Jacob ML, Norwood WL Jr: Fontan operation: Influence of modification on morbidity and mortality. Ann Thorac Surg 58:945–951, 1991.

Kawashima Y, Kitamura S, Matsuda H, et al: Total cavopulmonary shunt operation in complex cardiac anomalies: A new operation. J Thorac Cardiovasc Surg 87:74–81, 1984.

Kreutzer G, Galindez E, Bono H, et al: An operation for the correction of tricuspid atresia. J Thorac Cardiovasc Surg 66:613–621, 1973.

Mertens L, Hagler DJ, Sauer U, et al: Protein-losing enteropathy after the Fontan operation: An international multicenter study. J Thorac Cardiovasc Surg 115:1063–1073, 1998.

Norwood WI Jr, Jacobs ML, Murphy JD: Fontan's procedure for hypoplastic left heart syndrome. Ann Thorac Surg 54:1025–1029, 1992.

Pearl JM, Laks H, Drinkwater DC, et al: Modified Fontan procedure in patients less than 4 years of age. Circulation 86(suppl II):II-100–II-105, 1992.

Song JY, Choi JY, Ko JT, et al: Long-term aspirin therapy for hepatopulmonary syndrome. Pediatrics 97:917–920,1966.

Thompson LD, Petrossian E, McElhinney DB, et al: Is it necessary to routinely fenestrate an extracardiac Fontan? J Am Coll Cardiol 34:539–544, 1999.

Pulmonary Atresia

Alwi M, Geetha K, Bilkis AA, et al: Pulmonary atresia with intact ventricular septum percutaneous radiofrequency-assisted valvotomy and balloon dilatation versus surgical valvotomy and Blalock-Taussig shunt. J Am Coll Cardiol 35:468–476, 2000.

Bull C, de Leval MR, Mercanti C, et al: Pulmonary atresia and intact ventricular septum: A revised classification. Circulation 66:266–280, 1982.

Cheung YF, Leung MP, Chae AK: Usefulness of laser-assisted valvotomy with balloon valvoplasty for pulmonary valve atresia with intact ventricular septum. Am J Cardiol 90:438–442, 2002.

Hanley FL, Sade RM, Blackstone EH, et al: Outcomes in neonatal pulmonary atresia with intact ventricular septum: A multi-institutional study. J Thorac Cardiovasc Surg 105:406–427, 1993.

Kan JS, White RI Jr, Mitchell SE, et al: Percutaneous balloon valvuloplasty: A new method for treating congenial pulmonary-valve stenosis, N Engl J Med 307:540–542, 1982.

Hypoplastic Left Heart Syndrome

Chang AC, Farrell PE Jr, Murdison KA, et al: Hypoplastic left heart syndrome: Hemodynamic and angiographic assessment after initial reconstructive surgery and relevance to modified Fontan procedure. Pediatr Cardiol 17:1143–1149, 1991.

Douglas WI, Goldberg CS, Mosca RS, et al: Hemi-Fontan procedure for hypoplastic left heart syndrome: Outcome and suitability for Fontan. Ann Thorac Surg 68:1361–1368, 1999.

Glauser TA, Rorke LB, Weinberg PM, Clancy RR: Congenital brain anomalies associated with the hypoplastic left heart syndrome. Pediatrics 85:984–990, 1990.

Jacobs ML: Recent innovations in the Norwood sequence of operations. Cardiol Young 14(suppl 1): 47–51, 2004.

Kishimoto H, Kawahira Y, Kawata H, et al: The modified Norwood palliation on a beating heart. J Thorac Cardiovasc Surg 118:1130–1132, 1999.

Norwood WI, Lang P, Castaneda AR, et al: Experience with operations for hypoplastic left heart syndrome. J Thorac Cardiovasc Surg 82:511–519, 1981.

Starnes VA, Griffin ML, Pitlick PT, et al: Current approach to hypoplastic left heart syndrome: Palliation, transplantation, or both. J Thorac Cardiovasc Surg 104:189–195, 1992.

Ebstein's Anomaly

Cappato R, Schuter M, Weiss C, et al: Radiofrequency current catheter ablation of accessory atrioventricular pathways in Ebstein's anomaly. Circulation 94:376–383, 1996.

Carpentier A, Chauvaud S, Mace L, et al: A new reconstructive operation for Ebstein's anomaly of the tricuspid valve. J Thorac Cardiovasc Surg 96:92–101, 1988.

Danielson GK, Driscoll DJ, Mair DD, et al: Operative treatment of Ebstein's anomaly. J Thorac Cardiovasc Surg 104:1195–1202, 1992.

Shiina A, Sewer JB, Edwards WD, et al: Two-dimensional echocardiographic spectrum of Ebstein's anomaly: Detailed anatomic assessment. J Am Coll Cardiol 3:356–370, 1984.

Starnes VA, Pitlick PT, Bernstein D, et al: Ebstein's anomaly appearing in the neonate, J Thorac Cardiovasc Surg 101:1082–1087, 1991.

Truncus Arteriosus

Lenox CC, Debich DE, Zuberbuhler JR: The role of coronary artery abnormalities in the prognosis of truncus arteriosus. J Thorac Cardiovasc Surg 104:1724–1742, 1992.

Spicer RL, Behrendt D, Crowley DC, et al: Repair of truncus arteriosus in neonates with the use of a valveless conduit. Circulation 70(suppl I):I-26–I-29, 1984.

Williams JM, de Leeuw M, Black MD, et al: Factors associated with outcomes of persistent truncus arteriosus. J Am Coll Cardiol 34:545–553, 1999.

Single Ventricle

Douville EC, Sade RM, Fyfe DA: Hemi-Fontan operation in surgery for single ventricle: A preliminary report. Ann Thorac Surg 51:893–899, 1991.

Freedom RM, Benson LN, Smallhorn JF, et al: Subaortic stenosis, the univentricular heart, and banding of the pulmonary artery: An analysis of the courses of 43 patients with univentricular heart palliated by pulmonary artery banding. Circulation 73:758–764, 1986.

Newfeld EA, Niakidoh H: Surgical management of subaortic stenosis in patients with a single ventricle and transposition of the great vessels. Circulation 76(suppl III): III-29–III-33, 1987.

Sano S, Ishino K, Kawata M, et al: Right ventricle–pulmonary artery shunt in first-stage palliation of hypoplastic left heart syndrome. J Thorac Cardiovasc Surg 126:504–510, 2003.

Stein DG, Iaks H, Drinkwater DC, et al: Results of total cavopulmonary connection in the treatment of patients with a functional single ventricle. J Thorac Cardiovasc Surg 102:280–287, 1991.

Double-Outlet Right Ventricle

Belli E, Serraf A, Lacour-Gayet F, et al: Biventricular repair for double-outlet right ventricle: Results and long-term follow-up. Circulation 98:II-360–II-367, 1998.

Kirklin JW, Pacifico AD, Blackstone EH, et al: Current risks and protocols for operation for double-outlet right ventricle: Derivation from an 18 year experience. J Thorac Cardiovasc Surg 92:913–930, 1986.

Sridaromont S, Feldt RH, Ritter DG, et al: Double outlet right ventricle: Hemodynamic and anatomic correlation. Am J Cardiol 38:85–94, 1976.

Heterotaxia

Lamberti JJ, Waldman JD, Mathewson JW, et al: Repair of subdiaphragmatic total anomalous pulmonary venous connection without cardiopulmonary bypass. J Thorac Cardiovasc Surg 88:627–630, 1984.

Sapire DW, Ho SY, Anderson RH, et al: Diagnosis and significance of atrial isomerism. Am J Cardiol 58:342–346, 1986.

Van Mierop LHS, Gessner IH, Schiebler GL: Asplenia and polysplenia syndrome. Birth Defects Orig Artic Ser 8:36–44, 1972.

Persistent Pulmonary Hypertension of Newborn

Abman SH: Neonatal pulmonary hypertension: A physiologic approach to treatment. Pediatr Pulmonol Suppl 26:127–128, 2004.

Rudolph AM: High pulmonary vascular resistance after birth. I. Pathophysiologic considerations and etiologic classification. Clin Pediatr 19:585–590, 1980.

CHAPTER 15. VASCULAR RING

Huhta J, Gutgesell H, Latson L, et al: Two-dimensional echocardiographic assessment of the aorta in infants and children with congenital heart disease. Circulation 70:417–424, 1984.

Shuford WH, Sybers RG: The Aortic Arch and Its Malformation with Emphasis on the Angiographic Features. Springfield, Ill, Charles C Thomas, 1974.

CHAPTER 16. CHAMBER LOCALIZATION AND CARDIAC MALPOSITION

Huhta JC, Smallhorn IF, Macartney FJ: Two dimensional echocardiographic diagnosis of situs. Br Heart J 48:97–108, 1982.

Van Praagh R, Weinberg PM, Foran RB, et al: Malposition of the heart. In Adams FH, Emmanouilides GC, Riemenschneider TH (eds): Moss' Heart Disease in Infants, Children, and Adolescents, 4th ed. Baltimore, Williams & Wilkins, 1989.

CHAPTER 17. MISCELLANEOUS CONGENITAL CARDIAC CONDITIONS

Berthet K, Lavergne T, Cohen A, et al: Significant association of atrial vulnerability with atrial septal abnormalities in young patients with ischemic stroke of unknown cause. Stroke 31:398–403, 2000.

Gao Y, Burrows PE, Benson LN, et al: Scimitar syndrome in infancy. J Am Coll Cardiol 22:873–882, 1993.

Goldmuntz E: DiGeorge syndrome: New insights. Clin Perinatol 32:963–978, 2005.

Goldstein LB, Adams R, Alberts MJ, et al: Primary prevention of ischemic stroke: A guideline from the American Heart Association/American Stroke Association Stroke Council: Cosponsored by the Atherosclerotic Peripheral Vascular Disease Interdisciplinary Working Group; Cardiovascular Nursing Council; Clinical Cardiology Council; Nutrition, Physical Activity, and Metabolism Council; and the Quality of Care and Outcomes Research Interdisciplinary Working Group. Circulation 20;113:e873–e923, 2006.

Grifka RG, O'Laughlin MP, Nihill MR, Mullins CE: Double-transseptal, double-balloon valvuloplasty for congenital mitral stenosis. Circulation 88:123–129, 1992.

Guntheroth WG, Schwaegler R, Trent E: Comparative roles of the atrial septal aneurysm versus patient foramen ovale in systemic embolization with inference from neonatal studies Am J Cardiol 94:1341–1343, 2004.

Hara H, Virmani R, Ladich E, et al: Patent foramen ovale: Current pathology, pathophysiology, and clinical status. J Am Coll Cardiol 46:1768–1776, 2005.

Hirsch R, Landt Y, Porter S, et al: Cardiac troponin I in pediatrics: Normal levels and potential use in the assessment of cardiac injury. J Pediatr 130:872–877, 1997.

Lucas RV Jr, Krabill KA: Anomalous venous connections, pulmonary and systemic. In Adams FH, Emmanouilides GC, Riemenschneider TA (eds): Moss' Heart Disease in Infants, Children, and Adolescents, 4th ed. Baltimore, Williams & Wilkins, 1989.

Mas JL, Arquizan C, Lamy C, et al: Recurrent cerebrovascular events associated with patent foramen ovale, atrial septal aneurysm, or both. N Engl J Med 345:1740–1746, 2001.

Meissner I, Khandheria BK, Heit JA, et al: Patent foramen ovale: Innocent or guilty? Evidence from a prospective population-based study. J Am Coll Cardiol 47:440–455, 2006.

Overell JR, Bone I, Lees KR: Interatrial septal abnormalities and stroke: A meta-analysis of case-control studies. Neurology 55:1172–1179, 2000.

Reul RM, Cooley DA, Hallman GL, Reul GJ: Surgical treatment of coronary artery anomalies. Texas Heart Inst J 29:299–307, 2002.

Takeuchi S, Imamura H, Katsumoto K, et al: New surgical method for repair of anomalous left coronary artery from pulmonary artery. J Thorac Cardiovasc Surg 89:7–11, 1979.

Tashiro T, Todo K, Haruta Y, et al: Anomalous origin of the left coronary artery from the pulmonary artery. J Thorac Cardiovasc Surg 106:718–722, 1993.

Van Son JAM, Danielson GK, Schaff HV, et al: Congenital partial and complete absence of the pericardium. Mayo Clin Proc 68:743–747, 1993.

CHAPTER 18. PRIMARY MYOCARDIAL DISEASE

Anderson JL, Gilbert EM, O'Connell JB, et al: Long-term (2 year) beneficial effects of beta-adrenergic blockage with bucindolol in patients with idiopathic dilated cardiomyopathy. J Am Coll Cardiol 17:1373–1381, 1991.

Fazio S, Sabatini D, Capaldo B, et al: A preliminary study of growth hormone in the treatment of dilated cardiomyopathy. N Engl J Med 334:809–814, 1996.

Friedman RA, Moak JP, Garson A Jr: Clinical course of idiopathic dilated cardiomyopathy in children. J Am Coll Cardiol 18:152–156, 1991.

Helton E, Darragh R, Francis P, et al: Metabolic aspects of myocardial disease and a role for L-carnitine in the treatment of childhood cardiomyopathy. Pediatrics 105:1260–1270, 2000.

Iarussi D, Indolfi P, Casale F, et al: Anthracycline-induced cardiotoxicity in children with cancer: Strategies for prevention and management. Paediatr Drugs 7:67–76, 2000.

Ino T, Benson LN, Freedom RM, et al: Endocardial fibroelastosis: Natural history and prognostic risk factors. Am J Cardiol 62:431–434, 1988.

Katritsis D, Wilmshurst PT, Wendon JA, et al: Primary restrictive cardiomyopathy: Clinical and pathologic characteristics. J Am Coll Cardiol 18:1230–1235, 1991.

Lipshultz SE, Rifai N, Dalton VM, et al: The effect of dexrazoxane on myocardial injury in doxorubicin-treated children with acute lymphoblastic leukemia. N Engl J Med 351:145–153, 2004.

Lipshultz SE, Sanders SP, Goorin AM, et al: Monitoring for anthracycline cardiotoxicity. Pediatrics 93:433–437, 1994.

Marcus Fl, Fontaine GH, Guiraudon G, et al: Right ventricular dysplasia: A report of 24 adult cases. Circulation 65:384–398, 1982.

Maron BJ, Bonow RO, Cannon RO III, et al: Hypertrophic cardiomyopathy: Interrelations of clinical manifestations, pathophysiology, and therapy. I. N Engl J Med 316:780–789, 1987.

Maron BJ, Bonow RO, Cannon RO III, et al: Hypertrophic cardiomyopathy: Interrelations of clinical manifestations, pathophysiology, and therapy. II. N Engl J Med 316:843–852, 1987.

Maron BJ, McKenna WJ, Danielson GK, et al: American College of Cardiology/ European Society of Cardiology Clinical Expert Consensus Document on Hypertrophic Cardiomyopathy. J Am Coll Cardiol 42:1687–1713, 2003.

McElhinney DB, Colan SD, Moran AM, et al: Recombinant human growth hormone treatment for dilated cardiomyopathy in children. Pediatrics 114:e452–e458, 2004.

Ni J, Bowles NE, Kim YH, et al: Viral infection of the myocardium in endocardial fibroelastosis. Molecular evidence for the role of mumps virus as an etiologic agent. Circulation 95:133–139, 1997.

Pelliccia A, Maron BJ, Spataro A, et al: The upper limit of physiologic cardiac hypertrophy in highly trained elite athletes. N Engl J Med 324:295–301, 1991.

Shaddy RE: Beta-blocker therapy in young children with congestive heart failure under consideration for heart transplantation. Am Heart J 136:19–21, 1998.

Steinherz LJ, Graham T, Hurwitz R, et al: Guidelines for cardiac monitoring of children during and after anthracycline therapy: Report of the Cardiology Committee of the Children's Cancer Study Group. Pediatrics 89:942–949, 1992.

Vaillant MC, Chantepie A, Casasoprana A, et al: Transient hypertrophic cardiomyopathy in neonates after acute fetal distress. Pediatr Cardiol 18:52–56, 1997.

Yetman AT, McCrindle SW, MacDonald C, et al: Myocardial bridging in children with hypertrophic cardiomyopathy—A risk factor for sudden death. N Engl J Med 339:1201–1209, 1998.

CHAPTER 19. CARDIOVASCULAR INFECTIONS

Akagi T, Kato H, Inoue O, et al: Valvular heart disease in Kawasaki syndrome: Incidence and natural history. Am Heart J 120:366–372, 1990.

Baddour LM, Wilson WR, Bayer AS, et al: Infective endocarditis: diagnosis, antimicrobial therapy, and management of complications: A statement for healthcare professionals from the Committee on Rheumatic Fever, Endocarditis, and Kawasaki Disease, Council on Cardiovascular Disease in the Young, and the Councils on Clinical Cardiology, Stroke, and Cardiovascular Surgery and Anesthesia, American Heart Association: Endorsed by the Infectious Diseases Society of America. Circulation 111:e394–e433, 2005.

Dajani AS, Taubert KA, Wilson W, et al: Prevention of bacterial endocarditis: Recommendations by the American Heart Association. JAMA 277:1794–1801, 1997.

Drucker NA, Colan SD, Lewis AB, et al: Gamma-globulin treatment of acute myocarditis in the pediatric population. Circulation 89:252–257, 1994.

Durack DT, Lukes AS, Bright DK: New criteria for diagnosis of infective endocarditis: Utilization of specific echocardiographic findings. Am J Med 96:200–209, 1994.

Ferrieri P, Gewitz MH, Gerber MA, et al: Unique features of infective endocarditis in childhood. Pediatrics 109:931–943, 2002.

Harada K, Yamaguchi H, Kato H, et al: Indication for intravenous gamma globulin treatment for Kawasaki disease. In Takahashi M, Taubert K (eds): Proceedings of the Fourth International Symposium on Kawasaki Disease. Dallas, TX, American Heart Association, 1993.

Ishii M, Ueno T, Ikeda H, et al: Sequential follow-up results of catheter intervention for coronary artery lesions after Kawasaki disease: Quantitative coronary artery angiography and intravascular ultrasound imaging study. Circulation 105:3004–3010, 2002.

Kato H, Ichinose E, Yoshioka F, et al: Fate of coronary aneurysms in Kawasaki disease: Serial coronary angiography and long-term follow-up study. Am J Cardiol 49:1758–1766, 1982.

Kurotobi S, Nagai T, Kawakami N, Sano T: Coronary diameter in normal infants, children and patients with Kawasaki disease. Pediatr Int 44:1–4, 2002.

Li JS, Sexton DJ, Mick N, et al: Proposed modification to the Duke criteria for the diagnosis of infective endocarditis. Clin Infect Dis 30:633–638, 2000.

Lipshultz SE, Orav EJ, Sanders SP, Colan SD: Immunoglobulins and left ventricular structure and function in pediatric HIV infection. Circulation 92:2220–2225, 1995.

Melish ME: Kawasaki syndrome. Pediatr Rev 17:153–162, 1996.

Newburger JW, Fulton DR: Kawasaki disease. Curr Opin Pediatr 16:508–514, 2004.

Newburger JW, Takahashi M, Beiser AS, et al: A single intravenous infusion of gamma globulin as compared with four infusions in the treatment of acute Kawasaki syndrome. N Engl J Med 324:1633–1639, 1991.

Newburger JW, Takahashi M, Gerber MA, et al: Diagnosis, treatment, and long-term management of Kawasaki disease: A Statement for Health Professionals from the Committee on Rheumatic Fever, Endocarditis, and Kawasaki Disease, Council on Cardiovascular Disease in the Young, American Heart Association. Pediatrics 114:1708–1733, 2004.

Okada Y. Shinohara M, Kobayashi T, et al: Effect of corticosteroids in addition to intravenous gamma globulin therapy on serum cytokine levels in the acute phase of Kawasaki disease in children. J Pediatr 143:363–367, 2003.

Red Book: 2006 Report of the Committee on Infectious Disease, by Larry K. Pickering. American Academy of Pediatrics, Elk Grove Village, Ill, 2006.

Shapiro ED: Lyme disease. Pediatr Rev 19:147–154, 1998.

Starc TJ, Lipshultz SE, Kaplan S, et al: Cardiac complications in children with human immunodeficiency virus infection. Pediatrics 104:e14, 1999.

Williams RV, Wilke VM, Tani LY, Minich LL: Does abciximab enhance regression of coronary aneurysms resulting from Kawasaki disease? Pediatrics 109:E4, 2002.

CHAPTER 20. ACUTE RHEUMATIC FEVER

Dajani AS, Ayoub E, Bierman FZ, et al: Guidelines for the diagnosis of rheumatic fever: Jones criteria, updated 1992. JAMA 87:302–307, 1992.

Dajani A, Taubert K, Ferrieri P, et al: Treatment of acute streptococcal pharyngitis and prevention of rheumatic fever: A statement for health professionals. Committee on Rheumatic Fever, Endocarditis, and Kawasaki Disease of the Council on Cardiovascular Disease in the Young, the American Heart Association. Pediatrics 96:758–764, 1995.

Garvey MA, Snider LA, Leitman SF, et al: Treatment of Sydenham's chorea with intravenous immunoglobulin, plasma exchange, or prednisone. J Child Neurol 20:424–429, 2005.

Taranta A, Markowitz M: Rheumatic Fever, 2nd ed. Dordrecht, the Netherlands, Kluwer Academic, 1989.

Veasy LG, Tani LY: A new loot at acute rheumatic mitral regurgitation. Cardiol Young 15:568–577, 2005.

Vijayalakshmi IB, Mathravinda J, Deva ANP: The role of echocardiography in diagnosing carditis in the setting of acute rheumatic fever. Cardiol Young 15:583–588, 2005.

CHAPTER 21. VALVULAR HEART DISEASE

ACC/AHA 2006 guidelines for the management of patients with valvular heart disease. Circulation 114:e84–e231, 2006 or J Am Coll Cardiol 48:e1–e148, 2006.

Bisset GS III, Schwartz DC, Meyer RA, et al: Clinical spectrum and long-term follow-up of isolated mitral valve prolapse in 119 children. Circulation 62:423–429, 1980.

Levine RA, Stathogiannis E, Newell JB, et al: Reconsideration of echocardiographic standards for mitral valve prolapse: Lack of association between leaflet displacement isolated to the apical four chamber view and independent echocardiographic evidence of abnormality. J Am Coll Cardiol 11:1010–1019, 1988.

Levine RA, Triulzi MO, Harrigan P, et al: The relationship of mitral annular shape to the diagnosis of mitral valve prolapse. Circulation 75:756–767, 1987.

Lock JE, Khalilullah M, Shrivastava S, et al: Percutaneous catheter commissurotomy in rheumatic mitral stenosis. N Engl J Med 313:1515–1518, 1985.

Smith MS, Doroshow C, Womack WM, et al: Symptomatic mitral valve prolapse in children and adolescents: Catecholamines, anxiety, and biofeedback. Pediatrics 84:290–298, 1989.

Warth DC, King ME, Cohen JM, et al: Prevalence of mitral valve prolapse in normal children. J Am Coll Cardiol 5:1173–1177, 1985.

CHAPTER 22. CARDIAC TUMORS

Ludomirsky A: Cardiac tumors. In Garson A Jr, Bricker JT, McNamara DG (eds): The Science and Practice of Pediatric Cardiology. Philadelphia, Lea & Febiger, 1990.

McAllister HA, Fenoglio JJ Jr: Tumors of the Cardiovascular System: Atlas of Tumor Pathology, 2nd series. Washington, DC, Armed Forces Institute of Pathology, 1978.

Nir A, Tajik AJ, Freeman WK, et al: Tuberous sclerosis and cardiac rhabdomyoma. Am J Cardiol 76:419–421, 1995.

CHAPTER 23. CARDIAC INVOLVEMENT IN SYSTEMIC DISEASES

Bhakta D, Lowe MR, Groh WJ: Prevalence of structural cardiac abnormalities in patients with myotonic dystrophy type I. Am Heart J 147:224–227, 2004.

Caddell JL: Metabolic and nutritional diseases. In Adams FH, Emmanouilides GC, Riemenschneider TA (eds): Moss' Heart Disease in Infants, Children, and Adolescents, 4th ed. Baltimore, Williams & Wilkins, 1989.

Dangel JH: Cardiovascular change in children with mucopolysaccharide storage diseases and related disorders—Clinical and echocardiographic findings in 64 patients. Eur J Pediatr 157:534–538, 1998.

Duboc D, Meune C, Lerebours G, et al: Effect of perindopril on the onset and progression of left ventricular dysfunction in Duchenne muscular dystrophy. J Am Coll Cardiol 45:855–857, 2005.

Gott VL, Greene PS, Alejo DE, et al: Replacement of the aortic root in patients with Marfan's syndrome. N Engl J Med 340:1307–1313, 1999.

Jefferies JL, Eidem BW, Belmont JW, et al: Genetic predictors and remodeling of dilated cardiomyopathy in muscular dystrophy. Circulation 112:2799–2804, 2005.

Kim SY, Martin N, Hsia EC, et al: Management of aortic disease in Marfan syndrome: A decision analysis. Arch Intern Med 165:749–755, 2005.

Mohan UR, Hay AA, Cleary MA, et al: Cardiovascular changes in children with mucopolysaccharide disorders. Act Paediatr 91:799–804, 2002.

Pierpoint MEM, Moller JH: Cardiac manifestations of systemic disease. In Adams FH, Emmanouilides GC, Riemenschneider TA (eds): Moss' Heart Disease in Infants, Children, and Adolescents, 4th ed. Baltimore, Williams & Wilkins, 1989.

Shores J, Berger KR, Murphy EA, et al: Progression of aortic and the benefit of long-term β-adrenergic blockade in Marfan's syndrome. N Engl J Med 330:1335–1341, 1994.

Yetman AT, Bornemeier RA, McCrindle BW: Usefulness of enalapril versus propranolol or atenolol for prevention of aortic dilation in patients with the Marfan syndrome. Am J Cardiol 95:1125–1127, 2005.

CHAPTER 24. CARDIAC ARRHYTHMIAS

Ackerman MJ: The long QT syndrome. Pediatr Rev 19:232–238, 1998.

Alexander ME: Ventricular arrhythmias in children and young adults. In Walsh EP, Saul JP, Triedman JK: Cardiac Arrhythmias in Children and Young Adults with Congenital Heart Disease. Philadelphia, Lippincott Williams & Wilkins, 2001, pp 201–234.

Collins KK, Van Hare GF: Advances in congenital long QT syndrome. Curr Opin Pediatr 18:497–502, 2005.

Garson A Jr: How to measure the QT interval: What is normal? Am J Cardiol 72:14B–16B, 1993.

Goel AK, Berger S, Pelech A, Dhala A: Implantable cardioverter defibrillator therapy in children with long QT syndrome. Pediatr Cardiol 25:370–378, 2004.

Lerman BB, Belardinelli L: Cardiac electrophysiology of adenosine: Basic and clinical concepts. Circulation 83:1499–1509, 1991.

Martin AB, Perry JC, Robinson JL, et al: Calculation of QTc duration and variability in the presence of sinus arrhythmia. Am J Cardiol 75:950–952, 1995.

Pent JC, Fenrich AL, Hulse JE, et al: Pediatric use of intravenous amiodarone: Efficacy and safety in critically ill patients from a multicenter protocol. J Am Coll Cardiol 27:1246–1250, 1996.

Rochini AP, Chun PO, Dick M: Ventricular tachycardia in children. Am J Cardiol 47:1091–1097, 1981.

Schwartz PJ, Moss AJ, Vincent GM, Crampton RS: Diagnostic criteria for the long QT syndrome: An update. Circulation 88:782–784, 1993.

Seslar SP, Zimetbaum PJ, Berul CI, Josephson ME: Diagnosis of congenital long QT syndrome. UpToDate 14.2, April 2006 (www.uptodate.com).

Schwartz PJ: The long QT syndrome. Curr Probl Cardiol 22:297–351, 1997.

Towbin JA, Friedman RA: Long QT syndrome. In Walsh EP, Seal JP, Triedman JK (eds): Cardiac Arrhythmias in Children and Young Adults with Congenital Heart Disease. Philadelphia, Lippincott Williams & Wilkins, 2001, pp 235–270.

Yabek SM: Ventricular arrhythmias in children with an apparently normal heart. J Pediatr 119:1–11, 1991.

CHAPTER 25. DISTURBANCES OF ATRIOVENTRICULAR CONDUCTION

Eronen M, Siren M-K, Ekblad H, et al: Short- and long-term outcome of children with congenital complete heart block diagnosed in utero or as a newborn. Pediatrics 106:86–91, 2000.

Ross BA, Gillette PC: Atrioventricular block and bundle branch block. In Gillette PC, Garson A Jr (eds): Clinical Pediatric Arrhythmias, 2nd ed. Philadelphia, WB Saunders, 1999, pp 63–77.

CHAPTER 26. CARDIAC PACEMAKERS AND IMPLANTABLE CARDIOVERTER-DEFIBRILLATORS IN CHILDREN

Friedman RA: Pacemakers in children: Medical and surgical aspects. Tex Heart Inst J 19:178–184, 1992.

Gillette PC, Heinle JS, Zeigler VL: Cardiac pacing. In Gillette PC, Garson A Jr (eds): Clinical Pediatric Arrhythmias, 2nd ed. Philadelphia, WB Saunders, 1999, pp 190–220.

Gregoratos G, Abrams J, Epstein AE, et al: ACC/AHA/NASPE 2002 Guideline Update for Implantation of Cardiac Pacemakers and Antiarrhythmia Devices. Circulation 106:2145–2161, 2002 or www.acc.org/clinical/guidelines/pacemaker/pacemaker.pdf.

CHAPTER 27. CONGESTIVE HEART FAILURE

Amman M, Graham TP Jr: Guidelines for vasodilator therapy of congestive heart failure in infants and children. Am J Cardiol 113:994–1005, 1987.

Bruns LA, Chrisant MK, Lamour JM, et al: Carvedilol as therapy in pediatric heart failure: An initial multicenter experience. J Pediatr 138:505–511, 2001.

Buchhorn R, Bartmus D, Siekmeyer W, et al: Beta-blocker therapy of severe congestive heart failure in infants with left to right shunts. Am J Cardiol 98:1366–1368, 1998.

Friedman WF: New concepts and drugs in the treatment of congestive heart failure. Pediatr Clin North Am 31:1197–1227, 1984.

Montigny M, Davignon A, Fouron J-C, et al: Captopril in infants for congestive heart failure secondary to a large ventricular left-to-right shunt. Am J Cardiol 63:631–633, 1989.

Nir A, Nasser N: Clinical value of NT-ProBNT and BNT in pediatric cardiology. J Card Fail 11:S76–S80, 2005.

Park MK: The use of digoxin in infants and children with specific emphasis on dosage. J Pediatr 108:871–877, 1986.

Shaddy RE, Tani LY, Gidding SS, et al: Beta-blocker treatment of dilated cardiomyopathy with congestive heart failure in children: A multi-institutional experience. J Heart Lung Transplant 18:269–274, 1999.

CHAPTER 28. SYSTEMIC HYPERTENSION

Chobanian AV, Bakris GL, Black HR, et al: The Seventh Report of the Joint National Committee on Prevention, Detection, Evaluation, and Treatment of High Blood Pressure: The JNC 7 report. JAMA. 289:2560–2572, 2003.

Daniels SR, Meyer RA, Liang YC, Bove KE: Echocardiographically determined left ventricular mass index in normal children, adolescents, and young adults. J Am Coll Cardiol 12:703–708, 1988.

Feig DI, Johnson RJ: Hyperuricemia in childhood primary hypertension. Hypertension 42:247–252, 2003.

Flynn JT, Newburger JW, Daniels SR, et al: A randomized, placebo-controlled trial of amlodipine in children with hypertension. J Pediatr 145:288–290, 2004.

Frolich ED, Labarth DR, Maxwell MH, et al: Recommendations for human blood pressure determination by sphygmomanometers: Report of a Special Task Force appointed by the Steering Committee, American Heart Association. Circulation 77:501A–514A, 1988.

Hammond IW, Urbina EM, Wattigney WA, et al: Comparison of fourth and fifth Korotkoff diastolic blood pressures in 5 to 30 year old individuals. The Bogalusa Heart Study. Am J Hypertens 8:1083–1089, 1995.

Jago R, Harrell JS, McMurray RG, et al: Prevalence of abnormal lipid and blood pressure values among an ethnically diverse population of eighth grade adolescents and screening implications. Pediatrics 117:2065–2073, 2006.

Park MK: Blood pressure tables (Letter to the Editor). Pediatrics 115:826–827, 2005.

Park MK, Guntheroth WG: Accurate blood pressure measurement in children: A review. Am J Noninvas Cardiol 3:297–309, 1989.

Sever P: New hypertension guidelines from the National Institute for Health and Clinical Excellence and the British Hypertension Society. J Renin Angiotensin Aldosterone Syst 7:61–63, 2006.

The Fourth Report on the Diagnosis, Evaluation, and Treatment of High Blood Pressure in Children and Adolescents. National High Blood Pressure Education Program Working Group on High Blood Pressure in Children and Adolescents. Pediatrics 111:555–576, 2004.

Update on the 1987 Task Force Report on High Blood Pressure in Children and Adolescents: A Working Group Report from the National High Blood Pressure Education Program. Pediatrics 98:649–658, 1996.

CHAPTER 29. PULMONARY HYPERTENSION

Albersheim SG, Solimanu AJ, Sharma AK, et al: Randomized, double-blind, controlled trial of long-term diuretic therapy for bronchopulmonary dysplasia. J Pediatr 115:615–620, 1989.

Barst RJ, Ivy D, Dingemanse J, et al: Pharmacokinetics, safety, and efficacy of bosentan in pediatric patients with pulmonary arterial hypertension. Clin Pharmacol Ther 73:372–382, 2003.

Barst RJ, Langleben D, Badesch D, et al: Treatment of pulmonary arterial hypertension with the selective endothelin-A receptor antagonist sitaxsentan. J Am Coll Cardiol 47:2049–2056, 2006.

Barst RJ, Maislin G, Fishman AF: Vasodilator therapy for primary pulmonary hypertension in children. Circulation 99:1197–1208, 1999.

Dillon PW, Cilley RE, Mauger D, et al: The relationship of pulmonary artery pressure and survival in congenital diaphragmatic hernia. J Pediatr Surg 39:307–312, 2004.

Din-Xuan AT: Disorders of endothelium-dependent relaxation in pulmonary disease. Circulation 38(suppl V): V-81–V-87, 1993.

Game S: Pulmonary hypertension (grand rounds). JAMA 284:3160–3168, 2000.

Gorenflo M, Nelle M, Schnabel PA, Ullmann MV: Pulmonary hypertension in infancy and childhood. Cardiol Young 13:219–227, 2003.

Humpl T, Reyes JT, Holtby H, et al: Beneficial effect of oral sildenafil therapy on childhood pulmonary arterial hypertension. Twelve-month clinical trial of a single-drug, open-label, pilot study. Circulation 111:3274–3280, 2005.

King ME, Braun H, Goldblatt A, et al: Interventricular septal configuration as a predictor of right ventricular systolic hypertension in children: A cross-sectional echocardiographic study. Circulation 68:68–75, 1983.

Maiya S, Hislop AA, Flynn Y, Haworth SG: Response to bosentan in children with pulmonary hypertension. Heart 92:664–670, 2006.

McQuillan BM, Picard MH, Leavitt M, Weyman AE: Clinical correlates and reference intervals for pulmonary artery systolic pressure among echocardiographically normal subjects. Circulation 104:2797–2802, 2001.

Richardi MK, Knight BP, Martinet FJ, et al: Inhaled nitric oxide in primary pulmonary hypertension: A safe and effective agent for predicting response to nifedipine. J Am Coll Cardiol 32:1068–1073, 1998.

Rosenzweig EB, Ivy DD, Widlitz A, et al: Effects of long-term bosentan in children with pulmonary arterial hypertension. J Am Coll Cardiol 46:697–704, 2005.

Stevenson JG: Comparison of several noninvasive methods for estimation of pulmonary artery pressure. J Am Soc Echocardiogr 2:157–171, 1989.

CHAPTER 30. CHILD WITH CHEST PAIN

Driscoll DJ, Glichlich LB, Gallen WJ: Chest pain in children: A prospective study. Pediatrics 57:648–651, 1976.

Klone RA, Hale S, Alker K, Rezkalla S: The effects of acute and chronic cocaine use on the heart. Circulation 85:407–418, 1992.

Kocis KC: Chest pain in pediatrics. Pediatr Clin North Am 46:189–203, 1999.

Middleton D: Evaluating the child with chest pain. Emerg Med 22:23–27, 1990.

Rowe BH, Dulburg CS, Peterson RG, et al: Characteristics of children presenting with chest pain to a pediatric emergency department. Can Med Assoc J 143:388–394, 1990.

Selbst SM, Ruddy RM, Clark BJ: Pediatric chest pain: A prospective study. Pediatrics 82:319–323, 1988.

CHAPTER 31. SYNCOPE

Ackerman MJ: The long QT syndrome. Pediatr Rev 19:232–238, 1998.

Bar-Or O, Rowland TW: Pediatric Exercise Medicine: Cardiovascular Diseases. Champaign, Ill, Human Kinetics, 2005, pp 177–217.

Berul CI, Sweeten TL, Dubin AM, et al: Use of the rate-corrected JT interval for prediction of repolarization abnormalities in children. Am J Cardiol 74:1254–1257, 1994.

Blanc JJ, Mansourati J, Maheu B, et al: Reproducibility of a positive passive upright tilt test at a seven-day interval in patients with syncope. Am J Cardiol 72:467–471, 1993.

Connolly SJ, Sheldon R, Thorpe KE, et al: Pacemaker therapy for prevention of syncope in patients with recurrent severe vasovagal syncope: Second Vasovagal Pacemaker Study (VPS II): A randomized study. JAMA 289:2224–2229, 2003.

Grubb BP, Kosinski D: Tilt table testing: Concepts and limitations. Pacing Clin Electrophysiol 20(pt II): 781–787, 1997.

Lewis DA, Dhala A: Syncope in the pediatric patient. Pediatr Clin North Am 46:205–219, 1999.

O'Marcaigh AS, MacLellan-Tobert SG, Perter CP: Tilt-table testing and oral metoprolol therapy in young patients with unexplained syncope. Pediatrics 93:278–283, 1994.

Salim MA, Ware LE, Barnard M, et al: Syncope recurrence in children: Relation to tilt-test results. Pediatrics 102:924–926, 1998.

Schwartz PJ, Montemerlo M, Facchini M, et al: The QT interval throughout the first 6 months of life: A prospective study. Circulation 66:496–501, 1982.

Scott WA: Syncope and the assessment of the autonomic nervous system. In Allen HD, Gutgesell HP, Clark EB, Driscoll DJ (eds): Moss and Adams' Heart Disease in Infants, Children, and Adolescents, 6th ed. Philadelphia, Lippincott Williams & Wilkins, 2001, pp 443–452.

Sra JS, Jazayeri MR, Avitall B, et al: Comparison of cardiac pacing with drug therapy in the treatment of neurocardiogenic (vasovagal) syncope with bradycardia or asystole. N Engl J Med 328:1117–1121, 1993.

Steiper MJ, Campbell RM: Efficacy of alpha-adrenergic agonist therapy for prevention of pediatric neurocardiogenic syncope. J Am Coil Cardiol 22:594–597, 1993.

Strickberger SA, Benson W, Biaggioni I, et al: AHA/ACCF Scientific Statement on the Evaluation of Syncope. From the American Heart Association Council on Clinical Cardiology, Cardiovascular Nursing, Cardiovascular Disease in the Young, and Stroke, and the Quality of Care and Outcome Research Interdisciplinary Working Group; and the American College of Cardiology Foundation in Collaboration with the Heart Rhythm Society. Circulation 113:316–327, 2006.

CHAPTER 32. PALPITATION

Giala F, Raviele A: Diagnostic management of patients with palpitation of unknown origin. Ital Heart J 5:581–586, 2004.

CHAPTER 33. DYSLIPIDEMIA AND OTHER CARDIOVASCULAR RISK FACTORS

Cardiovascular Risk Factors and the Metabolic Syndrome

Ashen MD, Blumenthal RS: Clinical practice: Low HDL cholesterol levels. N Engl J Med 353:1251–1260, 2005.

Berenson GS, Srinivasan SR, Bao W, et al: Association between multiple cardiovascular risk factors and atherosclerosis in children and young adults. N Engl J Med 338:1650–1656, 1998.

Cook S, Weizman M, Auinger P, et al: Prevalence of a metabolic syndrome phenotype in adolescents: Findings from the third National Health and Nutrition Examination Survey, 1988–1994. Arch Pediatr Adolesc Med 157:821–827, 2003.

Fernandez JR, Redden DT, Pietrobelli A, Allison DB: Waist circumference percentiles in nationally representative samples of African-American, European-American, and Mexican-American children and adolescents J Pediatr 145:439–444, 2004.

Grundy SM: Editorial: Obesity, metabolic syndrome, and coronary atherosclerosis. Circulation 105:2696–1698, 2002.

Grundy SM, Hansen B, Smith SC Jr, et al: Clinical management of metabolic syndrome. Report of the American Heart Association/National Heart, Lung, and Blood Institute/American Diabetes Association Conference on Scientific Issues Related to Management. Circulation 109:551–556, 2004.

Hubert HB, Fenileib M, McNamara PM, et al: Obesity as an independent risk factor for cardiovascular disease: A 26-year follow-up of participants in the Framingham Heart Study. Circulation 67:968–977, 1983.

Jago R, Harrell JS, McMurray RG, et al: Prevalence of abnormal lipid and blood pressure values among an ethnically diverse population of eighth grade adolescents and screening implications. Pediatrics 117:2065–2073, 2006.

Kavey RW, Daniels SR, Lauer RM, et al: American Heart Association guidelines for primary prevention of atherosclerotic cardiovascular disease beginning in childhood. Circulation 107:1562–1566, 2003.

McGill HC Jr, McMahan CA, Herderick EE, et al: Obesity accelerates the progression of coronary atherosclerosis in young men. Circulation 105:2712–2718, 2002.

Singh GK: Metabolic syndrome in children and adolescents. Curr Treat Options Cardiovasc Med 8:403–413, 2006.

Strong JP, Malcom GT, Oalmann MC: Environmental and genetic risk factors in early human atherosclerosis: Lesions from the PDAY study. Pathobiological Determinants of Atherosclerosis in Youth. Path Int 45:403–408, 1995.

Dyslipidemia

Dennison BA, Kikuchi DA, Srinivasan RS, et al: Parental history of cardiovascular disease as an indication for screening for lipoprotein abnormalities in children. J Pediatr 115:186–194, 1989.

Gidding SS, Dennison BA, Birch LL, et al: American Heart Association; American Academy of Pediatrics. Dietary recommendations for children and adolescents: A guide for practitioners. Pediatrics 117:544–559, 2006.

Holmes KW, Kwiterovich PO Jr: Treatment of dyslipidemia in children and adolescents. Curr Cardiol Rep 7:445–456, 2005.

Lambert M, Lupien P-J, Gagne C, et al: Treatment of familial hypercholesterolemia in children and adolescents: Effect of lovastatin. Pediatrics 97:619–628, 1996.

National Cholesterol Education Program: Report of the Expert Panel on Blood Cholesterol Levels in Children and Adolescents. US Department of Health and Human Services. NIH Publication No. 91-2732, September 1991.

Srinivasan SR, Myers L, Berenson GS: Distribution and correlates of non-high-density lipoprotein cholesterol in children. Pediatrics 110:e20, 2002.

Stein EA, Illingworth DR, Kwiterovich PO Jr, et al: Efficacy and safety of lovastatin in adolescent males with heterozygous familial hypercholesterolemia. JAMA 281:137–144, 1999.

Tershakovec AM, Rader DJ: Disorders of lipoprotein metabolism and transport. In Berhman RE, Kliegman RM, Jenson HB (eds): Nelson Textbook of Pediatrics, 16th ed. Philadelphia, WB Saunders, 2000, pp 387–398.

Third Report of the National Cholesterol Education Program (NCEP) Expert Panel on Detection, Education, and Treatment of High Blood Cholesterol in Adults (Adult Treatment Panel III) final report. Circulation 106:3143–3421, 2002.

Wiegman A, Hutten BA, de Groot E, et al: Efficacy and safety of statin therapy in children with familial hypercholesterolemia. JAMA 292:331–337, 2004.

Winter W, Schatz D: Pediatric Lipid Disorders in Clinical Practice. www.emedicine.com/ped/ CARDIOLOGY.HTM, last updated January 19, 2005.

Obesity

Becque MD, Katch VL, Rocchini AP, et al: Coronary risk incidence of obese adoloscents: Reduction by excercise plus diet intervention. Pediatrics 81:605–612, 1988.

Dietz WH: Health consequences of obesity in youth: Childhood predictors of adult disease. Pediatrics 101:518–525, 1998.

Gortmaker SL, Must A, Sobol AM, et al: Television viewing as a cause of increasing obesity among children in the United States, 1986–1990. Arch Pediatr Adolesc Med 150:356–362, 1996.

Gutin B, Manos TM: Physical activity in the prevention of childhood obesity. Ann NY Acad Sci 699:115–126, 1993.

Hannan WJ, Wrate RM, Cowen SJ, Freeman CP: Body mass index as an estimate of body fat. Int J Eat Disord 18:91–97, 1995.

Hedley AA, Ogden CL, Johnson CL, et al: Prevalence of overweight and obesity among US children, adolescents and adults, 1999–2002. JAMA 291:2847–2850, 2004.

Krebs NF, Baker RD, Greer FR, et al: Policy statement. Prevention of pediatric overweight and obesity. Committee on Nutrition. Pediatrics 112:424–430, 2003.

Ogden CL, Carroll MD, Curtin LS, et al: Prevalence of overweight and obesity in the United States, 1999–2004. JAMA 295:1549–1555, 2006.

Srinivasan SR, Myers L, Berenson GS: Temporal association between obesity and hyperinsulinemia in children, adolescents, and young adults: The Bogalusa Heart Study. Metabolism 48:928–934, 1999.

Smoking

Lu JT, Creager MA: The relationship of cigarette smoking to peripheral arterial disease. Rev Cardiovasc Med 5:189–193, 2004.

Marshall L, Schooley M, Ryan H, et al: Youth tobacco surveillance, United States; 2001–2002. MMWR Surveill Summ 9:55(3):1–56, 2006.

Rigotti NA, Lee JE, Wechsler H: U.S. college students' use of tobacco products: Results of a national survey. JAMA 284:699–705, 2000.

Williams CL, Hayman LL, Daniels SR, et al: Cardiovascular health in childhood. A statement for health professionals from the Committee on Atherosclerosis, Hypertension, and Obesity in the Young (AHOY) of the Council on Cardiovascular Disease in the Young, American Heart Association. Circulation 106:143–160, 2002.

CHAPTER 34. ATHLETES WITH CARDIAC PROBLEMS

36th Bethesda Conference: Eligibility recommendations for competitive athletes with cardiovascular abnormalities. J Am Coll Cardiol 45:1313–1375, 2005.

Bonow RO, Cheitlin MD: Bethesda Conference Report. Task Force 3: Valvular heart disease. J Am Coll Cardiol 45:1334–1340, 2005.

Kaplan NM, Deverauz RB, Miller HSJ: Task Force 4: Systemic hypertension. J Am Coll Cardiol 24:885–888, 1994.

Kaplan NM, Gidding SS, Pickering TG, Wright JT Jr: Task Force 5: Systemic hypertension. J Am Coll Cardiol 45:1346–1348, 2005.

Maron BJ: Sudden Cardiac Death in the Young Athlete and the Preparticipation Cardiovascular Evaluation. New York: Churchill Livingstone, 2000.

Maron BJ, Ackerman MJ, Towbin JA: Bethesda Conference Report. Task Force 4: HCM and other cardiomyopathies, mitral valve prolapse, myocarditis, and Marfan syndrome. J Am Coll Cardiol 45:1340–1345, 2005.

Maron BJ, Shirani J, Poline LC, et al: Sudden death in young competitive athletes: Clinical, demographic and pathological profiles. JAMA 276:199–208, 1996.

Maron BJ, Thompson PD, Puffer JC, et al: Cardiovascular preparticipation screening of competitive athletes: A statement for health professionals from the Sudden Death Committee (clinical cardiology) and Congenital

Cardiac Defects Committee (cardiovascular disease in the young), American Heart Association. Circulation 94:850–856, 1996.

Maron BJ, Zipez DP: Bethesda Conference Report. Introduction: Eligibility recommendations for competitive athletes with cardiovascular abnormalities—General Considerations. J Am Coll Cardiol 45:1318–1321, 2005.

McCaffrey FM, Braden DS, Strong WB: Sudden cardiac death in young athletes: A review. Am J Dis Child 145:177–183, 1991.

Mitchel JH, Haskel W, Snell P, Van Camp SP: Task Force 8: Classification of sports. J Am Coll Cardiol 45:1364–1367, 2005.

Pelliccia A, Maron BJ, Spataro A, et al: The upper limit of physiologic cardiac hypertrophy in highly trained elite athletes. N Engl J Med 324:295–301, 1991.

Risser WL, Anderson SJ, Bolduc SP, et al: Athletic participation by children and adolescent who have systemic hypertension. Pediatrics 99:637–638, 1997.

Risser WL, Anderson SJ, Bolduc SP, et al: Cardiac dysrhythmias and sports. Pediatrics 95:786–788, 1995.

Washington RL, Bernhardt DT, Brenner JS, et al: Promotion of healthy weight-control practices in young athletes. Pediatrics 116:1557–1564, 2005.

Zipes DP, Ackerman MJ, Estes NA 3rd, et al: Task Force 7: Arrhythmias. J Am Coll Cardiol 45:1354–1363, 2005.

CHAPTER 35. CARDIAC TRANSPLANTATION

Backer CL, Mavroudis C: Pediatrics transplantation, Part A: Heart transplantation. In Stuart FP, Abecassis MM, Kaufman DB, eds: *Organ transplantation,* Georgetown, Texas, Landes Bioscience, 2000.

Bailey L, Concepcion W, Shattuck H, et al: Method of heart transplantation for treatment of hypoplastic left heart syndrome. J Thorac Cardiovasc Surg 92:1–5, 1986.

Bailey LL, Gundry SR, Razzouk AJ, et al: Bless the babies: One hundred fifteen late survivors of heart transplantation during the first year of life. J Thorac Cardiovasc Surg 105:805–815, 1993.

Boucek MM, Mathis CM, Boucek RJ, et al: Prospective evaluation of echocardiography for primary rejection surveillance after infant heart transplantation: Comparison with endomyocardial biopsy. J Heart Lung Transplant 13:66–73, 1994.

Canter CE: Pediatric cardiac transplantation. In Moller JH, Hoffman RE (eds): Pediatric Cardiovascular Medicine. New York, Churchill Livingstone, 2000, pp 942–952.

Gabrys CA: Pediatric cardiac transplants: A clinical update. J Pediatr Nurs 20:139–143, 2005.

Kuhn MA, Jutzy KR, Derming DD, et al: The medium-term findings in coronary arteries by intravascular ultrasound in infants and children after heart transplantation. J Am Coll Cardiol 36:250–254, 2000.

Pahl E, Fricker FJ, Armitage J, et al: Coronary arteriosclerosis in pediatric heart transplant survivors: Limitation of long-term survival. J Pediatr 116:177–183, 1990.

Perlroch MG, Reitz BA: Heart and heart-lung transplantation. In Braunwald E (ed): Heart Disease: A Textbook of Cardiovascular Medicine, 5th ed. Philadelphia, WB Saunders, 1997, pp 515–533.

Seipelt IM, Crawford SE, Rodgers S, et al: Hypercholesterolemia is common after pediatric heart transplantation: Initial experience with pravastatin. J Heart Lung Transplant 23:317–322, 2004.

INDEX

Note: Page numbers followed by f indicate figures; those followed by t indicate tables; and those followed by b indicate boxed material.